LEININGER'S   Third Edition

Culture Care Diversity and Universality

A WORLDWIDE NURSING THEORY

Marilyn R. McFarland, PhD, RN, FNP-BC, CTN-A
Professor, Department of Nursing School of
University of Michigan–Flint
Flint, Michigan

Hiba B. Wehbe-Alamah, PhD, RN, FNP-BC, CTN-A
Associate Professor, Department of Nursing School of Health Professions
and Studies
University of Michigan–Flint
Flint, Michigan

D1112089

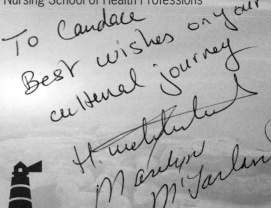

To Candace
Best wishes on your
cultural journey
Hi, meltstenture
Marilyn
M'Farland

JONES & BARTLETT
LEARNING

World Headquarters
Jones & Bartlett Learning
5 Wall Street
Burlington, MA 01803
978-443-5000
info@jblearning.com
www.jblearning.com

Jones & Bartlett Learning books and products are available through most bookstores and online booksellers. To contact Jones & Bartlett Learning directly, call 800-832-0034, fax 978-443-8000, or visit our website, www.jblearning.com.

Substantial discounts on bulk quantities of Jones & Bartlett Learning publications are available to corporations, professional associations, and other qualified organizations. For details and specific discount information, contact the special sales department at Jones & Bartlett Learning via the above contact information or send an email to specialsales@jblearning.com.

Production Credits

Executive Publisher: William Brottmiller
Senior Editor: Amanda Martin
Associate Acquisitions Editor: Teresa Reilly
Editorial Assistant: Rebecca Myrick
Production Editor: Keith Henry
Senior Marketing Manager: Jennifer Stiles
VP, Manufacturing and Inventory Control: Therese Connell

Rights Clearance Editor: Amy Spencer
Composition: Cenveo Publisher Services
Cover Design: Kristin E. Parker
Cover Image: © Pavel Klimenko/123RF
Printing and Binding: Edwards Brothers Malloy
Cover Printing: Edwards Brothers Malloy

Library of Congress Cataloging-in-Publication Data
McFarland, Marilyn R., author.
    [Culture care diversity and universality]
    Leininger's culture care diversity and universality : a worldwide nursing theory / Marilyn R. McFarland and Hiba B. Wehbe-Alamah.—Third edition.
        p. ; cm.
    Preceded by Culture care diversity and universality : a worldwide nursing theory / [edited by] Madeleine M. Leininger, Marilyn R. McFarland. 2nd ed. c2006.
    Includes bibliographical references and index.
    ISBN 978-1-284-02662-7 (pbk.)
    I. Wehbe-Alamah, Hiba B., author. II. Title.
    [DNLM: 1. Cultural Competency. 2. Transcultural Nursing—methods. 3. Nursing Methodology Research. 4. Nursing Theory. WY 107]
    RT86.54
    610.73'01—dc23
                          2014010415
6048

Printed in the United States of America
18 17 16 15 14   10 9 8 7 6 5 4 3 2 1

Contents

Chapter 8 An Examination of Subculture as a Theoretical Social Construct Through an Ethnonursing Study of Urban African American Adolescent Gang Members 255

Edith J. Morris

Chapter 9 Synopsis of Findings Discovered Within a Descriptive Metasynthesis of Doctoral Dissertations Guided by the Culture Care Theory with Use of the Ethnonursing Research Method 287

Marilyn R. McFarland
Hiba B. Wehbe-Alamah
Helene B. Vossos
Mary Wilson

Chapter 20 Transcultural Nursing Certification: Its Role in Nursing Education, Practice Administration, and Research 579

Priscilla Limbo Sagar

Foreword

I have dedicated my life to establishing transcultural nursing as a legitimate and essential area of formal study. The Theory of Culture Care Diversity and Universality and the ethnonursing research method, created and refined over the last 60 years, have been used to discover covert and embedded culture and care phenomena which are essential for the provision of quality health care. The theory is based on transcultural nursing research findings from many cultures that support the discipline and practice of nursing. Healthcare providers from different professional disciplines may use applications from both the theory and the method to assist diverse cultures in receiving culturally competent and congruent care.

Dr. Marilyn McFarland and Dr. Hiba Wehbe-Alamah along with their graduate students recently completed a major metasynthesis of ethnonursing studies guided by the culture care theory and wrote an outstanding and highly laudatory report of significant findings from many diverse cultures. The metasynthesis demonstrates many values and benefits from the use of the theory and the method which continue to be valued and used widely in the United States and in many countries worldwide.

I have entrusted Dr. McFarland and Dr. Wehbe-Alamah to co-author this and future editions of the 2006 theory book. Dr. McFarland has been my student, colleague, co-author, research partner, and co-presenter at many national and international venues. Likewise, Dr. Wehbe-Alamah has shared similar roles and responsibilities with Dr. McFarland. Together, they will continue to teach students, conduct research, and travel the world to share their understanding and promote the application of the culture care theory and the ethnonursing research method. I am very pleased to pass the torch for writing this excellent text and recommend it to all nurses and other healthcare providers in clinical practice, education, research, administration, and consultation.

Dr. Madeleine Leininger
Omaha, Nebraska
Summer 2012

Preface

Marilyn R. McFarland
Hiba B. Wehbe-Alamah

The purpose of this text is to present the reader with recent developments, new applications, and future directions related to the Theory of Culture Care Diversity and Universality and the ethnonursing research method. The goal of this edition is to promote the delivery of culturally congruent care to individuals, families, communities, and organizations in diverse contexts worldwide.

Since the first edition of this text authored in 1991 by Dr. Madeleine Leininger, and the subsequent second edition in 2006 by Drs. Leininger and McFarland, there have been several changes to further develop and clarify both the theory and the method. Nurses are using the culture care theory and the ethnonursing research method to study diverse culture care phenomena in the areas of research, education, clinical practice, and administration. The theory and method have been used by undergraduate and graduate nursing students to guide diverse educational and research projects and by nursing faculty to structure international and local service-learning and study-abroad experiences.

The authors have incorporated feedback from students and seasoned researchers, educators, and practitioners who have used the theory and research method to develop this new edition. This text includes all new and original chapters to present the expanded development and application of the culture care theory and ethnonursing research method. Most importantly, all previous, updated, and newly developed culture care constructs and ethnonursing research enablers have been included in this edition.

The authors have emphasized the importance of discovering in-depth culture care universalities/similarities and diversities/differences related to insider/emic and outsider/etic knowledge. It is also imperative to discover generic and professional care beliefs and practices to fully grasp the care phenomena under study and to guide application to practice by integrating the three culture care modes for nursing decisions and actions. The ethnonursing method with newly developed, revised, and original enablers can be used to systematically study diverse care phenomena related to the culture care theory. Exemplar studies are included in this revised edition with new researchers presenting their scholarly discoveries with local and global clinical and educational applications.

Chapters in this edition are primarily focused on updates and future directions of the culture care theory including new culture care constructs such as collaborative care and father protective care as well as the ethnonursing and meta-ethnonursing research methods and enablers. Also presented are original discoveries of the culture care of Lebanese and Syrian Muslims, Mauritian childbearing families in Australia, and urban African American adolescent gang members.

New directions in applying the culture care theory and ethnonursing research method in the development of curricula for undergraduate and graduate transcultural courses are presented with local U.S. and global applications in Italy, Greece, Australia, Taiwan, and Kenya. Furthermore, unique chapters describe the use of culture care theory to guide a translational research project, the collaborative preparation and implementation of a grant-funded university-based cultural competency project, and the development process for the examinations for transcultural nursing certification.

The authors predict the reader will appreciate this presentation of the newly-expanded worldview of the culture care theory and ethnonursing research method which will lead to further innovations and creative directions in building the theory and applying the method to discover and provide culture-specific and universal care. The chapters in this text also encourage nurses to value not only the uniqueness of cultures but also the commonalities among cultures in the world that bind us together as a human family in our growing multicultural world.

Dedication

Madeleine M. Leininger
July 13, 1925–August 10, 2012

This text is dedicated to the memory of the late Dr. Madeleine Leininger—nurse, researcher, theorist—whose visionary aspirations and unflagging inspirations continue to sustain and motivate us—the authors, her followers, colleagues, peers, and transcultural nurses everywhere—as we continue the leadership work she began through the creation of the Theory of Culture Care Diversity and Universality with the ethnonursing research method and the Sunrise Enabler, the establishment of the International Transcultural Society and the *Journal of Transcultural Nursing*, and her innumerable speeches and writings in books, articles, and newsletters across six decades. It has been a long journey with a long, interesting, and rich story that will endure far into the future. The sun rises every morning and the transcultural caring work of my mentor, leader, teacher, colleague, and friend goes on—just as predictably as the sun rises, Madeleine planned and prepared for us to do just that.

I remember my days at Wayne State in the early 1990s as the Golden Years of work with the culture care theory with that famous Sunrise and qualitative methods. From the mid-1980s to the mid-1990s, we were a community of committed scholarly graduate students working on our dissertation studies guided by Dr. Leininger and her theory with the use of the ethnonursing method. Madeleine was a strong leader, and she cared for us and she inspired us to develop our research within the qualitative paradigm. In fact, her leadership was so strong that we graduate students who worked with her often compared her entrance into a room of faculty, administrators, and students with all of us trailing behind her to Moses parting the Red Sea. All of us knew how important a strong dissertation chair was (and still is) for the successful completion of a doctoral study. Well, we had Madeleine and there was no stopping her students at the water's edge; we all finished our dissertations and graduated according to plan!

Among these early transcultural nursing scholars were the late Dr. Fran Wenger who studied caring and the Amish, was the first student at Wayne to finish her PhD with Madeleine, and I still consider her dissertation the outstanding exemplar of those early studies; Dr. Linda Luna who did her study of care with the Lebanese American community, and I view her study as the best example using Leininger's Phases of Ethnonursing Analysis of Qualitative Data; Dr. Joan McNeil who traveled to Uganda to study the Bagandan grandmothers who were caring for orphan children whose parents had died of AIDS; the late Dr. Marjorie Morgan who studied the prenatal care of African Americans in the urban North and rural South of the United States; and Dr. Eddie Morris, Madeleine's last graduate student at Wayne, who wrote about her discovery of the unique caring and compassion of urban gang members. Under Madeleine's guidance, more than 40 doctoral and master's students at Wayne discovered caring knowledge of diverse cultures, contributed that knowledge to our discipline, and made that knowledge known for nurses and other healthcare professionals to use in their practices.

I think back to those late nights working in Madeleine's office both as her teaching and her research assistant. She convinced her secretaries and office assistants, and any graduate students she could entice to put in long hours. We all have many fond memories of the famous regulated and limited breaks (Madeleine was never one to condone the waste of time!), late-night adventures of scurrying across the street to the local greasy spoon for a quick bite to eat, getting a *TCN Journal* to press, and working on analyzing research data into the wee hours of the morning. In fact, that rising sun in her theory was often viewed out of the east windows of her corner office after a long night's work! We even worked Sundays; she told us it was okay because it was the Lord's work, and we bought it! One faculty member at Wayne declared that when everyone else went to lunch, Madeleine wrote another book! It was sort of true. She was the most productive of all the faculty: She taught more classes, chaired more dissertation committees, spoke at more events, conducted more research, and published more than anyone else!

When graduation was over, in the same month we celebrated Madeleine's retirement from Wayne State, but there was no rest. The work continued! Somehow she talked me into becoming the editor of the *Journal of Transcultural Nursing*. We wrote together and published articles, books, and DVDs; we traveled the world together (Sweden, England, Australia, Canada, and all over the United States) speaking and spreading the transcultural word and her culture care theory and ethnonursing method for nursing practice, education, and research.

This mentorship journey with Madeleine and others has always been very much a shared and reciprocal experience. My colleague, Dr. Sandra Mixer, traveled to Omaha to take a postdoctoral course from Madeleine; I then had the privilege, along with Dr. Marge Andrews, of mentoring Sandy through her dissertation on the topic of teaching culture care. I also mentored my co-author, Dr. Hiba Wehbe-Alamah, through both her master's thesis and dissertation research on the caring practices of Lebanese and Syrian Muslims living in the United States. Now Sandy and Hiba are both mentoring graduate and undergraduate students who will carry on Madeleine's work and our work in transcultural nursing.

I want to mention one more accomplishment in my professional life where I have used Madeleine's theory and transcultural care concepts and principles. Rather late in my career, I became a family nurse practitioner. In addition to my academic appointment, I practice in a nurse-managed clinic at a local health department that serves the poor and uninsured. When I informed Madeleine about this, I think she thought I was straying from the theory and research fold; however, I know she came to realize that her theory and work informs my practice as well as my research and teaching. I put my hands on people, I provide culturally congruent care for them, and I contribute to their healing. There is not always a cure, but always care. Just like you taught me, Madeleine!

Madeleine gave us "the light" to see in the form of the culture care theory and her famous Sunrise that depicts the theory and informs our practice! I offer my caring theme that *"Care is continuing the important work of Dr. Madeleine Leininger."* The sun rises and just as predictably her work continues; we stand on her shoulders. She taught, inspired, nurtured, and cared for us and now we do the same for others. That was her plan all along and it is working! Thank you, Madeleine!

Marilyn R. McFarland

To Dr. Leininger:
 Just like the words *Open Sesame* unlocked Ali Baba's cave of treasures,
 Your work and theory have paved the way to discovering transcultural
 wonders. . . .
Thank you so much!

Hiba B. Wehbe-Alamah

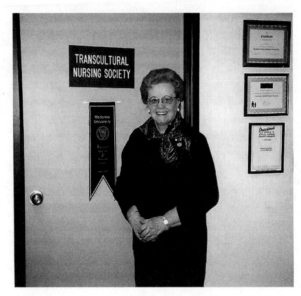

Figure 1 Dr. Madeleine Leininger on a visit to Madonna University, Detroit,
Michigan, circa 1999.
Source: The Madeleine M. Leininger Collection on Human Caring and Transcultural Nursing,
ARC-008, Photo 03, Archives of Caring in Nursing, Florida Atlantic University, Boca Raton,
Florida.

Special Acknowledgments

We would like to acknowledge our spouses and children (pet and human) for their support, patience, and love as we disappeared from the social fabric of their lives while working on this book. To them, we have these words: Brace yourselves: We have more books to come!

We would like to thank the staff at the Archives of Caring at the Christine E. Lynn College of Nursing at Florida Atlantic University, Boca Raton for their invaluable assistance during the writing of this book. We would especially like to express our heartfelt appreciation to Joanna Kentolall and to Claire Hanson for their unwavering support and dedication and to Claire for scanning the hundreds of documents from the Madeleine M. Leininger Collection on Human Caring and Transcultural Nursing (circa 1950–2012) located in the Archives of Caring in Nursing. This and other collections are accessible by visiting http://nursing.fau.edu/archives.

Finally, we wish to thank our colleague, Marilyn Eipperle, for her thoughtful and precise editing; for her gracious communications with us, the Jones & Bartlett staff, and all our contributors; and for her knowledge of and dedication to the integrity of the culture care theory and the work of the late Dr. Madeleine Leininger. Marilyn, we could not have done this book without you! We are truly grateful.

Marilyn and Hiba

About the Authors

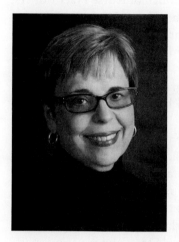

Marilyn R. McFarland, PhD, RN, FNP-BC, CTN-A is a Professor, Department of Nursing, School of Health Professions and Studies, at the University of Michigan–Flint. Dr. McFarland earned her PhD in Nursing with a focus in Transcultural Nursing from Wayne State University, Detroit, Michigan; her master of science in nursing from Wayne State with a major in Medical Surgical nursing and minors in Teaching in Nursing, Gerontological Nursing, and Transcultural Nursing; and her Bachelor of Science in Nursing also from Wayne State. Her family nurse practitioner certificate was earned from Saginaw Valley State University in 2005.

As a Certified Transcultural Nurse and Transcultural Nursing Author and Scholar, Dr. McFarland has been nationally and internationally recognized for her contributions to transcultural nursing by the Transcultural Nursing Society, receiving the 1993 Leininger Award for Excellence in Transcultural Nursing from the Society. She was also the 1994 recipient of the Leininger Transcultural Nursing Award for Excellence and Creative Leadership in Transcultural Nursing and Human Care from Wayne State University, College of Nursing, Detroit, Michigan. In addition to individually publishing numerous book chapters and articles, Dr. McFarland coauthored two texts with Dr. Madeleine Leininger, *Culture Care Diversity and Universality: A Worldwide Nursing Theory* (2006) and *Transcultural Nursing:*

Concepts, Theories, Research, & Practice (2002) which was the recipient of the 2003 American Journal of Nursing's Book of the Year Award.

Dr. McFarland is a past editor of the *Journal of the Transcultural Nursing*, a past chair of the Transcultural Nursing Certification Commission whose members developed a revised certification examination process under her guidance, has been a member of the TCNS Board, has served on numerous Society committees, and co-presented the Keynote Address with Dr. Leininger in 2011 at the 37th Annual TCNS International Conference in Las Vegas, Nevada. She is also a member of the National Organization of Nurse Practitioner Faculties, Michigan Council of Nurse Practitioners, American Nurses' Association, the Michigan Nurses' Association, and ANA-Michigan (formerly RN-AIM). As a career-long member of Sigma Theta Tau International, she is active in the local Pi Delta chapter based at UM–Flint.

Dr. McFarland has taught at the undergraduate level in the areas of gerontology, fundamentals of nursing, and health assessment. She currently teaches nursing at the graduate level focusing on transcultural health care, advanced practice nursing role development, and graduate translational research projects. She has served on many doctoral nursing dissertation committees nationally as well as on many master's theses committees statewide. Her clinical practice is focused on caring for the underinsured at a local health department family planning clinic. As a leader in transcultural nursing, Dr. McFarland has studied, practiced, consulted, and lectured throughout the United States and in various parts of Europe, Kenya, Taiwan, and Australia. She has conducted transcultural research studies focused on Polish, Anglo American, African American, Mexican American, and German American elders using Leininger's Theory of Culture Care Diversity and Universality. Dr. McFarland recently co-participated in a metasynthesis of culture care theory research studies guided by the Theory of Culture Care Diversity and Universality. Her scholarly interests include the Scholarship of Teaching and Learning (SOTL), the translation of evidenced-based research into clinical practice, and the integration of transcultural nursing theory into nurse practitioner practice in diverse settings

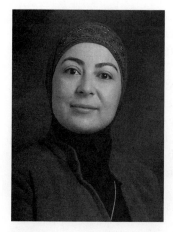

Hiba B. Wehbe-Alamah, PhD, RN, FNP-BC, CTN-A, is Associate Professor, Department of Nursing, School of Health Professions and Studies, at the University of Michigan–Flint. Dr. Wehbe-Alamah earned her PhD and post-master's certificate in Transcultural Nursing from Duquesne University in Pittsburgh, Pennsylvania; she also earned her Master of Science in Nursing (Family Nurse Practitioner) and Bachelor of Science in Nursing from Saginaw Valley State University in Saginaw, Michigan. She holds an advanced-level certification in transcultural nursing and was recognized by the Transcultural Nursing Society (TCNS) as a Transcultural Nursing Scholar in 2011.

A member of the Transcultural Nursing Society (TCNS), National American Arab Nurses' Association, National Organization of Nurse Practitioner Faculties, American Association of Nurse Practitioners, Michigan Council of Nurse Practitioners, Michigan Nurses' Association, and a career-long member of Sigma Theta Tau International, Dr. Wehbe-Alamah has presented, guest-lectured, and/or published in the United States, Australia, Europe, Asia, and the Middle East. Dr. Wehbe-Alamah was actively involved in the planning and implementation of a three-year federally funded Nurse Education, Practice, and Retention project at the University of Michigan–Flint entitled *Developing Nurses' Cultural Competencies: Evidence-Based and Best Practices*. Through this project, she played a key role in providing cultural competence training to registered nurses, advanced practice nurses, nursing faculty, nursing students, and diverse healthcare providers in 35 states across the United States.

Dr. Wehbe-Alamah led an interdisciplinary project involving faculty and students from the Nursing, Computer Science, and Art departments at the University of Michigan–Flint that created the first transcultural computer-based simulation game, *CultureCopia*. As a member of the Transcultural Nursing Society's Transcultural Nursing Certification Commission, she co-developed an international online certification exam for advanced transcultural nurses and contributed test questions to the basic transcultural nursing certification exam for registered nurses. She teaches nursing at the undergraduate, master's and doctoral levels focusing on women's health and transcultural health care; conducts and chairs doctoral dissertations and capstone projects with graduate nursing students; and advises students enrolled in undergraduate, master's, and doctoral programs. Her clinical practice centers on women's health and the underinsured at a local community health department.

Dr. Wehbe-Alamah's scholarly and research interests include obesity; women's health; mental health; primary care; creative teaching methodologies; computer simulation games; technology use in the academic setting; Asian, African American, and Middle Eastern health and wellbeing; health disparities; cultural healers and generic/folk beliefs and practices; and cultural competence for diverse healthcare providers, nursing students, practicing nurses, and nursing faculty.

Contributors

Margaret Andrews, PhD, RN, CTN-A, FAAN
Director and Professor of Nursing
Department of Nursing
School of Health Professions and Studies
University of Michigan–Flint

John Collins, MS, BSN, RN
Continuing Education Specialist
Office of Extended Learning
University of Michigan–Flint

Renee Courtney, DNP, RN, FNP-BC, CTN-B
Nursing Faculty
Department of Nursing
School of Health Professions and Studies
University of Michigan–Flint

Lana M. deRuyter, PhD, RN
Dean, Allied Health, Emergency Services and Nursing
Delaware County Community College
Media, Pennsylvania

Marilyn K. Eipperle, MSN, RN, FNP-BC, CTN-A
Nursing Faculty
Department of Nursing
School of Health Professions and Studies
University of Michigan–Flint

Linda D'Appolonia Knecht, MSN, RN
Assistant Professor
Department of Nursing
School of Health Professions and Studies
University of Michigan–Flint

Colleen Knecht Sabatine, MSN, RN, ANP-BC, CTN-B
Adult Nurse Practitioner
Traverse City, Michigan

Muriel Larson, MA, RN
Assistant Professor
Department of Nursing
Augustana College
Sioux Falls, South Dakota

Madeleine M. Leininger, PhD, LHD, DS, RN, CTN-A, FRCNA, FAAN
Theorist
Founder TCN Society
Sutton, Nebraska

Marilyn R. McFarland, PhD, RN, FNP-BC, CTN-A
Professor
Department of Nursing
School of Health Professions
and Studies
University of Michigan–Flint

Sandra J. Mixer, PhD, RN, CTN-A
Assistant Professor of Nursing
University of Tennessee
Knoxville, Tennessee

Edith J. Morris, PhD, RN, PNP-BC, CCHP
Associate Professor of Clinical Nursing
University of Cincinnati, Ohio

Akram Omeri, OAM, PhD, RN, CTN-A, FCNA
Transcultural Nursing & Healthcare Consulting, Ltd.
Homebush South, New South Wales, Australia

Lynette Mary Raymond, PhD, RN, RM, Dip. App. Counselling, Cert IV TAA
Community Health Nurse
NSW Health
Moss Vale, New South Wales, Australia

Priscilla Limbo Sagar, EdD, RN, ACNS-BC, CTN-A
Professor of Nursing
Mount Saint Mary College
Newburgh, New York

Melanie Turk, PhD, RN
Assistant Professor
School of Nursing
Duquesne University
Pittsburgh, Pennsylvania

Helene B. Vossos, DNP, RN, ANP-BC, PMHNP-BC
Assistant Professor
Department of Nursing
School of Health Professions and Studies
University of Michigan–Flint

Hiba B. Wehbe-Alamah, PhD, RN, FNP-BC, CTN-A
Associate Professor
Department of Nursing
School of Health Professions and Studies
University of Michigan–Flint

Mary Wilson, MSN, RN, ANP-BC
Nurse Practitioner
Waller Wellness Center
Rochester Hills, Michigan

Susan Wolgamott, DNP, RN, FNP-C, CEN, CTN-B
Nursing Faculty
Department of Nursing
School of Health Professions and Studies
University of Michigan–Flint

Rick Zoucha, PhD, APRN-BC, CTN-A
Coordinator, Transcultural Certificate/International Nursing Programs
Professor
School of Nursing
Duquesne University
Pittsburgh, Pennsylvania

Chapter 1

The Theory of Culture Care Diversity and Universality

Marilyn R. McFarland
Hiba B. Wehbe-Alamah

> *Understanding the why of culture care differences and simi-*
> *larities among and between cultures would offer explanatory*
> *power to support nursing as an academic discipline and prac-*
> *tice profession . . . Using the theory, then, could help to estab-*
> *lish the nature, essence, meanings, expressions, and forms of*
> *human care or caring—a highly unique, credible, reliable, and*
> *meaningful body of knowledge for nursing.*
>
> (Leininger, 1991, p. 35)

INTRODUCTION

Leininger's (2006a) Theory of Culture Care Diversity and Universality is the outcome of original thinking, an awareness of an ever-changing world, and more than 6 decades of using, building, and refining the theory. It is not a borrowed theory but has been developed as a nursing theory highly relevant to discover the care and health needs for persons, families, groups, and institutions from similar and diverse cultures. This chapter is based on the seminal works of the late Dr. Madeleine Leininger, her past experiences and creative thinking, and the work from all the dedicated scholars, research-ers, educators, and administrators from the discipline of nursing who have used her work to continue to build the culture care theory so that it remains relevant and useful for nursing and other healthcare fields. The development, growth, and expansion of the theory over a period of 6 decades reflect Dr. Leininger's early practice in hospitals, clinics, and community settings, and her studies of many cultures and the studies of her students and followers worldwide. In the late 1940s, patients often expressed their appreciation to the theorist for healing them through her caring actions. Many direct observations and experiences with clients of diverse cultures with a variety of health conditions led her to realize that the human care from nurses, other professionals, families, and friends was important for recovery from illnesses and maintaining health and wellbeing. Most importantly, a caring nurse who understood and could provide therapeutic care to people of diverse cultures was a critical and long-standing need in nursing and all health practices (Leininger, 1978, 1991, 2006a).

HISTORY OF THE CULTURE CARE THEORY

In the early 1950s, Madeleine Leininger worked as a clinical mental health specialist in a child guidance center with mildly disturbed children of diverse cultural backgrounds. It was during this time she saw challenges and noncaring actions in the care of children and realized that only limited research had been conducted in relation to care within specific cultures and in health institutions. It was evident to her that nurses and other health professionals had failed to recognize and appreciate the important role of culture in healing, in caring processes, and in healthcare treatment practices. Culture and care were identified by Leininger as major dimensions missing in nursing and healthcare services (Leininger, 1978, 1995). The theorist tried to use psychoanalytic and other mental health ideas popular after World War II to help patients, but these practices were woefully inadequate to explain or help children and adults of diverse cultural backgrounds. The theorist's interest continued to grow along with her many questions about the interface of culture and care. Leininger decided that understanding and responding appropriately and therapeutically to clients from different cultures was a critical need that merited theoretical explanations and research investigations to discover beneficial outcomes.

Given that the theorist had no substantive knowledge about cultures and care in her basic and advanced nursing education and no preparation in cultural anthropology, Leininger decided to pursue a PhD in anthropology at the University of Washington in Seattle in the early 1960s, first conducting a field research study in the Eastern Highlands of Papua New Guinea and later making a return visit in 1985 to do a follow up study

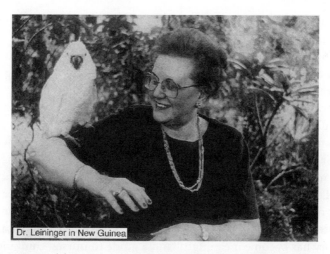

Dr. Leininger in New Guinea

Figure 1-1 Dr. Madeleine Leininger in New Guinea, circa 1985.
Source: The Madeleine M. Leininger Collection on Human Caring and Transcultural Nursing, ARC-008, Photo 49, Archives of Caring in Nursing, Florida Atlantic University, Boca Raton, Florida.

(**Figure 1-1**). Her goal was to become knowledgeable about different cultures and the theories with research findings related to caring and diverse cultures. During her doctoral study, the Theory of Culture Care Diversity and Universality was developed with a specific focus on nursing care and health. Leininger's goal was to provide a sound theory in nursing but also one that could be used in other health-related disciplines. She envisioned a new field of transcultural nursing as an important discipline for study and practice in the mid-1950s. Through creative thinking and the discovery of the close relationship between culture and care phenomena, Leininger began to envision her theory. Bringing culture and care together into a new conceptual and theoretical relationship was a challenging endeavor due to the lack of studies and limited interest by nurses in the idea. However, the need became more and more apparent in Leininger's clinical observations and studies. Gradually the theorist envisioned the Theory of Culture Care Diversity and Universality as a new way to discover caring ways to help people. Both culture and care needed to be studied in-depth and worldwide with a comparative focus. Leininger envisioned that such knowledge could greatly transform nursing and health care in both education and practice worldwide. Care research with a theoretical base was definitely needed, and care meanings and actions were vague and limitedly understood (Leininger, 1978, 1991, 2002c, 2006a). In the period following World War II, many immigrants and refugees from diverse cultures were leaving their homes and native countries and moving to the United States and to other places worldwide. There was also the need to bring knowledge related to care, culture, and health into nursing as a sound basis for the new discipline of transcultural nursing.

After 6 decades of study and research, the Theory of Culture Care Diversity and Universality has been established as a major nursing theory. It has been recommended for use by other health-related disciplines to provide transcultural care to people of diverse cultures (McFarland, Mixer, Wehbe-Alamah, & Burk, 2012). Most importantly, transcultural nursing has become a recognized field of study and practice. Knowledge of cultures with their care needs using the culture care theory has become a major and unique emphasis in nursing as a means to know and help diverse cultural groups (Leininger, 1978, 1991, 2002c, 2006a). Culturally-based care factors are recognized as influences on human care expressions, beliefs, and practices related to health, illness, and wellbeing or to face death and disabilities. The theory has become meaningful and a guide to nurses' thinking, practices, and research. The process of envisioning and reconceptualizing care as the essence of nursing from a holistic care perspective is an important way of knowing and understanding people (Leininger, 2006a).

Epistemologically and ontologically, Leininger held that care was the essence of nursing or what made nursing what it is or could be in healing, in wellbeing, and to help people face disabilities and death. Leininger held that care is nursing, care is health, care is curing, and care is wellbeing (1991, 2002c, 2006a). The theorist also postulated that *human care* is what makes people human, gives dignity to humans, and inspires people to get well and to help others (Leininger, 1978, 2002c, 2006a). She further held and predicted that there could be no curing without caring, but caring could exist without curing (Leininger, 1991, p. 45; 2006a, p. 18). This was a profound theoretical hunch predicting that care was a powerful and central dominant force for healing and wellbeing. This statement continues to be studied with a transcultural focus (Andrews, 2006; McFarland, 2002). Research focused on culture care as a phenomenon interrelated with health and the environmental context was crucial to identify and advance nursing and health care. Care has come to be viewed as meaningful, explicit, and beneficial. Care is a powerful and dynamic force to understand the totality of human behavior within the context of health and illness worldwide.

Culture care decision and action modes related to care that are culturally based and maintained have led to beneficial health outcomes (Leininger, 1991, 2002c, 2006a). Leininger (1978, 1991, 2006a) held that culture was the broadest, most comprehensive, holistic, and universal feature of human beings and care was predicted to be embedded in culture. She also maintained both had to be understood to discover clients' care needs. Caring was held as the action mode to help people of diverse cultures while care was the phenomenon to be understood and to guide actions. Culture care together was predicted to be a powerful theoretical construct essential to human health, wellbeing, and survival. Knowledge of the specific culture care values, beliefs, and lifeways of human beings within life's experiences was held as important to unlock a wealth of new knowledge for nursing and health practices. These ideas have been studied in-depth or from a transcultural comparative perspective (Andrews, 2006; McFarland, 2002). Culturally-based care was held by Leininger (1994) as essential and long overdue to help people of diverse cultures in healing, in recovery, and to face death and disabilities.

Leininger predicted that culture and care were embedded in each other and needed to be teased out and understood within a cultural context. Most importantly, she predicted this knowledge would contribute to transcultural nursing as a discipline and practice field. The culture care theory and transcultural nursing are closely related as bases for being human, but also for health and wellbeing. The embedded phenomenon of culturally-based care is significant and has been studied and the research findings used to provide transcultural nursing care. Such care has been supported as culturally meaningful, therapeutic, congruent, and safe for people of diverse and similar cultures (Andrews, 2006; Gunn & Davis, 2011; Leininger, 2002a, 2006a, 2006d; McFarland, 2002, 2014; McFarland, Wehbe-Alamah, Wilson, & Vossos, 2011; Morris, 2012; Schumacher, 2010). Using culturally-based research findings to provide care has been done to lead to healing, recovery, wellbeing, and healthy lifeways. This goal remains a major challenge for healthcare professionals. These ideas and predictions continue to need to be rigorously studied transculturally in order to guide nurses and other health professionals in their caring actions and decisions. Care and culture are both important, and neither should be neglected. The idea of culture care as a synthesized dominant and central construct within the theory of Culture Care Diversity and Universality continues to be the major focus of the theory (Andrews, 2006; Gunn & Davis, 2011; Leininger, 2002a, 2006a, 2006d; McFarland, 2002, 2014; McFarland et al., 2011; Morris, 2012; Schumacher, 2010). Most importantly, Leininger has challenged nurses to discover both cultural diversity and universality about care worldwide (Andrews, 2006; Gunn & Davis, 2011; Leininger, 2002a, 2006a, 2006d; McFarland, 2002, 2014; McFarland et al., 2011; Morris, 2012; Schumacher, 2010).

PURPOSE OF THE CULTURE CARE THEORY

The purpose of the Theory of Culture Care Diversity and Universality is to discover, document, know, and explain the interdependence of care and culture phenomena with differences and similarities between and among cultures. Such knowledge is essential for current and future professional nursing care practice and for other healthcare providers. A new body of research-based culture care knowledge was envisioned as opening ways to practice nursing and provide healthcare services. This body of knowledge is changing and transforming nursing and health care with benefits to people of similar and diverse cultures. Most importantly, this supports the discipline of transcultural nursing envisioned by Leininger and has led to therapeutic health outcomes.

GOAL OF THE THEORY

From the beginning, the goal of the culture care theory has been to use culture care research findings to provide culture-specific and/or generic care that would be culturally congruent, safe, and beneficial to people of diverse or similar cultures for their health, wellbeing, and healing, and to help people face disabilities and death (Leininger, 1991, 2002d, 2006a; Mixer, 2011; Morris, 2012; Schumacher, 2010; Webhe-Alamah, 2011). The Theory of Culture Care Diversity and Universality has been a major breakthrough for research-based knowledge discovered from direct field experiences to support the discipline of transcultural nursing over the past many decades.

Next, we offer some brief statements about the philosophical basis, theoretical tenets, and major assumptions of the Theory of Culture Care Diversity and Universality.

PHILOSOPHICAL AND THEORETICAL ROOTS

Given that the theory was developed independently without any particular persons or schools of thought, Leininger's philosophy of life, extensive professional nursing experiences, anthropological and other relevant knowledge, diverse intellectual scholarly interests, and spiritual insights and beliefs were used as its foundation. As a spiritual person, the theorist believed that a Superior Being created all human beings. Nursing was viewed as a unique caring profession to serve others worldwide. It is influenced by ethnohistory, culture, social structure, and environmental factors in different geographic areas and by the different needs of people (Leininger, 1991, 2006a). Nursing is a dynamic field of study and practice that takes into account culture, religion, social change, and multiple factors that influence health and wellbeing. It is a profession with discipline knowledge to help people, whether ill or well, with their diverse care needs (Leininger, 1991, 2006a).

The theorist's intellectual and educational interest in religious beliefs and in the humanities and diverse philosophies of life were all important in developing the theory. Leininger's preparation in the biological sciences, philosophy, mental health, nursing, anthropology, psychology, and the many diverse and broad life experiences of her 80-plus years all influenced ongoing development of the theory. Her more than 60 years as a professional nurse clinician and educator, as well as her extensive experience in nursing administration, education, and research, were reflected upon in developing the theory. Leininger was interested in developing new practices for nursing to meet diverse cultural needs and to provide therapeutic care practices. The complexity of human beings and diverse cultural lifeways challenged her thinking about the provision of comprehensive and holistic care practices. Thus, she contended that the medical model of focusing on diseases, symptom relief, and pathological conditions was far too narrow for a caring discipline. Holistic and broad worldviews respecting the sacredness and uniqueness of humans and their culturally-based values were imperative to surpass traditionally narrow medical and past nursing perspectives. The culture care theory thus had to be broad, holistic, and yet culture-specific with research-based knowledge to transform nursing and traditional medicine (Leininger, 1991, 2006a). The discipline of transcultural nursing remains as an essential field of study and practice and especially to serve neglected cultures (Leininger, 2006a).

Theoretical Tenets and Predictions

Tenets are the positions one holds or are givens that the theorist uses with a theory. In developing the culture care theory, Leininger conceptualized and formulated four major tenets:

- Culture care expressions, meaning, patterns, and practices are diverse and yet there are shared commonalities and some universal attributes;
- The worldview, multiple social structure factors, ethnohistory, environmental context, language, and generic and professional care are critical influencers of cultural care patterns to predict health, wellbeing, illness, healing, and ways people face disabilities and death;
- Generic emic (folk) and etic (professional) health factors in different environmental contexts greatly influence health and illness outcomes; and
- From an analysis of the above influencers, three major actions and decision guides were predicted to provide ways to give culturally congruent, safe, and meaningful health care to cultures. The three

culturally-based action and decision modes were *culture care preservation and/or maintenance; culture care accommodation and/or negotiation;* and *culture care repatterning and/or restructuring.* Decision and action modes based on culture care were key factors predicted for congruent and meaningful care. Individual, family, group, or community factors are assessed and responded to in dynamic and participatory nurse–client relationships (Leininger 1991, 2006a).

Assumptive Premises of the Theory

These major theoretical tenets and predictions of the theory led to the formation of specific theoretical hunches or assumptions that the researcher could use in Western and non-Western cultures over time and in different geographic locations. The theoretical assumptive premises (assumed givens) were the following (Leininger, 2006a, pp. 18–19):

- Care is the essence and the central dominant, distinct, and unifying focus of nursing;
- Humanistic and scientific care is essential for human growth, well-being, health, survival, and to face death and disabilities;
- Care (caring) is essential to curing or healing, for there can be no curing without caring; this assumption was held to have profound relevance worldwide;
- Culture care is the synthesis of two major constructs that guide the researcher to discover, explain, and account for health, wellbeing, care expressions, and other human conditions;
- Culture care expressions, meanings, patterns, processes, and structural forms are diverse but some commonalities (universalities) exist among and between cultures;
- Culture care values, beliefs, and practices are influenced by and embedded in the worldview, social structure factors (e.g., religion, philosophy of life, kinship, politics, economics, education, technology, and cultural values), and the ethnohistorical and environmental contexts;
- Every culture has generic (lay, folk, naturalistic; mainly emic) and usually some professional (etic) care to be discovered and used for culturally congruent care practices;
- Culturally congruent and therapeutic care occurs when culture care values, beliefs, expressions, and patterns are explicitly known and used appropriately, sensitively, and meaningfully with people of diverse or similar cultures;

- Leininger's three theoretical modes of care offer new, creative, and different therapeutic ways to help people of diverse cultures;
- Qualitative research paradigmatic methods offer important means to discover largely embedded, covert, epistemic, and ontological culture care knowledge and practices; and
- Transcultural nursing is a discipline with a body of knowledge and practices to attain and maintain the goal of culturally congruent care for health and wellbeing.

CENTRAL CONSTRUCTS IN THE CULTURE CARE THEORY

For several decades, transcultural nursing has been defined as a discipline of study and practice focused on comparative culture care differences and similarities among and between cultures in order to assist human beings to attain and maintain meaningful and therapeutic healthcare practices that are culturally based (Leininger, 1991, 2002c, 2006a). Transcultural nursing continues to identify and use comparative care discoveries, skills, and standards to help human beings of diverse or similar cultures in beneficial ways. As stated earlier, transcultural nursing came into being as an essential and imperative field of study and practice to meet societal and global needs of people of diverse and similar cultures.

Several central constructs used in the culture care theory have been described and defined (Leininger, 1991, 2006a). These constructs and their orientational definitions were adapted within several published research studies, such as Farrell (2006), Luna (1998), McFarland (1997), McFarland and Zehnder (2006), and Schumacher (2010). Thus theory definitions are orientational (not operational) to encourage the researcher to discover new qualitative knowledge and to avoid being focused on the researcher's quantitative definitions. Cultures usually have their own definitions and uses of their terms. This is another major difference between the culture care theory and other nursing theories that have prescribed definitions which usually reflect the researchers' interests or viewpoints.

- *Care* refers to both an abstract and/or a concrete phenomenon. Leininger has defined care as those assistive, supportive, and enabling experiences or ideas toward others (Leininger, 1995, 2002b, 2006a). Caring refers to actions, attitudes, and practices to assist or help others toward healing and wellbeing (Leininger, 1995, 2002b, 2006a). Care as a major construct of the theory includes both folk and professional care which are major parts of the theory and have been predicted to influence and explain the health or wellbeing of diverse cultures. Based on the findings from current research, care is largely an embedded, invisible, and often taken for granted phenomenon that is difficult for nurses to quickly identify or grasp with in-depth meaning. However, over the past 6 decades many books, articles, and research studies have become available enabling nurses to discover and know differential care meanings of diverse cultures (Leininger, 1978, 1991, 2002b, 2006a). Nurses are also learning that care is more than doing or performing physical action tasks. Care has cultural and symbolic meanings such as care as protection, care as respect, and care as presence. These care linkages are essential to provide culture-specific care and are often gender linked. Many master's and doctoral research studies have discovered transcultural care meanings within and between cultures (**Table 1-1**). Most of these studies have been conducted by doctorally-prepared transcultural nurse researchers who have teased out covert and in-depth meanings of care in scientific and authentic ways for clinical care practices.

- *Culture* as the other major construct central to the Theory of *Culture* Care Diversity and Universality has been equally as important as care and is therefore not an adverb or adjective modifier to care. Leininger conceptualized culture care as synthesized and closely linked phenomena with interrelated ideas. Both culture and care require rigorous and full study with attention to their embedded and constituted relationship to each other as a human care phenomenon. Leininger (1991, 2002b, 2006a) defined culture as the learned, shared, and transmitted values, beliefs, norms, and lifeways of a particular culture that guide thinking, decisions, and actions in patterned ways. From an anthropological perspective, culture is usually viewed as a broad and most comprehensive means to know, explain, and predict people's lifeways over time and in different geographic locations. Moreover, culture is more than social interaction and symbols. Culture can be viewed as the blueprint for guiding human actions and decisions and includes material and nonmaterial features of any group or individual. It has been a major construct in anthropology for nearly a century. Culture is more than ethnicity or social relationships. Culture phenomena distinguish human beings from nonhumans. Transculturally prepared nurses are advancing culture knowledge in many ways by uniting culture and care together conceptually and for research purposes. This approach in nursing is encouraging. Social scientists are also learning

Table 1-1 Care/Caring Constructs of the Culture Care Theory, 1991–2013

1. Acceptance	36. Concern for/about/with
2. Accommodating	37. Congruence with
3. Accountability	38. Connectedness
4. Action (ing) for/about/with	39. Consideration of
5. Adapting to	40. Consultation (ing)
6. Affection for	41. Controlling
7. Alleviation (pain/suffering)	42. Communion with another
8. Anticipation (ing)	43. Cooperation
9. Assist (ing) others	44. Coordination (ing)
10. Attention to/toward	45. Coping with/for
11. Attitude toward	46. Creative thinking/acts
12. Being nonassertive	47. Culture care (ing)
13. Being aware of others	48. Cure (ing)
14. Being authentic (real)	49. Dependence
15. Being clean	50. Direct help to others
16. Being genuine	51. Discernment
17. Being involved	52. Doing for/with
18. Being kind/pleasant	53. Eating right foods
19. Being orderly	54. Enduring
20. Being present	55. Embodiment
21. Being watchful	56. Emotional support
22. Bribing	57. Empathy
23. Care (caring)	58. Enabling
24. *Caritas* (charity)	59. Engrossment in/about
25. Cleanliness	60. Establishing harmony
26. Closeness to	61. Experiencing with
27. Cognitively knowing	62. Expressing feelings
28. Collaborative care*	63. Faith (in others)
29. Collective care*	64. Family involvement
30. Comfort (ing)	65. Family support
31. Commitment to/for	66. Father protective care*
32. Communication (ing)	67. Feeling for/about
33. Community awareness	68. Filial love
34. Compassion (ate)	69. Generosity toward others
35. Compliance with	70. Gentle (ness) & firmness

(continues)

Table 1-1 Care/Caring Constructs of the Culture Care Theory, 1991–2013 (*continued*)

71. Giving to others in need	106. Ministering to others—filial love
72. Giving comfort to	107. Need fulfillment
73. Group assistance	108. Nurturance (nurture)
74. Group awareness	109. Obedience to
75. Growth promoting	110. Obligation to
76. Hands on	111. Orderliness
77. Harmony with	112. Other care (ing)/nonself-care
78. Healing	113. Patience
79. Health instruction	114. Performing rituals
80. Health (wellbeing)	115. Permitting expressions
81. Health maintenance	116. Personalized acts
82. Helping self/others	117. Physical acts
83. Helping kin/group	118. Praying with
84. Honor (ing)	119. Presence (being with)
85. Hope (fullness)	120. Preserving (preservation)
86. Hospitality	121. Prevention (ing)
87. Improving conditions	122. Promoting
88. Inclined toward	123. Promoting independence
89. Indulgence from	124. Protecting (other/self)
90. Instruction (ing)	125. Purging
91. Integrity	126. Quietness
92. Interest in/about	127. Reassurance
93. Intimacy/intimate	128. Receiving
94. Involvement with/for	129. Reciprocity
95. Kindness (being kind)	130. Reflecting goodness
96. Knowing of culture	131. Reflecting with/about
97. Knowing (another's reality)	132. Rehabilitate
98. Know cultural values/taboos	133. Regard for
99. Limiting (set limits)	134. Relatedness to
100. Listening to/about	135. Respect for/about lifeways
101. Loving (love others)—Christian love	136. Respecting
102. Maintaining harmony	137. Respecting privacy/wishes
103. Maintaining privacy	138. Respecting sex differences
104. Maintaining reciprocity	139. Responding appropriately
105. Mentoring/comentoring*	140. Responding to context

Table 1-1 Care/Caring Constructs of the Culture Care Theory, 1991–2013 (*continued*)

141.	Responsible for others	160.	Symbols (ing)
142.	Restoration (ing)	161.	Sympathy
143.	Sacrificing	162.	Taking care of environment
144.	Saving face	163.	Technical skills
145.	Self-reliance (reliance)	164.	Techniques
146.	Self-responsibility	165.	Tenderness
147.	Sensitivity to others' needs	166.	Timing actions/decisions
148.	Serving others (*caritas*)	167.	Touch (ing)
149.	Sharing with others	168.	Trust (ing)
150.	Silence (use of)	169.	Understanding
151.	Speaking the language	170.	Use of folk foods/practices
152.	Spiritual healing	171.	Use of limit setting
153.	Spiritual relatedness	172.	Using nursing knowledge
154.	Stimulation (ing)	173.	Valuing another's ways
155.	Stress alleviation	174.	Watchfulness
156.	Succorance	175.	Wellbeing (health)
157.	Suffering with/for	176.	Wellbeing (family)
158.	Support (ing)	177.	Wholeness approach
159.	Surveillance (watch for)	178.	Working hard

* Indicates new care constructs since 2006 publication of table.

Source: Adapted from Leininger, M. M. (2006d). Selected culture care findings of diverse cultures using culture care theory and ethnomethods. In M. M. Leininger & M. R. McFarland (Eds.), *Culture care diversity and universality: A worldwide nursing theory* (2nd ed., pp. 302–304). Sudbury, MA: Jones & Bartlett.

the importance of transcultural nurse research. The powerfulness of the culture care dual construct to discover and understand illness, wellness, and other human health expressions remains a new thrust in nursing. The theorist has held that culture care phenomena conceived and linked together have great power to explain health and/or illness.

- The constructs *emic* and *etic* care are another major part of the culture care theory. Leininger wanted to identify differences and similarities among and between cultures and to differentiate the client's insider knowledge in contrast with the researcher's outsider or professional knowledge. It was believed desirable to know what is universal [or common] and what is different [or diverse] among cultures with respect to care. The term *emic* refers to the local, indigenous, or insider's cultural knowledge and view of specific phenomena; *etic* refers to the outsider's or stranger's views and often health professionals' views and the institutional knowledge of phenomena (Leininger, 1991, 2002b, 2006a). The terms emic and etic were derived from linguistics but were reconceptualized by Leininger within her theoretical perspectives to discover contrasting culture care phenomena. These two dual constructs, emic and etic, have been invaluable in explicating the differences and similarities among cultural informants' and professional nurses' knowledge and practices over the past several decades (Leininger, 1991, 2002b, 2006a). Emic and etic are formally defined as:

- Generic (emic) care refers to the learned and transmitted lay, indigenous, traditional, or local folk (emic) knowledge and practices to provide assistive, supportive, enabling, and facilitative acts for or toward others with evident or anticipated health needs in order to improve wellbeing or to help with dying or other human conditions (Leininger, 2002b, 2006a).
- Professional (etic) nursing care refers to formal and explicit cognitively learned professional care knowledge and practices obtained generally through educational institutions [usually nongeneric]. They are taught to nurses and others to provide assistive, supportive, enabling, or facilitative acts for or to another individual or group in order to improve their health, prevent illnesses, or to help with dying or other human conditions (Leininger, 2002b, 2006a).
- *Culturally congruent care* refers to culturally-based care knowledge, acts, and decisions used in sensitive and knowledgeable ways to appropriately and meaningfully fit the cultural values, beliefs, and lifeways of clients for their health and wellbeing, or to prevent illness, disabilities, or death (Leininger, 2006a). To provide culturally congruent and safe care has been the major goal of the culture care theory.
- *Care diversity* refers to the differences or variabilities among human beings with respect to culture care meanings, patterns, values, lifeways, symbols, or other features related to providing beneficial care to clients of a designated culture (Leininger, 2002c, 2006a). More recently, the term *cultural disparities* has been used by people with

limited transcultural insights. It is not an acceptable term to use in transcultural nursing because of its negative connotations and narrow viewpoint.

- *Culture care universality* refers to the commonly shared or similar culture care phenomena features of human beings or a group with recurrent meanings, patterns, values, lifeways, or symbols that serve as a guide for caregivers to provide assistive, supportive, facilitative, or enabling people care for healthy outcomes (Leininger, 2006a).
- *Health* refers to a state of wellbeing that is culturally defined, valued, and practiced, and which reflects the ability of the individuals or groups to perform their daily role activities in culturally expressed, beneficial, and patterned lifeways (Leininger, 1991, p. 48); a state of wellbeing restorative state that is culturally constituted, defined, valued, and practiced by individuals or groups that enables them to function in their daily lives (Leininger, 2002c, p. 84).
- *Ethnohistory* is another construct of the theory. Ethnohistory comes from anthropology but the theorist reconceptualized it within a nursing perspective. The theorist defines ethnohistory as the past facts, events, instances, and experiences of human beings, groups, cultures, and institutions that occur over time in particular contexts that help explain past and current lifeways about culture care influencers of health and wellbeing or the death of people (Leininger, 1991, 2002c, 2006a). Ethnohistory is another guide to attain culturally congruent care. Special past and current events and conditions within the historical context of cultures and their caring modalities over time are important data for transcultural nursing knowledge and caring practices, especially when studied within the context of care and wellbeing.
- *Environmental context* refers to the totality of an event, situation, or particular experience that gives meaning to people's expressions, interpretations, and social interactions within particular geophysical, ecological, spiritual, sociopolitical, and technologic factors in specific cultural settings (Leininger, 1989, 1991, 2002c, 2006a).
- *Worldview* refers to the way people tend to look out upon their world or their universe to form a picture or value stance about life or the world around them (Leininger, 1978, 1991, 2002c, 2006a). Worldview provides a broad perspective of one's orientation to life, people, or groups that influence care or caring responses and decisions. Worldview guides one's decisions and actions, especially related to health and wellbeing as well as care actions.

Culture Care Decision and Action Modes

In the culture care theory, Leininger predicted three culture care decision and action modes for providing culturally congruent nursing care. The three modes were highly innovative and unique in nursing and health care. Leininger (1994) held that nurses needed creative and different approaches to make care and culture needs meaningful and helpful to clients. These three theoretically predicted decision and action modes of the culture care theory were defined as:

- Culture care preservation and/or maintenance referred to those assistive, supportive, facilitative, or enabling professional acts or decisions that help cultures to retain, preserve, or maintain beneficial care beliefs and values or to face handicaps and death;
- Culture care accommodation and/or negotiation referred to those assistive, accommodating, facilitative, or enabling creative provider care actions or decisions that help cultures adapt to or negotiate with others for culturally congruent, safe, and effective care for their health, wellbeing, or to deal with illness or dying; and
- Culture care repatterning and/or restructuring referred to those assistive, supportive, facilitative, or enabling professional actions and mutual decisions that would help people to reorder, change, modify, or restructure their lifeways and institutions for better (or beneficial) healthcare patterns, practices, or outcomes (Leininger, 2006a).

The modes have substantively guided nurses to provide culturally congruent nursing care and thereby fostered the development of culturally competent nurses. Nurses practicing in large urban centers typically care for clients from many different cultures or subcultures. Leininger's culture care theory provides practicing nurses with an evidence-based, versatile, useful, and helpful approach to guide them in their daily actions and decisions regardless of the number of clients under their care or complexity of their care needs.

The three modes based on research findings are essential for caring and are to be used with specific research care data discovered with the theory. The culture care theory has challenged nurses to discover specific and holistic care as known and used by the cultures over time in different contexts. Both care and culture are held to be central and critical for the discipline and practice of nursing. Leininger's theory was the first theory directed toward discovering and using culturally-based research care knowledge in nursing practice. *Nursing interventions* is a term that is seldom used in the culture care theory or in transcultural nursing. This term has often been used inappropriately and is viewed by several cultures as too controlling or all knowing. When used by nurses, this term may lead to interferences through words or actions with the cultural lifeways, values, and practices of others. This is because it sometimes is viewed as or represents cultural imposition nursing practices used when providing care to clients which may be offensive or in conflict with their lifeways (Leininger, 2006a).

Leininger proposed that culture care preservation and/or maintenance should in most circumstances be considered first, as many times people are doing meaningful and acceptable care for their families and others that leads to beneficial health outcomes. Many nurses from Western cultures are focused on intervening for change and believe that care should be based on professional nursing knowledge. However, it is important to first consider what people are doing right in caring for themselves and their families. Many times people are giving exquisite care in their homes or in institutional settings such as hospitals or nursing homes for their children or elderly relatives (Gunn & Davis, 2011; McFarland, 1997; McFarland & Zehnder, 2006; Wehbe-Alamah, 2011) and these caring actions should be maintained and supported by nurses. In international service-learning courses, considering preserving and/or maintaining care that is therapeutic is essential for nurses and nursing students. They need to be guided by the care modes and in most circumstances to consider first what caring actions should be maintained or preserved; then to consider what should be accommodated or negotiated; and only as a final decision consider what should be changed or repatterned or restructured (Leininger, 1991, pp. 39, 41–44; M. M. Leininger, personal communication, fall 2005). Studies that have effectively demonstrated the discovery of culture-specific care modes include those by "first generation" [taught by Leininger] ethnonursing researchers Morris (2012) and Ehrmin (2005)—the last dissertations overseen or chaired by Leininger—and those by "second generation" ethnonursing researchers such as Schumacher (2010) and Mixer (2011) who were supervised by "first generation" ethnonursing researchers McFarland and Zoucha.

Cultural and Social Structure Factors

Cultural and social structure factors are other major features of the culture care theory (Leininger, 1978). Social structure phenomena provide broad, comprehensive, and special factors influencing care expressions and meanings. Social structure factors of clients include religion (spirituality); kinship (social ties); politics; legal issues; education; economics; technology; political factors; philosophy of life; and cultural beliefs and values with gender and class differences. The theorist has predicted that these diverse factors must be understood as they directly or indirectly influence health and wellbeing. In the past, social structure factors were not explicitly studied in nursing nor in reference to care until the advent of transcultural nursing (Leininger, 1978, pp. 61–62). The use of Leininger's theory has helped nurses to study these dimensions for a holistic or total view of clients. The study of these factors has provided a wealth of invaluable insights about culturally-based care leading to health, wellness, or illness.

BASIC THEORETICAL DIFFERENCES

Philosophically and professionally many questions about culture, care, and nursing were raised within nursing but few nursing research studies were available as resources. Many nurses viewed *care* as an important word to use in teaching and practice but few possessed substantive care knowledge or could explain care within a culture. Care knowledge that had scientific and accurate data about cultures with care meanings, expressions, and beneficial outcomes was missing. Indeed, many nurses in the 1950s and 1960s were absorbed in studying medical diseases, symptoms, and regimens of treatment for many diseases.

While working on her theory, it became apparent to Leininger that the Theory of Culture Care Diversity and Universality would be very different from existing ideas or emerging nursing theories in several respects. First, the central domain of the theory was focused on culture and care relationships. This theory was directed mainly toward discovering largely unknown or vaguely known ideas about care and culture. For Leininger, care should not and was not to be taken for granted or remain as an invisible, covert, and unknown dimension (Leininger, 1991, 2006a). It was time that care became explicit, confirmed, and documented within and among cultures.

Second, some theorists used the terms theories and models in the same way. But as one studies the constructs of *theory* and *models*, it becomes apparent that they are different. Theories should predict and lead to discovery of unknown or vaguely known truths about some phenomena. Such theoretical knowledge should explain and guide nurses' thinking, actions, and decisions. Models are mainly pictorial diagrams of some idea, but they are not theories because they usually fail to show predictive relationships. Different kinds of theories are used by different disciplines to generate knowledge. However, all theories have as their primary goal to discover new phenomena or explicate vaguely known knowledge (Leininger, 1991).

Third, theorists have hunches and predictions about the interrelationships of the major phenomena or variables under study. The culture care theory was open to the discovery of new ideas that were vague or largely unknown but influenced people's culture care outcomes related to their health and wellbeing. No other theorist had focused explicitly on synthesized culture care using an open discovery process. Some researchers focused on a few specific variables to be measured. However, Leininger's theory focused on culture care as a broad yet holistic phenomenon and the central domain of care inquiry with multiple factors or influencers on care and culture.

Fourth, Leininger valued an open discovery and naturalistic process to explore different aspects of care and culture in natural or familiar living contexts and in unknown environments.

Fifth, Leininger developed a specific research method—namely, the ethnonursing method—to systematically and rigorously discover the domain of inquiry (DOI) concerning culture care. This method was new and unknown in nursing and was different from other qualitative methods including ethnography. The ethnonursing method was designed as an open, natural, and qualitative inquiry mode seeking informants' ideas, perspectives, and knowledge about care and culture. Leininger did not want a method that controlled, reduced, or manipulated culture and care as with the quantitative methods. Studying only a few variables selected by the researcher was not acceptable. To discover entirely new or different phenomena, it was necessary for the researcher to hear informants tell stories about their health and cultural lifeways. Indeed, narrow hypotheses with reductionistic goals could greatly limit obtaining holistic and unknown culture and care knowledge, and would curtail the discovery of complex, covert, and embedded phenomena about culture and care (Leininger, 1991, 2006a).

Comparison with the Traditional Nursing Metaparadigm

The culture care theory was focused on obtaining in-depth knowledge of care and culture constructs from key and general informants related to health or wellbeing, dying, or disabilities. Again, nurse theorists in the 1950s and 1960s were very few and most of them focused on a few concepts to be measured. They followed the quantitative paradigm and philosophy. In contrast, Leininger's theory and method followed the qualitative paradigm and was used to tease out largely unknown or vaguely known data about culture care. Most importantly, Leininger's theory differed considerably from other nurses' work or thinking in the mid-1980s as the few nurse leaders concerned with theory development relied on the four metaparadigm concepts of person, environment, health, and nursing to explain nursing. These concepts were proclaimed as the definitive metaparadigm of nursing

(Fawcett, 2000). However, Leininger (1991, 2006a) found these four concepts were too limited to fully discover nursing and especially ideas bearing on transcultural nursing. She was greatly concerned that care and culture were unfortunately excluded from the metaparadigm. It is not logical to use nursing to explain nursing—it is a theoretical and logical contradiction to use the same term to explain or predict the same phenomenon. Leininger held that such illogical and inappropriate reasoning violated scholarly research and discovery principles.

Most importantly, Leininger's early definition of nursing had become known and was desired by many nurses. Nurses were beginning to study human care as an area of interest to them. The absence of care in the metaparadigm demonstrated limited nurses' interest or value in studying care as a nursing phenomenon needing to be explained. Leininger had defended nursing as a ". . .learned humanistic and scientific profession and discipline which is focused on human care phenomena and activities in order to assist, support, facilitate, or enable individuals or groups to maintain or regain their wellbeing (or health), in culturally meaningful and beneficial ways or to help people face handicaps or death" (Leininger, 1991, p. 47). This definition was held by academically prepared and perceptive nurses as giving credence to the true nature of nursing. However, only a few nurses identified care and culture as worthy of study. *Why were care and culture excluded from nursing? Did it reflect a lack of knowledge and interest in these two major phenomena? Was it a failure to envision the great relevance and potential for nursing?* The culture care theory explicitly focused on care and culture because they were the missing phenomena that had been long neglected and needed to be discovered in order to grasp the full nature of nursing or to explain nursing. Indeed, the culture care theory was the earliest theory focused on developing a new knowledge for the discipline of transcultural nursing. There was evidence that nurses needed to provide care to diverse cultures worldwide but were unable to do so without a base of culture care research knowledge (Leininger, 1978, 1991, 2002d, 2006a).

Leininger (1978, 1991, 2002d, 2006a) saw culture and care knowledge as critical societal and global needs for sustaining and maintaining nursing as a profession. Culturally congruent care for the health or wellbeing of humans was largely undiscovered. Her theory with its focus on culture and care was in its infancy until the 1980s and long overdue for study by nursing. Care and culture were held by Leininger as the heart and soul of nursing and essential for developing new transcultural nursing knowledge and practices and to move nursing into a predicted multicultural and global world (Leininger, 1991, 2002d, 2006a).

Decision and Action Modes

Yet another major difference in Leininger's theory in comparison with other nursing ideas was that this theory predicted three action modalities or decision modes for providing culturally congruent nursing care. These three decision and action culture care modes were unique and were not found in other theories or in current nursing and health practices. Leininger (1994) held that nurses needed creative and different approaches to make care and culture needs meaningful and helpful to clients. In turn, she defined the three theoretically predicted action and decision modes of the culture care theory (Leininger, 1991, 2002d).

Furthermore, Leininger held that the three modes based on research data were essential for caring and to be used with specific research care data discovered from the theory. The culture care theory challenged nurses to discover specific and holistic care as known and used by cultures over time in different contexts. Leininger's theory was the first theory directed toward discovering and using culturally based or derived research care knowledge in nursing obtained from cultural informants.

Emic and Etic Knowledge

To achieve this goal, both emic (insider) and etic (outsider) knowledge were two new and important constructs in the theory introduced by Leininger to differentiate the informants' inside knowledge from the researcher's outsider or professional knowledge. This was another unique difference from other theorists' or nurses' work. The cultural informants' emic knowledge about care was deeply valued. Both emic and etic data were studied as integral parts of the theory to obtain comparative and contrasting care knowledge. Such insider (emic) and outsider (etic) knowledge gave valuable insights to nurses caring for cultures, and to date has led to many new ideas about culture care that nurses need to know and understand.

Person

Another concern with the four metaparadigm concepts (Fawcett, 2000) was the use of the word *person*. Based on transcultural knowledge, *person* may not be used and may not be the central, meaningful, or dominant term in some cultures (Leininger, 1991, 2002d, 2006a). Instead, the linguistic terms of *human beings, families, clans,* and *collective groups* are frequently used transculturally because these terms have cultural meanings and are often used by the people. These terms in many cultures are spiritually derived. Moreover, in non-Western cultures, *person* or *individual* may be culturally taboo and not used as these terms are too egocentric and do not fit the philosophy of people. This practice sharply contrasts with American, Canadian, European, and other Western cultures where person and individualism tend to dominate thoughts and communication modes.

Environmental Context

The concept of environment was a complex and multifaceted dimension in all cultures. It varied transculturally and required very broad geophysical and social knowledge. Understanding ecologies and different environments in which people live and survive or die is important. Leininger (1991) valued the phenomenon of environment, and it was included in the theory as depicted in the Sunrise Enabler.

Environment as a major construct of the culture care theory had to be systematically examined. As an influencer on health and caring, *environment* refers to the totality of geophysical situation(s) or the lived-in geographic and ecological settings of cultures. Special environmental meanings, symbols, and commonly shared views and values exist as part of the environmental context. The environmental context includes multiple factors such as the physical, ecological, spiritual, sociopolitical, kinship, or technological dimensions that influenced culture care, health, and wellbeing. The environmental context gives clues about care expressions, meanings, and patterns of living for individuals, groups, and families (Leininger, 2006a). Holistic cultural context knowledge provides for different environments as care settings for self or others living in culturally specific ways, such as woodlands, plains, wet lands, or arid areas. Such holistic dimensions of environment go beyond the common biophysical and emotional foci as used by nurses and extend to broad areas of grasping living and caring contexts. The environmental context also provides information about birthing and dying rituals in one's environmental context (Leininger, 1991, 2002c, 2006a).

Health

The concept of health has remained important in the culture care theory but was predicted as an outcome of using and knowing culturally-based care, rather than solely on biophysical or medical procedures and treatments. Leininger defined health as ". . . a state of wellbeing that is culturally defined and constituted. . . . Health is a state of being to maintain and the ability to help individuals or groups to perform their daily role activities in culturally expressed beneficial care and patterned lifeways" (1991, p. 48; 1995, p. 106).

All cultures have both different and similar patterns and ways to maintain health. Observing and following cultural rules for wellness is culturally known. By using the culture care theory, the nurse researcher discovers what constitutes health with its meanings and symbols, and ways cultures know, transmit, and practice health care including intergenerational practices with both differences and similarities. The focus on human care rather than health alone has challenged nurses to discover health and care together and to explore how this knowledge has been preserved, maintained, and restored for health outcomes through use of culture care theory. Many nurse theorists have focused only on health as the outcome without knowledge of cultural care influences. Leininger held that care and caring knowledge and actions can explain and lead to the health or wellbeing of people in different or similar cultures (Leininger, 1991, 2002c, 2006a). The theorist predicted that one can explain health in diverse contexts and also discover the commonalities or universalities transculturally. Thus, the culture care theory was significantly different from other nursing theories that focused on health or a few specific physical illnesses or conditions to arrive at nursing activities. These theorists failed to study the importance, power, or major influence of care to explain health or wellbeing. For Leininger (1991, 2002b, 2006a), care beliefs, values, and practices were predicted to be the powerful explanatory means to discover and understand health as well as to explain nonhealth or predict illness conditions. Transcultural nursing studies have found that the terms *health and wellbeing* are often used interchangeably when explaining health and care (Leininger, personal communication, 2006).

Such terms often explained health promoting and maintenance attributes in many cultures (Leininger, 1991, 2002b, 2006a). Most importantly, health was discovered as an often restorative attribute, whereas wellbeing implied a quality of life or a desired state of existence in most cultures studied (Leininger, 1991, 2002b, 2006a). The Theory of Culture Care Diversity and Universality has given primary emphasis to care as the essence and central dominant construct of nursing since 1960. Since the 1980s, nurses such as Gaut (1984), Ray (1987), Watson (1985), and others have studied, valued, and stressed care as important to nursing (Leininger, 1984, 1988a, 1988b, 1988c, 1997). In fact, several current nurse researchers are actively explicating new care phenomena (Gunn & Davis, 2011; Mixer, 2011; Morris, 2012; Schumacher, 2010; Wehbe-Alamah, 2011).

THE RELATIONSHIP OF THE CULTURE CARE THEORY AND THE ETHNONURSING RESEARCH METHOD

The ethnonursing research method was explicitly designed by Leininger (1985) to fit the Theory of Culture Care Diversity and Universality and to fit the purposes of qualitative research methods. Leininger developed the ethnonursing research method for nurse researchers to study and advance nursing phenomena from a human science philosophical perspective with the qualitative analytical lens of culture and care (Leininger, 2002b, 2002d, 2006a, 2006b, 2006c; Leininger & McFarland, 2002, 2006). The method was developed with the Theory of Culture Care Diversity and Universality to study the nursing dimensions of culture care which include care phenomena, research enablers, social structural factors (e.g., kinship and social; cultural values, beliefs, and lifeways; religious and philosophical; economic; educational; political/legal systems; technological; and, environmental context, language, and ethnohistory), and the three modes of care decisions and actions (Leininger, 2002c, 2006a, 2006c; McFarland, 2002; McFarland et al., 2012; Ray, Morris, & McFarland, 2013). It was developed as an important means to tap into vague, largely complex, covert, and unknown care and cultural phenomena in order to generate fresh data as a basis for culturally congruent care. Findings from use of the culture care theory and the ethnonursing research method are analyzed in detail to improve care to clients of diverse cultures (Leininger, 1978, 1991, 2006a, 2006c). Ethnonursing is a rigorous, systematic, and in-depth method for studying multiple cultures and care factors within familiar environments of people and to focus on the interrelationships of care and culture to arrive at the goal of culturally congruent care services (Leininger, 1991, 2002c, 2006a, 2006c).

Sunrise Enabler

The culture care theory is a highly rewarding and valuable theory and the ethnonursing research method fits the theory. The Sunrise Enabler (**Figure 1-2**) and other enablers were developed by Leininger as research guides to obtain broad, yet specific, in-depth knowledge bearing on the goal of the theory and researchers' domains of inquiry. The six enablers cover multiple factors influencing care patterns and expressions.

The Sunrise Enabler has been widely used and valued to expand nurses' views and discoveries. The Sunrise Enabler is not the theory per se, but depicts multiple factors predicted to influence culture care expressions and their meanings (Leininger, 1991, 2002c, 2006a). The Sunrise Enabler serves as a cognitive map to discover embedded and multiple factors related to the theory, tenets, and assumptions with the specific domain of inquiry under study. This visual diagram reminds the researcher to search broadly for diverse factors influencing care within any culture under study.

Leininger's enablers do not neglect professional or etic medical knowledge about human beings in illness and health such as biophysical, social,

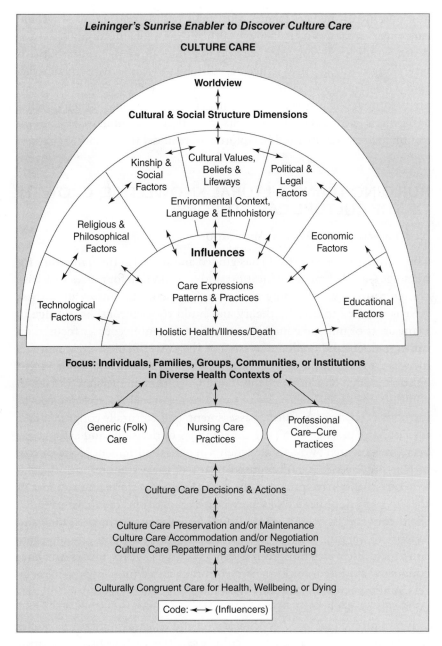

Figure 1-2 Leiniger's Sunrise Enabler to Discover Culture Care
Modified with permission from © M. Leininger 2004, by McFarland and Wehbe-Alamah.

and nursing or medical factors, but focus mainly on total lifeways and care or caring factors influencing health and/or wellbeing, disabilities, and death. Traditional emic medical and nursing knowledge exists but it is often lodged within social structure, ethnohistory, and environmental factors. These emic sources of knowledge (limitedly discovered in the past) are now providing very rich and new insights about people in their familiar and general cultural holistic contexts with specific cultural needs. The ethnonursing research method is explored more in-depth in another chapter.

BUILDING TRANSCULTURAL KNOWLEDGE: GROWTH OF THE CULTURE CARE THEORY

New Directions for Theory Application

The culture care theory (CCT) has guided and provided the framework for nursing research, practice, education, and consultation for nurses who have chosen to work with Leininger's theory. Transcultural nurses and others have continued to use the theory and build transcultural knowledge in many areas of nursing education including designing courses focused on undergraduate and graduate nursing in the areas of culture care and faculty care, international service learning within the context of underserved cultural groups, and local and international cultural immersion courses. In addition, the use of the theory to guide translational research projects to introduce culture care, cultural assessment, and culturally congruent care into nursing practice using the three modes of decisions and actions has been implemented by doctoral students in partial fulfillment of the Doctor of Nursing Practice (DNP) degree. The use of the assumptions of the culture care theory have provided the bases for these efforts and support of these assumptions has led to theory-based applications that have extended the theory and have built transcultural knowledge for the discipline and practice of nursing. Many of these research efforts have substantiated care constructs discovered by Leininger and other transcultural nurses who have conducted studies or implemented culturally-based nursing practice projects. A number of new care constructs have been discovered since 1991 and 2006 and some innovative uses of the theory have been developed.

International and local service-learning and cultural immersion courses have been developed based on the culture care theory. Knecht and Sabatine (2015) state that short-term international service-learning experiences provide opportunities for nursing students to develop cultural understanding and competency, grow personally and professionally, and become engaged citizens within a multicultural society. These authors provide examples of how the culture care theory can be used for planning, implementing, and evaluating an international service-learning course. Using the culture care theory as the guiding framework in an international service-learning course provides students opportunities to gain cultural competence congruent with the purpose of the cultural care theory. Larson (2015) developed a cultural immersion course for undergraduate students to gain an understanding of cultural competence and the roots and history of Western civilization with their significance to U.S. history, their relationships to health care, and relevance to the cultural and social structure dimensions of Leininger's Theory of Culture Care Diversity and Universality. Zoucha and Turk (2015) developed a transcultural and global health perspectives course for DNP students based on the culture care theory that included a cultural immersion component with research-oriented fieldwork and a series of readings and practical exercises.

Courtney and Wolgamott (2015) have described a translational research project using the framework of Leininger's Theory of Culture Care Diversity and Universality and her theoretical construct of collaborative care to facilitate and support the ongoing cultural competence education of a multidisciplinary healthcare team in an urban clinic for underserved individuals and groups. This project utilized a formal educational process as a means to expand the cultural awareness of healthcare providers and clinic staff members and to integrate cultural assessment into the documentation of each clinical encounter. Leininger's collaborative care construct was used as a guide to assist clinic staff to work together to develop materials for instruction and to help the clinic staff in learning how to tease out multiple social, cultural, and environmental dimensions of patients and families for cultural assessments and providing culturally congruent care (Leininger & McFarland, 2011).

Wehbe-Alamah and McFarland (2015) have shared core content, transcultural exercises, outlines, and syllabi of their undergraduate, graduate, and international transcultural nursing courses. One exemplar module presents transcultural nursing theories and models beginning with Leininger's Theory of Culture Care Diversity and Universality. Faculty are especially encouraged to address professional and generic care as well as the three culture care modes of decisions and actions and to advocate for their inclusion in clinical care planning.

In a unique application of the culture care theory, Andrews and Collins (2015) described the ways that Leininger's Theory of Culture Care Diversity and Universality was used as the organizing framework for a federally-funded cultural competence project and served as an example for those wanting to write grant proposals using the culture care theory and/or the ethnonursing research method. Leininger's theory guided the project toward increasing nurses' and other healthcare providers' holding knowledge about diverse cultures they commonly encounter.

Mixer (2011) conducted an ethnonursing research study that extended the culture care theory into the context of nursing education. The purpose of this ethnonursing research study was to discover nursing faculty care practices that support teaching students to provide culturally congruent care within baccalaureate programs in urban and rural universities in the Southeastern United States. Mixer reported a new professional care construct—mentoring/comentoring—as a form of reciprocal care but also as a distinct care construct in that the caring takes place over a sustained period of time and involves faculty members making a significant impact on one another's professional career (2011).

Care Constructs and the Culture Care Theory

More than 6 decades of transcultural nursing research using the ethnonursing research method and culture care theory led to the discovery of 175 care constructs from 58 cultures (Leininger, 2006d). These care constructs have helped nurses understand the meaning of care to people. Additional study and the discovery of new care constructs by Leininger and others in the past decade have facilitated further knowing the epistemic roots of caring and health phenomena.

The idea for a father protective care construct was originally discovered by Leininger in her New Guinea study of Gadsup cultures (Leininger, 2006b, 2011, 2015). She reported that father protective care focuses on the use of protective care in the socialization and enculturation of young boys, adolescents, and older adults. Leininger (2011, 2015) offered several theoretical premises that have been developed to stimulate new lines of inquiry guided by the culture care in addition to identifying the potential therapeutic benefits and practices of father protective care. Specifically, she proposed father protective care could become a major guide in assisting young males, adolescents, and older adults in the prevention of illness and maintenance of healthy outcomes. Father protective care was investigated by Leininger in three Western cultures (Anglo American, Mexican American, and Old Order Amish living in the mid-United States) over a 5-year period to provide a comparative perspective to further develop the father protective care construct (Leininger, 2011, 2015). The researcher's experiences and observations with these diverse cultures provided evidence that father protective care could be extremely beneficial in child rearing, and especially with young males, adolescents, and older adults (Leininger, 1995, 2006b, 2006c, 2011, 2015).

Leininger proposed the construct of collaborative care as part of the culture care theory in 2011 describing a collaborative care approach as those values, meanings, and expressions by persons that reveal a desire for working together in order to maintain and preserve health and wellbeing for others (Leininger & McFarland, 2011). She explained that through the collaborative care process persons involved could potentially be relieved of cultural stresses, conflicts, and threats. She stated that to use this collaborative care approach, the researcher needs to first identify the individual values of the person or persons being studied or cared for and then follow the culture care theory for culture care decisions and actions to best help individuals.

The purpose of sharing these most recent care constructs is to update the list of care constructs discovered by researchers in studies guided by the culture care theory. Leininger's original question in the mid-1950s—*What is universal and diverse about human care/caring?*—has been only partially answered by the care constructs listed in Table 1-1. The updated care constructs also are offered to encourage nurses to do further work with these constructs to add to the body of transcultural knowledge and to discover the epistemic roots of culture care and health phenomena in many subcultures and cultures that have yet to be studied for care meanings with the culture care theory. In addition, sharing how some studies guided by the culture care theory have substantiated the assumptive premises of the theory and contributed to the body of culture care knowledge has also demonstrated the manner in which growth of the theory does and should occur.

The editors/authors of this text and a team of collaborating nurse researchers have yet to complete a series of comparative syntheses about care knowledge drawing from the care constructs of diverse cultures in light of the tenets and assumptive premises of culture care theory. The project will build on the previous descriptive metasynthesis of doctoral dissertations guided by the culture care theory using the ethnonursing research method and will lead to further discoveries of universal and diverse care meanings, practices, and structures of care. This discovered knowledge will ultimately be used for clinical practices, curricular development, and teaching in nursing education, administrative efforts, and further research (McFarland, 2011) and serve as a sound knowledge base for the discipline and practice of nursing in the 21st century and beyond.

CONCLUSION

In this chapter, the nature, importance, and major features of the Theory of Culture Care Diversity and Universality were presented. The ethnonursing research method and the enablers were briefly reviewed to show the fit between the theory and the method. Knowledge of both the theory and the method are needed before launching an ethnonursing study. Fully understanding the theory and method leads to obtaining credible and meaningful research findings. Transcultural research becomes meaningful, exciting, rewarding, and understandable as the researcher develops confidence and competence in the use of the theory and method.

The Theory of Culture Care Diversity and Universality has become increasingly valued worldwide. With slight modifications, other disciplines have been encouraged to use the theory and method (McFarland et al., 2012). Nurses who use the theory and method over time frequently communicate how valuable and important it is to discover new ways to know and practice nursing and health care. Practicing nurses can now use holistic, culturally-based research findings to care for clients of diverse and similar cultures or subcultures in different countries. Contrary to some views, the theory is not difficult to use once the researcher understands the theory and method and has available mentorship guidance if needed. Newcomers to the theory and method can benefit from experienced and expert mentors in addition to studying published transcultural research conducted using the theory and method.

Researchers have found ethnonursing to be a very natural and humanistic research method to use in nursing studies and to assist researchers to gain fresh insights about care, health, and wellbeing. The theory will continue to evolve and remain useful in the future to guide the provision of culture care in our increasingly diverse world. The research and theory provide unique and distinctive pathways to advance the profession of nursing and the body of transcultural knowledge for application in nursing education, research, consultation, and clinical practices worldwide.

DISCUSSION QUESTIONS

1. Discuss the difference between *emic* and *etic* care.
2. Discuss the meanings of and nursing applications for: care; caring; culturally congruent care; and cultural competence.
3. Discuss how knowledge of the culture care theory has changed your own worldview.
4. Discuss the importance of your own personal cultural lifeways; with family; with friends or acquaintances; and with strangers.
5. Discuss how having knowledge of the culture care theory will change your own current or future nursing practice. Be specific.

REFERENCES

Andrews, M. M. (2006). The globalization of transcultural nursing theory and research. In M. M. Leininger & M. R. McFarland (Eds.), *Culture care diversity and universality: A worldwide nursing theory* (2nd ed. pp. 91–110). Sudbury, MA: Jones & Bartlett.

Andrews, M. M., & Collins, J. (2015). Using the culture care theory as the organizing framework for a federal project on cultural competence. In M. M. McFarland & H. B. Wehbe-Alamah (Eds.), *Culture care diversity and universality: A worldwide theory of nursing* (3rd ed.). Burlington, MA: Jones & Bartlett Learning.

Courtney, R., & Wolgamott, S. (2015). Using Leininger's theory as the building block for cultural competence and cultural assessment for a collaborative care team in a primary care setting. In M. M. McFarland & H. B. Wehbe-Alamah (Eds.), *Culture care diversity and universality: A worldwide theory of nursing* (3rd ed.). Burlington, MA: Jones & Bartlett Learning.

Ehrmin, J. T. (2005). Dimensions of culture care for substance-dependent African American women. *Journal of Transcultural Nursing, 16*(2), 117–125.

Farrell, L. S. (2006). Culture care of the Potawatomi Native Americans who have experienced family violence. In M. M. Leininger & M. R. McFarland (Eds.), *Culture care diversity and universality: A worldwide nursing theory* (2nd ed., pp. 207–238). Sudbury, MA: Jones and Bartlett.

Fawcett, J. (2000). The structure of contemporary nursing knowledge. In J. Fawcett, *Analysis and evaluation of contemporary nursing knowledge: Nursing models and theorists* (pp. 3–33). Philadelphia, PA: F. A. Davis.

Gaut, D. (1984). A theoretical description of caring as action. In M. M. Leininger, *Caring: The essence of nursing and health* (pp. 17–24). Thorofare, NJ: Charles B. Slack.

Gunn, J., & Davis, S. (2011). Beliefs, meanings, and practices of healing with botanicals re-called by elder African American women in the Mississippi Delta. *Online Journal of Cultural Care in Nursing and Healthcare, 1*(1), 37–49.

Knecht, L., & Sabatine, C. (2015). Application of culture care theory to international service-learning experiences in Kenya. In M. M. McFarland & H. B. Wehbe-Alamah (Eds.), *Culture care diversity and universality: A worldwide theory of nursing* (3rd ed.). Burlington, MA: Jones & Bartlett Learning.

Larson, M. A. (2015). The Greek connection: Discovering the cultural and social structure dimensions of the Greek culture using Leininger's theory of culture care: A model for a baccalaureate study abroad experience. In M. M. McFarland & H. B. Wehbe-Alamah (Eds.), *Culture care diversity and universality: A worldwide theory of nursing* (3rd ed.). Burlington, MA: Jones & Bartlett Learning.

Leininger, M. M. (1978). Towards conceptualization of TCN healthcare systems: Concept and a model. In M. M. Leininger (Ed.), *Transcultural nursing: Concepts, theories, & practices* (pp. 53–74). New York, NY: John Wiley & Sons.

Leininger, M. M. (1984). *Reference sources for transcultural health and nursing.* Thorofare, NJ: Slack.

Leininger, M. M. (1985). *Qualitative research methods in nursing.* Orlando, FL: Grune & Stratton.

Leininger, M. M. (1988a). *Care: The essence of nursing and health.* Detroit, MI: Wayne State University Press.

Leininger, M. M. (1988b). *Caring: An essential human need.* Detroit, MI: Wayne State University Press.

Leininger, M. M. (1988c). Leininger's theory of nursing: Culture care diversity and universality. *Nursing Science Quarterly, 2*(4), 152–160.

Leininger, M. M. (1989). Transcultural nursing: Quo vadis (Where goeth the field?). *Journal of Transcultural Nursing, 1*(1), 33–45.

Leininger, M. M. (1991). The theory of culture care diversity and universality. In M. M. Leininger (Ed.), *Culture care diversity and universality: Theory of nursing* (pp. 5–68). New York, NY: National League for Nursing.

Leininger, M. M. (1994). *Transcultural nursing: Concepts, theories, & practices.* Columbus, OH: Greyden Press.

Leininger, M. M. (1995). *Transcultural nursing concepts, theories, research & practices.* Columbus, OH: McGraw-Hill Custom Series.

Leininger, M. M. (1997). *An essential human need.* Detroit, MI: Wayne State University Press.

Leininger, M. M. (2002a). Culture care assessments for congruent competency practices. In M. M. Leininger & M. R. McFarland (Eds.), *Transcultural nursing: Concepts, theories, research, & practice* (3rd ed., pp.117–143). New York, NY: McGraw-Hill.

Leininger, M. M. (2002b). Essential transcultural nursing care concepts, principles, examples, and policy statements. In M. M. Leininger & M. R. McFarland (Eds.), *Transcultural nursing: Concepts, theories, research, & practice* (3rd ed., pp. 45–69). New York, NY: McGraw-Hill.

Leininger, M. M. (2002c). Part I: The theory of culture care and the ethnonursing research method. In M. M. Leininger & M. R. McFarland (Eds.), *Transcultural nursing: Concepts, theories, research, & practice* (3rd ed., pp. 71–116). New York, NY: McGraw-Hill.

Leininger, M. M. (2002d). Transcultural nursing and globalization of health care: Importance, focus, and historical aspects. In M. M. Leininger & M. R. McFarland (Eds.), *Transcultural nursing: Concepts, theories, research, & practice* (3rd ed., pp. 3–43). New York, NY: McGraw-Hill.

Leininger, M. M. (2006a). Culture care diversity and universality theory and evolution of the ethnonursing method. In M. M. Leininger & M. R. McFarland (Eds.), *Culture care diversity and universality: A worldwide nursing theory* (2nd ed., pp. 1–41). Sudbury, MA: Jones and Bartlett.

Leininger, M. M. (2006b). Culture care of the Gadsup Akuna of the Eastern highlands of New Guinea. In M. M. Leininger & M. R. McFarland (Eds.), *Culture care diversity and universality: A worldwide nursing theory* (2nd ed., pp. 115–157). Sudbury, MA: Jones and Bartlett.

Leininger, M. M. (2006c). Ethnonursing research method and enablers. In M. M. Leininger & M. R. McFarland (Eds.), *Culture care diversity and universality: A worldwide nursing theory* (2nd ed., pp. 43–81). Sudbury, MA: Jones and Bartlett.

Leininger, M. M. (2006d). Selected culture care findings of diverse cultures using culture care theory and ethnomethods. In M. M. Leininger & M. R. McFarland

(Eds.), *Culture care diversity and universality: A worldwide nursing theory* (2nd ed., pp. 281–305). Sudbury, MA: Jones and Bartlett.

Leininger, M. M. (2011). Leininger's reflection on the ongoing father protective care research. *Online Journal of Cultural Competence in Nursing and Healthcare, 1*(2), 1–13.

Leininger, M. M. (2015). Leininger's father protective care. In M. M. McFarland & H. B. Wehbe-Alamah (Eds.), *Culture care diversity and universality: A worldwide theory of nursing* (3rd ed.). Burlington, MA: Jones & Bartlett Learning.

Leininger, M. M., & McFarland, M. R. (Eds.). (2002). *Transcultural nursing: Concepts, theories, research, & practice* (3rd ed.). New York, NY: McGraw-Hill.

Leininger, M. M., & McFarland, M. R. (Eds.). (2006). *Culture care diversity and universality: A worldwide theory of nursing* (2nd ed.). Sudbury, MA: Jones and Bartlett.

Leininger, M. M. (via videotape), & McFarland, M. R. (2011, October 21). *The culture care theory and a look to the future for transcultural nursing.* Keynote address presented at the 37th Annual Conference of the International Society of Transcultural Nursing, Las Vegas, NV.

Luna, L. (1998). Culturally competent health care: A challenge for nurses in Saudi Arabia. *Journal of Transcultural Nursing, 9*(2), 8–14.

McFarland, M. R. (1997). Use of culture care theory with Anglo and African American elders in a long-term care setting. *Nursing Care Quarterly, 10*(4), 186–192.

McFarland, M. R. (2002). Part II: Selected research findings from the culture care theory. In M. M. Leininger & M. R. McFarland (Eds.), *Transcultural nursing: Concepts, theories, research, & practice* (3rd ed., pp. 99–116). New York, NY: McGraw-Hill.

McFarland, M. R. (2014). Culture care theory of diversity and universality. In M. A. Alligood (Ed.), *Nursing theorists and their work* (8th ed., pp. 417–441). St. Louis, MO: Elsevier/Mosby.

McFarland, M. R., Mixer, S., Wehbe-Alamah, H., & Burk, R. (2012). Ethnonursing: A qualitative research method for studying culturally competent care across disciplines. *International Journal of Qualitative Methods, 11*(3), 259–279.

McFarland, M., Wehbe-Alamah, H., Wilson, M., & Vossos, H. (2011). Synopsis of findings discovered within a descriptive metasynthesis of doctoral dissertations guided by the culture care theory with use of the ethnonursing research method. *The Online Journal of Cultural Competence in Nursing and Healthcare, 1*(3), 24–39.

McFarland, M. R., & Zehnder, N. (2006). Culture care of German American elders in a nursing home context. In M. M. Leininger & M. R. McFarland (Eds.), *Culture care diversity and universality: A worldwide nursing theory* (2nd ed., pp. 181–205). Sudbury, MA: Jones and Bartlett.

Mixer, S. (2011). Use of the culture care theory to discover nursing faculty care expressions, patterns, and practices related to teaching culture care. *Online Journal of Cultural Competence in Nursing and Healthcare, 1*(1), 3–14.

Morris, E. J. (2012). Respect, protection, faith, and love: major care constructs identified within the subculture of selected urban African American Adolescent gang members. *Journal of Transcultural Nursing, 23*(3), 262–269.

Ray, M. (1987). Technological caring: A new model in critical care. *Dimensions of Critical Care Nursing, 6*(3), 166–173.

Ray, M. D., Morris, E. M., & McFarland, M. R. (2013). Qualitative nursing methods: Ethnonursing. In D. E. Polit & C. T. Beck (Eds.), *Nursing research: Generating and assessing evidence for nursing practice* (8th ed.). Philadelphia, PA: Wolters Kluwer/ Lippincott, Williams, & Wilkins.

Schumacher, G. (2010). Culture care meanings, beliefs, and practices in rural Dominican Republic. *Journal of Transcultural Nursing, 21*(2), 93–103.

Watson, J. (1985). *Human science and human care: A theory of nursing.* Norwalk, CT: Appleton Century Crafts.

Wehbe-Alamah, H. (2011). The use of culture care theory with Syrian Muslims in the Mid-western United States. *Online Journal of Cultural Competence in Nursing and Health-care, 1*(3), 1–12.

Webhe-Alamah, H. B., & McFarland, M. R. (2015). Transcultural nursing course outline, educational activities, and syllabi using the culture care theory. In M. M. McFarland & and H. B. Wehbe-Alamah (Eds.), *Culture care diversity and universality: A worldwide theory of nursing* (3rd ed.). Burlington, MA: Jones & Bartlett Learning.

Zoucha, R., & Turk, M. (2015). Using the culture care theory as a guide to develop and implement a transcultural global health course for doctor of nursing practice students for study in Italy. In M. M. McFarland & H. B. Wehbe-Alamah (Eds.), *Culture care diversity and universality: A worldwide theory of nursing* (3rd ed.). Burlington, MA: Jones & Bartlett Learning.

Chapter 2

The Ethnonursing Research Method

Hiba B. Wehbe-Alamah
Marilyn R. McFarland

> *In developing the theory of Culture Care, I saw the need for the ethnonursing research method in order to enter into the people's world and let the people tell me first hand their ideas and experiences related to culturally based care. I wanted **people to teach me** about culture care meanings, symbols, and practices in their cultures.*
>
> (Leininger, 1995, pp. 97–98)[*]

INTRODUCTION

The ethnonursing research method was explicitly designed by Leininger to fit the Theory of Culture Care Diversity and Universality [also known as the culture care theory (CCT)] and to obtain meaningful data with a qualitative approach. Both theory and method were developed and refined over the course of 5 decades. While the CCT was intended for use with the ethnonursing research method, it can and has been used with other qualitative research methods such as ethnography and phenomenology. The ethnonursing research method, in contrast, can be used only under the theoretical guidance of the CCT.

The ethnonursing research method was viewed by Leininger as an important means to tap into vague, largely complex, covert, and unknown care and cultural phenomena in order to generate fresh data as a basis for culturally congruent care (Leininger, 1991a, 1991c, 1993a, 1993b, 2006a). It was

---

[*]Leininger, M. M. (1995). *Transcultural nursing: Concepts, theories, research & practices.* Columbus, OH: McGraw-Hill Companies, Inc.

designed as an open, natural, and qualitative inquiry mode seeking informants' stories about their health and cultural lifeways, ideas, perspectives, and knowledge about care and culture to systematically and rigorously discover the domain of inquiry (DOI) concerning culture care (Leininger, 2006a). Ethnonursing is a rigorous, systematic, and in-depth method for studying multiple cultures and care factors within familiar environments of people, focusing on the interrelationships of care and culture to arrive at the goal of providing culturally congruent care services.

The ethnonursing method was designed so the researcher could discover both macro and micro phenomena, depending on the researcher's stated domain of inquiry within the tenets of the culture care theory. The theory, with its broad holistic focus, can provide both particular and general care data in relation to social structure and other factors. Both rich descriptive subjective and objective culture care phenomena are the informants' authentic truths to explain care and culture phenomena within their world. Detailed observations and shared information from key and general informants provide researchers with scientific and humanistic data as macro or micro findings when using the qualitative ethnonursing method, its paradigm enablers, and the culture care theory as a guiding theoretical framework.

Researchers using the theory and method discovered social structure factors related to specific care phenomena such as kinship and religious ideas that explain care and care practices. Care constructs such as comfort, succorance, nurturance, presence, comfort, respect, and many other specific care expressions have been discovered over the past many decades largely by using the ethnonursing research method and enablers (Leininger, 1991a, 1991c, 1997b, 2002, 2006a). Although the ethnonursing method was designed to focus on culture care phenomena, many new insights and findings have been discovered with the method and theory related to nursing, care, and health–illness practices. Credible and accurate data are sought from informants using verbatim statements and other data, along with symbolic referents and ways to heal and care for people of specific cultures. Such findings provide both depth and breadth of research knowledge about human care phenomena (Leininger, 1985b, 1991a, 1991c, 1995, 1997a, 2002, 2006a).

Leininger developed several enablers to tease out extensive care and culture knowledge from informants living in different cultural contexts. These enablers, discussed in the next chapter, serve as research guides to obtain broad, yet specific, in-depth knowledge bearing on the goal of the theory and researchers' domains of inquiry, and cover multiple factors influencing care patterns and expressions.

In this chapter, the authors present the historical development, purpose, rationale, and philosophy of the ethnonursing research method. Specific features of the method are addressed along with the research process, as well as principles for evaluating qualitative research findings and other aspects of the method. The chapter serves as a background framework for several research studies that follow and demonstrate the use of the method with the culture care theory.

DEFINITION

The ethnonursing method is a qualitative nursing research method focused on naturalistic, open discovery, and largely inductive [emic] modes and processes with diverse strategies, techniques, and enabling guides to document, describe, explain, and interpret people's worldview, meanings, experiences, symbols, life experiences, and other related aspects as they bear on actual or potential nursing care phenomena (Leininger, 1978, 1985b, 1991a, 1995, 2002, 2006a). This method is valuable for discovering both *emic* (generic, folk) and *etic* (professional) data. It is a natural and familiar people-centered method that informants enjoy—finding the open and informal discovery process comfortable and natural. Researchers conducting a study using the ethnonursing methodology incorporate diverse strategies and enablers to document, describe, and understand people's experiences as well as care meanings and symbols related to their care, health, and cultural beliefs, values, and lifeways (Leininger, 2005).

HISTORICAL DEVELOPMENT OF THE ETHNONURSING RESEARCH METHOD

Ethnonursing is the first nursing research method developed specifically to fit a nursing theory (Shapiro, Miller, & White, 2006). Although developed specifically for nursing, both the theory and the method were envisioned by Leininger for use by other healthcare fields as well as nursing (Leininger, 2006a, 2006b). However, while most ethnonursing research conducted to date involves nursing, culture care research guided by the CCT and ethnonursing research method continues to be encouraged within and across healthcare disciplines such as physical, occupational, and speech therapy; social work; pharmacy; medicine; and other fields that aim to provide optimal culturally congruent and sensitive health outcomes (McFarland, Mixer, Wehbe-Alamah, & Burke, 2012).

It was in the 1950s that Leininger realized the need for a theory and research method focused on discovery of care and health needs of diverse cultures—two major and significant phenomena in nursing that lacked formal and systematic study (Leininger, 1997a). At that time, nurse-researchers often borrowed quantitative research methods and tools from other disciplines to investigate nursing phenomena. Leininger developed the culture care theory and the ethnonursing research method in the early 1960s to address the need for a people- and culture-centered approach to discover transcultural nursing phenomena from a qualitative perspective (Leininger, 2002; Shapiro et al., 2006, as cited by Leininger, 1991b).

Leininger began conceptualizing the culture care theory and ethnonursing research method while observing children of diverse cultural backgrounds in a mental health setting and while conducting a study of the Gadsup Akuna of New Guinea (**Figure 2-1**) for her anthropology PhD study. The evolution of both theory and method is documented in Leininger's numerous publications, beginning with her work in nursing and anthropology (Leininger, 1970; McFarland et al., 2012) and culminating with this third edition of her culture care theory book. The Leininger Collections at Wayne State University (Detroit, Michigan) and Archives of Caring in Nursing, Christine E. Lynn College of Nursing, Florida Atlantic University (Boca Raton, Florida) provide interested readers with numerous resources

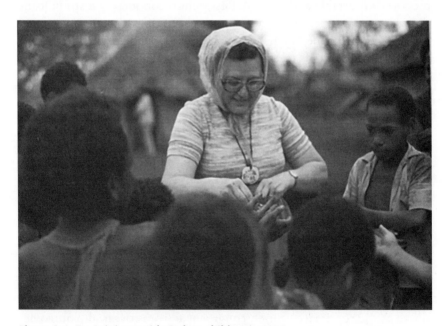

Figure 2-1 Dr. Leininger with Gadsup children in 1977.
Source: The Madeleine M. Leininger Collection on Human Caring and Transcultural Nursing, ARC-008, Photo 2013-01, Archives of Caring in Nursing, Florida Atlantic University, Boca Raton, Florida.

that showcase earlier versions and consequent refinement of the culture care theory and the ethnonursing research method. A brief review of earlier papers and publications of Leininger's work revealed that as she developed the ethnonursing research method, the theorist was greatly inspired by ethnomethods used in anthropology, including ethnoscience and ethnography (Leininger, 1985c, 1994).

Purpose

The central purpose of the ethnonursing research method is to establish a naturalistic and largely *emic* open inquiry discovery method to explicate and study nursing phenomena related to the Theory of Culture Care Diversity and Universality. This research method was designed to tease out complex, elusive, and largely unknown or vaguely known nursing dimensions from people's local viewpoints, such as human care, wellbeing, health, and environmental influencers, as well as noncaring practices potentially leading to illness, disability, or death (Leininger, 2006b). The goal of the ethnonursing research method is to discover culture-specific beliefs, values, expressions, lifeways, and emic worldviews in order to offer culturally congruent care to individuals, families, communities, and organizations through cultural care decisions and actions.

Rationale

In the 1950s and 1960s, Leininger had already identified human care as central to nursing, and recognized a critical need to discover the meanings, expressions, patterns, functions, and structure of human care and caring. She strongly believed that without such knowledge, nursing could not support or justify its existence as a profession or a discipline. How people knew and experienced human care was, in her opinion, essential for nurses to describe, document, and explain so that this knowledge could ultimately guide nursing practices. Leininger held that nurses needed research methods to establish the scientific, humanistic, epistemic, and ontologic bases for nursing's unique discipline perspectives especially focused on human care (Leininger, 1969). She viewed the practice of borrowing research methods from different disciplines to study human caring from a transcultural perspective as highly inadequate. Leininger maintained that the quantitative methods heavily used by the scientific community at the time provided only a limited understanding of human care and nursing care meanings, practices, and processes, and lacked the openness needed to examine subjective, intersubjective, spiritual, or supernatural experiences as well as the caring experiences lived by cultures. She identified the need for a nursing research method that would enable researchers to fully discover, understand, and explain the nature, essence, and characteristics of human care and of actual or perceived nursing phenomena (Leininger, 2006b).

The ethnonursing research method was conceived and developed to overcome the limitations and philosophical tenets of logical positivism, the use of the prevailing scientific method, and other conventional features and goals of the quantitative paradigm to study nursing phenomena. Nursing was different from many established disciplines and its researchers needed better ways to discover its distinctive body of care knowledge. Thus, the ethnonursing method was viewed as the answer to discover the true essence, nature, patterns, and expressions of human care among others to advance nursing care knowledge (Leininger, 1969, 1978, 1981, 1984, 2006b).

From an anthropological perspective, Leininger realized that care was embedded in the worldview, social structure, and cultural values of a particular culture. She maintained that revealing undiscovered care phenomena required an inductive and open inquiry research method that was familiar to human groups and would permit people to share their ideas about care in a spontaneous and informative way with nurse-researchers. Such a research method would assist nurse-researchers to discover, document, preserve, and accurately interpret care meanings and experiences of different cultural groups, and would help nurses fully understand the many elusive, culture-specific, and unknown ideas about human care and caring. The idea of an ethnonursing research method that was people-centered rather than researcher-centered seemed necessary to know human care and its influence on the health and wellbeing of people from different cultures in the world. The ethnonursing inductive and naturalistic research method was needed to discover the nature, essence, and distinguishing features of human care in different life contexts and cultures (Leininger, 2006b).

Another major reason to establish the ethnonursing research method was interest in discovering differences between generic or native folk (naturalistic) care—informally learned indigenous knowledge—and professional nursing care—learned through formal educational systems in nursing—among different cultures. In the early 1960s, during her field study with the Gadsup of the Eastern Highlands of New Guinea, Leininger realized that discovering generic or naturalistic care was essential to know and to use in developing meaningful, congruent, and acceptable professional nursing care practices (Leininger, 1966). However, generic care was unknown and had not been considered for systematic discovery in professional nursing prior to the 1960s. Leininger predicted that differences between generic and professional care existed, but a research method was needed to uncover the subtle and elusive aspects of these sources of care (Leininger, 1970, 1976, 1978, 1981, 2006b).

In the late 1950s, Leininger ran across Pike's (1954) use of the terms emic and etic in linguistic studies and thought that they would be most helpful to explicate and understand human care from a transcultural perspective. These terms were unknown in nursing at the time, and had not been used in anthropological field research. According to Pike, *emic* referred to the local informant's or insider's views of people, whereas *etic* referred to the outsider's views of a culture. Leininger incorporated these concepts in her study with the Gadsup Akuna of New Guinea and found they greatly helped to reveal the meanings of ideas regarding the values, beliefs, norms, rituals, and symbols of care, health, and illness (Leininger, 1966, 1970, 2006b). She came to the conclusion that the emic view was needed to discover human care with other cultures regarding their history, social structure, environment, biological, ecological, and many other factors. Etic knowledge about professional nursing views was also needed to obtain a full understanding about human caring or care. As a result, Leininger incorporated emic, etic, generic, and professional care concepts in her developing ethnonursing research method to study care and other nursing phenomena.

MAJOR FEATURES

The ethnonursing research method, conceptualized from a nursing perspective, was the first qualitative research method developed to study nursing phenomena (Leininger, 1978, 1985a, 1987, 1991a, 2006b). The prefix *ethno-* was chosen to refer to *people* or a *particular culture* with a focus on their worldview, ideas, and cultural practices related to nursing phenomena. Ethnonursing was developed as a research method to help nurses systematically document and gain greater understanding of the meaning of the people's daily life experiences related to human care, health, and wellbeing in different or similar environmental contexts (Leininger, 1980, 1985a, 1987, 1991a, 2006b).

Leininger's anthropological experiences with ethnography, ethnoscience, and ethnology in the early 1960s provided some rich insights into ways to study people and a basis to develop the ethnonursing method. People-centered research with an emic focus required a friendly naturalistic approach that permitted people to share their ideas, beliefs, and experiences with researchers or investigators who were unknown to the people being studied. It also was clear that the goals, purposes, and phenomena of anthropological research were different from those of nursing. As a result, the ethnonursing method was focused on the discovery of nursing's central interests or phenomena within the scope of human caring. New holistic (biophysical and psychocultural) insights and care perspectives from diverse cultures were needed to establish professional nursing within a discipline that is both humanistic and scientific (Leininger, 1978, 1985b, 1991a).

Establishing the ethnonursing research method required an approach radically different from the traditional quantitative paradigm (Leininger, 1985b). In the early 1960s, while the qualitative and quantitative paradigms and their features were largely unknown to nurses, their attributes were becoming identifiable. The ethnonursing method was designed to discover how things really were and the way people knew and lived in their world. The method focused on learning from the people through their eyes, ears, and experiences and how they made sense out of situations and lifeways that were familiar to them. The method required direct naturalistic observations, participant experiences, reflections, and checking back with the people to understand what the researcher observed, heard, or experienced. It required that the ethnonurse-researcher enter into a largely unknown world, remaining with the people of concern for an extended time, to learn firsthand meaningful constructions specific to the natural context or lived environment of people. It meant that the realities of individuals, families, groups, organizations, or communities were developed over time by enculturation or socialization processes and influenced by a variety of cultural and environmental factors.

With the ethnonursing method, there were no a priori judgments, scientific hypotheses, or testing of the researcher's interests or variables; instead, the researcher had to suspend or withhold fixed judgments and predetermined truths to let the people's ideas come forth and be discovered and documented (Leininger, 1985a, 1987, 2006b). Exploring the informants' world to discover vaguely known or unknown ideas about human care and other nursing phenomena was a dominant focus. The researcher had to be sensitive and responsive to people's ideas and to interpret ideas that give meaning to the informants' views and cultural lifeways about human care or noncaring, along with the factors influencing the phenomena discovered.

Beginning in the mid-1950s, Leininger perceived *care* as the essence of nursing, which distinguished nursing from other health professions (Leininger, 1967, 1970, 1976, 1980, 1984). However, she also realized that *human care* required systematic investigation with a method appropriate to discover the full subjective and objective human meanings, patterns, and values of care in different cultures. Because nurses claimed to care for all people, a research method was needed to discover what was universal or diverse about human care transculturally. Generic- or people-based care could only be fully known by studying care from people in their natural contexts such as the home, workplace, or wherever people lived and functioned each day and night, and in different cultures. Thus, the ethnonursing method functioned as a means to obtain new foundational or substantive nursing knowledge to establish human care as the discipline's knowledge base and to guide nursing care decisions and actions in professional practices.

In the early 1960s, Leininger realized that care, wellbeing, health, illness, and other related aspects of nursing were largely embedded in worldview and complex social structure factors related to kinship, cultural values, religion, environment, politics, economy, education, technology, and language expressions. These dimensions had to be explicated and fully known in nursing. To obtain care knowledge from such broad dimensions of social structure and other factors required an inductive ethnonursing approach to grasp the totality of cultural care and to ultimately establish holistic nursing care practices over those traditionally derived from the fragmented, ethnocentric, predetermined, disease, and symptom medical model then in use (Leininger, 1978, 1980, 2006b). The ethnonursing method, combined within the tenets of the culture care theory, provided the broadest and most comprehensive holistic means to discover care and related nursing knowledge.

Leininger began developing and refining the ethnonursing research method largely from her ongoing research experiences and with graduate students whom she encouraged to study care from a transcultural nursing viewpoint. It is of historical interest to note that the method was initially conceptualized before she went to the Eastern Highlands of New Guinea. Leininger maintained that she developed the earlier versions of some of her enablers, such as the Stranger–Friend Enabler and the Observation–Participation–Reflection Enabler (discussed in *Leininger's Enablers for Use with the Ethnonursing Research Method* chapter), in preparation for her study with the Akuna and Arona people of New Guinea (2006b):

> These enablers helped guide me in entering and remaining with the people to study their lifeways in relation to nursing care phenomena in a systematic and reflective way. The Stranger–Friend Model became an important part of the ethnonursing method and has been an essential guide for the researcher to obtain accurate and credible data. It was a fascinating and rewarding research experience to discover rich and meaningful data by entering the people's world as a co-participant. I soon realized that the ethnonursing method was important to discover caring ways of feeding infants, dealing with pain and anxiety, supporting people in lifecycle events and crises, finding different ways to help people, and instructing people to maintain their wellbeing. (Leininger, 2006b, p. 50)

In Leininger's view, nurse-researchers who were firmly entrenched within logical positivism and the quantitative scientific methods in the 1950s and 1960s regarded the ethnonursing qualitative method as too *soft*. It did not have measurable and statistical outcomes, as required by the received view of the logical positivists (Carter, 1985; Leininger, 1985a, 1987, 1991a; Watson, 1985). Moreover, the idea of nursing developing its own method to study nursing phenomena was not acceptable in those early days. Nursing as a profession was then trying to become "scientific" by joining the league of other "hard-core" quantitative scientists and emulating their ways.

Epistemic and Philosophical Values That Support the Ethnonursing Method

Philosophically, the term *ethnonursing* was purposefully coined for this research method because *ethno* comes from the Greek word ethos and refers to *the people* or culture with their lifeways. The suffix *nursing* was essential to focus the research on nursing's phenomena concerned primarily with the humanistic and scientific aspects of human care, wellbeing, and health in different environmental and cultural contexts (Leininger, 1978, 1980, 1984, 1985a, 1988, 2006b). The ethnonursing research method was designed to discover how people knew and experienced these major but insufficiently explored areas of nursing phenomena from a transcultural context and perspective in relation to the Theory of Culture Care Diversity and Universality. Discovering such a potentially large base of nursing knowledge, Leininger thought, would provide the epistemic, historic, and ontological roots as well as contemporary sources of nursing's discipline knowledge (Leininger, 1980, 1984, 1991a).

Philosophically and epistemologically, the sources of ethnonursing knowledge were held to be grounded with the people as the knowers about human care and other nursing knowledge. It was the ethnonurse-researcher's task to learn from the people nursing phenomena and the factors influencing care and health from the local knowers' viewpoints and daily and nightly lived experiences. The knowers were teachers who could share their experiences, insights, and other knowledge of interest with the researcher. Grounded data discoveries had long been part of ethnographic methods as a way of knowing and generating theoretical data, at least since the early creative work of Bronislaw Malinowski (1922) with the Trobrianders in the mid-19th century and Franz Boas (1924) and his detailed work with the North American Indians (Leininger, 1991b). These pioneers established the idea of grounded, detailed, and epistemic sources of knowledge from *the people* long before the work of Glaser and Strauss (1967, as cited by Leininger,

1991b) and other later qualitative methodologists. While the ethnonursing method aims to discover full, rich data directly from people about human care and related nursing phenomena, it uses both emic (local) and etic (nonlocal) methods to obtain a more complete understanding of the phenomena of interest to nursing. This philosophical posture—namely, that indigenous or local people are able to cognitively describe, know, explain, interpret, and even predict human care patterns—was an entirely new perspective to nurses in the 1960s. Leininger (2006a, 2006b) affirmed that a combination of professional and indigenous (generic) knowledge is needed to guide culturally congruent nursing decisions and actions.

The ethnonursing method, therefore, was a way of discovering, knowing, and confirming people's knowledge about care, and ways to keep well, or how they become ill or disabled. For the ethnonurse-researcher, the challenge was to be an interested friend of the people and to participate with them in discovering their past and current cultural beliefs, values, and ideas about human care, health, wellbeing, and other nursing dimensions. The ethnonurse-researcher had to develop skills in teasing out or explicating the people's ideas about human care meanings, expressions, forms, patterns, and general care experiences as lived. This required the use of relaxed, open-ended inquiry modes approached in nonaggressive or nonconfrontational ways. It also required a genuinely interested mode of listening to and confirming informants' ideas. This approach was held to be essential for informants to become the primary sharers and definers of ideas in discussion with the researcher which could ensure accurate and meaningful interpretation of those ideas. Being a humble and open learner is vital to this research method. In addition, keeping an open mind and suspending personal beliefs, past professional experiences, and research experiences are essential attributes of the method and philosophy.

When launched in the early 1960s, the ethnonursing research method was presented with several general philosophical and research features to study ideas related to the Theory of Culture Care Diversity and Universality (Leininger, 1966, 1970, 1978, 1985b, 1987, 1991a, 2006b). First, the method required the researcher to move into familiar and naturalistic people-centered settings to study human care and related nursing phenomena. The use of contrived or artificially controlled settings was not acceptable to obtain credible and accurate people-based data. Likewise, a tightly or rigidly controlled research design was not desired; instead, the nurse-researcher was expected to *move with the local people or situation* as the informants told their past or present stories, events, or lived experiences. The researcher was challenged to enter the emic or local world and to gradually become an active and genuinely interested learner. The ethnonursing method guided the researcher to move with the people or local informants in their lifeways and their patterns of knowing and sharing ideas bearing on human caring within their local environmental context, human ecology, or framework.

Second, by necessity, the ethnonursing method reflected detailed observations, reflections, descriptions, participant experiences, and data derived from largely unstructured open-ended inquiries, or from enabler strategies. Open statements such as "What can you tell me about your views, ideas, or experiences about caring for others or self, in this setting or culture?" are used (Leininger, 1985a, 1987, 1991a). An open-ended question framing such as "I would appreciate it if you would tell me more about. . ." [whatever is being shared] is also used. In addition, emic local folktales, stories, or spontaneous narratives are elicited as well as etic ones to show any contrasts and similarities. Many additional examples of inquiry modes are given in other works (Leininger, 1984, 1985a; Wehbe-Alamah, 2008; Wenger, 1985, as cited in Leininger, 1991b). In addition, learning to enter into a strange world requires some willingness to risk uncertainties and to become comfortable with strangers. It means developing skills to be an astute observer, listener, reflector, and accurate interpreter by taking a learner's role in the most naturally possible way. Being able to tolerate highly ambiguous, uncertain, subjective, or vaguely known complex sets of ideas requires patience, time, and genuine interest in others as essential features of the ethnonursing method.

Third, the ethnonursing method requires that the researcher's biases, prejudices, opinions, and pre-professional interpretations be withheld, suspended, or controlled so that informants can present their emic ideas and interpretations rather than those of the researcher. Learning to value and respect the people's views and experiences when well, sick, with a disability, oppressed, dying, or whatever human condition they are experiencing is an important skill with the method. Being cognizant of the researcher's views and any prejudices requires centering on the informant, active listening, and self-reflection, often with a research mentor. Informants can share ideas that make sense to them and are important to them whether ill or well. Avoiding an interpretation of the informant's ideas to fit professional knowledge and expectations is important. As such, research mentors prepared in the method are extremely valuable for the conduct of this method. Experienced ethnonurse-researchers who have lived through and used the method can deal with novice researchers' tendencies related to ethnocentrism, biases, prejudice, and reinterpretation and assist them in obtaining accurate and credible ethnonursing knowledge. Mentors (preferably with certification as an advanced transcultural nurse) experienced in the ethnonursing method are extremely important to assess ethical and moral issues related to informant "secrets," confidentiality, the process of obtaining consent, and recording of detailed people data. They are especially useful in teasing out generic and professional care findings from large volumes of qualitative data and in analyzing all data collected.

Fourth, the ethnonursing method requires that the researcher focus on the cultural context of whatever phenomena are being studied. The cultural context refers to the totality of the situation or lifeway at hand (Leininger, 1970, 1987, 1991a). The discovery and full understanding of cultural context requires an examination of both contemporary and ethnohistorical underpinnings. Grasping the full meaning of cultural context means examining historical, biosocial, cultural values, language expressions, technology, material, and symbolic referents in the environment of the people being studied. Any removal of cultural contextual data, or "surgical pruning," can markedly reduce the credibility, accuracy, and meaning of what was seen, heard, or experienced. The qualitative criterion of meaning-in-context emphasizes the importance of describing and detailing diverse factors impinging on the meanings of human care, health, or wellbeing of cultures. Indeed, inclusion of cultural context remains an essential aspect of ethnonursing research. Contextual data also provide thick descriptions to establish the study's credibility. Thick descriptions about human care with multiple external or internal cultural factors, symbols, and beliefs help the researcher identify embedded "truths" about human care, wellbeing, and the lifeways of the people. However, teasing out contextual data from the social structure and worldview takes time, patience, and cultural sensitivity.

Encouraging the people themselves to come forth and take control of their knowledge and experiences by sharing their emic cultural viewpoints, values, and lifeways is important. The inductive emic approach helps to prevent researchers from using preconceived judgments or a priori views of modifying informants' ideas. In general, obtaining full, rich, and detailed accounts of cultural care situations, events, or happenings through direct observations, participation, and interviews over time is critical to confirm and establish meaningful patterns of culture care. The ethnonurse-researcher remains a co-participant with informants to discover these detailed accounts and to see how the people practice human care in their daily lives.

With ethnonursing research, it is important to obtain in-depth particularistic or diverse accounts while searching for commonalities (Leininger, 1988, 1989, 2006b). Ideographic or particularized patterns and situations are usually considered more important than broad sweeping generalizations with qualitative studies (Lincoln & Guba, 1985; Reason & Rowan, 1981, as cited by Leininger, 1991b, p. 88). Arriving at generalizations to be applied to large numbers of people or population groups is not the goal of qualitative or ethnonursing research; ethnonursing research and the goals of this research are therefore very different from quantitative research goals (Leininger, 1985a, 1991a; Lincoln & Guba, 1985, as cited by Leininger, 1991b). Simply stated, the goal of ethnonursing research is to know as fully as possible actual or potential nursing phenomena such as the meanings and expressions of human caring in different or similar contexts.

By focusing on some phenomena, the researcher often discovers new insights and ways people interpret and explain their world of knowing. For example, one of the authors discovered that there were gender differences between Lebanese and Syrian men and women regarding provision of care. Lebanese and Syrian men had different ways to provide care that contributed to the wellbeing of nuclear and extended family members when compared to their female counterparts. They typically offered physical assistance with household activities whenever their spouses were physically ill, and provided financial assistance including, but not limited to, paying for a housekeeper to relieve their wives from certain duties and wiring money to extended family overseas on a regular basis. Lebanese and Syrian women, by comparison, were mostly in charge of providing emotional and physical care (Wehbe-Alamah, 2006, 2008, 2011). Similarly, while conducting her study with the Gadsup Akuna of New Guinea, Leininger discovered that the Gadsup did not follow Erikson's (1963) stipulated stages of growth and development. Instead, the Gadsup experienced several phases of human development that were part of Gadsup caring and nurturance and surveillance through the life cycle (Leininger, 1966). Leininger maintained that these comparative emic and etic differences provided refreshing new lifecycle insights that Gadsup care expressions, meanings, and interpretations were different from those in U.S./Western culture; moreover, many New Guinea findings were not generalizable to other cultures, but were more culture specific or relativistic to the Gadsups due largely to enculturation, social structure, and ethnohistorical factors. Accordingly, findings of a particular culture may provide in-depth quality data, rather than generalized data about an unknown group of people.

An important consideration in the use of the ethnonursing method is to give attention to the sequence of events or the ethnohistory of how care lifeways and patterns developed over time. Discovering how human care was traditionally viewed and how it may have changed with individuals and groups often provides fresh insights about cultural changes and variabilities in the culture. The use of ethnohistorical data from anthropologists or social science historians can be useful as background information to show how changes have occurred over time and under different circumstances. It is the task of the nurse-researcher, however, to focus specifically on nursing phenomena in relation to ethnohistorical data. For example, human care practices often change drastically due to certain cultural events, such as major wars, feuds, coups, or major migrations to a new culture. The people's interpretations or explanations of these changes can provide meaningful insights into the dynamic aspects of the culture. Such interpretations of current events often contrast sharply with the findings of quantitative studies; during the latter studies, these events are viewed as threats to the validity and reliability of a study and must be avoided or controlled (Polit & Hungler, 1983).

In conducting an ethnonursing study, the researcher uses the Theory of Culture Care Diversity and Universality as a broad theoretical framework to guide the study. The researcher remains active to identify whether the data support or refute the general or specific theoretical premises and remains alert to the theoretical assumptions or presuppositions of the study. The Theory of Culture Care Diversity and Universality helps the researcher reflect on the theoretical tenets as well as the assumptions and major components of the theory such as worldview, social structure, cultural care values and beliefs, environment, and other dimensions held to influence human care. The theoretical framework serves as an important guide in the search for holistic and particular cultural factors about human care and caring. Accordingly, Leininger (2006b) developed a specific method of data analysis as part of the ethnonursing method to provide systematic data analysis in relation to theoretical assumptions, as well as enablers to explicate or tease out data related to the social structure and other components of the theory.

General Ethnonursing Principles to Support the Research Method

Leininger (2006b) developed the following general summative principles to guide the nurse-researcher in using the ethnonursing research method:

- The first principle the ethnonursing-researcher requires is to maintain an open discovery, active listening, and a genuine learning attitude in working with informants in the total context in which the study is conducted. The researcher's attitude and willingness to be an active learner and to discover as much as possible from the informants and the culture are extremely important for a sound ethnonursing study. The researcher remains an active learner about the people's world by becoming involved in and showing a willingness to learn from the people. Discovering and learning about the meanings, expressions, values, beliefs, and patterns of human care also require active listening, suspended judgments, and reflection about informants' ideas. Informants are usually willing to respond to an active listener who is genuinely interested in their lifeways and viewpoints. Learning from the knowers (informants) may be difficult for some nurse-researchers who are skilled clinicians, administrators, or in other roles where subject-matter expertise prevails. The nurse-researcher, therefore, needs to be aware of ethnocentric views and biases. Being a humble learner is not always easy, especially if female nurses are eager to assert their rights and knowledge to patriarchal informants. Learning from strangers and respecting what is shared without moral (right or wrong) judgments and respecting cultural secrets are essential.

- The second principle the ethnonurse-researcher requires is to maintain an inquisitive attitude and an active and curious posture about the "why" of whatever is seen, heard, or experienced, and with appreciation for whatever informants share with the researcher. Being an active participant and reflector about phenomena means becoming sensitive to the local emic viewpoints and reflecting on etic professional ideas. Searching for the "why" means remaining interested in the informant's views whether they are different or similar to the views of the nurse. It requires a willingness to explore new or different ideas about human caring from folk (generic) and professional viewpoints. Observing and pondering the "why" of care expressions and action modes from both indigenous and professional caregivers often provide new insights about unknown aspects of care. Exploring caring behaviors related to care constructs such as touch, assisting others, protection, support, comfort, and other largely undiscovered culture-specific care concepts necessitates time, patience, and teasing out of vague ideas to get to the epistemics or knowledge sources. The ethnonurse becomes an unrelenting researcher to obtain specific meanings, functions, and expressions of care in relation to well-being, health, illness, death, or any other human condition.

- The third ethnonursing principle is to record whatever is shared by informants in a careful and conscientious way with full meanings, explanations, or interpretations to preserve informant ideas. To satisfy this principle, the nurse-researcher needs to value whatever is shared and try to grasp the diverse and common linkages about human caring. It also means that informants and others in the culture usually are able to interpret and make sense out of their beliefs, experiences (subjective and real), and decision modes if permitted to do so by the researcher. Sometimes it is difficult for the researcher to make sense out of cultural data that he or she sees and hears, but the more the researcher trusts local informants, the more he or she can learn about cultural care and health patterns or experiences. Patience and a willingness to listen and reflect on informant ideas are essential to comprehend and fully understand care and related phenomena. For example, the researcher often records deviant, ambiguous, or questionable ideas with interpretations suspended or withheld until their meanings become understandable with help from informants' diverse expressions. Such diverse expressions must be preserved as well. Not only do they provide significant help in understanding informant ideas but often they are indicators of cultural changes, areas of conflict, or special modes of expressing cultural care practices.

- The fourth ethnonursing principle is to seek a mentor who has experience with the ethnonursing research method to act as a guide. An experienced mentor who has conducted ethnonursing studies can be most helpful in examining the research process at hand. He or she also can help to reduce biases, prejudices, prejudgments, and questionable interpretations that do not support grounded data. Guidance from a knowledgeable research mentor provides an opportunity for the researcher to reflect on the findings and to make meaningful linkages with diverse and similar findings. Moreover, a seasoned qualitative mentor can help process large amounts of qualitative data when the researcher feels overwhelmed and not able to move or "get hold of the data." Often, when cultural linkages may be difficult to make, the researcher mentor can reflect on the ideas in a way that facilitates the researcher's analysis. Finally, the research mentor can be very helpful in presenting and publishing ethnonursing research findings, which are often issued in long, detailed reports.
- The fifth ethnonursing principle is to clarify the purposes of additional qualitative research methods if they are combined with the ethnonursing method, such as combining life histories, ethnography, phenomenology, or ethnoscience. Such combinations are possible, but the reasons and purposes for combining several methods must be made clear at the outset and with the domain of inquiry, the theory, and the research purposes. It is recommended that nurse-researchers do not use additional research methods unless absolutely necessary; if another method is used, however, it should fit the paradigm and study purposes. Nurses who have not been well prepared in qualitative research methods may fail to realize that the qualitative and quantitative paradigms have very different goals and purposes (Leininger, 1985b; Lincoln & Guba, 1985).

Leininger (2006b) asserted that ethnomethods and paradigms should not be mixed. Leininger (1987, 1990) stated that one can mix methods within a paradigm, but not mix methods of different paradigms as doing so violates the purposes and integrity of each paradigm. If methods are used from different paradigms, then the researcher cannot hope to fully understand the purposes and philosophy of each paradigm. A host of serious problems arise when nurses use triangulation, mixing both qualitative and quantitative methods and paradigms with only limited rationale stated. As a consequence, much confusion prevails and such study results are very questionable and have limited credibility. Leininger (2006b) maintained that it is possible to use qualitative or quantitative studies sequentially but it is not possible to simultaneously merge methods and paradigms.

Domain of Inquiry

Discoveries within the CCT and ethnonursing research method (which are developed with a close fit) begin with the researcher making a statement of the domain of inquiry (DOI). This domain must be carefully stated and then rigorously and fully examined with the theory tenets using the six criteria for evaluation of ethnonursing research findings (discussed later in this chapter). Each researcher's enabler is designed to cover every aspect (words or ideas) stated in the DOI, and is focused primarily on the researcher's major hunches and general interests about care and culture. At all times, the researcher keeps focused on the DOI and the general tenets of the culture care theory and the theory goal (Leininger, 1991a, 1991c; Leininger & McFarland, 2002). The following is an example of a DOI: ". . .The generic and the professional care meanings, beliefs and practices related to health and illness of Syrian Muslims living in several urban communities in the Midwestern United States" (Wehbe-Alamah, 2011).

Ethnonursing Research Enablers

Leininger developed several enablers as research guides to obtain broad, yet specific, in-depth knowledge bearing on the goal of the theory and researchers' domains of inquiry and to assist the researcher to discover care and culture knowledge from informants living in different cultural contexts: Sunrise Enabler; Observation–Participation–Reflection Enabler; Stranger to Trusted Friend Enabler; Acculturation Health Care Assessment Guide for Cultural Patterns in Traditional and Nontraditional Lifeways Enabler; Life History Health Care Enabler; Leininger's Phases of Ethnonursing Data

Analysis Guide Enabler; Leininger's Open-Ended Inquiry Guide Enabler for Use with the Ethnonursing Research Method; and Leininger–Templin–Thompson Ethnoscript Coding Enabler. These enablers cover multiple factors influencing care patterns and expressions and are discussed in detail in the next chapter.

Key and General Informants

Selecting key and general informants in any ethnonursing research study for interviewing, observation, and in-depth study is very important. The ethnonurse-researcher does not have samples, objects, subjects, or cases from which to choose (Leininger, 1985a), but works instead with key and general informants such as individuals, families, and groups of people in diverse contexts, institutions, or communities. Key and general informants become a major source for nurse-researchers to learn about people and their cultural care, wellbeing, health, illness, and general lifeways as influenced by a variety of factors. When use of the term "informant" does not fit with the DOI, research design, or setting, the researcher may use the term "participant" instead.

Criteria for Selection of Informants

The selection criteria for informants often include that the informant

- Is associated or identifies with or is a member of the culture being studied;
- Is willing to participate in the study and be interviewed;
- Speaks English or a language understood and spoken by the researcher or by an interpreter hired by the researcher;
- Volunteers time to be observed and interviewed by the researcher; and
- Has lived in the community or country for at least 5 to 10 years.

The researcher may adapt the last criterion to suit the DOI if indicated and/or add more criteria as needed. For example, a researcher may choose to add the criterion that informants must be at least 18 years of age.

Identification of Key and General Informants

Key informants are persons who have been thoughtfully and purposefully selected (often by people in the culture or subculture) to be most knowledgeable about the domain of inquiry of interest to the nurse-researcher. Key informants are held to reflect the norms, values, beliefs, and general lifeways of the culture, and are usually interested in and willing to participate in the study. Key informants are the main source with whom to check and recheck data collected as to its internal (emic) and external (etic) relevance, meanings, accuracy, and dependability along with the researcher's direct observations and participant experiences.

General informants, like key informants, are thoughtfully and purposefully selected. They usually are not as fully knowledgeable about the domain of inquiry as key informants but do have general ideas about the domain under study and are willing to share their ideas and offer relevant reflections and cultural insights. Typically, after the researcher has involved key informants in several sessions, general informants are used to reflect on how similar or different their ideas are from those of key informants. Such information from key and general informants helps to identify the diversity or universality of ideas about human care and other nursing phenomenon. Several interview sessions of approximately 1 to 2 hours are usually needed with key informants to obtain in-depth insights, full meanings, interpretations, and other data that are often embedded in diverse social structure factors and in different human care experiences (Leininger, 1989, 1991a, 2006a, 2006b). Because general informants provide reflective information and are not key informants, less time is given to them. Ethnonursing studies in which the researcher spends limited time with key informants can result in unreliable and inaccurate data. As a result, the researcher does not get backstage or access the "cultural secrets" of informants, and the findings may be questionable.

Number of Informants Related to Maxi- and Mini-ethnonursing Studies

A mini- or micro-ethnonursing study is one that is conducted on a smaller scale and requires approximately 6 to 8 key informants and 12 to 16 general informants who are interviewed and observed over approximately 6 to 8 months. A maxi- or macro-ethnonursing study is research conducted on a larger scale and necessitates approximately 12 to 15 key informants and 24 to 30 general informants. A ratio of 1:2 is the general rule to follow for key to general informants, with two to five lengthy sessions being held with key informants and one session with general informants. The researcher spends approximately 30 minutes with general informants in their home or other familiar settings. Key informants are visited more often than general informants and also observed more often. The length of time spent with key informants may vary until in-depth and accurate data have been obtained, as stated in the DOI.

The numbers of key and general informants were established by Leininger following many decades of research and in accord with other nurse-researchers. Leininger maintained that large numbers of informants alone are not the basis of the rule; instead, the focus is on obtaining comprehensive knowledge to understand fully the phenomena under study

(Leininger, 1985b, 1987; Lincoln & Guba, 1985, as cited in Leininger, 1991b). The use of a large sample of informants for qualitative studies generally leads to superficial knowledge, less credibility for interpretations and explanations, and limited insights about the why and how of particular care phenomena. The researcher's ultimate goal is to search for exhaustive knowledge about care and confirm ideas with a small number of individuals.

Human Subjects Considerations

Voluntary consent to talk with the informants is obtained at the outset and reaffirmed throughout the study (Leininger, 2002, p. 94). Both key and general informants are always free to withdraw from the study at any time without negative consequences. If the study is conducted in a hospital, clinic, or community setting, it is necessary to obtain agency as well as individual consent to protect both informant and agency rights. Written consent is usually preferred but verbal consent may occasionally be more culturally appropriate, as may be the case with Muslim (Luna, 1989, 1994) or Amish (Wenger, 1988) informants.

Language Skills

The ethnonursing method requires that the nurse-researcher possess appropriate language skills to communicate with people in the culture and to interpret ideas and written documents. The researcher must be able to cue into what informants are talking about relative to the topic under discussion. This may require nurses to learn the language of a culture to study cultural care phenomena, as language and culture are closely linked. Language becomes the means to understand meanings, patterns, and other emic or etic expressions and interpretations that are critical to ethnonursing studies. Many different meanings, types, and patterns of care are often found in special language expressions that must be carefully written out with detailed interpretations.

Ethnohistorical data about care, health, wellbeing, or illnesses also are expressed in special language statements over different time spans that the researcher must know how to explore with informants in written and spoken language. Most importantly, the nurse-researcher needs to be aware of not imposing professional or personal language ideas on the data and not interpreting the data using the researcher's linguistic expressions, professional viewpoints, or phrases. When this occurs, one can anticipate less accurate knowledge of culture care meanings from the people. In general, language skills with attention to the informants' ways of expression are essential to conduct a successful, accurate, and credible ethnonursing study.

Field Journal

Keeping a field journal with condensed and expanded notes with focus on the theory and the Sunrise Enabler components is essential to a comprehensive ethnonursing study (Leininger, 1985a, 1988, 1990). The field journal offers the researcher the means to record data directly from the people in both condensed and expanded forms. The Sunrise Enabler serves as a comprehensive guide to the nurse-researcher while recording grounded or raw field data and when checking on areas not fully explored. The Sunrise Enabler also serves as a cognitive map that covers the major components of the theory while collecting and analyzing the findings. The field journal covers data related to the worldview, social structure, ethnohistorical, environmental factors, folk, and professional features as areas to be explored to discover potential influencers of human care. It is considered a primary data source, along with computer data processing of all field data.

CRITERIA TO EVALUATE ETHNONURSING RESEARCH FINDINGS

Because qualitative and quantitative paradigms have very different purposes, goals, and predicted outcomes, the nurse-researcher must be knowledgeable about and use qualitative criteria to evaluate findings from ethnonursing studies. In qualitative research, the researcher is challenged to discover diversities and universalities in relation to the theory and the qualitative paradigm (Leininger, 1987, 1991a, 2006b citing Guba, 1990; Lincoln & Guba, 1985; Reason & Rowan, 1981). As the purpose of ethnonursing research studies is to discover the nature, essence, attributes, meanings, characteristics, and understandings of particular phenomena under study, use of qualitative criteria is imperative.

With the culture care theory and the ethnonursing method, qualitative criteria were chosen to explicate largely covert, detailed, and meaningful data on care, culture, and nursing. After rigorous study of many diverse qualitative research methods and evaluation criteria, Leininger identified and defined six qualitative research criteria to fit the theory goals and the new ethnonursing method (Leininger, 1985b, 1991a, 1995; Leininger & McFarland, 2002). These criteria were designed to systematically examine and discover in-depth care and culture meanings and interpretive findings for qualitative paradigmatic investigations, and are presented here (Leininger, 1970, 1978, 1989, 1991a, 2006a, 2006b):

- **Credibility**: Refers to the "truth," accuracy, and believability of findings that have been mutually established between the researcher and the informants as accurate, believable, and credible about the experiences and knowledge of phenomena. These truths, beliefs, and values (largely from emic findings) have been substantiated through the researcher's observations and with documentation of meanings-in-contexts, specific situations, or events. In addition, direct experiences of the researcher with the people over time and the people's interpretations or explanations are used to substantiate this criterion.

- **Confirmability**: Refers to repeated direct and documented objective and subjective data confirmed with the informants, primarily through observed and primary informant source data, and recurrent explanations or interpretive data from informants about certain phenomena. Confirmability means reaffirming what the researcher has heard, seen, or experienced with respect to the phenomena under study. It reflects evidence of the informants restating or reaffirming ideas or instances that have occurred over time in familiar and natural living contexts. Audit trails (Lincoln & Guba, 1985, as cited by Leininger, 2006b) or confirmed informant checks (Leininger, 1991a) with direct people feedback are ways to establish confirmability.

- **Meaning-in-context**: Refers to findings that are understandable to informants studied within their natural and familiar environmental context(s). Data are understandable with relevant referents or meanings to the informants or people studied in different or similar environments. This criterion focuses on the significance of interpretations and understanding of the actions, symbols, events, communication, and other human activities within specific or total contexts in which something occurred or happened.

- **Recurrent patterning**: Refers to repeated instances, patterns of expressions, sequences of events, experiences, or lifeways that tend to reoccur over a period of time in designated ways and contexts. Repeated experiences, expressions, events, or activities that reflect identifiable sequenced patterns of behavior over time are used to substantiate this criterion.

- **Saturation**: Refers to the exhaustive search from informants of data relevant to the domain of inquiry in which no new findings are forthcoming from informants. Saturation means that the researcher has conducted an exhaustive exploration of whatever is being studied and there are no further data or insights forthcoming from informants or observed situations. A redundancy of information is observed in which the researcher gets the same (or similar) information, and the informants contend there is no more to offer, as they have said or shared everything. Data reveal duplication of content with similar ideas, meanings, experiences, descriptions, and other expressions from the informants or from repeated observations of some phenomena.

- **Transferability**: Refers to whether particular findings from a qualitative study can be transferred to another similar context or situation and still preserve the particularized meanings, interpretations, and inferences of the completed study. While the goal of qualitative research is not intended to produce generalizations but rather to obtain in-depth knowledge of a particular study, this criterion looks for any general similarities of findings under similar environmental conditions, contexts, or circumstances that one might make from the findings. The researcher is responsible for establishing whether this criterion can be met in a new research context. Transferability is the most difficult to use of all the criteria and often necessitates a good mentor to prevent inappropriate uses.

Each these criteria meets the purposes and philosophy of qualitative research analysis and the purposes of the ethnonursing method. While some numerical informant data are included, they are used primarily to confirm data or for directional findings alone. Numbers may be used for weighing interpretive statements or the extent of influences as provided by the informants. The preceding six criteria address internal and external dimensions of discovering care phenomena but must not be dichotomized or reduced to numbers without qualitative indicators. Currently, these six qualitative criteria can be studied more fully in other early publications (Leininger, 1991a; Lincoln & Guba, 1985) as well as in the many published nurse-research studies. Leininger noted that although Lincoln and Guba (1985, as cited by Leininger, 2006b) used the criteria of transferability, credibility, dependability, and confirmability, they failed to identify the importance of meaning-in-context, saturation, and recurrent patterning. Leininger held the latter criteria to be extremely important to establish the soundness of most qualitative studies; she viewed the use of internal and external validity or reliability measurements as inappropriate, as they cannot be used meaningfully with qualitative studies because the purposes and goals of the qualitative and quantitative paradigms are very different.

ETHNONURSING RESEARCH PROCESS

Nurse-researchers need to envision the general research process of conducting an ethnonursing study. With the previously discussed philosophy,

Phases:	1 ⟶	2 ⟶	3 ⟶	4
	Primary *Observation and Active Listening* (no active participation)	Primary *Observation* with limited participation	Primary *Participation* with continued observations	Primary *Reflection and Reconfirmation* of findings with informants

Figure 2-2 Leininger's Observation–Participation–Reflection Enabler

rationale, and enablers in mind, Leininger's Phases of the Ethnonursing Research Process Enabler (**Figure 2-2**) is presented as a visual guide to the general sequence of an ethnonursing research process. While this sequence offers general guidelines, the researcher may modify the process to fit with the research setting or context. Most importantly, the ethnonursing process needs to remain flexible so that the researcher can move with the people and in accordance with the naturalistic developments and human research conditions. As the researcher moves from a stranger to a trusted friend to collect and process data, flexibility and modifications in the research plan often are needed. Nonetheless, the ethnonursing research process helps the researcher to perceive himself or herself when entering, remaining in, or leaving informants as part of the research sequence, whether in the hospital, community agency, urban street clinic, rural community, or other places. Careful use of the ethnonursing research process helps the researcher to ensure a complete and comprehensive study by being attentive to areas that need to be considered to systematically and fully discover the domain of inquiry. Any credible research method contains desired ways to carry out a sound method of investigation for a complete, rigorous study, and this process is offered to help the researcher attain this goal.

The following is a brief description of the ethnonursing research process depicted in Appedix 2-A at the end of this chapter:

1. The first step in preparing for an ethnonursing study is to develop the domain of inquiry or area of interest for investigation, as well as the purpose and goal of the study. Typically, the purpose of an ethnonursing study is related to discovery of knowledge associated with the DOI. For example, a purpose for an ethnonursing study conducted by one of the authors is ". . .to discover, describe and analyze the influences of worldview, cultural context, technological, religious, political, educational, and economic factors on the traditional Syrian Muslims' generic and professional care meanings, beliefs, expressions, and practices" (Wehbe-Alamah, 2011, p. 2).

The goal of an ethnonursing research is usually action-oriented and addresses application of findings to clinical practice, nursing education, management, theory development, and/or research. An example of a goal developed for an ethnonursing study is ". . .to assist nurses with provision of culturally congruent and sensitive care to Syrian Muslims living in urban communities in the Midwestern United States through incorporation of cultural care decisions and actions in their clinical practice" (Wehbe-Alamah, 2011).

2. The researcher identifies the potential significance of the proposed study to advance the nursing profession and discipline. In this section, the researcher discusses how findings from his or her study could increase the body of nursing knowledge, address identified gaps in the literature, and advance or effect nursing research, education, and/or clinical practice.

3. The researcher reviews the available literature to gather relevant information about the DOI under study, examine past and current research about the area of interest, and develop a better understanding of the culture care theory and ethnonursing research method. In addition, it is recommended that the researcher appraise other studies conducted using the theory and method, as discoveries from these studies could later be compared with the researcher's own findings when presenting and discussing the study results.

4. The researcher conceptualizes a research plan that addresses selection, entry, and exit from the research site; identification of facilitators (e.g., researcher speaks same language as informants; researcher secured a mentor who is an expert in both theory and method); and plans or measures for anticipated barriers (e.g., researcher does not speak same language as informants and plans to hire a bilingual interpreter or transcriptionist). The researcher considers human subjects considerations and files for appropriate institutional review board approval. He or she identifies the appropriate gatekeeper who will facilitate (or prohibit) entry into the research site. In the community setting, a gatekeeper is typically a person who is respected by community members and holds a leadership status. In an organizational setting, the gatekeeper may be a member of the management team. The researcher develops selection criteria for key and general informants and seeks gatekeeper assistance with recruitment of informants. Snowball sampling is a technique commonly used in ethnonursing studies to recruit potential informants.

With assistance from a mentor (when available), the researcher decides which enablers will be used in the study. It is recommended that researchers incorporate in their study design use of the Sunrise Enabler; Stranger to Trusted Friend Enabler; Observation–Participation–Reflection Enabler; Leininger's Phases of Ethnonursing Data Analysis Guide Enabler; Leininger's Suggested Inquiry Guide for Use with the Sunrise Enabler to Assess Culture Care and Health Enabler; and Leininger–Templin–Thompson Coding Ethnoscript Enabler. All of these enablers are designed to be adapted by the researcher to fit the DOI of the study. Use of these enablers, under the guidance of the expert mentor, can facilitate the ongoing process of observation, active data analysis, reflection (both by the researcher and with informants), journaling, coding, and computer processing. Data from in-depth interviews and direct and indirect observations of informants are documented and used to confirm findings. Both material and nonmaterial evidence such as informant biographies, photos, written or verbal stories, and other kinds of qualitative data are used to confirm the findings for the ethnonursing method. Qualitative data analysis computer software, such as NVivo, assists the researcher with processing large amounts of data. While the computer software does not analyze the data per se, it helps the researcher categorize, code, and organize the data for ongoing analysis. As the data are analyzed and patterns and themes are identified, the researcher needs to keep Leininger's six criteria for evaluation of qualitative findings in mind and confirm and reconfirm findings with informants to check the credibility and confirmability of those findings.

5. Although data analysis is ongoing, a major review and analysis of data occur once saturation is reached and the study is completed. The research mentor can provide guidance and assistance in this process.

6. A study is not truly complete until its findings are disseminated, as doing so will help achieve the stated (action-oriented) goal of the research. The researcher is encouraged to present the study findings at local, national, and international conferences and to persist (because initial rejection of a manuscript is not uncommon) in submitting a paper for publication at an appropriate peer-reviewed scholarly journal.

7. When applicable, the researcher can help implement the findings with nurses and others interested in findings. In this case, the researcher becomes a consultant and mentor to practicing nurses or others interested in applying study findings and recommendations. **Figure 2-3** shows Dr. Leininger with a group of nurses from Papua

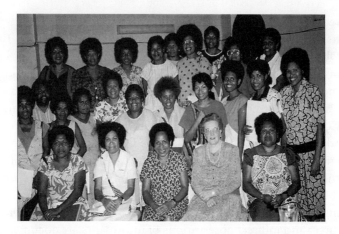

Figure 2-3 Dr. Leininger with Papua New Guinea nurses in Port Moresby, Papua New Guinea, July 1992.
Source: The Madeleine M. Leininger Collection on Human Caring and Transcultural Nursing, ARC-008, Photo 47, Archives of Caring in Nursing, Florida Atlantic University, Boca Raton, Florida.

New Guinea years following her original study with the Gadsup Akuna and Arona of the Highlands of New Guinea.

8. The researcher identifies plans for future studies or areas in need of exploration based on the researcher's personal experience with conducting the ethnonursing study and recognized needs, personal interests, or gaps in the literature. This stage is also where ideas for transferability of research design and findings can be explored.

9. Once the researcher becomes confident in his or her skills and knowledge (of culture care theory and ethnonursing method), he or she becomes a mentor for other novice researchers in the area of research design and implementation and/or the investigated DOI.

Throughout the research process, the theory tenets, predictions, and goals should remain foremost in the researcher's mind. Leininger has always maintained that the use of the word tested is inappropriate for qualitative paradigmatic studies; instead, she recommends using the phrases *in-depth examination of data or confirming the findings*. Detailed, supportive data are used to report findings with qualitative methods such as ethnonursing (Leininger, 2006a). Most ethnonursing studies usually cover an extended period of time, often 6 months to a few years. Much depends on the scope of the domain of the inquiry and whether the researcher desires to conduct a maxi-, mini-, or longitudinal study. The ethnonursing researcher seeks to grasp the world of the informants and the totality of their culture with care meanings and life experiences. The Sunrise and other enablers focus on theory tenets to provide a full and accurate picture of the domain of inquiry. Diverse and similar findings must be documented to remain within the theory tenets. The theory findings often provide rich practical ideas but may also encompass data that explain meanings and practices. Symbolic and abstract data may be discovered in a culture and studied for their care meanings. Most importantly, the criteria of credibility, confirmability, and meaning-in-context must be used from the beginning to the end of the study with documentation. Rich and meaningful truths from cultural informants are largely emic data. The cultural truths are known and held by the informants over time which gives them constancy and credibility. All data obtained are discussed, confirmed, and even analyzed with the informants for accuracy and to fulfill the confirmability criterion.

Data are sought from informants in naturalistic ways (largely informal modes) without the researcher controlling the informants' views. The informants are encouraged to be open and spontaneous in sharing their knowledge. The researcher encourages informants to *tell their stories* from their life experiences. Several interviews and observations are done with key and general informants in their natural and familiar living or working contexts. The researcher relies on open-ended questions or open frames related to all areas identified and related to the stated domain of inquiry (DOI). Open-ended questions such as "Tell me about . . ." must be thoughtfully used to ensure the researcher covers the DOI and fully assesses the acculturation and lifestyle patterns of the informant(s).

RESEARCH FINDINGS FROM THE FIRST TRANSCULTURAL NURSING STUDY

The first transcultural nursing research was an ethnonursing and ethnographic study conducted by Leininger over a 2-year span with the Gadsup people of the Eastern Highlands of New Guinea in the early 1960s (Leininger, 1996, 1991a, 1994; Leininger & McFarland, 2002). Leininger made a few visits to the Gadsup people in subsequent decades (1970s–1990s) to discover culture changes in care beliefs and practices (**Figure 2-4**). Culture care findings, beliefs, and values with major care meanings and cultural action modes of the Gadsup were initially discovered in the 1960s. Several informants were subsequently assessed over time to determine changes in what they believed and practiced. The findings from the Gadsup study have been and continue to be used in nursing practice and education today.

From an exhaustive study over time the researcher-theorist found the following dominant Gadsup core care meanings and practices: *Respect;*

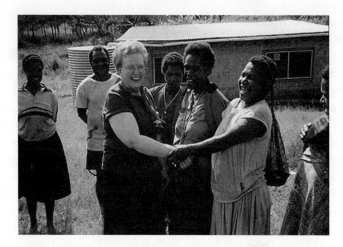

Figure 2-4 Dr. Leininger among the Gadsup of New Guinea in 1992.
Source: The Madeleine M. Leininger Collection on Human Caring and Transcultural Nursing, ARC-008, Photo 48, Archives of Caring in Nursing, Florida Atlantic University, Boca Raton, Florida.

succorance; differential gender roles; nurturance (ways to help people grow and survive); *watchfulness and surveillance nearby and at a distance; male protective caring with women and children in nurturant modes; prevention as care from illnesses and to prevent death; touching as caring;* and *presence.* In addition, nearly 35 transcultural care practices were observed in the culture. The meanings of *cultural pain, suffering, cultural touch, spiritual care,* and many other transcultural care principles and practices were discovered. Leininger (2006a) discovered a very rich body of new knowledge for nursing and healthcare personnel while living in this non-Western culture. These findings were within the culture's special ethnodemographic living context in the Eastern Highlands of New Guinea. Many social structure factors influenced care, but especially mother and father care roles, kinship, and strong cultural values. This was the first maxi transcultural nursing study; Leininger later reported having studied approximately 25 Western and non-Western cultures (Leininger, 1991a, 1995).

The New Guinea findings were a major breakthrough in nursing and health knowledge from a non-Western culture. The care constructs gave new hope for the discovery of the beliefs within a specific culture and for seeing cultural values preserved over many years. The care values were assets and contributed to the health and wellbeing of the Gadsup. The theory tenets were confirmed using the ethnonursing method with the Gadsup people.

Since the early 1960s, nearly 100 definitive care constructs within the meanings and practices of diverse cultures have been discovered (Leininger, 1991a, 1995). Most importantly, the care meanings were largely embedded in kinship, politics, gender roles, cultural values, environment, politics, economic, and historical factors. These factors were major influencers of care patterns and outcomes for healing, helping others, and maintaining or preserving healthy lifeways, as confirmed by the informants and researchers' repeated observations (Leininger & McFarland, 2002). A wealth of other findings also emerged from the use of the theory and method from the Gadsup and many other cultures (1960 to 2012). Leininger and others continued to study and compare culture care findings in Western and non-Western (nontechnological cultures), looking at similarities and differences among and between cultures. Such studies and others have confirmed care phenomena with some unique cultural attributes, adding to the body of transcultural nursing knowledge and practice.

These care meanings and dominant care constructs were unknown in nursing and health services. This new knowledge for transcultural nursing and for nursing education and practices transformed the discipline of nursing. Since Leinigner conducted the first New Guinea transcultural nursing study nurses have been studying culturally-based care. This first study was also a major breakthrough in encouraging nurses to study cultures in-depth and over time for their culture care values, beliefs, and practices in both Western and non-Western cultures. More nurses than ever before are using the theory and the ethnonursing method to study complex and embedded care practices with different cultures in order to provide culturally congruent and sensitive care. Additionally, other healthcare disciplines are becoming interested in the theory and the ethnonursing method. The enablers and the qualitative criteria for congruent care knowledge and practices are being adopted by many health researchers. Qualitative data are becoming more widely used and more highly valued in the research arena and in healthcare services. Other disciplines are finding that the theory and method are natural ways to relate to cultures and can lead to a wealth of meaningful data to improve care to people from cultures that have been neglected in many health institutions and ensure client satisfaction. The theory and method can be used by other health disciplines if they focus on the distinct features of care, culture, and health/wellbeing in their specific discipline. The reader is encouraged to read the full text/primary source of cited and other published studies using the CCT and the ethnonursing research method.

CONCLUSION

In this chapter, the authors have provided an overview of the ethnonursing research method within the qualitative paradigm to show how this method can be used to systematically study cultures using the culture care theory. While it is possible that culture care theory studies can be conducted using other qualitative methods, the ethnonursing method has been designed to be used with the CCT to explicate largely unknown and elusive aspects of human care from transcultural perspectives (Leininger, 2006a). Nursing phenomena such as *care, wellbeing, healing, health, environmental contexts*, and other undiscovered or vaguely discovered nursing phenomena remain a challenge to document fully in regard to their epistemic, ontological, and culturally relevant forms. Over the past 6 decades, Leininger made several revisions and refinements to the theory, the ethnonursing method, and the Sunrise and other enablers so as to better explicate human care and related nursing phenomena. As a result, a new and different way of discovering, knowing, and interpreting humanistic and scientific care is now available. Humanistic and scientific dimensions of care are being established with research findings largely obtained with the use of the ethnonursing research method and other methods within the qualitative paradigm. Unquestionably, the ethnonursing method has become one of the most rigorous and relevant ways to discover human care and many other untapped nursing phenomena. Knowledge of both the theory and the method is needed before launching an ethnonursing study. Fully understanding the theory and method leads to obtaining credible and meaningful research findings. Transcultural research becomes meaningful, exciting, rewarding, and understandable as the researcher develops confidence and competence in the use of the theory and method.

The Theory of Culture Care Diversity and Universality has become valued worldwide. With slight modifications, other disciplines have found the theory and method most helpful and valuable for the provision of care and for conducting research. Nurses who use the theory and method over time frequently communicate how valuable and important it is to discover new ways to know and practice nursing and health care. Practicing nurses can now use holistic, culturally-based research findings to care for clients of diverse and similar cultures or subcultures in different countries. Contrary to some views, the theory and method are not difficult to use once understood and with some expert guidance. Newcomers to the theory and method can benefit from the expertise of experienced mentors in addition to studying published transcultural research conducted using the theory and method. The ethnonursing method is a very natural and humanistic method to use in nursing that helps the researcher to gain fresh, new insights about care, health, and wellbeing. Use of the theory is predicted to grow in the future due to our increasingly multicultural world. The research and theory provide new pathways to advance the profession of nursing and the body of transcultural knowledge for application in nursing education, research, and clinical consultation practices worldwide.

DISCUSSION QUESTIONS

1. Explain purpose and goal of the ethnonursing research method.
2. Differentiate between emic and etic care; provide examples to support your explanation.
3. Discuss the historical development of the ethnonursing research method.
4. Discuss three philosophical underpinnings that support the ethnonursing research method.
5. Explain importance of using criteria for evaluation of qualitative research findings. Analyze use of these criteria in a published ethnonursing research study.

APPENDIX 2-A: UPDATED PHASES OF THE ETHNONURSING RESEARCH METHOD

1. Identify the general intent of your study. Develop the domain of inquiry or phenomenon under study, purpose(s) and goal(s) of the study, and research questions to be addressed.
2. Identify the potential significance of the study to advance nursing knowledge, research, education, and practices.
3. Review available literature on the domain or phenomena being studied, the culture care theory, the ethnonursing research method, and studies conducted using both theory and method.
4. Conceptualize a research plan from beginning to end with the following general phases or sequence factors in mind:
   a. Consider the research site, community, and people to study the phenomena.
   b. Deal with the informed consent expectations and human subjects considerations.
   c. Explore and gradually gain entry (with essential permissions) to the community, hospital, institution, or country where the study is being done.
   d. Anticipate potential barriers and facilitators related to gatekeepers' expectations, language, political ramifications, location, and other factors.

    e. Select and appropriately use relevant ethnonursing enablers with the research process (e.g., Leininger's Stranger–Friend Enabler and Observation–Participation–Reflection Enabler). The researcher may also develop other specific enablers or guides for their study.

    f. Develop selection criteria and choose key and general informants.

    g. Maintain trusting and favorable relationships with the people while continuously conferring with ethnonurse-research mentor expert(s) to prevent unfavorable developments.

    h. Collect and confirm data with observations, interviews, participant experiences, and other data. (This is a continuous process from beginning to end and requires the use of qualitative research criteria to confirm findings and credibility factors.)

    i. Maintain continuous and ongoing active data analysis, reflection, and processing using computers, field journals, and discussions with research mentor(s). Qualitative data analysis computer software is a helpful means to process large amounts of qualitative data. Data coding can be greatly facilitated through the use of an adaptation of Leininger-Templin-Thompson's Ethnoscript Coding Enabler.

    j. Frequently present and reconfirm findings with the people studied to check the credibility and confirmability of findings.

    k. Make plans to leave the field site or community by informing people in advance.

5. Do final analysis and writing of the research findings soon after completing the study.

6. Disseminate the research process and findings via publications in appropriate journals and presentations at local, national, and/or international conferences.

7. Help implement the findings with nurses and others interested in findings.

8. Plan future studies related to this domain or other new ones.

9. Mentor other researchers in the ethnonursing research process.

References

Boas, F. (1924). The methods of ethnology. *American Anthropologist, 22*(4), 311–321.

Carter, M. (1985). The philosophical dimensions of qualitative nursing science research. In M. M. Leininger (Ed.), *Qualitative research methods in nursing* (pp. 27–32). Orlando, FL: Grune & Stratton.

Erikson, E. H. (1963). *Childhood and society* (2nd ed.). Toronto, ON: W. W. Norton.

Glaser, G., & Strauss, L. (1967). *The discovery of grounded theories: Strategies for qualitative research*. Chicago, IL: Aldine.

Guba, E. (1990). *The paradigm dialog*. Newbury Park, CA: Sage.

Leininger, M. M. (1966). *Convergence and divergence of human behavior: An ethnopsychological comparative study of two Gadsup villages in the Eastern Highlands of New Guinea* (Unpublished doctoral dissertation). University of Washington, Seattle.

Leininger, M. M. (1967). The culture concept and its relevance to nursing. *Journal of Nursing Education, 6*(2), 27–39.

Leininger, M. M. (1969). Nature of science in nursing. Conference on the Nature of Science in Nursing. *Nursing Research, 18*(5), 388–389.

Leininger, M. M. (1970). *Nursing and anthropology: Two worlds to blend*. New York, NY: John Wiley & Sons.

Leininger, M. M. (1976). Caring: The essence and central focus of nursing. American Nurses' Foundation. *Nursing Research Report, 12*(1), 2, 14.

Leininger, M. M. (1978). *Transcultural nursing: Concepts, theories, & practices*. New York, NY: John Wiley & Sons.

Leininger, M. M. (1980). Care: A central focus of nursing and health care services. *Nursing and Health Care*, 135–143.

Leininger, M. M. (1981). *Care: An essential human need*. Detroit, MI: Wayne State University Press.

Leininger, M. M. (1984). *Care: The essence of nursing and health*. Detroit, MI: Wayne State University Press.

Leininger, M. M. (1985a). *Ethnography and ethnonursing: Models and modes of qualitative data analysis*. In M. M. Leininger (Ed.), *Qualitative research methods in nursing* (pp. 33–72). Orlando, FL: Grune & Stratton.

Leininger, M. M. (Ed.). (1985b). *Qualitative research methods in nursing*. Orlando, FL: Grune & Stratton.

Leininger, M. M. (1985c). *The role of ethnomethods in the development of nursing theories*. Paper presented at the second Nursing Science Colloquium, Boston School of Nursing. The Madeleine M. Leininger Collection on Human Caring and Transcultural Nursing Archives of Caring in Nursing, Christine E. Lynn College of Nursing, Florida Atlantic University, Boca Raton, FL.

Leininger, M. M. (1987). Importance and uses of ethnomethods: Ethnography and ethnonursing research. In M. Cahoon (Ed.), *Recent advances in nursing* (pp. 17, 23–25). London, UK: Churchill Livingston.

Leininger, M. M. (1988). Leininger's theory of nursing: Culture care diversity and universality. *Nursing Science Quarterly, 2*(4), 152–160.

Leininger, M. M. (1989). Ethnonursing: A research method to generate nursing knowledge. Unpublished paper of the Proceedings of Qualitative Summer Research Conferences. Detroit, MI: Wayne State University.

Leininger, M. M. (1990). Ethnomethods: The phiolosophic and epistemic basis to explicate transcultural nursing knowledge. *Journal of Transcultural Nursing, 1*(2) 40–51.

Leininger, M. M. (1991a). *Culture care diversity and universality: Theory of nursing*. New York, NY: National League for Nursing.

Leininger, M. M. (1991b). Ethnonursing: A research method with enablers to study the theory of culture care. In M. M. Leininger (Ed.), *Culture care diversity and universality: Theory of nursing* (pp. 73–116). New York, NY: National League for Nursing.

Leininger, M. M. (1991c). The theory of culture care diversity and universality. In M. M. Leininger (Ed.), *Culture care diversity and universality: Theory of nursing* (pp. 5–68). New York, NY: National League for Nursing.

Leininger, M. M. (1993a). Culture care theory: The comparative global theory to advance human care nursing knowledge and practice. In D. Gaut (Ed.), *A global agenda for caring* (pp. 3–19). New York, NY: National League for Nursing.

Leininger, M. M. (1993b). Quality of life from a transcultural nursing perspective. *Nursing Science Quarterly, 7*(1), 22–28.

Leininger, M. M. (1994). *Transcultural nursing: Concepts, theories, & practices.* Columbus, OH: Greyden Press.

Leininger, M. M. (1995). *Transcultural nursing: Concepts, theories, research, & practices.* Columbus, OH: McGraw-Hill Custom Series.

Leininger, M. M. (1997a). Overview of the theory of culture care with the ethnonursing method. *Journal of Transcultural Nursing, 8*(2), 32–52.

Leininger, M. M. (1997b). Transcultural nursing research to transform nursing education and practice: 40 years. *Image, 29*(4), 341–347.

Leininger, M. M. (2002). Part 1. The theory of culture care and the ethnonursing research method. In M. M. Leininger & M. R. McFarland (Eds.), *Transcultural nursing: Concepts, theories, research, & practice* (3rd ed., pp. 71–116). New York, NY: McGraw-Hill.

Leininger, M. M. (2005). *Overview of Leininger's ethnonursing research method and process.* PowerPoint lecture presentation. University of Nebraska Medical Center, College of Nursing, Omaha, NE.

Leininger, M. M. (2006a). Culture care diversity and universality theory and evolution of the ethnonursing research method. In M. M. Leininger & M. R. McFarland (Eds.), *Culture care diversity and universality: A worldwide nursing theory* (2nd ed., pp. 1–42). Sudbury, MA: Jones and Bartlett.

Leininger, M. M. (2006b). Ethnonursing research method and enablers. In M. M. Leininger & M. R. McFarland (Eds.), *Culture care diversity and universality: A worldwide nursing theory* (2nd ed., pp. 43–82). Sudbury, MA: Jones and Bartlett.

Leininger, M. M., & McFarland, M. R. (2002). *Transcultural nursing: Concepts, theories, research, & practices* (3rd ed.). New York, NY: McGraw-Hill.

Lincoln, Y., & Guba, G. (1985). *Naturalistic inquiry.* Beverly Hills, CA: Sage.

Luna, L. J. (1989). *Care and cultural context of Lebanese Muslims in an urban US community: An ethnographic and ethnonursing study conceptualized within Leininger's theory* (p. 89). Doctoral dissertation. Available from ProQuest Dissertations and Theses database (UMI No. 9022423).

Luna, L. J. (1994). Care and cultural context of Lebanese Muslim immigrants: Using Leininger's theory. *Journal of Transcultural Nursing, 5*(20), 12–20.

Madeleine M. Leininger Collection, ARC-008. Archives of Caring in Nursing, Christine E. Lynn College of Nursing, Florida Atlantic University, Boca Raton, FL. Retrieved from http://nursing.fau.edu/archives/index. php?main=6&nav=536

Malinowski, B. (1922). *Argonauts of the Western Pacific*. New York, NY: E. P. Dutton.

McFarland, M. R., Mixer, S., Wehbe-Alamah, H., & Burk, R. (2012). Ethnonursing: A qualitative research method for all disciplines. *International Journal of Qualitative Methods, 11*(3), 259–279.

Pike, K. (1954). *Language in relation to a unified theory of the structure of human behavior*. Glendale, CA: Summer Institute of Linguistics.

Polit, D. F., & Hungler, B. P. (1983). *Nursing research: Principles and methods*. Philadelphia, PA: Lippincott.

Reason, P., & Rowan, J. (1981). *Human Inquiry: A sourcebook of new paradigm research*. New York, NY: John Wiley & Sons.

Shapiro, M., Miller, J., & White, K. (2006). Community transformation through culturally competent nursing leadership: Application of theory of culture care diversity and universality and tri-dimensional leader effectiveness model. *Journal of Transcultural Nursing, 17*(2), 113–118.

Walter P. Reuther Library, Madeleine M. Leininger Collection, Wayne State University, Detroit, MI. Accession number WSP000725.

Watson, J. (1985). *Nursing: Human science and human care: A theory of nursing*. Norwalk, CT: Appleton-Century-Crofts.

Wehbe-Alamah, H. (2006). *Generic care of Lebanese Muslims in the Midwestern United States*. In M. Leininger & M. McFarland (Eds.), *Culture Care Diversity and Universality Theory and ethnonursing research method* (pp. 307–325). Sudbury, MA: Jones and Bartlett.

Wehbe-Alamah, H. (2008). *Culture care of Syrian Muslims in the Midwestern USA: The generic and professional health care beliefs, expressions, and practices of Syrian Muslims and implications to practice*. Saarbrucken, Germany: VDM Verlag Dr. Muller.

Wehbe-Alamah, H. (2011). The use of culture care theory with Syrian Muslims in the Mid-western United States. *Online Journal of Cultural Competence in Nursing and Healthcare, 1*(3), 1–12.

Wenger, A. (1985). Learning to do a mini ethnonursing research study: A doctoral student's experience. In M. M. Leininger (Ed.), *Qualitative research methods in nursing* (pp. 283–316). Orlando, FL: Grune & Stratton.

Wenger, A. F. Z. (1988). *The phenomenon of care in a high context culture: The Old Order Amish* (p. 74). Doctoral dissertation. Available from ProQuest Dissertations and Theses database (UMI No. 8910384).

Chapter 3

Leininger's Enablers for Use with the Ethnonursing Research Method

Hiba B. Wehbe-Alamah
Marilyn R. McFarland

> *Both the theory and method are creative contributions to nursing and society which took several years to perfect and systematically examine. Discovering what is universal and diverse remains most timely in nursing as nursing becomes a truly global profession and discipline with substantive transcultural research knowledge to guide teachers and practitioners of nursing. By the year 2020 I have predicted that nursing must become a transcultural discipline and profession. When this occurs, the pioneering work I have begun with the theory and ethnonursing method will be more fully recognized and used worldwide.*
>
> (Leininger, 1997, p. 51)[*]

INTRODUCTION: ETHNONURSING RESEARCH ENABLERS TO DISCOVER HUMAN CARE AND RELATED NURSING PHENOMENA

Over the course of several decades, Leininger developed and refined the Theory of Culture Care Diversity and Universality (also known as *culture care theory*) and the ethnonursing research method with the goal of using

---

[*]Leininger, M. M., *Journal of Transcultural Nursing* 8(2), pp.32–52, copyright 1997 by Sage Publications. Reprinted by Permission of SAGE Publications.

qualitative culture care research findings to provide specific and/or general care that would be culturally congruent, safe, and beneficial to people of diverse or similar cultures for their health, wellbeing, and healing, and to help people face disabilities and death (Leininger, 1963, 1991a, 1991b, 1994a, 1995, 2006a). Leininger (2006b) held that in accordance with any given method, the methodologist develops not only the major features of the method, but also techniques, strategies, and ways that can be used with the method to attain envisioned purposes. She maintained that it is the methodological features with specific techniques and guides that differentiate one research method from another (Leininger, 2006b). In the late 1950s and before conducting her first ethnonursing and ethnographic study with the Gadsup Akuna and Arona of the Highlands of New Guinea, Leininger conceived the idea of *enablers* as ways to explicate, probe, or discover in-depth phenomena that seemed as complex, elusive, and ambiguous as human care. She disliked use of the terms *tool* or *instrument* as she felt that they were too impersonal, mechanistic, and more fitting with objectification, experimentation, and other methods and logical features of the quantitative paradigm. Her vision of enablers and friendly researchers communicated a participatory and cooperative way to obtain ideas that were often difficult to know without the researcher gently probing informants who were willing to share their cultural secrets. Leininger viewed the use of enablers as congruent with the qualitative paradigm and as a means to explicate cultural care.

The research enablers, as part of the ethnonursing method, have been extremely valuable for teasing out hidden and complex data. The enablers, as the name implies, facilitate the discovery of informants' ideas and stories in natural and unstructured ways. With the ethnonursing method, the researcher is expected to adapt the enablers to fit the domain of inquiry (or area) about culture and care to be studied. The enablers are facilitators, and not models per se. They are also not tools or scales, but are ways to examine the major tenets of the theory and the domain of inquiry (DOI). The most commonly used of Leininger's enablers are:

- Sunrise Enabler
- Stranger-to-Trusted-Friend Enabler
- Observation-Participation-Reflection Enabler
- Leininger's Semi-Structured Inquiry Guide Enabler to Assess Culture Care and Health
- Leininger's Acculturation Healthcare Assessment Enabler for Cultural Patterns in Traditional and Nontraditional Lifeways

- Leininger's Phases of Ethnonursing Data Analysis Enabler for Qualitative Data
- Leininger-Templin-Thompson (LTT) Ethnoscript Coding Enabler
- Life History Healthcare Enabler

Enablers do not neglect professional or *etic* medical knowledge about human beings in illness and health such as biophysical, social, and nursing or medical factors, but focus mainly on total lifeways and care or caring factors influencing health and/or wellbeing, disabilities, and death. Traditional *emic* medical and nursing knowledge exist but are often lodged in social structure, ethnohistory, and environmental factors. These emic sources of knowledge (limitedly discovered in the past) are now providing very rich and new insights about people in their familiar and general cultural holistic contexts with specific cultural needs (Leininger, 2006a).

Although Leininger developed several unique enablers over the past 6 decades, the authors present in this chapter only those of major importance that are frequently used by ethnonurse-researchers to study comparative culture care. The ethnonursing research studies that follow this chapter have used some of these common enablers, and some researchers have developed their own specific enablers for a particular focus of their study.

MAJOR ENABLERS TO FACILITATE ETHNONURSING RESEARCH DISCOVERY

The Sunrise Enabler

The Sunrise Enabler (**Figure 3-1**), also known as Leininger's Sunrise Enabler to Discover Culture Care, has been widely used and valued to expand nurses' views and culture care discoveries. Originally developed as a model, and later refined into an enabler, the Sunrise Enabler is not the theory per se, but depicts multiple factors predicted to influence culture care expressions and their meanings (Leininger, 1988, 1991a, 1991b, 1994b, 1995, 1997, 2002, 2006a). It serves as a *cognitive map* to discover embedded and multiple factors related to the theory, tenets, and assumptions with the specific domain of inquiry under study. It is a visual diagram that reminds the researcher to search broadly for diverse factors influencing care within any culture under study and is used as a major guide throughout the study to explore comprehensive and multiple influences on care and culture.

The Sunrise Enabler assists the researcher in identifying factors that could potentially influence human care phenomena including but not limited to technology; religion and philosophy; kinship; cultural values, beliefs,

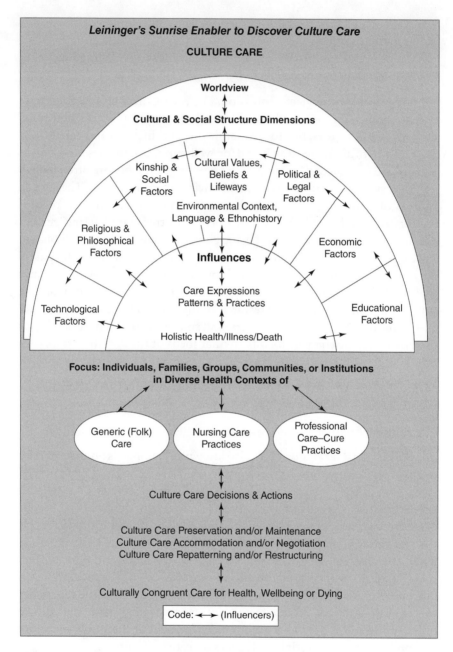

Figure 3-1 Leininger's Sunrise Enabler to Discover Culture Care
Modified with permission from © M. Leininger 2004, by M.R. McFarland and Wehbe-Alamah

and lifeways; politics; economy; and education. Leininger (2002) held that with the Sunrise Enabler to be:

> . . . a true holistic and comprehensive picture can be discovered to reflect the totality of knowing people in their lifeworld or culture. . . Researchers . . . discover hidden, obvious, and unexpected factors influencing care meanings, patterns, symbols, and practices in different cultures. *Let the sun shine and rise* figuratively means to have nurses open their minds to informants to discover many different factors influencing care in their culture with their meanings, and the ways they influence the health and wellbeing of people. (p. 81)

Dr. Leininger's vision encompassed the accessibility and sharing not only of her theory and method but also the enablers. Her only requirement was that researchers, authors, and students cite the full title of each enabler, giving full credit to Dr. Leininger and crediting the source from which each enabler was obtained (Leininger, 2006a, p. 65).

The Stranger-to-Trusted-Friend Enabler

This enabler may be seen in the literature in the following abbreviated form: Stranger–Friend Enabler. This was one of the first enablers developed by Leininger before conducting her ethnonursing and ethnography field study in the Eastern Highlands of New Guinea in the early 1960s (Leininger, 1985a). She further refined this enabler as she studied both Western and non-Western cultures around the globe. Leininger maintained that although some aspects of the enabler were stimulated from reading Berreman's (1962) paper *Behind Many Masks*, it was reconceptualized with new practical indicators to help researchers move from a stranger to friend role when studying people to discover nursing phenomena.

The purpose of the Stranger–Friend Enabler (**Figure 3-2**) is to serve as an assessment or reflection guide for the researcher to become consciously aware of one's own behaviors, feelings, and responses as one moves with informants and works to collect data for confirmation of cultural "truths" (Leininger, 1985a). Each of the indicators or characteristics for the stranger or friend is used and studied over time to identify patterned behaviors and expectations of people-centered studies. These discovered truths have been established as credible and reliable indicators with multiple cultures over many years (Leininger, 1985a, 1985c, 2006b). In using the enabler, the goal is to move from stranger to friend in order to help ensure a credible, meaningful, and accurate study. The enabler can be used by the researcher in hospital settings, community contexts, and many other places where

The purpose of this enabler is to facilitate the researcher (or it can be used by a clinician) to move from mainly a distrusted stranger to a trusted friend in order to obtain authentic, credible, and dependable data (or establish favorable relationships as a clinician); The user assesses him or herself by reflecting on the indicators as he/she moves from stranger to friend.

Indicators of Stranger (Largely *etic* or outsider's views) Informant(s) or people are:	Date Noted	Indicators as a Trusted Friend (Largely *emic* or insider's views) Informant(s) or people are:	Date Noted
1. Active to protect self and others. They are "gatekeepers" and guard against outside intrusions. Suspicious and questioning.		1. Less active to protect self. More trusting of researchers (their 'gatekeeping' is down or less'). Less suspicious and less questioning of researcher.	
2. Actively watch and are attentive to what researcher does and says. Limited signs of trusting the researcher or stranger.		2. Less watching the researcher's words and actions. More signs of trusting and accepting a new friend.	
3. Skeptical about the researcher's motives and work. May question how findings will be used by the researcher or stranger.		3. Less questioning of the researcher's motives, work, and behavior. Signs of working with and helping the researcher as a friend.	
4. Reluctant to share cultural secrets and views as private knowledge. Protective of local lifeways, values and beliefs. Dislikes probing by the researcher or stranger.		4. Willing to share cultural secrets and private world information and experiences. Offers most local views, values, and interpretations spontaneously or without probes.	
5. Uncomfortable to become a friend or to confide in stranger. May come late, be absent, and withdraw at times from researcher.		5. Signs of being comfortable and enjoying friends and a sharing relationship. Gives presence, on time, and gives evidence of being a 'genuine friend.'	
6. Tends to offer inaccurate data. Modifies 'truths' to protect self, family, community, and cultural lifeways. *Emic* values, beliefs, and practices are not shared spontaneously.		6. Wants research 'truths' to be accurate regarding beliefs, people, values, and lifeways. Explains and interprets *emic* ideas so researcher has accurate data.	

*Developed and used since 1959: Leininger.

Figure 3-2 Leininger's Stranger-to-Trusted-Friend Enabler

nurses study nursing phenomena but requires consistent use from the beginning of the research until its completion (Leininger, 1991a, 1991b; Leininger & McFarland, 2002). Leininger (2006b) viewed this enabler as a powerful means for self-disclosure, self-reflection, and assessment and a means for providing high reliability and confirmability with informants as the researcher carefully moves from a stranger role to becoming a trusted research friend.

The enabler was designed with the philosophical belief that the researcher should always assess and gauge the relationships with the people being studied in order to enter or get close to the people or situation under study. It was anticipated that the researcher needed to move from a stranger or distrusted person to a trusted and friendly person during the ethnonursing research process to obtain truthful, sensitive, meaningful, and credible data. Leininger held that researchers usually viewed by informants as etic strangers (outsiders) needed to be trusted before they would be able to obtain any accurate, reliable, or credible data. Initially, most cultures or informants find the researcher to be an outsider or a distrusted stranger until proven otherwise and someone to watch in regard to actions, motives, and behaviors. During the time that researcher remains a distrusted stranger, the people are generally quite reluctant to share their ideas with the researcher; therefore, research data are often superficial, inaccurate, and incomplete (Leininger, 1970, 1978, 1985c). Informants often want to protect themselves, their people, and their ideas until they get to know and trust the researcher(s). The pattern of moving from stranger to trusted friend can be identified in all research studies that have been published over the past six decades (Leininger, 1970, 1978, 1985a, 1985c, 2006b).

The Stranger–Friend Enabler also serves to gauge the researcher's progress, with some researchers remaining in the distrusted role longer than others. The enabler assists the researcher in becoming reflective of and honest about one's own behavior as he/she moves from a stranger to a trusted friend. Becoming aware of self-behavior as a researcher as well as observing those being studied is a major task for the researcher while actively participating with the people. If one remains a stranger to informants, mistrust prevails, and limited personal, intimate, reliable, and accurate details and data are shared by informants (Leininger, 2002a, 2006b).

The Stranger–Friend Enabler is a valuable means for mentoring transcultural nursing students as they perfect their transcultural nursing clinical skills. It is also especially useful as nurses study nurse–client, nurse–group, and nurse–family relationships in the hospital or home. Researchers using this enabler learn to appraise the progress in the study by remaining sensitive to verbal feedback or responses from the people. This enabler is essential to all people-centered investigations, and can be used by many non-nurse researchers involved in humanistic qualitative studies to facilitate the research process, get close to people, and obtain accurate data in a sensitive and skilled manner within different life contexts.

The Observation-Participation-Reflection Enabler

The Observation-Participation-Reflection (OPR) Enabler (**Figure 3-3**) guides the researcher to obtain focused observations of the informants in their familiar and natural living or working environments. Leininger developed this enabler in the early 1960s, and refined and used it for six decades along with many graduate students (Leininger, 1978, 1985a, 1990, 2006a, 2006b). The OPR Enabler was partially derived from the traditional participant-observation approach used in anthropology, but was modified in several ways with the added focus on reflections to fit the philosophy, purposes, and goals of the ethnonursing method. The enabler is different from the conventional anthropological participant-observation approach in that the process was reversed. With the OPR Enabler, the researcher is expected to devote a period of time making observations before becoming an active participant. This *resequenced role* serves the important function of allowing the nurse-researcher to become fully cognizant of the situation or context before becoming a full participant or *doer*. In addition, the reflection phase was added to obtain important and essential confirmatory data from the people being studied. Reflection occurs throughout the research process, but especially during the last phase of research. The four phases in the OPR Enabler were especially conceptualized and developed to fit with the people-centered nursing ways in which professional nurses are expected to work throughout their daily client encounters or experiences.

Users find that the enabler provides a most helpful and systematic way to enter into, remain with, and conclude an ethnonursing study with individuals, groups, communities, and cultures related to human caring and nursing. This enabler helps the researcher get close to the people, study

Phases:	1 →	2 →	3 →	4
	Primary *Observation and Active Listening* (no active participation)	Primary *Observation* with limited participation	Primary *Participation* with continued observations	Primary *Reflection and Reconfirmation* of findings with informants

Figure 3-3 Leininger's Observation-Participation-Reflection Enabler

their total context, and obtain accurate data from them. The most difficult phase for most nurse-researchers is the first phase of observation, because most nurses find it difficult to remain in a focused observer role before becoming a participant. Nurses who are active doers and who have not learned to do sustained observing before acting find that this enabler helps them learn about the importance of observing for a period of time before becoming an active participant.

The researcher gradually moves from the observation to participation phase and still later to full reflection and confirmation of data obtained from informants. The researcher continually confirms findings during and after each observation period with informants. These sequenced phases help ensure sound data collection to obtain a full and accurate database from informants. Each phase is essential and builds upon the preceding phase. It is important not to move into the participation phase until the researcher is trusted by and sensitive to the informants. The extensive observations in the first phase help the researcher to later become a trusted participant with informants and provide confidence for data collection in subsequent phases. This enabler can facilitate highly reliable client care cultural assessments. Throughout the research study this enabler becomes a valuable guide for obtaining detailed and systematic observations with informants. The observations are essential as the basis for sound and accurate reflections in the last phase. Reflections are done with the informants to verify the accuracy of their views or the information obtained, and especially to confirm what was observed, as well as to help to identify any gaps and research biases related to the domain of inquiry.

Reflection is an integral part of the ethnonursing method. Reflection on the phenomena observed or ideas heard helps the nurse to focus on all contextual aspects of the research before proclaiming or interpreting an idea or experience. At the conclusion of the study, the researcher reflects back on all findings to recheck and confirm them, primarily with key informants. Reflection on small and large segments of the data is essential at every phase of the research process as it helps one to study meanings-in-context and other aspects of the data. The OPR phases are a critical and important feature of the ethnonursing research method to ensure accurate and systematic observations and interpretations of findings.

Leininger's Semi-Structured Inquiry Guide Enabler to Assess Culture Care and Health

Leininger's Semi-Structured Inquiry Guide Enabler to Assess Culture Care and Health (**Figure 3-4**) was previously known as Leininger's Suggested

Instructions: The purpose of this ethnonursing guide is to enter the world of the client and discover information to provide holistic, culture-specific care. Use broad and open inquiry modes rather than direct confrontational questions. Move with the client (or informant) to make the inquiry natural and familiar. These inquiry areas are examples for the inquiry and not exhaustive. Identify at the outset if assessing an individual, family, group, institution or community. (This inquiry guide focuses on the individual). Identify yourself and the purpose of the inquiry to the client, i.e., to learn from the client about his/her lifeway to provide nursing care that will be helpful or meaningful.

Domains of Inquiry: Suggested Inquiry Modes

1. Worldview — I would like to know how you see the world around you. Could you share with me your views of how you see things are for you?

2. Ethnohistory — In nursing we can benefit from learning about the client's cultural heritage, (e.g., Korean, Philippine, etc). Could you tell me something about your cultural background? Where were you born and where have you been living in the recent past? Tell me about your parents and their origins. Have you and your parents lived in different geographic or environmental places? If so, tell me about your relocations and any special life events or experiences you recall that could be helpful to understand you and your needs. What languages do you speak? How would you like to be referred to by friends or strangers?

3. Kinship and Social Factors — I would like to hear about your family and/or close social friends and what they mean to you. How have your kin (relatives) or social friends influenced your life and especially your caring or healthy lifeways? Who are the caring or non-caring persons in your life? How has your family (or group) helped you to stay well or become ill? Do you view your family as a caring family? If not, what would make them more caring? Are there key family responsibilities to care for you or others when ill or well? (Explain) In what ways would you like family members (or social friends) to care for you? How would you like nurses to care for you?

4. Cultural Values, Beliefs, and Lifeways — In providing nursing care, your cultural values, beliefs, and lifeways are important for nurses to understand. Could you share with me what values and beliefs you would like nurses to know to help you regain or maintain your health? What specific beliefs or practices do you find most important for others to know to care for you? Give me some examples of "good caring" ways based on your care values and beliefs.

Figure 3-4 Leininger's Semi-Structured Inquiry Guide Enabler to Assess Culture Care and Health
Source: Leininger, M. M. (2002). Culture Care Assessments for Congruent Competency Practices. In M. M. Leininger, & M. R. McFarland (Eds.), *Transcultural nursing: Concepts, theories, research, & practices* (3rd ed., pp. 117–143). New York: McGraw-Hill Companies, Inc.

5. Religious/ Spiritual/ Philosophical Factors	When people become ill or anticipate problems, they often pray or use their religion or spiritual beliefs. In nursing we like to learn about how your religion has helped you in the past and can help you today. How do you think your beliefs and practices have helped you to care for yourself or others in keeping well or to regain health? How does religion help you heal or to face crisis, disabilities or even death? In what ways can religious healers and nurses care for you, your family or friends? What spiritual factors do we need to incorporate into your care?
6. Technological Factors	In your daily life are you greatly dependent upon "high-tech" modern appliances or equipment? What about in the hospital to examine or care for you? (Explain) In what ways do you think technological factors help or hinder keeping you well? Do you consider yourself dependent upon modern technologies to remain healthy or get access to care? (Give some example)
7. Economic Factors	Today, one often hears "money means health or survival." What do you think of that statement? In what ways do you believe money influences your health and access to care or to obtain professional services? Do you find money is necessary to keep you well? If not, explain. How do you see the cost of hospital care versus home care cost practices? Optional: Who are the wage earners in your family? Do they earn enough to keep you well or help you if sick?
8. Political and Legal Factors	Our world seems full of ideas about politics and political actions that can influence your health. What are some of your views about politics and how you and others maintain your wellbeing? In your community or home what political or legal problems tend to influence your wellbeing or handicap your lifeways in being cared for by yourself or others? (Explain)
9. Educational Factors	I would like to hear in what ways you believe education contributes to your staying well or becoming ill. What educational information, values or practices do you believe are important for nurses or others to care for you? Give examples. How has your education influenced you to stay well or become ill? How far did you go with formal education? Do you value education and health instruction? (Explain)
10. Language and Communication Factors	Communicating with and understanding clients is important to meet care needs. How would you like to communicate your needs to nurses? What language(s) do you speak or understand? What barriers in language or communication influence receiving care or help from others. What verbal or nonverbal problems have you seen or experienced that influences caring patterns between you and the nursing staff? In what ways would you like people to communicate with you and why? Have you experienced any prejudice or racial problems through communication that nurses need to understand? What else would you like to tell me that would lead to good or effective communication practices with you?

(continues)

11. Professional and Generic (folk or lay) Care Beliefs and Practices	What professional nursing care practices or attitudes do you believe have been or would be most helpful to your wellbeing within the hospital or at home? What home remedies, care practices or treatments do you value or expect from a cultural viewpoint? I would like to learn about your home healers or special healers in your community and how they help you. What does health, illness or wellness mean to you and your family or culture? What professional and/or folk practices make sense to you or are most helpful? Could you give some examples of healing or caring practices that come from your cultural group? What folk or professional practices and food preferences have contributed to your wellness? What foods are taboo or prohibited in your life or in your culture? In what ways have your past or current experiences in the hospital influenced your recovery or health? What other ideas should I know about what makes you well through good caring practices?
12. General and Specific Nursing Care Factors	In what ways would you like to be cared for in the hospital or home by nurses? What is the meaning of care to you or your culture? What do you see as the link between good nursing care and regaining or maintaining your health? Tell me about some of the barriers or facilitators to good nursing care. What values, beliefs or practices influence the ways you want nursing care? What stresses in the hospital or home need to be considered in your recovery or in staying well? What else would you like to tell me about ways to care for you? What community resources have helped you get well and stay well? Give some examples of non helpful care nursing practices. What environmental or home community factors should nurses be especially aware of to give care to you and your family? What cultural illnesses tend to occur in your culture? How do you manage pain and stress? (Clarify) What else would you like to tell me so that you can receive what you believe is good nursing care? Give specific and general examples.

Figure 3-4 Leininger's Semi-Structured Inquiry Guide Enabler to Assess Culture Care and Health (*continued*)

Inquiry Guide for Use with the Sunrise Model to Assess Culture Care and Health. This enabler was developed by Leininger to assist researchers to enter the world of informants, hear their stories, and make holistic and culture-specific discoveries. This enabler correlates closely with the culture care theory (CCT) and includes the following 12 domains of inquiry derived from the Sunrise Enabler: Worldview; ethnohistory; kinship and social factors; cultural values, beliefs, and lifeways; religious/spiritual/philosophical factors; technological factors; economic factors; political and legal factors; educational factors; language and communication factors; professional and generic (folk or lay) care beliefs and practices; and general and specific nursing care factors (Leininger, 2002a, pp. 137–139).

When using this enabler, researchers develop several open-ended questions for each DOI using an adaptation of the questions suggested in this enabler. Using semi-structured open-ended questions generally elicits more information than closed-ended inquiries during interviews and cultural assessments. Such questions are flexible rather than rigid in content, order, and method of questioning. This type of question allows researchers to remain respectful active listeners, learners, and reflectors throughout the entire research process. Researchers can collaborate with informants, use indirect probing techniques that focus on areas of inquiry, and encourage informants to share their personal stories and life experiences. Nurse-researchers who have moved from the stranger to the trusted friend status find this enabler very helpful in tapping informants' cultural secrets and in collecting truthful and credible data (Leininger, 2002a).

Leininger's Acculturation Healthcare Assessment Enabler for Cultural Patterns in Traditional and Nontraditional Lifeways

The purpose of this enabler (**Figure 3-5**) is to help assess the extent of acculturation of an individual or group with respect to a particular culture or subculture and to identify the extent to which informants are more traditionally or nontraditionally oriented toward their culture (Leininger, 1991a; 1991b, pp. 98–103; 2002, p. 92). Leininger's Acculturation Healthcare Assessment Enabler for Cultural Patterns in Traditional and Nontraditional Lifeways was developed as part of the ethnonursing research method to identify cultural variability or universality features of individuals or groups of a particular culture along major lines of differentiating cultural experiences (Leininger, 1978, 1991b). Since the early 1960s, this enabler has been used, modified, confirmed, and perfected with many informants and in diverse contexts in that acculturation factors such as social structure, worldview, and human care factors were added.

With this enabler, the researcher can obtain a profile of the extent and areas of acculturation with respect to traditional and nontraditional cultural orientations. Data from this enabler are analyzed and reported in the study findings in different creative ways such as pictorial graphs, bar graphs, narratives, or informant or group profiles. There is provision for written narrative statements to support the cultural assessments in each area. The researcher may want to use percentages or simple numerical data to show the direction or degree of acculturation, which is in keeping with qualitative analysis. The acculturation enabler has shown high credibility, reliability,

Name of Assessor: _____ Date: _____

Informants or Code No.: _____ Sex: _____ Age: _____

Place or Context of Assessment: _____

Directions: This enabler provides a general qualitative profile or assessment of traditional or nontraditional orientation of informants of their patterned lifeways. Health care influencers are assessed with respect to worldview, language, cultural values, kinship, religion, politics, technology, education, environment, and related areas. This profile is primarily focused on *emic* (local) information to assess and guide health personnel in working with individuals and groups. The *etic* (or more universal view) also may be evident. In Part I, the user observes, records, and rates behavior on the scale below from 1 to 5 with respect to traditional or nontraditionally oriented lifeways. Numbers are plotted on the summary Part II to obtain a qualitative profile to guide decisions and actions. The user's brief notations on each criterion should be used to support ratings and reliable profile. This enabler was not designed for quantitative measurements, but rather as a qualitative enabler to explicate data from informants.

Part I: Rating of Criteria to Assess Traditional and Nontraditional Patterned Cultural Lifeways or Orientations

Rating indicators:	Mainly Traditional 1	Moderate 2	Average 3	Moderate 4	Mainly Nontraditional 5	Rater Value No.

Cultural Dimensions to Assess Traditional or Nontraditional Orientations

1. Language, Communication and Gestures (Native or Nonnative). Notations: _____
   _____
   _____

2. General Environmental Living Context (Symbols, material and nonmaterial signs).
   Specify: _____
   _____
   _____

3. Wearing Apparel and Physical Appearance. Notations: _____
   _____
   _____

4. Technology Being Used in Living Environment. Notations: _____
   _____
   _____

5. Worldview (How person looks out upon the world). Notations: _____
   _____
   _____

6. Family Lifeways (Values, beliefs and norms). Notations: _____
   _____
   _____

Figure 3-5 Leininger's Acculturation Health Care Assessment Enabler for Cultural Patterns in Traditional and Nontraditional Lifeways

Rating indicators:	Mainly Traditional 1	Moderate 2	Average 3	Moderate 4	Mainly Nontraditional 5	Rater Value No.

7. General Social Interactions and Kinship Ties. Notations: _____

8. Patterned Daily Activities. Notations: _____

9. Religious (or Spiritual) Beliefs and Values. Notations: _____

10. Economic Factors (Rough cost of living estimates and income). Notations: _____

11. Educational Values or Belief Factors. Notations: _____

12. Political or Legal Influencers. Notations: _____

13. Food Uses and Nutritional Values, Beliefs, and Taboos. Specify: _____

14. *Folk* (Generic or Indigenous) *Health Care (-Cure)* Values, Beliefs & Practices. Specify: _____

15. *Professional Health Care (-Cure)* Values, Beliefs and Practices. Specify: _____

16. Care Concepts or Patterns that.guide actions, (i.e., concern for, support, presence, etc.): _____

17. Caring Patterns or Expressions: _____

18. Views of Ways to: a) Prevent illnesses: _____
    b) Preserve or maintain wellness or health: _____
    c) Care for self or others: _____

19. Other Indicators to support more traditional or nontraditional lifeways: _____

(*continues*)

Part II: Acculturation Profile from Assessment Factors

Directions: Plot an X with the value numbers rated on this profile to discover the orientation or acculturation gradient of the informant. The clustering of numbers will give information of traditional or nontraditional patterns with respect to the criteria assessed.

Criteria	1 Mainly Traditional	2 Moderate	3 Average	4 Moderate	5 Mainly Nontraditional
1. Language and Communication Modes					
2. Physical Environment					
3. Physical Apparel and Appearance					
4. Technology					
5. World View					
6. Family Lifeways					
7. Social Interaction and Kinship					
8. Daily Lifeways					
9. Religious Orientation					
10. Economic Factors					
11. Educational Factors					
12. Political and Legal Factors					
13. Food Uses					
14. Folk (Generic) Care-Cure					
15. Professional Care-Cure Expressions					
16. Caring Patterns					
17. Curing Patterns					
18. Prevention/ Maintenance Factors					
19. Other Indicators					

Note: The assessor may total numbers to get a summary orientation profile. Use of these ratings with written notations provide a wholistic qualitative profile. More detailed notations are important to substantiate the ratings.

Figure 3-5 Leininger's Acculturation Health Care Assessment Enabler for Cultural Patterns in Traditional and Nontraditional Lifeways (*continued*)

and confirmability as it has been used with many cultures over the past six decades to identify specific characteristics or patterns of a culture bearing on cultural lifeways, worldview, beliefs, values, care practices, and related nursing phenomena. It is one of the few major acculturation enablers available in nursing, anthropology, and the social sciences (Leininger, 2006b).

Leininger's Phases of Ethnonursing Data Analysis Enabler for Qualitative Data

A major concern for qualitative researchers is to find ways to systematically analyze large amounts of field data. To meet this challenge, Leininger developed and refined the Phases of Ethnonursing Data Analysis (**Figure 3-6**) as

---

Fourth Phase (Last Phase)

Major Themes, Research Findings, Theoretical Formulations, and Recommendations

This is the highest phase of data analysis, synthesis, and interpretation. It requires synthesis of thinking, configuration analysis, interpreting findings, and creative formulation from data of the previous phases. The researcher's task is to abstract and confirm major themes, research findings, recommendations, and sometimes make new theoretical formulations.

Third Phase

Pattern and Contextual Analysis

Data are scrutinized to discover saturation of ideas and recurrent patterns of similar or different meanings, expressions, structural forms, interpretations, or explanations of data related to the domain of inquiry. Data are also examined to show patterning with respect to meanings-in-context and along with further credibility and confirmation of findings.

Second Phase

Identification and Categorization of Descriptors and Components

Data are coded and classified as related to the domain or inquiry and sometimes the questions under study. *Emic* or *etic* descriptors are studied within context and for similarities and differences. Recurrent components are studied for their meanings.

First Phase

Collecting, Describing, and Documenting Raw Data (Use of Field Journal and Computer)

The researcher collects, describes, records, and begins to analyze data related to the purposes, domain of inquiry, or questions under study. This phase includes: Recording interview data from *key* and *general* informants; making observations, and having participatory experiences; identifying contextual meanings; making preliminary interpretations; identifying symbols; and recording data related to the DOI or phenomenon under study mainly from an *emic* focus. Attention to *etic* ideas is also recorded. Field data from the condensed and full field journal can be processed directly into the computer and coded, ready for analysis.

Figure 3-6 Leininger's Phases of Ethnonursing Data Analysis Enabler for Qualitative Data

another enabler to facilitate the research process. This enabler was refined during the past 6 decades as a part of the ethnonursing method to provide rigorous, in-depth, and systematic analysis of qualitative ethnonursing research data, especially research findings bearing on the cultural care theory and the ethnonursing research method (Leininger, 1987).

The Phases of Ethnonursing Data Analysis Enabler offers four sequenced phases of analysis. The researcher begins data analysis on the first day of research and continues with regular data coding, processing, and analysis until all data are collected (saturation). The data are continuously processed and reflected on by the researcher during each phase. In Phase I, the researcher collects, records, describes, and begins to analyze detailed raw data related to the purposes, domain of inquiry, or questions under study. Raw data include interviews from key and general informants, researcher's observations, accounts of participatory experiences, descriptions of contextual meanings, preliminary interpretations, identification of symbols, and data recordings related to the DOI or phenomenon under study mainly from an emic focus. In Phase II, the researcher identifies, codes, and categorizes the descriptors, indicators, and raw data collected in Phase I. In Phase III, the researcher identifies the recurrent patterns from the data derived from Phases I and II. In Phase IV, themes of behavior and other summative research findings are abstracted from the data derived from the three previous phases. At all times, research findings from the data analysis can be traced back to each phase and to the raw data in Phase I (Leininger, 1987). This interphase check is essential to preserve emic data and to confirm findings by checking back on the findings at each phase. This detailed and rigorous process of data analysis is essential to understand the data and to be able to trail back on the findings or conclusions as well as to show how the researcher met the criteria of qualitative analysis including but not limited to credibility, recurrent patterning, confirmability, and meaning-in-context.

Data from ethnonursing interviews and the enablers such as the Observation–Participant–Reflection Enabler, Stranger–Friend Enabler, Healthcare Life History Enabler, and others are integrated into the total ethnonursing mode of data collection and analysis. The culminating abstraction and identification of themes in Phase IV constitute the highest level of data analysis. This phase also presents the most difficult level of analysis as it requires critical examination of all data and keen intellectual abilities to synthesize and abstract meanings from all four phases so that conclusions are credible and understandable. Additionally in Phase IV, findings related to contextual factors, cultural interpretations, language analysis, social structure, and other influencers of human care and wellbeing are also included in the data analysis.

To conduct an accurate synthesis, the researcher must be fully immersed into and familiar with the data. The researcher must carefully preserve relevant verbal statements, meanings, and interpretations from informants in a meaningful way and not reduce data to spurious or questionable themes. Attention is given to special linguistic terms, verbatim statements (quotes), and subjective and experiential data of emic and etic content. In addition, the key informants' interpretations of diverse themes and universalities (commonalities) are identified. Ethnohistorical facts, artistic expressions, worldviews, material cultural items, values and beliefs, and many other aspects influencing culture care and health are integral elements for analysis. Each phase of analysis builds on and supports previous phases so that accurate and meaningful findings are evident.

It is important to note that research assistants and nurses who have had no preparation with the ethnonursing method may have difficulty processing and analyzing vast amounts of data using these phases unless assisted by a teacher or a mentor experienced with the method. For those prepared in the method, this enabler offers a highly rewarding process to make sense out of large or small volumes of ethnonursing qualitative data. Studies presented in this book provide examples of detailed and rigorous analyses of data using the four phases of Leininger's data analysis. These studies have provided new knowledge and insights about culture care transculturally.

The Leininger–Templin–Thompson Ethnoscript Coding Enabler

To facilitate the previously described systematic mode of data collection, processing, and analysis, the Leininger–Templin–Thompson Ethnoscript Qualitative Software was developed around 1985 (Leininger, 1990). The LTT Software was designed as a tailor-made means to process large amounts of ethnonursing data for the culture care theory (Leininger, 1987). This software was initially used for ethnonursing data analysis in that the researcher could directly process large amounts of detailed qualitative data using computer technology. It assisted with coding and processing data focusing on the worldview; social structure; cultural values; language; environmental context; historical facts; folk and professional healthcare systems; specific caring modes; key and general informants; field observations; and other data (Leininger, 1990). The LTT Ethnoscript Qualitative Software Program was developed, refined, and tested by several doctoral nursing students under Dr. Leininger's mentorship—namely, Marie Gates, Teresa

Thompson, Linda Luna, Cynthia Cameron, Zenaida Spangler, and Rauda Gelazis (Leininger, Templin, and Thompson, 1991, p. 3).

As part of the software program, a coding system was developed for Leininger's Theory of Culture Care Diversity and Universality. This coding system followed the general and specific domains of the Sunrise Enabler and included six categories that correlate with the CCT. Although the LTT Ethnoscript Qualitative Software is no longer used, the coding system originally developed for it has become an *enabler* designed to assist researchers using diverse qualitative research software in their quest to code their data. The Leininger–Templin–Thompson Ethnoscript Coding Enabler (**Figure 3-7**) has been used by many researchers conducting ethnonursing

---

Code Numbers, Categories, and Domains of Information: (Includes processing of observations, interviews, interpretations, material, and nonmaterial data)

Code Numbers	Categories and Domains of Information

Category I: General Cultural and Holistic Domains of Inquiry

1	Worldview
2	Cultural–social lifeways and activities (typical day/night)
3	Ethnohistorical (includes chrono-data, acculturation, cultural contacts, etc.)
4	Environmental contexts (i.e., physical, ecological, cultural, social)
5	Linguistic terms and meanings
6	Cultural foods related to care, health, illness, and environment
7	Material and nonmaterial culture (includes symbols and meanings)
8	Ethnodemographics (numerical facts, dates, population size, and other numerical data)
9	*

Category II: Domain of Cultural and Social Structural Data
(Includes normative values, patterns, functions, and conflicts)

10	Cultural values, benefits, norms
11	Economic factors
12	Educational factors
13	Kinship (family ties, social network, social relationships, etc.)
14	Political and legal factors
15	Religious, philosophical, and ethical values and beliefs
16	Technological factors
17	Interpersonal relationships (individual groups or institutions)
18	*
19	*

Figure 3-7 Leininger–Templin–Thompson Ethnoscript Coding Enabler
Source: Adapted as an enabler by Wehbe-Alamah, H.B., & McFarland, M.R. from the original document by Leininger, M.; Templin, T.; Thompson, F. (1991). *The Leininger–Templin–Thompson Ethnoscript Qualitative Software Program User's Handbook* (pp. 16–19), Wayne State University (MI), the Madeleine M. Leininger Collection on Human Caring and Transcultural Nursing (ARC-008, Folder 6–29). Retrieved from the Archives of Caring in Nursing, Christine E. Lynn College of Nursing, Florida Atlantic University, Boca Raton, FL.

Code Numbers	Categories and Domains of Information

Category III: Care, Cure, Health (Wellbeing), and Illness of Folk and Professional Lifeways and Systems

20	Folk (includes popular health and illness benefits, values, and practices)
21	Professional health
22	Human care/caring and nursing (general beliefs, values, and practices)
23	Folk care/caring (emic or indigenous beliefs, values, and lifeways)
24	Professional care/caring (etic beliefs, values, lifeways)
25	Professional nursing care/caring (etic and emic) lifeways (congruence and conflictareas)
26	Noncare/caring beliefs, values, and practices
27	Human cure/curing beliefs, values, and practices
28	Folk and generic cure/curing (etic beliefs, values, and practices)
29	Professional cure/curing (etic and emic perspectives)
30	Alternative or emerging care/cure systems
31	*
32	*
33	*
34	*

Category IV: Health Care, Social Structure Institutions/Systems
(Includes administrative norms, beliefs, and practices with meanings-in-context)

35	Cultural–social norms, beliefs, values, and context
36	Political–legal factors
37	Economic factors
38	Technological factors
39	Environmental factors
40	Educational factors (formal and informal)
41	Social organization or structural factors
42	Decisions and action patterns
43	Inter and multidisciplinary norms, values, and collaborative practices
44	Nursing specialties and features
45	Non-nursing specialties and features
46	Ethical/moral care-cure factors
47	*
48	*
49	*

Category V: Life Cycle with Inter- and Intragenerational Patterns
(Includes ceremonies, beliefs, and rituals)

50	Life cycle male and female enculturation and socialization processes
51	Infancy and early childhood years
52	Adolescence (or transitions) to adulthood
53	Middlescence years
54	Advanced years
55	Cultural life-cycle values, beliefs and practices
56	Cultural life-cycle intra and intergenerational conflict areas
57	Special life-cycle subcultures and groups
58	Life passages (includes birth, marriage, death)
59	*
60	*

(continues)

Code Numbers	Categories and Domains of Information
Category VI: Methodological, Reflections, Issues, and Research Features	
61	Specific methods or techniques used
62	Key informants
63	General informants
64	Enabling tools or instruments used
65	Problem areas, concerns or conflicts
66	Strengths, favorable and unanticipated outcomes of researcher or informants, subjective data and questions
67	Unusual incidents, interpretations, questions, etc.
68	Factors facilitating or hindering the study (time, staff, money, etc.)
69	Emic data methodological issues
70	Etic data methodological issues
71	Dialogue by interviewer
72	Dialogue by someone other than informant or interviewer
73	Additional contextual data (includes nonverbal symbols, total view, environmental features, etc.)
74	Informed consent factors
75–100	*

*Denotes areas where researcher adds own additional codes and descriptions

Figure 3-7 Leininger–Templin–Thompson Ethnoscript Coding Enabler (*continued*)

and metasynthesis studies (McFarland, 1995; McFarland, Mixer, Wehbe-Alamah, & Burke, 2012; McFarland, Wehbe-Alamah, Wilson, & Vossos, 2011).

The Life History Healthcare Enabler

The Life History Healthcare Enabler (**Figure 3-8**) is a guide to obtaining longitudinal data from selected informants of *their lived experiences across their lifespan* with focus on care and caring (or related nursing aspects). Life histories have long been of value in anthropology. Ideas for this enabler were derived from several authors' experiences and from anthropological life histories (MacNeil, 1994). Nurses are now learning how to use full life histories to study nursing and healthcare practices.

It is of interest that clients and families often enjoy talking about their life history accounts, especially middlescent and elderly adults. Hence, this enabler was designed to obtain a full and systematic account from informants about their caring healthy—or less healthy—lifeways and how care beliefs and practices influenced their wellbeing. Enormously rich and detailed data have been obtained from the use of this enabler especially with respect to human caring and health values, expressions, and meanings (Leininger,

1. Introduce yourself and explain that you would like to obtain the person's life and health history. Indicate how such a history could be helpful to health personnel and of interest to him or her. Answer questions or clarify concerns of the individual. Obtain written permission from the individual for the autobiographical or biographical health history study (clarify the differences in these methods).

2. If the individual wishes to write his or her own life history (an autobiography), encourage him to write in his own style, but ask him to include his views and experiences about health, care, and illness patterns in order to help him and others benefit from such knowledge. Clarify how you plan to use the research findings.

3. If you are writing the individual's health and care history biographical account, proceed as follows:

    A. Plan to record the information *before* initiating the interview. Use unobtrusive materials so that you do not distract the informant in celling his history. If you are using a tape recorder, choose one hour tapes to prevent distruption in the flow of the life history with the informant. Written permission must be obtained from the informant prior to any recording (follow the requirements of the committee for human subjects research). If you use ethnographic field notes, you may wish to use the guidelines already described by the author in this book, or use Spradley's suggestions for record keeping (Spradley, 1979, 1980). It is important to note that some informants are not comfortable with having their life history taped and their request must be respected. If an informant consents to taping, offer him or her a copy of the tape without cost. (Usually the informant does want a copy.) If taping is not agreed to, use a stenographer's pad and record words and an outline of what you are observing and talking about. *Immediately* after the history taking, write in detail what you observed, heard, and talked about. Do not wait hours or days, as recall is difficult and accuracy decreases.

    B. Use primarily the ethnographic open-ended type of interview method described in this book or in Spradley's book (1979) to encourage and promote an open flow of information. The researcher's introductory comment might be, "I would like to learn about you and how you have known and experienced health, caring, illness, or disabilities." "As a nurse, I am interested in your past and present lifeways so I can learn what has made you healthy or less healthy, and who you believe have been caring persons in your life." "Feel free to offer special stories or events as you recall ideas important to you." (Clarify as needed how this information may be helpful to nurses to improve nursing care.)

    C. Suggest some life history domains or topic areas on which to focus, using with lead-in statements with a sequence, such as the following:

        (1) "Let us talk about where you were born and what you remember about your early days of growing up, keeping well, or experiencing illness."

        (2) "Can you recall special events, experiences, and health practices during childhood and adolescent years that were especially important to you in keeping well, or that limited your wellness or healthiness?"

(continues)

Figure 3-8 The Life History Health Care Enabler
Source: Leininger, M. M. (1985). Life History Health Care Enabler. In J. MacNeil, (1994) *Culture care: Meanings, patterns and expressions for Baganda women as AIDS caregivers within Leininger's theory* (pp. 144–146). (Doctoral dissertation). Available from ProQuest Dissertations and Theses database. (UMI No. 9519922)

(3) "Let us talk about your speical health care experiences that were particularly clear and pleasant (or unpleasant) to you regarding these periods in your life" (encourage use of folk stories, humorous tales, and descriptions of special events):

    a. Early childhood days
    b. Adolescent years
    c. Mid-life years
    d. Older years

(4) "Give some examples of healthy caring activities or ways of living by your family, cultural group, or significant people who helped you."

(5) "As you think about your life experiences to date, what do you recall about these experiences and what did you value most or least about":

    a. Going to school (primary, secondary, and college days) and your health status.
    b. Employment experiences and how you viewed or experienced them as healthy or less healthy.
    c. Marriage or remaining single throughout life (stresses or nonstresses).
    d. Sudden (or gradual) death of loved persons and how such experiences influenced your thinking and health status.
    e. Accident or illness events to you, your family, or friends and the care expressions.

(6) "I would like to hear about your general philosophy of keeping well and how you believe your religion, political, and cultural values have helped (or hindered) your life goals and health. Can you tell me what beliefs or values have especially guided you to remaining well or become ill?" (Give examples.)

(7) "Can you recall special folk or professional health and caring experiences that were most important to you during your life regarding the following topics?"

    a. Staying well (or becoming ill).
    b. Becoming disabled (and maintaining/ getting well).
    c. Experiencing or dealing with healthy patterns of living.
    d. Recovering from a traumatic experiences as perceived by you.

(8) "Can you recall who you believe were 'good caretakers in the past (and today) and what made them such good caretakers? What noncaring persons influenced your lifestyle or made life difficult or unhealthy for you? What caregivers were important in your life and what made them so? Can you tell me about nurses as caretakers?"

(9) "Throughout your life, what factors seemed to keep you going, living, or establishing healthy patterns of living for yourself and others?"

(10) "What have been some of the greatest rewards or joys in your life? The least rewarding and why? How are these joys related to health or illness?"

(11) "Feel free to tell me other aspects of your life so I can understand it as fully as possible. You can tell me stories, jokes, healing practices, and any special events you believe I should know about to understand you."

Figure 3-8 The Life History Health Care Enabler (*continued*)

D. *Writing and Checking the History.* Covering the above life history points (and others the researchers wishes to include) will take several sessions–usually three to four. Upon completion of the history, you should carefully review and check the history, and then clarify vague points immediately while fresh in the mind of informant. Use the informants own words and account as much as possible. Thank the information and make plans to confirm and share the written (biographical) account. If the account is autobiographical, return and go over the written account to be sure it is understandable and readable, suitable for reproduction as a written document. Express appreciation for the informant's time and information. Present a copy of the tape(s) to the informant. Be sure to provide sufficient time after you have written the account to clarify, confirm, reexamine, or explicate ideas from the informant.

E. *Analysis of Data.* Analyzing the data is a creative art and skill in that the researcher must consciously preserve the informant's statements, but still identify salient themes and synthesize life events in context. It is also an art and skill to both write a health and care life history and keep it accurate and interesting. The verbatim and sequenced account is preserved. Generally thematic, semantic, contexual, and general textual analyses of the data are done with life histories as part of the researcher's separate but special analysis. (See other chapters in this book on these methodological approaches.) Try to identify and analyze patterns of health, care, and illness (if present) so that a synthesis of ideas can be readily identified and used by research consumers. The researcher may wish to present the raw biographical data to the informant and retain theoretical and complex data for the researcher, still sharing dominant findings with the informant at the end of the study.

Figure 3-8 The Life History Health Care Enabler (*continued*)

1985b). Nurse-researchers using the ethnonursing method are encouraged to use this enabler to tease out historical insights about healthcare values and practices, especially related to generic and professional care patterns and practices throughout the lifespan. The life history guide has been useful in obtaining longitudinal narratives about informants' special experiences in folk and professional health care at home and in institutional settings.

Leininger's Ethnodemographic Enabler

This enabler is used as a guide to tap into general ethnographic data about key informants with respect to their environment, history, and related factors. Ethnodemographic factors include social and cultural factors, ethnic orientation, gender, and geographic locations where the informants are living or have lived. Family data, the geographic area, and general environmental factors such as water supply, buildings, and other factors may be included. Specific ethnodemographic facts of different cultures and within a historical context can help to understand the meaning of care and care practices. This enabler is generally used during interviews with key and general informants and while talking to informants about their family origins, general history, and current or past living and working environments; the present and past history are part of the data obtained during these open-ended interviews (Leininger, 2006b). Many researchers fold this enabler into their adaptation of Leininger's Semi-Structured Inquiry Guide Enabler to Assess Culture Care and Health.

Other Enablers Developed by Leininger

Over time, Leininger developed other enablers for use with specific studies. Some of these enablers were eventually folded into some of the enablers described previously in this chapter. Examples of such enablers include: Cultural Care Values and Meanings; Culturalogical [Cultural] Care Assessment Guide; Audio-Visual Guide; Generic and Professional Care Enabler Guide; Cross-Cultural Interview Guide to Study Ethnonursing, Caring, and Related Aspects; and Ethnonursing Field Research Data Form (Leininger, 1985a, 1988).

CONCLUSION

In addition to using an adaptation of any of the enablers presented in this chapter, Leininger encouraged researchers using the ethnonursing method to study diverse cultures in different domains of inquiry to develop their own additional enablers related to cultural care theory as needed. In developing the culture care theory, ethnonursing research method, and enablers, Leininger's ultimate goal was the discovery of new knowledge that could assist nurses and other healthcare professionals to deliver culturally congruent, sensitive, and meaningful care to people worldwide. Although she is no longer with us, Leininger's passion and vision for transcultural nursing remain ignited as a powerful driving force in transcultural nursing thanks to student and seasoned researchers using her theory, method, and enablers.

DISCUSSION QUESTIONS

1. What are enablers and why/how are they used in ethnonursing research?
2. Discuss use of the Stranger-to-Trusted-Friend Enabler. Provide examples that could indicate reaching *trusted friend* status.
3. Develop interview questions using an adaptation of Leininger's Semi-Structured Inquiry Guide Enabler to Assess Culture Care and Health.
4. Discuss the process of ethnonursing data analysis.

REFERENCES

Berreman, G. (1962). *Behind many masks.* Ithaca, NY: Society for Applied Anthropology.

Leininger, M. M. (1963). *Transcultural nursing: A new field to be developed.* Address to Minnesota League for Nursing, Northfield, MN.

Leininger, M. M. (1970). *Nursing and anthropology: Two worlds to blend.* New York, NY: John Wiley & Sons.

Leininger, M. M. (1978). *Transcultural nursing: Concepts, theories, and practices.* New York, NY: John Wiley & Sons.

Leininger, M. M. (1985a). Ethnography and ethnonursing: Models and modes of qualitative data analysis. In M. M. Leininger (Ed.), *Qualitative research methods in nursing* (pp. 33–72). Orlando, FL: Grune & Stratton.

Leininger, M. M. (1985b). Life health care history: Purposes, methods and techniques. In M. M. Leininger (Ed.), *Qualitative research methods in nursing* (pp. 119–132). Orlando, FL: Grune & Stratton.

Leininger, M. M. (Ed.). (1985c). *Qualitative research methods in nursing.* Orlando, FL: Grune & Stratton.

Leininger, M. M. (1987). Importance and uses of ethnomethods: Ethnography and ethnonursing research. In M. Cahoon (Ed.), *Recent advances in nursing* (pp. 17, 23–25). London, UK: Churchill Livingston.

Leininger, M. M. (1988). *Care: The essence of nursing and health.* Detroit, MI: Wayne State University Press.

Leininger, M. M. (1990). *Leininger–Templin–Thompson Ethnoscript Qualitative Software Program: User's handbook.* Detroit, MI: Wayne State University.

Leininger, M. M. (1991a). *Culture care diversity and universality: Theory of nursing.* New York, NY: National League for Nursing.

Leininger, M. M. (1991b). The theory of culture care diversity and universality. In M. M. Leininger (Ed.), *Culture care diversity and universality: Theory of nursing* (pp. 73–117). New York, NY: National League for Nursing.

Leininger, M. M. (1994a). *Nursing and anthropology: Two worlds to blend.* Columbus, OH: Greyden Press. [Original work published 1970; New York, NY: Wiley & Sons.]

Leininger, M. M. (1994b). *Transcultural nursing: Concepts, theories, & practices.* Columbus, OH: Greyden Press.

Leininger, M. M. (1995). *Transcultural nursing: Concepts, theories, research, & practices.* Columbus, OH: McGraw-Hill Custom Series.

Leininger, M. M. (1997). Classic article: Overview of the theory of culture care with the ethnonursing method. *Journal of Transcultural Nursing, 8*(2), 32–52.

Leininger, M. M. (2002a). Culture care assessments for congruent competency practices. In M. M. Leininger & M. R. McFarland (Eds.), *Transcultural nursing: Concepts, theories, research, & practices* (3rd ed., pp. 117–143). New York, NY: McGraw-Hill.

Leininger, M. M. (2002). The theory of culture care and the ethnonursing research method. In M. M. Leininger & M. R. McFarland (Eds.), *Transcultural nursing:*

Concepts, theories, research, & practices (3rd ed., pp. 71–116). New York, NY: McGraw-Hill.

Leininger, M. M., & McFarland, M. R. (Eds.). (2002). *Transcultural nursing: Concepts, theories, research, & practice* (3rd ed.). New York, NY: McGraw-Hill.

Leininger, M. M. (2006a). Culture care diversity and universality theory and evolution of the ethnonursing method. In M. M. Leininger & M. R. McFarland (Eds.), *Culture care diversity and universality: A worldwide nursing theory* (2nd ed., pp. 1–41). Sudbury, MA: Jones and Bartlett.

Leininger, M. M. (2006b). Ethnonursing research method and enablers. In M. M. Leininger & M. R. McFarland (Eds.), Culture care diversity and universality: A worldwide nursing theory (2nd ed., pp. 42–81). Sudbury, MA: Jones & Bartlett.

Leininger, M. M., Templin, T., & Thompson, F. (1991). *The Leininger–Templin–Thompson Ethnoscript Qualitative Software Program: User's handbook*. Detroit, MI: Wayne State University. Retrieved from the Madeleine M. Leininger Collection on Human Caring and Transcultural Nursing (ARC-008, Folder 6-29). Archives of Caring in Nursing, Christine E. Lynn College of Nursing, Florida Atlantic University, Boca Raton, FL.

MacNeil, J. M. (1994). *Culture care: Meanings, patterns and expressions for Baganda women as AIDS caregivers within Leininger's theory*. Doctoral dissertation. Available from ProQuest Dissertations and Theses database (UMI No. 9519922).

Madeleine M. Leininger Collection. (ARC-008). Archives of Caring in Nursing, Christine E. Lynn College of Nursing, Florida Atlantic University, Boca Raton, FL. http://nursing.fau.edu/archives/index.php?main=6&nav=536

McFarland, M. R. (1995). *Cultural care of Anglo and African American elderly residents within the environmental context of a long-term care institution*. Doctoral dissertation. Available from ProQuest Dissertations and Theses database (UMI No. 9530568).

McFarland, M., Mixer, S., Wehbe-Alamah, H., & Burk, R. (2012). Ethnonursing: A qualitative research method for all disciplines. *International Journal of Qualitative Methods, 11*(3), 259–279.

McFarland, M., Wehbe-Alamah, H., Wilson, M., & Vossos, H. (2011). Synopsis of findings discovered within a descriptive meta-synthesis of doctoral dissertations guided by the culture care theory with use of the ethnonursing research method. *Online Journal of Cultural Competence in Nursing and Health Care, 1*(2), 24–39.

Spradley, J. (1979). *The ethnographic interview*. New York: Holt, Rinehard and Winston.

Spradley, J. (1980). *Participant observation*. New York, NY: Holt, Rinehart and Winston.

Chapter 4

The Benefits of the Culture Care Theory and a Look to the Future for Transcultural Nursing

Madeleine M. Leininger

Dr. Leininger drafted this chapter shortly before her death in August 2012. It is a revised update of the chapter she authored for *Culture Care Diversity and Universality: A Worldwide Nursing Theory* by Leininger and McFarland (2006) with integrated elements from her speech to the 37th Annual Conference of the International Transcultural Nursing Society held in Las Vegas, Nevada, in October 2011. We are grateful to have this, her last work, to share with our readers.

Marilyn R. McFarland

Hiba B. Wehbe-Alamah

Care is an essential human need and the essence of nursing
(Leininger, 2002, p. 46)[*]

INTRODUCTION

It is extremely important that any profession—and especially a discipline—look to the future and plan for future goals or directions to maintain its stature and scholarship. Transcultural nursing as a recognized and growing discipline needs to keep these thoughts and goals foremost in mind

---

[*]Leininger, M. M. (2002). Essential transcultural nursing care concepts, principles, examples, and policy statements. In M. M. Leininger & M. R. McFarland (Eds.), *Transcultural nursing: Concepts, theories, research, & practice* (3rd ed., p. 46). New York, NY: McGraw-Hill Companies, Inc.

with regard to the current and distant future of transcultural nursing. The 21st century is well under way with many world leaders discussing their thoughts and plans for the coming decades. Identifying and strategizing to meet discipline goals are not only prudent but essential for the growth of any discipline and for the interests of the membership. Indeed, a legitimate discipline with members from respected professional fields needs to think ahead and plan for future goals. This means giving serious thought about developing plans to project the future of the field and envision ways to reach desired goals. It also means identifying major areas of emphasis with the goals.

Wise leaders and their members usually generate much excitement and enthusiasm as they discuss their thoughts and plans to reach future goals or possibilities with ways that such goals might be realized or achieved in the future. Moreover, wise leaders and futuristic members let their imagination explore broadly and deeply into their ideas as they envision the future goals and directions. Most futurists become excited to plan for the future and to offer ways to reach their goals. As futurists let their imaginations explode or dreams with their desired goals dominate their thinking and plans, they often imagine almost endless possibilities and then share their ideas with respected leaders and expected potential followers or students. Indeed, very few leaders and their followers succeed unless they discuss their ideas and goals with other persons who can ignite the thinking of these people and send the ideas further. In the history of great leaders, as futurists, these leaders not only ignite flames of possible realities but also make plans as they visualize possibilities. Dynamic futurists get people thinking far ahead, envision future possibilities, and plan ways to make these ideas or goals come into reality. There is a dynamism in their talk and enthusiasm for ideas to make these ideas become real and possible. These dynamic leaders as *futurists* want members of any organization to become excited and feel hopeful that their ideas will move forward into reality.

Futurists are goal sellers, promoters, and dynamic planners who emphasize that projected ideas and opportunities will become alive as possibilities, realities, and opportunities that can be attained and realized. Futurists are the true leaders of any organization, and their thoughts, predictions, opportunities, and possibilities become contagious or real. Moreover, futurist leaders in professions and organizations often gain power, respect, and noteworthy recognition for their dynamic and futuristic thinking, ideas, plans, and action-oriented possibilities as goals. Several of these futurists exist as transcultural nurses, and their ideas need to be tapped and given serious thought.

TRANSCULTURAL NURSING

We as transcultural nurses are extremely pleased that transcultural nursing has a growing membership, many dynamic leaders, with many action-oriented planners and practitioners. I contend that transcultural nursing today is in a unique position to lead the transformation of health care across the 21st century and beyond. I believe we are at a point in our evolutionary development to support the futuristic ideas and practices of transcultural nursing and move the discipline forward not only within the United States but worldwide. It is time for innovative breakthroughs globally throughout health care and transcultural nurses can provide the guiding leadership for such breakthroughs.

Transcultural health care with a focus on *culture care-based theory, research, and practice for a healthy world is a realistic goal.* This goal is needed in the United States and in many other places in the world. I believe transcultural nurse-leaders can initiate and sustain the momentum toward this goal. Indeed, in the United States futurists recognize the need to stimulate some entirely new and different ideas about health care to serve Americans, the many cultures within and outside the United States, and for all people in the world. Transcultural nurse-leaders are capable of spearheading this goal with a focus on *culture care*. This could be the powerful breakthrough to *transform* health care not only in the United States but worldwide. It is a noteworthy goal much needed and in demand to improve and provide quality-based health care. Transcultural nurses can stimulate other health-care professionals to become cooperative to achieve this goal. Their wisdom, knowledge, and demonstrated transcultural practices can be powerful guides for our colleagues, as they work to fulfill this goal.

INTERDISCIPLINARY GOAL SETTING

Currently in the United States and in several other countries, I find there are many leaders, scientists, philosophers, and futurists who are actively discussing transcultural health care as a major goal to meet the need for and transform health services. They need transcultural nurse-leaders to help them achieve this goal as their future contribution to society and to the world. Some of these healthcare professionals want transcultural nurses to demonstrate such leadership. While some consider this idea desirable, others think it impossible. Therefore, transcultural nurses need to transform bold, wise, and almost unthinkable predictions—the sign of a true futurist—into realistic goals and practices.

Moreover, I believe that transcultural nurses with our professional colleagues can be coleaders to make such goals or major breakthroughs into distinguished contributions to health care in the United States and globally. *Why not?* Transcultural nurse-leaders can propose such bold future directions with plans and become powerful leaders to *transform health care* with a focus on *culture care* to provide effective, wellness-based, and culturally congruent outcomes.

Most importantly, this multidisciplinary healthcare goal with plans for the 21st century should have shared values, shared visions, shared actions, and noteworthy shared health goals to provide care and promote healthy citizens and prevent illness or negative outcomes. Transcultural nurses are indeed in a unique position to impact on this shared and desired goal to transform health care within the United States and globally.

Shared goals can provide positive health care to some cultures which have been neglected or overlooked in the past. Yes, and still today there are cultures in the United States and globally who are hoping for health care that fits or is congruent with their cultural beliefs, values, and practices. These cultures welcome transcultural care to support their culture. Many of these cultures will welcome transcultural nursing that integrates their cultural values into health care. Moreover some of these cultures, I predict, will soon demand beneficial transcultural care as essential for quality and health-promoting care. Such expectations are a human right and culture care can no longer be neglected or not provided. Transcultural care that is culturally-based can impact favorably on the people for healthy outcomes and to prevent illnesses. Transcultural nursing is in a good position to make this a reality and transform healthcare practices in many countries and within the United States. In addition, with transcultural nursing research focused on culture care theory and practice, one can predict some transformation of health outcomes in the near future. Research findings with many cultures will be important to realize this future trend and to support this new national and global goal.

Transcultural nurses, however, must continue to build upon our traditional and current goals. We must expand the number of cultures to be served and incorporate other cultures and professional personnel as we move forward in this new endeavor. Unquestionably, we have made noteworthy progress over the past 50 years, but we need to greatly expand our thoughts and research and unite other health personnel with transcultural nurses. We also need to consider some bold and new strategies for collaboration that are worthy of our consideration with other disciplines in the near future. We need to ask ourselves: *What noteworthy contributions, collaborations, or united actions can transcultural nursing make as we expand our goals and endeavors and unite our services with colleagues to reach culturally congruent health outcomes based on transcultural nursing theory and research?*

As we collaborate on transcultural care services with other disciplines, we need to focus on selected areas as we build transcultural nursing across the 21st century.

FUTURE TRENDS AND GOAL AREAS

Future Vision

In this chapter, I offer some potential future trends to stimulate the thinking of transcultural nurses about the future goals not only in the United States but also globally. And, as we collectively consider *selected areas* where we believe transcultural nurses can make some meaningful and significant contributions and transform healthcare services to become culturally based in the United States and with some impact globally, we recognize these ideas will still need multidisciplinary debate and discussion before being realized.

But as we do futuristic thinking and planning, let us maintain a strong theory and research focus to our explorations, expansions, and collaborations. Given that the Theory of Culture Care Diversity and Universality has been quite effective to guide many nurses to plan and provide culturally congruent health care, I believe we need to use this theory. Dr. McFarland, Dr. Wehbe-Alamah, and their research students have completed a metasynthesis of the culture care theory with many transcultural nursing research studies and findings and produced an outstanding and highly laudatory report of significant findings in many cultures (McFarland, Wehbe-Alamah, Wilson, & Vossos, 2011). This is an excellent starting point. The metasynthesis discovered many values and benefits in the use of the culture care theory. The theory with the ethnonursing research method continues to be widely used in the United States and in many countries around the world. The Theory of Culture Care Diversity and Universality, based on transcultural nursing research findings in many cultures, supports substantive culture care beneficial outcomes to the people studied (Leininger, 2006). This metasynthesis of transcultural nursing research with the theory and the method can be built upon, expanded, strengthened, and reaffirmed with new culture care findings to advance transcultural nursing knowledge and skills. These are positive signs of nursing contributions from Dr. McFarland's large metasynthesis investigation that can be built upon and used to engage collaborative interdisciplinary research participation. Uniting our efforts with nursing and interdisciplinary colleagues will be important.

Moreover, with the Certification Examination being offered worldwide, we can strengthen transcultural theory services, nursing skills, research, and practices. We can also use the culture care theory and ethnonursing research method to generate more comparative, meaningful data to transform health care and to establish effective transcultural nursing collaborative actions and communication modes worldwide. Indeed, health care can be transformed by making transcultural human care with a culture care focus essential for effective quality care practices. Thus this goal seems realistic, feasible, and attainable as well as sustainable for the future.

Future Goals

For the second part of this chapter, some futuristic trends must be considered about where transcultural nursing might head in the 21st century: Our minds and thinking must be open. In preparation of this chapter, I identified 50 future trends, but I reduced this number to eight major ones to consider. Some trends may appear unbelievable, some impossible, some possible, and some not too quickly possible or beyond your capabilities and resources (financial and human) to consider. Nonetheless, it is essential to present the trends to expand nurses' thinking and to consider possible other areas or goals for transcultural nursing to consider. Of course, some trends may be beyond our scope, interests, or imaginations, or just be impossible. Nevertheless, we need to keep these trends alive in our minds, as they may become real possibilities or future realities. So, as I identify and briefly discuss some of the dominant future trends for transcultural nursing, let your thoughts be ignited by these possibilities before tossing them aside. In the meantime, keep in mind our valued and established transcultural nursing goal to provide culturally congruent care to cultures we serve now and in the future that will lead to health, wellbeing, and meaningful care for all cultures.

And as these future trends are identified, you will realize there are many influencing factors with each future trend. Time and space will not permit me to discuss these influencers. Nevertheless, such influencing factors are essential to discuss, debate, and explore before deciding on any specific domains, goals, or directions. Most of all, permit yourself to consider such possibilities and then allow your imagination to dream about them, and keep open the possibilities or feasibilities of each trend.

Undoubtedly, it will be difficult to consider global trends as it requires global thinking, global possibilities, and global considerations. This is difficult to envision fully or even partially. However, if we fail to consider global trends, we may be missing important possibilities for transcultural nursing. And, while hearing and thinking about exploring the unexplored future possibilities, one needs the *freedom to choose* potential areas and to think *possible* and *if not, why not*. The freedom to select barely known areas is important for these may be the great possibilities and potential realities. And, one should not wait too long to identify such possibilities as other futurists may soon select these goals which might not be congruent with transcultural nursing goals.

Concluding these preliminary comments, let me now go on to identify a few futuristic trends for transcultural nurses to consider as possibilities, goals, or directions for transcultural nursing in the future.

Trend 1: Globalization of Health Care

The first futuristic and almost inevitable future trend is the globalization of health care. This is familiar language to transcultural nurses, as health care is a global human phenomenon and a cultural right and expectation. We know that we live, exist, practice, and function in a global world for survival. The ways humans stay well, become ill, and/or survive in a global world are only partially known to us, but not fully known or understood. There are endless cultural possibilities and multiple care modalities or practices with different cultures. It is difficult to comprehend globalization in its fullest perspective—as it is conceptually too big for our current conceptual and thinking modes. But, as we think about globalization as a future trend, our thoughts must be worldwide and include and engage many possible cultures and subcultures. We also need to think about the many diverse cultural groups with different languages who live in many different geographic locations under different and changing political, economic, social, and religious environments within different cultural contexts and climates. This is very difficult to consider, almost mind boggling and beyond human abilities; nevertheless, we must try to think within a very broad worldview. There are many dimensions to grasp about globalization, but we must struggle with these dimensions. *What views or areas might transcultural nurses envision, hold, or choose to know about globalization while remaining mindful not to have our particular views be incongruent with these global ideas?*

To grasp globalization of transcultural nursing within and outside the United States one must continually look for the broadest scope or worldview with care diversities and similarities which are major constructs of the culture care theory. We must also view globalization as broad in geographic scope with great diversity and complexity of cultures and to incorporate these ideas into transcultural nursing. I would suggest, however, that we begin by selecting a smaller dimension with a specific feature that might be considered for future globalization.

Of course, transcultural nursing multicultural values, practices, beliefs, and lifeways are also to be considered with globalization, but again I believe we might identify aspects of cultures or more limited areas related to globalization. For example, one might consider the Pacific Islander culture care practices and then study cultures with different languages who live in many different geographic locations under different and changing political, economic, social, and religious environments within different cultural contexts and climates. To teach and practice transcultural care skills related to specific research ideas, a smaller perspective might be important to consider rather than a *too big* view of the larger Pacific Islander culture; instead choose a specific island culture on which to focus the study about a globalization-related phenomena.

And as I discovered from my global research, there were *universal culture care values* and *diverse values* which could be focused upon as an aspect of globalization. Some of the major universal culture care values identified from my research were *respect, kindness,* and *attention*; these all needed in-depth study for their meanings. There were also many culture care diversities that could be studied as an aspect of globalization or from a comparative health outcome perspective for future globalization. *Globalization means attention to local, regional, and international culture care values and practices in large or smaller culture areas.*

The comparative focus leads to a synthesis of differences and similarities to guide transcultural nursing care practices. Culture care beliefs and practices in many regions of the world, such as the Oceanic culture, Arctic area, Europe, Near East, and many other regions, countries, or territories including five ocean areas worldwide, merit study. Discovering the *culture care meanings and expressions of cultures requires extensive and intensive emic and etic contrasts.* Such care differences and similarities would be a major new thrust to advance transcultural nursing care. Again, the culture care theory would be helpful to discover care from regional globalization aspects. One would also need to consider geographic areas, climate, historical and geographic shifts, and other topographic factors. This would require considerable study to delineate particular care phenomena or domains. However, many selected regions and their cultures could be considered or chosen; one could also collaborate on such research with other disciplines such as anthropologists who have worked in diverse regions and countries for many years.

Transcultural care tenets might need to be expanded with globalization as one includes historical, political, economic, and social changes along with climate differences in geographic regions. A related focus on regional or smaller dimensions of globalization could include the prevention of illnesses, death, and accidents. Climate and economic changes would be important parts of culture care globalization. Other areas that might be considered could be child deformities, elder illnesses, or health conditions of subcultures. The Sunrise Enabler would be most helpful with these foci to explicate culture care values, expressions, and practices. Religious, ethical, and other related factors that might prevent such illnesses along with care values could be studied and would be valuable transcultural care research data.

Most importantly, anthropological historical and current demographic data would be important to include as foci with globalization. Transcultural nurse researchers could consult and unite with scholars in different disciplines to define and refine specific care areas for globalization. Transcultural Nursing Society members should retain transcultural nursing philosophy and interests such as the lifespan and the elderly with globalization. There are many valuable potential areas to study with culture care worldwide—many areas which are still unknown or unexplored. Members of some disciplines, especially social and geographic scientists, have already identified their domains of interest for globalization such as population needs and healthcare services. Some scientists may have chosen major geographic culture areas such as Poland, the Arctic, Asia, Russia, and the Middle East as their focus. Collaborative or shared research-based knowledge will be important to consider in globalization studies. Knowledge of climate changes in the world will also be important with the elderly and special groups such as the homeless or immigrants. And, as transcultural nurses expand their work, they will need research-based data about culture care phenomena with knowledge of *culture climate changes* and healthcare environments for children and the elderly for meaningful, comparative globalization findings.

And with the increased migration of immigrants and refugees settling in or leaving diverse places in the world, our knowledge of these migrations with respect to *health care* is critical to discover how culturally congruent care can decrease or increase culture conflicts, stresses, killings, and criminal acts. *Will transcultural nurses pursue study of immigration and healthcare practices or lack of culture caring with migration that may lead to illnesses, increased culture care conflicts, culture care stresses, and unfavorable illness outcomes? Will illnesses be more evident among selected migrations and why? Are there cultures that have healthy migrations?* Transcultural nurses will want to be knowledgeable about and sensitive to culture care expressions and caring (or noncaring) acts to help immigrants and refugees survive migrations. *In the future, will migration groups become an integral part of larger cultures and adjust to similarities and differences or will they remain isolated and at high risk for illnesses or untimely death?*

Trend 2: Managing Population Increases and Decreases

Another major future trend is increased populations worldwide. A marked increase in world populations has been predicted for the 21st century. Data estimates are overwhelming with facts and predictions that change almost daily. As a consequence, the new future trend is labeled *managing population increases and decreases*. Now, this is a mind-boggling future trend and is almost too difficult to fully comprehend. The term *managing* seems overwhelming to consider, let alone handle its implications. I doubt if this trend will be one chosen by transcultural nurses. Nevertheless, the predicted population increase or decrease merits our consideration as the population increases will influence globalization and healthcare outcomes. Transcultural nurses and healthcare providers worldwide need to work together to consider this as a major influencer upon healthcare outcomes. *How will transcultural nurses and the world cope with increased populations?*

Most assuredly, population changes will have a major impact on health, illnesses, wellbeing, and accidents among cultures. Economic, environmental, food, and human resources will be affected by population changes across all ages and cultures. Population increases will influence small and large families, small and large cultures as well as organizations and institutions. Currently, many futurists, scientists, researchers, therapists, and population specialists are writing about and discussing their predictions for population trend increases. It is currently a *hot and inevitable trend* to be faced. *If transcultural nurses decide to focus on population changes and/or managing populations, what aspect will they consider? In what ways will growing populations locally, regionally, and worldwide impact nurse shortages and especially transcultural nurses? What role will transcultural nurses have with this major trend? How will healthcare resources be rendered with increased populations?* These are urgent and important questions to answer or consider before the problem becomes too severe.

Trend 3: Transportation and Communication

Another inevitable and major future trend will be *rapid transportation and communication factors worldwide*. It has been predicted that in the 21st century, human beings will witness and directly experience many new, diverse, and rapid transportation and communication modes worldwide. Many technological transportation and communication innovations are already under development in the United States and in other countries. New types of airplanes, cars, buses, and mobile modes of transportation will exist almost everywhere in airways, oceans, mountain areas, and remote geographic areas. Accordingly, many new kinds of transportation and communication *products* will soon be on the market in different sizes and forms. It is difficult to fully imagine the diverse responses and impact of rapid and diverse transportation and communication technologies on humans. All forms of electronic media such as televisions, cellular telephones, and computers with wireless and nonwireless communication technologies are already on the market with many more yet to be developed. Such technological diversities will challenge transcultural nurses, health personnel, and all human beings to understand and use effectively and skillfully in their work.

These modern technologies will impact upon the abilities of humans to fully understand these products and to influence their proper and safe uses in health care, illnesses, accidents, and diverse life stresses. Transcultural nurses will be challenged to know and learn how to use these products safely, effectively, and skillfully. Healthcare institutions will need to address this trend as well. It was Dr. Margaret Mead who envisioned and predicted this trend in her early writings and speeches in the 1920s. She stated that modern technologies in the future would be so rapid, diverse, and difficult for humans to understand and use that most people would be overwhelmed with them and their proper uses in their homes, hospitals, or wherever they live (Mead, 1955). Many diverse technological accidents related to communication and transportation will occur with these modern technologies. Improper use of them in homes, health institutions, hospitals, or wherever modern technologies are used will prevail. People will be in states of confusion and experience problems while learning to use or interface with many of these technologies. Undoubtedly, transcultural nurses will be greatly influenced by modern technologies that are already in use and whose impact is being felt in health and wellness care areas. *Will transcultural nurses help people and cultures become prepared to respond to and consider modern technologies in their daily practices? Will transcultural nurses help clients of diverse cultures prevent accidents and destructive outcomes? Will the Transcultural Nursing Society develop policies, principles, or guidelines to help cultures use modern technologies safely and effectively?*

Transcultural nurses need to study and urgently consider ways modern technologies will be used in order to prevent major accidents, conflicts, mental confusion, and harmful acts and influence negative or positive care patterns. Most of all, non-Western cultures may fall prey to modern technologies and technology products in health services with unfortunate outcomes. *What role will transcultural nurses play to prevent technology accidents and misuses in health services? Will nurses be prepared for modern technologies of the*

21st century to prevent harmful uses of technologies and especially technologies that will be strange and confusing to many non-Western cultures?

Trend 4: Illnesses, Accidents, and Other Threats to Humans

Still another future and major trend will be an *increase in illnesses, disabilities, accidents, and threats to human lives* largely due to people living closely together and in limited spaces and with limited resources and access to services. Modern technologies, use of commercial products, and food shortages, along with many stresses and conflicts related to limited personal space, living too closely together, and other environmental changes, will be evident. Housing patterns will change creating different living patterns among and between cultures. Diverse modes of living among cultures will be a big problem in the 21st century for many cultures. Cultures will encounter new, unknown, strange, and unexpected contacts with people from diverse cultures that will lead to mental stresses, illnesses, diseases, accidents, and criminal acts. Cultures will also show signs of strange and unknown illnesses. Unfortunately, there will be limited medical and nursing knowledge to help prevent these *new and strange illnesses and accidents. What will or should be transcultural nurses' responses to this trend of more illnesses, accidents, and short- and long-term disabilities with perhaps insufficient numbers of nurses to care for these clients?*

It is anticipated that many of these illnesses will be related to changing climates, travel contacts, and close living and working environments among different and unknown cultures living in close quarters in post-disaster or political refugee camps with limited sanitation, food, and health resources. Work conditions, seasonal climate changes, compromised air and water quality, and food shortages will increase and lead to illnesses and increased tensions. The lack of early and adequate assessment and diagnosis in addition to these food shortages will be a major concern. I predict that many emergency and field clinics will need to be established to cope with malnutrition, dehydration, and many illnesses, accidents, and disease conditions. One can predict there will be many illnesses that may not be treatable due to lack of medical research, proper healing methods, and appropriate treatments or medicines. Professional personnel will be overwhelmed to discover these conditions, especially with limited caring and healing resources. Undoubtedly many illnesses will be precipitated or influenced by cultural factors such as cultural tensions, threats, and conflicts and absence of culture care practices by professional staff. *Will transcultural nurses work actively to prevent or decrease this trend?* It will be a disturbing trend of great concern to health professionals and for national and global professional groups and institutions.

Trend 5: Intercultural Diversity Issues

One can envision another major trend as being related to *human diversities among and between cultures as manifested by cultural stresses, genocides, poverty and political/economic oppression, and mental and physical illnesses. Will transcultural nurses help to ameliorate or prevent these intercultural diversity challenges?* This is another major area in which research studies bearing on culture care are urgently needed, and soon, to prevent such health problems. *Will transcultural nurses step forward to help prevent health problems and to prevent negative, unhealthy consequences before these expressions, actions, or conditions occur?*

Trend 6: Intercultural Competition for Human Resources

Still another trend can be identified as *intercultural competition for human resources, especially related to food, water, money, modern equipment, and resources for daily living.* Food and water shortages will be of greatest concern. Competition for food and water for all humans for their survival will prevail—with criminal acts to procure food and water. This may precipitate severe crises especially with poverty and political oppression and corruption that affect displaced refugees and other neglected cultures and culture groups. Intense food and water shortages will lead to major neglect resulting in crimes and thefts to maintain a subsistent human existence. Cultures will be overwhelmed by the need to obtain enough food supplies for their families. Some large families and especially immigrants and refugees will find this trend overwhelming and disturbing and may lead to genocides. One can predict that many crimes and the killing of endangered and other animals for food will continue to occur for human survival. Intercultural competition for such resources will be intense, serious, and disturbing. Limited ethical and moral behavior to curtail criminal acts will be evident but overlooked due to their goal to survive. In fact, ethical and moral awareness will be almost disregarded for the survival of family members, groups, and special individuals. Such intercultural competition will increase across the 21st century and it will be difficult to predict consequences. Migratory people, especially starving families, will compete and steal food, water, produce, and agricultural supplies. Farm supplies will be limited due to fewer farmers or producers of food. Thus, adequate food supplies for families will become inadequate by the end of the 21st century.

What role could or should transcultural nurses have with this trend? Will nurses develop policies, principles, or strategies to lessen or decrease intercultural competition and destructive acts, and to increase ways humans can seek health in caring ways? The need to provide adequate food for the world's population and decrease criminal acts for food and water will be major concerns.

Trend 7: Rise in Cultural Minorities

The *rise in the number of culture minorities* will be significant in the future and needs to be identified as a future trend. Socio- and culture care—*justice care*—will be in great demand. The increased percentages of minorities and majorities will markedly shift in the 21st century and lead to cultural tensions and cultural, social, and economic injustices that will challenge nurses, transcultural nurses, and other healthcare personnel worldwide. Ethical, moral, and religious strategies will challenge nurses along with pressure by groups to meet minority needs.

Trend 8: Rise in Mental Illness

Another major anticipated trend is the *increase in mental illness*. Different cultures and subcultures will demonstrate different expressions of mental illnesses that will be precipitated by culture contact with unknown cultures or strange cultures leading to *cultural conflict*. Some of these cultural conflicts will add to violent acts such as suicides, mass genocides, and shootings at homes, schools, and workplaces. Many cultural forms of mental illness will be unknown because the cultural expressions and behavioral acts are not yet known or understood and therefore cannot be anticipated. Transcultural nurses will struggle to develop mental health principles and practices and to *discover culture care factors to decrease and transform these conditions*. New and better ways to help these clients will be expected and needed. In addition, mental illness problems and age-related mental conditions will show great variability among cultures. The way transcultural nurses respond to these mental health trends and expressions will be of concern. These trends and others need to be considered now as transcultural nurses select and develop appropriate roles to help cultures. Many psychiatrists and psychologists will also struggle to diagnose and understand these culturally-based mental illnesses due to culture variances and lack of culture knowledge of these cultural groups by these scientists.

CONCLUSION

The major future trends identified might sound rather frightening but nonetheless these future trends need to be considered. We need to expand our thinking and give thought to such possibilities as well as the roles transcultural nurses will take with these trends. Unquestionably, culture care factors will play a major role in each of these future trends, to try to keep cultures healthy and prevent illnesses. It is wise to study and ponder now on these trends and their potentials that transcultural nurses may encounter and need to consider.

In summary, it is wise and imperative to give thought to these future trends with ways to study and address such trends. Most importantly, research studies on *prevention strategies and appropriate culture care decisions and actions* will no doubt be *in demand to guide culturally beneficial care along with transcultural practice skills*. I believe and recommend that transcultural nursing needs to establish *field research stations* that are focused on teaching, research, and practice in the United States and other countries. Transcultural nursing centers worldwide could develop these field stations in the future. These field stations will be important to initiate, nurture, and support research studies and also to facilitate education and care practices that deal with the future trends cited. These field stations need to be located in diverse cultural areas; they also need to be envisioned and developed soon in order to evolve and support transcultural nursing for the future. As identified, most of these outlined future trends should be discussed, debated, and considered soon for the future of transcultural nursing. We need to consider our special interests, skilled areas, and also collaborative care practices to facilitate transcultural nursing and to plan with different disciplines and healthcare providers for *collaborative health care*. Collaborative and united care efforts will be essential to facilitate transcultural nursing efforts and to provide culturally congruent care that is effective and helpful not only for national health care but also global care.

Undoubtedly, other future trends will occur and will influence health care in the future. Most importantly, we need to maintain an open discovery attitude as well as identify strategies and plans to transform health care. I believe we will see many new emergency healthcare clinics focused on preventive care related to suicide, homicides, mass killings, and other concerns of the 21st century. Plans to transform destructive behavior, accidents, illnesses, and mental confusions will challenge transcultural nurses' thinking, decisions, and actions. Reinforcing favorable care approaches will be essential to alter, modify, or respond to unexpected and unpredicted trends. Accordingly, transcultural nurses will need to prepare a core of transcultural nurse specialists to deal with transformation processes, models, principles, and guidelines in order for successful transformation to occur in relation to future trends.

Many of these identified major trends are likely to occur during the 21st century and they may indeed seem overwhelming and disturbing. One may want to deny that these predictions might occur, but we need to expand and explore them as possibilities. Some of these trends are already occurring in the United States and worldwide. Unquestionably, these trends and others will play a major role in health care and will require transcultural consideration and action soon.

Some signs of these trends are already evident in various places in the world, and they are disturbing and alarming. Transcultural nurses need to ponder on these trends soon and consider the potential influences on health care and what their own role will be in regard to these trends. Ethical and moral concerns will influence nurses' critical thinking and nursing care decisions and actions. I believe that transcultural nurses need to align themselves with other disciplines in a collaborative and unified manner to provide professional services and cope with these trends. Perhaps my most recent innovation of *collaborative culture care* will be beneficial.

Lastly, one can predict that cultures will promote and establish their own indigenous or traditional caring, curing, and health practices for survival. Indeed, traditional care and healing models, which are becoming more evident in the United States and in other countries, will increase in numbers. Fortunately, some transcultural nurses have been working with traditional healers and caregivers. Traditional *cure* will be supported with an increased number of traditional healers and caregivers. Nurses with transcultural nursing preparation and anthropological preparation will be in a good position to respond to this cultural trend. However, nurses need to give serious thought to unite and work with traditional healers, diverse health personnel, and established medical care providers. This will be a good way to transform transcultural nursing and health care in the United States and globally. Collaborative or united care may be the most essential and promising trend to consider. *If so, recognition for leadership needs to be given to indigenous healers and to trends to unite and combine collaborative and traditional modes with transcultural nursing care.* Transforming trends into effective and beneficial practices will be essential and will require thoughtful plans and diverse strategies by transcultural nurse leaders with traditional healers and caretakers.

Most importantly, all of the described future trends and others will also be influenced by persons skilled in diverse languages and cultural value understandings of Western and non-Western cultures. In addition, an understanding of the cultural context for care and cure practices will be imperative. Transcultural leaders, teachers, practitioners, and administrators will soon need to speak in diverse languages, function with more cultures, and use available research from members of other disciplines such as anthropology, sociology, and psychology as well as others—many who have spent numerous years studying and working with indigenous and diverse cultures.

Lastly, I will leave you with one of my traditional sayings from the 1950s:

> To look is one thing.
> To understand what you observe is another.
> To understand as fully as possible what you have seen or heard is essential.
> To learn what you saw and what you understand is even more critical.
> But most important, is to act upon what you have seen and understood, and what appears to be important to cultures or human beings.
> These are the ingredients of a professional person.

Desire goals as transcultural nurses and function to provide beneficial and health-promoting care in the 21st century. This saying merits thought and should be a major challenge and an exciting goal not only for nurses in the United States but for *all* nurses to be able to function effectively and professionally in our global world.

Transcultural nursing and the 21st century seem very promising partners to establish and transform health care in new and promising directions in the United States and globally. Our creative ideas and decision and action modes will be visibly used with promising success. We shall succeed in the future just as we have succeeded in the past with the beginning of transcultural nursing.

DISCUSSION QUESTIONS

1. Discuss how transcultural nursing/nurses may approach the trends identified by Dr. Leininger in this chapter.
2. Discuss the questions posed by Dr. Leininger in the chapter.
3. Identify other possible global trends; discuss whether they are appropriate for transcultural nursing/nurses to address, and if so, how.
4. Discuss what individual transcultural nurses, or small transcultural nursing groups or chapters, can do to address these trends locally, nationally, and globally.

REFERENCES

Leininger, M. M. (2002). Essential transcultural nursing care concepts, principles, examples, and policy statements. In M. M. Leininger & M. R. McFarland (Eds.), *Transcultural nursing: Concepts, theories, research, & practice* (3rd ed., p. 46). New York, NY: McGraw-Hill.

Leininger, M. M. (2006). Ethnonursing research method and enablers. In M. M. Leininger & M. R. McFarland (Eds.), *Culture care diversity and universality: A worldwide nursing theory* (2nd ed., p. 51). Sudbury, MA: Jones and Bartlett.

Leininger, M. M., & McFarland, M. R. (Eds.). (2006). *Culture care diversity and universality: A worldwide nursing theory* (2nd ed.). Sudbury, MA: Jones and Bartlett.

McFarland, M. R., & Leininger, M. M. (2011, October 21). *The culture care theory and a look to the future for transcultural nursing.* Keynote address jointly presented (Leininger via videotape) at the 37th Annual Conference of the International Society of Transcultural Nursing, Las Vegas, NV.

McFarland, M., Wehbe-Alamah, H., Wilson, M., & Vossos, H. (2011). Synopsis of findings discovered within a descriptive meta-synthesis of doctoral dissertations guided by the culture care theory with use of the ethnonursing research method. *Online Journal of Cultural Competence in Nursing and Healthcare, 1*(2), 24–39.

Mead, M. (1955). *Cultural patterns and technical change.* Westport, CT: Greenwood Press. Reprinted 1985.

Chapter 5

Leininger's Father Protective Care

Madeleine M. Leininger
Revised by Hiba B. Wehbe-Alamah

INTRODUCTION

Three Western cultures and one non-Western culture were investigated in order to obtain in-depth knowledge about father protective care beliefs and practices. Protective care/caring refers to specific ways to help individuals, groups, families, institutions, and communities to maintain well-being and health and to prevent destructive or harmful acts toward self or others. Protective care is a critical factor in the prevention of destructive acts or ways that could threaten the life, health, or survival of human beings directly or indirectly. The three Western cultures observed were mid-American Old Order Amish, Anglo American, and Mexican American, and the non-Western culture was the indigenous Gadsup of the Eastern Highlands of New Guinea. In this chapter, reflections and descriptions of extended ethnonursing qualitative care research utilizing the Theory of Culture Care Diversity and Universality or the culture care theory (CCT) with the goal of discovering the expressions and characteristics of *father protective care* are discussed.

Given that the phenomenon of protective care is manifested differently in Western and non-Western cultures, this research focused on the subtle, hidden, obscure, and diverse expressions and examples of father protective

Revised reprint from Leininger, M. (2011). Leininger's reflection on her ongoing father protective care research. *Online Journal of Cultural Competence in Nursing and Healthcare, 1*(2), 1–13.

care in both types of cultures. While protective care was more readily identified, practiced, and held as an expected cultural norm in the non-Western culture studied, its presence was also identifiable in the Western cultures. Protective care was especially evident with regard to young children, adolescents, and older adults. The benefits to recipients of father protective care were identified in addition to the impact on the health, wellbeing, illness, and ease of death.

DISCOVERY OF THE FATHER PROTECTIVE CARE PHENOMENON

The father protective care phenomenon was initially discovered in the early 1960s while investigating the culture of the Gadsup from the Eastern Highlands of New Guinea. This discovery was made through immersed living in the culture in addition to direct observations of the villagers and their geographic homeland. The confirmation of this kind of care came through interviews with Gadsup fathers, discussions of their actions, verbal statements, and storytelling. Father protective care was discovered to be essential for the growth and survival of the Gadsup people. Protective care was valued for the young males, teenagers, and older adults for their health benefits. At the same time, each father's protective care practices reaffirmed and increased the importance of the father and his self-esteem. A father's enthusiasm and confidence about providing protective care allowed for theorization about the actual and potential benefits of father protective care for health, protection, and wellbeing of the Gadsup. Identifying the actual and potential benefits of father protective care was important as it could have significant impact on the health and wellbeing of individuals from all cultural backgrounds.

Father protective care has nurturing and protective attributes that can keep the young and the old away from dangers, illnesses, accidents, and even death. From anthropological and nursing views, one could envision that protective care had played a role in the long history of Gadsup human survival. While father protective care was clearly evident among the Gadsup of New Guinea, the concept had not been identified or recognized with indigenous or other specific cultures. Although the idea of *father* protective care has been overlooked, different gender roles have been noted in diverse cultures as well as geographical locations. Specifically, in the Western cultures that were under observation, the nurturing role of mothers and mother substitutes such as grandmothers and kinswomen had been clearly identified. However, the role of fathers in providing protective care had not been identified or discussed in most Western cultures. Protective care appears to be institutionalized and less evident in Western cultures due to social and cultural differences.

DEFINITION OF PROTECTIVE CARE

After a mini-pilot study of the three Western cultures and one non-Western (Gadsup) culture, the following definition of protective care was formulated and guided the researcher: Protective care/caring refers to assistive, supportive, and facilitative acts for and with specific ways to help individuals, groups, families, institutions, and communities to maintain wellbeing and health and to prevent destructive or harmful acts toward self or others. This definition was developed as originally defined with the culture care theory (Leininger, 1977).

Theoretically, protective care was held and predicted to be a critical factor in the prevention of destructive acts or ways that could threaten the life, health, or survival of human beings directly or indirectly. Discovery of the themes and patterns of protective care was held to be essential in order to understand the phenomenon and to discover the nature of this kind of care. Additionally, it was essential to document the phenomenon as a way to promote the growth and development of human beings in a cultural environment and in different life situations.

The researcher observed the Gadsup fathers' affirmed stance that they played an important role in providing and maintaining protective care to the villagers. Father protective care, however, had to be explicated and demonstrated by the fathers and reaffirmed with examples of qualitative data to substantiate the phenomenon. From the researcher's view, protective care could not be "taken for granted" or assumed to be a reality or practiced by fathers unless observed and verified by the researcher.

IMPORTANCE OF FATHER PROTECTIVE CARE

Father protective care focuses on the use of protective care across the lifespan as well as in the socialization and enculturation of young boys, adolescents, and older adults. Several theoretical premises have been developed and are offered in this chapter to stimulate new lines of inquiry in addition to identifying the potential therapeutic benefits and practices of father protective care. The initial forecast and theoretical viewpoint predicted that if father protective care was fully identified, practiced, and known transculturally, new benefits would be achieved, especially for young boys and older adults. Specifically, father protective care could become a major guide in assisting young males, adolescents, and older adults in the prevention of illness and maintenance of healthy outcomes.

Direct clinical observations of children and adults receiving culturally-based care revealed many positive outcomes by transculturally prepared nurse clinicians (Leininger, 2006b). However, culture-based care practices that lead to healthy lifeways, prevent mental disturbances, thwart adolescent conflicts, and impede death have been sparsely addressed. The thought of human care attitudes, actions, and practices of protective care as *culturally-constituted practices* and as *prevention modes* is important in order to initiate and maintain health and wellbeing. The researcher's experiences and observations with diverse cultures provided evidence that father protective care could be extremely beneficial in childrearing, and especially with young males, adolescents, and older adults (Leininger, 1995, 1997, 2006b). These hunches reinforced the search for culturally-based care in several cultures and with the three Western cultures included in this study for comparative purposes.

OVERVIEW OF SELECTED CULTURES

The three Western cultures (Anglo American, Mexican American, and Old Order Amish living in the Midwestern United States) were investigated over a 5-year period. The informants from the Western cultures understood English but were very proud of their specific cultural heritage, values, and beliefs. The non-Western culture investigated was the Gadsup of the Eastern Highlands of New Guinea. Two Gadsup villages, also known as *Gadsup peoples*, were analyzed for comparative purposes over a 2-year period. The Gadsup were selected because of their very limited exposure to Western influences and because they represented *a very old culture with traditional lifeways* (Leininger, 1966). In both villages of approximately 200 people each, the Gadsup lived in bamboo huts without modern technologies, electric lights, running water, or other Western conveniences (Leininger, 1994). In her role as principal investigator, the author studied and interviewed all key and general informants from these villages, maintained daily documentation, and observed the villagers and their lifeways (**Figure 5-1**).

When the researcher initially arrived in the Gadsup villages, the language had not been recorded or translated into English. As a result, she used Melanesian Pigeon or a *turn-talk* as the principal communication mode. A villager who spoke English volunteered to assist in clarification or reaffirmation of Gadsup words, stories, and verbal expressions. Kinship, political activities, and provision of different kinds of protective care from within

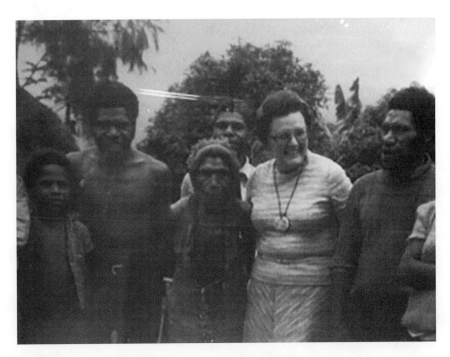

Figure 5-1 Dr. Leininger with Gadsup fathers and children in 1977.
Source: The Madeleine M. Leininger Collection on Human Caring and Transcultural Nursing, ARC-008, Photo 2013-01, Archives of Caring in Nursing, Florida Atlantic University, Boca Raton, Florida.

and outside the villages were discovered to be important for the Gadsup who were mainly a patriarchal culture with the fathers being leaders of the villages, clans, and sub-clans. As clan fathers, they were viewed as strong men and fierce fighters as well as protectors of the villagers (Leininger, 1966). Older Gadsup women worked daily in the gardens, cooked, and kept the children from harm. The Gadsup fathers provided protective care so that no harm came to the women while working the gardens. It is through the recurrent observations, interviews, and direct living immersion experiences with the Gadsup that the initial discovery of the phenomenon of father protective care was made.

The following is a sample of the researcher's observations that describes social, economic, environmental, and technological factors, and lifeways of the Gadsup of the Eastern Highlands of New Guinea:

> They [Gadsup] live in a forested and grassland environment in bamboo huts with no electricity or running water in their huts or villages. The Gadsup are known as a sweet potato culture for this is their major

food source that is essential for their survival. Sweet potatoes of a great variety are raised in Gadsup village gardens. The Gadsup like all kinds of greens and occasionally have seasonal fruits and nuts. Fresh meat and milk are not available. It is only on very special occasions that a wild pig is killed and roasted in an earth oven for a ceremonial feast. This seems to be a joyous occasion and often is talked about in the villages. The Gadsup hunt birds and selected insects, which are cooked and eaten as protein foods, but these are scarce foods. Since there are no cows or milk sources, the Gadsup consume water from a nearby stream. Modern Western drinks such as soda or sweetened "pops" or commercial juices are not consumed as they have no money for them. Most importantly, the Gadsup have very limited income and no money to buy Western foods and products. The women are the garden workers and also take care of the coffee trees, small pigs, children, and the older adults. Their only income is from their coffee grown in the villages. The women wear grass skirts and the men wear khaki shorts bought from their limited monies. Girls wear handmade grass skirts and boys are mostly bare-skinned except for coverings of their genitalia. (Leininger, 2011, p. 4)

Because the Gadsup had no modern Western living conveniences, they contrasted very sharply with the Anglo American culture as well as the other cultures studied by the researcher.

RESEARCH DESIGN

In keeping with the ethnonursing research method used in this study, 25 key informants and 40 general informants from each of the cultures were selected based on the following criteria: Lived in their culture for at least 5 to 8 years; spoke their native language, such as English, Gadsup, or Spanish; and firmly identified that they belonged to the culture being studied. This number of informants was sufficient to support the ethnonursing research method and to obtain in-depth qualitative and credible data of the cultures (Leininger, 2006a, 2006b). The purpose of the study was explained to all informants when their consent to participate in the research was solicited. In addition, they were instructed that they were free to withdraw from the study at any time, if they chose; however, none of them did so.

Key informants were selected because they were held to be the most knowledgeable about the culture, while general informants provided confirmation that the findings by the researcher were generally well known and affirmed by the majority of culture informants. All key informants had elementary school education, while a few also had high school education. Virtually none of the informants of the cultures studied had college or special trade preparation. The age range for the father informants in each culture was from 15 to 80 years and for the adolescent informants 14 to 21 years. In each culture, 10 children and 25 elders from ages 55 to 70 years were also selected. The children and older adults were observed and interviewed by the researcher for their views in addition to being asked to confirm examples of father protective care.

All interviews with informants occurred in their natural and familiar living context. The majority of the interviews were made during the daytime, but some interviews occurred in the evening in order to study day and night cultural practices. All data collected were coded and maintained in an ethnonursing field diary and kept in a locked box in the researcher's hut and/or office.

RATIONALE AND POTENTIAL IMPORTANCE OF FATHER PROTECTIVE CARE CONSTRUCT

Given that the phenomenon of father protective care as a construct had not been explicated or documented in most cultures, it was determined that the discovery and understanding of fathers' protective care could be an important and essential baseline of knowledge to substantiate human care. It was imperative to identify whether protective care promoted and maintained the health and wellbeing of young boys, adolescents, and older adults. Choosing a non-Western culture such as the Gadsup was significant as it facilitated the discovery and documentation of natural and established care practices. This nontechnological culture allowed the researcher to obtain a "fresh look" at a culture that had experienced limited changes and Western cultural influences. This perspective was desired to grasp natural and humanistic care practices in a traditional culture. While the research focused on father care modes, Gadsup mothers and their care roles were noted as well. The data from the Gadsup mothers clearly revealed a nurturing care role with children and adults that supported the health and wellbeing of their children. The mother's nurturing role was complementary to the father's protective care role, which the villagers valued. The Gadsup in both villages loved their children and offered them surveillance, protection, and direct help as needed. The average Gadsup family had three to five children who were protected and cared for until about the age of 15 years, which is when they were considered eligible for marriage.

The Gadsup study concluded that the young males of that culture become adults with limited conflicts and destructive acts. Additionally, the research also established that the Gadsup older adults were able not only to maintain their health and wellness, but also live a long life of approximately 65 years. It was because of the fathers' protective care of older adults during the daytime and at night that older adults were protected from daily accidents and especially from sorcerers and strangers that could lead to illness or even death. The fathers were also very attentive to the protection of the young male children, especially from birth through adolescence. A common daily practice of the Gadsup fathers was to walk around the entire village. This daily practice was held to be good surveillance over all villagers. The fathers repeatedly explained during interviews:

> We walk about to be sure there is no trouble coming to our children and the elders. We must watch for potential sorcerers and strangers who come into the village who might cause them harm. We watch for dangerous animals that might harm them and especially powerful male sorcerers who can bring sickness to children and older adults and which can lead to death of both children and elders. (Leininger, 2011, p. 6)

The father protective care "walk-about" gave much reassurance to the Gadsup and alleviated their daily anxiety and danger concerns.

The fathers also described ways they protected the villagers from destructive storms such as tornadoes, earthquakes, and windstorms which occurred frequently in both villages. The researcher noted:

> The fathers spoke proudly of the wealth of knowledge told by their deceased Gadsup fathers in the villages about storm protection. Their ancestors were proud of their ways to protect the people from frequent drastic weather conditions. Both villages had sudden and frequent torrential rain storms and earthquakes, especially in the "rainy season." It was the fathers who watched for cloud changes and other signs of storms. They would watch for dark cloud formations, humidity changes, wind flows and dark wind clouds. Accordingly, the fathers would quickly warn the villagers by calling loudly to the villagers that the storm was coming and what to do. The fathers guided the villagers where to go that was safe before the storms hit the villages. The fathers knew what strong winds, heavy rainstorms and earthquakes could do to their fragile bamboo huts, their gardens and how they could kill or injure the villagers. (Leininger, 2011, p. 6)

Protective care was essential and greatly valued. The villagers depended on the fathers for their quick protective care actions and their wisdom, guidance, and general protective advice. All key village informants praised the fathers for

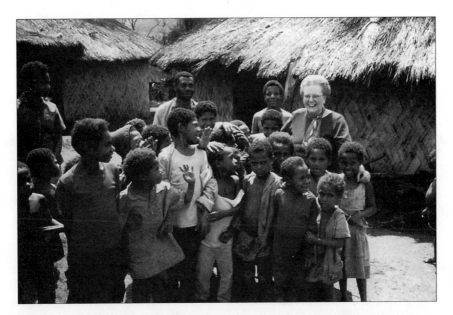

Figure 5-2 Dr. Leininger among the Gadsup of New Guinea in 1992.
Source: The Madeleine M. Leininger Collection on Human Caring and Transcultural Nursing, ARC-008, Photo 50, Archives of Caring in Nursing, Florida Atlantic University, Boca Raton, Florida.

such important protective care actions. It was an excellent example of "protective community village care" (**Figure 5-2**). The fathers would spontaneously tell the researcher of these weather protective care actions. The villagers also affirmed that the fathers' protection was effective and that they were confident of such protection in the villages. They reported many times that the people were not killed or hurt due to father care. Approximately 40 accounts of protective care actions were collected. While observing, listening to, and discovering the father's role as a protective care provider, the fathers' accounts were validated by practically all key and general informants for their actions and role behavior.

After completing the Gadsup study in 1965, the Anglo American, Mexican American, and Old Order Amish Western cultures were studied in order to establish a contrast with the Gadsup father protective care. During interviews with key Anglo American father informants, 10 key informant fathers spoke about their failure to guide and help their young boys, especially the adolescents. Specifically, they spoke openly and hopelessly about being too punitive, too harsh, and too abusive in their talks with their sons. In addition, those informants described how their own fathers had severely punished them physically if they were disobedient. The informants explained how their fathers addressed them frequently with demeaning statements such as "You will never amount to anything."

These fathers believed that rapid changes in the American culture "were the cause" of their sons' problems. One informant stated: ". . . it is our responsibility to punish our sons in order that they obey and to avoid future problems." Another informant added that such "harsh punishment did not seem to work." Many of the fathers were sad and reported that they felt helpless and hopeless about their male sons but did not know what to do to address these issues. Five key informants added that they regretted saying demeaning words and giving harsh punishments because ". . . it didn't help them and made their sons angry toward them." Three fathers shared that such actions lessened their sons' self-esteem and confidence. These fathers also held that their negative statements to their older adults were harmful as opposed to helpful. Hence, verbal and physical abuse by Anglo American fathers was held as ineffective. These fathers maintained that they would not use such measures again and believed that their harsh words and punishment often led their sons to become depressed and resentful of them. In general, these father informants felt guilty to have used harsh statements and punishments and would not recommend such actions to others.

Ten of the Mexican American father informants said ". . . physical punishment and hard direct talk" were believed to be essential to guide their sons, and especially when ". . . they disobeyed their father" (Zoucha, 1998). Ten Old Order Amish father informants maintained that they preferred to talk to their sons and to show them by their actions how they needed to be obedient to their fathers. In general, Anglo American fathers were most concerned about their sons and said they felt helpless about ways to raise them in the American culture. The idea of protective father care was of interest to them but they were "sure this would not be effective with adolescent males in the American culture."

USE OF THE CULTURE CARE THEORY DECISION AND ACTION MODES AND ACCULTURATION ENABLER

Decision and Action Modes

The culture care theory decision and action modes can guide nurses and healthcare providers as they strive to provide culturally congruent care to the cultural groups investigated in this study. These three decision and action modes include culture care preservation and/or maintenance; culture care accommodation and/or negotiation; and culture care repatterning and/or restructuring (Leininger, 2006a, 2006b). These decision and action modes were discussed with the fathers as potential ways the fathers might incorporate their cultural values and practices into their ways of helping their sons.

Even though the Old Order Amish is a Western culture, these informants exhibited similar behaviors to the Gadsup in terms of father protective care. All key Gadsup and Old Order Amish father informants and the majority of general informants maintained that their cultural values, practices, and beliefs of protective care should be preserved to promote the health and wellbeing of their people, and especially of young males, teenagers, and older adults. A father's protective care role in these cultures was viewed as positive, beneficial, visible, and culturally congruent to support and maintain health and wellbeing. Many Gadsup and Old Order Amish maintained that this was the first time they had openly shared their cultural stories, beliefs, and practices with others.

The culture care theory empowered informants to be open about the cultural values they would like to uphold and maintain. Culture care preservation and/or maintenance were strongly reaffirmed with the Old Order Amish and the Gadsup, as these cultures wanted to keep their practices and beliefs as healthy lifeways. These cultures wanted to help male youths, adolescents, and older adults remain well and active so there was no desire to change their values and practices.

Culture care accommodation and/or negotiation was identified and confirmed by 10 Anglo American male adolescents and by the majority of the key father informants. The areas of identified need for change for fathers and adolescents were the following:

- Anglo American adolescents did not want their fathers to demean or harshly punish them in the future.
- The Anglo American and Mexican American fathers wanted to accommodate selected practices that would be good as long as these practices caused no harm to self, the family, and community and were acceptable to other fathers in the community, with Anglo Americans fathers being uncertain what would be the best changes to make.
- Both Anglo American and Mexican American fathers wanted to find ways to transmit spiritual and religious knowledge to their sons in order to guide their sons' thinking and future goals.
- The Old Order Amish fathers and adolescents reaffirmed that they did not wish to change their own values, especially their religious and traditional life practices, but would learn to use technological advancements. The Amish fathers wanted help to prevent destructive acts that might negatively influence their strong Amish communities (Wenger, 1991).

- The Old Order Amish fathers wanted to abolish shunning, as it was viewed as too destructive to young males. However, they still planned to give verbal guidance to their younger males (Wenger, 1991) throughout their lifetime as this is an Amish father's obligation and responsibility.
- The Gadsup fathers and adolescent males wanted to have electricity and running water in their homes in the future "like the Europeans have in their modern homes."
- The Gadsup fathers, 10 adolescent males, and several Old Order Amish teenagers were interested in Anglo American modern technologies such as phones, radios, and television sets. They realized that "some [technologies] did not fit their culture" as they were against their religious beliefs. They also wondered if these technologies would be harmful to their people.
- The Mexican American male teenagers were eager and ready to use modern technologies but shared that they had limited money to buy such items. Mexican American fathers relied on Catholic religious beliefs to protect their adolescent and young children, and hoped that these beliefs would be emphasized and taught more in schools and churches.

Culture care repatterning and/or restructuring decisions and actions seemed very difficult for the informants to consider. Five Gadsup fathers said that Americans and Europeans could help them to repattern some of their lifeways, but they did not want their "good lifeways" changed. The Gadsup and Old Order Amish did not want to change most of their lifeways and values, and they strongly wanted to keep the fathers' role of protection with their teenagers and the older adults. Five key Old Order Amish informants said they would like to change some lifeways but they could not change their religious beliefs and daily living patterns. They were interested in selected modern technologies but feared harm from their use. In general, they were content with their values and lifeways (Wenger, 1991).

Acculturation Enabler

Leininger's Acculturation Enabler was used with the cultures investigated in this study during its early phase (Leininger, 1995, 2006b). This enabler helped to assess whether members of each culture were more traditionally or nontraditionally oriented in their values, beliefs, and lifeways. The Gadsup, Old Order Amish, Mexican Americans, and Anglo Americans identified their traditional or established values as old values that they wanted to uphold. The Gadsup and the Old Order Amish had strong traditional values, beliefs, and practices whereas the Anglo American father informants were ambivalent and uncertain about their cultural values and especially their practices. Throughout the study, the firmly expressed values and practices of the cultures were reaffirmed by the majority of the general and key informants. The more traditional the culture, the more hesitant informants were about changing their values and lifeways through acculturation. The transmission of cultural values intergenerationally was strongest and most evident with the cultures that held firmly to their values, practices, and beliefs—namely, the Old Order Amish and the Gadsup.

CRITERIA USED TO EXAMINE THE QUALITATIVE DATA

It is important to state that the criteria used to examine the qualitative data collected in this study were congruent with the qualitative research method (Leininger, 1985, 2006b). Quantitative criteria were not used, as they did not fit with the research method used in this study. The following criteria were used:

- Credibility: This referred to the "truths" held by key informants as they expressed and confirmed the ideas they spoke about or demonstrated.
- Meaning-in-context: This referred to the meaning given by the informants about the subject under discussion and often confirmed by the majority of key informants.
- Confirmability: This referred to data shared by key informants and strongly affirmed and reaffirmed by the general informants.
- Recurrent patterning: This referred to the repeated practices that occur over time in daily living and in the patterned lifeways of the informants.
- Saturation: This referred to the repeated expressions and practices by key informants. Comments such as "I have no more to tell you—I told you all," as well as repetition and recurrence of similar ideas and practices with key informants with no new information becoming evident, indicated that saturation was reached.

RESULTS

In this chapter the beliefs, values, and practices of protective care were identified by fathers from diverse cultural backgrounds. Examples of actions, stories, and observations were also documented. Because protective care has been virtually unknown, the qualitative findings helped to discover dominant themes, attributes, characteristics, patterns, practices, and values about father protective care. The findings from the four cultures—namely, Anglo American, Mexican American, Old Order Amish, and the Gadsup of the Eastern Highlands of New Guinea—revealed many differences but also some commonalities in their expressions of father protective care and its benefits.

The major commonalities or benefits of protective care were that protective care by fathers' knowledge, practices, and (especially) actions contributed to male courage, hope, confidence, self-esteem, and wellbeing. It also gave males direction and guidance for the male role in the future. The fathers firmly believed that by their examples, actions, demonstrations, and verbal guidance, protective care reduced thoughts of suicide, destructive acts, and other crime activities in the cultures studied.

Findings from this study identified several themes and benefits to male youths, adolescents, and the older adults: *Protective care gave confidence; protective care gave courage; protective care gave hope;* and *protective care gave guidance on future direction* as well as *increased self-esteem to male fathers, boys, and older adults.* The following patterns supported the identified themes and can assist nurses and other healthcare providers when providing care to the members of the cultures investigated in this study:

- The indigenous Gadsup father's examples, stories, and firm and confident manner with actions and overt demonstrations were dominant features of father protective care which allowed the male sons to observe and learn protective care. Father protective care was also identified in the investigated Western cultures, but the values and benefits were not as strongly identified when compared to the indigenous Gadsup fathers.

- For the Gadsup of New Guinea, protective father care incorporated culturally-based practices and values to help young boys, teenagers, and older adults maintain healthy lifeways and to prevent older adults from having accidents and illnesses.

- Protective Gadsup father care helped young boys and male adolescents to gain confidence, hope, courage, self-esteem, and care practice in their daily living context by relying on the fathers' guidance and action-based practices.

- Protective father care meant practicing by actions or demonstrations and explicit ways to promote and maintain protective care for healthy lifeways. Several practices were identified in all cultures, but were not readily seen in practice or with firm confirmation in Anglo Americans and Mexican Americans. Anglo Americans had limited protective care measures with the older adults and male youths.

- Father protective care had many positive benefits to young males and to older adults in the Western cultures studied, but especially with the Gadsup. These positive benefits included prevention of illness and death and promotion of health and wellbeing. Action-based father protective care was important to demonstrate and practice with the Gadsup for health benefits to male youths.
- Father protective care appeared to be essential for health maintenance and wellbeing. This care construct was especially evident with the Gadsup older adults who relied on father protective care to prevent common accidents, depression, and unexplained deaths. The Gadsup of New Guinea and the Old Order Amish were quick to offer and demonstrate protective elder care; whereas the Anglo Americans remained unsure and ambivalent about elder protective care.
- Father protective care was most reassuring to the Gadsup older adults as this care protected them from village accidents, falls, illnesses, sorcerers, and terrible or sudden storms.
- Father protective care had been taught and transmitted through several generations by the fathers, grandfathers, clan leaders, and elders of the Gadsup and Old Order Amish, who viewed this practice as a responsibility and moral obligation. There was much pride and pleasure in telling about ancestor and father protective care by key and general Gadsup informants.
- Protective father care expressions and daily actions for different life events were viewed as essential to intergenerationally teach and to guide young males in order to promote and maintain healthy older adults' lifeways. The Gadsup fathers were action-oriented role models to the villagers who relied on them to demonstrate and practice protective care in daily living situations.
- Father protective care was discovered not to be unique to human beings, as examples with animals such as horses and cattle and other species demonstrated protective care.

CONCLUSION

This study focused on father protective care with four cultures for comparative viewpoints to discover the nature, characteristics, dominant expressions, themes, and benefits of father protective care. Leininger's Theory of Culture Care Diversity and Universality was used with the qualitative ethnonursing research method. The purpose of the study was to discover overt, subtle, and covert expressions exhibited by father protective care as documented and confirmed by key and general informants in the cultures studied. Diversities and several commonalities regarding father protective care were identified through in-depth observations and interviews and by the researcher living in the villages or near the investigated cultures.

The identification of fathers providing and knowing protective care was a significant discovery. Father protective care was identified as important for male socialization and to promote the health and wellbeing of the villagers and cultures studied. This study highlighted the importance as well as the vital role of fathers with respect to guidance, support, and facilitation of positive ways to help young males' and older adults' protective care practices. To date, the identification of father protective care had been limitedly known, valued, and documented. This transcultural investigation which focused on gender-based male care could stimulate health personnel to investigate the benefit and possibilities for protective care to prevent illness, death, and accidents.

The many benefits of father protective care need to be studied in all cultures for comparative outcomes. The challenge is to identify and nurture father protective care and to make the fathers' role more visible, rewarded, and known in diverse cultures. The global use of father protective care appears encouraging, gives hope, and supports social justice for humans and their health and wellbeing. Protective care appears vital to young males and older adults to prevent illnesses and destructive behaviors and, therefore, could be a major approach to actively promote prevention and health maintenance practices.

From this investigation, several principles were identified that can be used as guidelines to parents, teachers, health personnel, and others interested in applying protective care in childrearing and handling difficult adolescent problems and conflicts. The three modes of culture care decisions and actions can be helpful in discussing and guiding personnel to think creatively about ways to provide culturally sensitive and appropriate protective care practices in nursing and in selected cultures. The identification of the father's role in caring offers support for and recognition of the father's important role to serve people, especially young males and the older adults, in positive ways.

Since the evolution of transcultural nursing as a formal area of study and practice in the 1950s, it has been the author's hope and dream that someday all cultures will be fully studied and documented to discover and understand culturally-based care beliefs, practices, and lifeways. Culturally-based care is a powerful means to prevent illness and to nurture health, maintain wellness, and promote healing. Most importantly, prevention with a care focus should become the powerful and new healing approach in the future. Preventive healthcare practices need to be documented with cultures and used in all healthcare settings. This approach supports the researcher's view that care is curing and healing in many health–illness events. I predict that care knowledge and explicit care practices will become the dominant cure and healing mode in the future. The benefits from protective caring offer a new direction in health care for the future.

Cultures have a right to receive culturally appropriate care that fits their values and beliefs. The discovery of father protective care could reduce health costs and prevent serious illnesses and even death. Learning about and discovering the nature of protective human care seems an urgent need if we are to serve people of many diverse cultures in a sensitive, humanistic, and ethical way and with social and cultural justice. The growing multicultural world makes this challenge imperative. The discovery of father protective care is, therefore, most encouraging and is a promising means to reinforce the father's role in diverse cultures. The Gadsup and the Old Order Amish provide excellent examples of father wisdom, knowledge, and practice of protective care. It is, indeed, important to pursue, understand, and use this knowledge with great wisdom and with keen sensitivity to indigenous values, beliefs, and practices from the long history of diverse cultures worldwide.

DEDICATION

This chapter is dedicated to the late Dr. Madeleine Leininger, who authored the original article in the *Online Journal of Cultural Competence in Nursing and Healthcare.*

DISCUSSION QUESTIONS

1. What is *protective care* and how can it affect health and wellbeing?
2. What are the father protective care themes discovered in this study?
3. How can knowledge of these themes be incorporated in clinical practice?
4. Discuss how the construct of father protective care will influence your own practice or practice in your care setting.

REFERENCES

Leininger, M. M. (1966). Convergence and divergence of two Gadsup villages in the Eastern Highlands of New Guinea. *Dissertation Abstracts International: Section B. Sciences and Engineering, 27*(6), 1704.

Leininger, M. M. (1977). Caring: The essence and central focus of nursing. *Nursing Research Foundation Report, 12*(1), 2–14.

Leininger, M. M. (1985). *Qualitative research methods in nursing.* Orlando, FL: Grune & Stratton.

Leininger, M. M. (1994). *Transcultural nursing*. Columbus, OH: Greyden Press.

Leininger, M. M. (1995). *Transcultural nursing concepts, theories, research & practice*. Columbus, OH: McGraw Hill College Custom Series.

Leininger, M. M. (1997). Transcultural nursing research to transform nursing education and practice: 40 years. *Journal of Nursing Scholarship, 29*(4), 341–347.

Leininger, M. M. (2006a). Culture care diversity and universality theory and evolution of the ethnonursing method. In M. M. Leininger & M. R. McFarland (Eds.), *Culture care diversity and universality: A worldwide nursing theory* (2nd ed., pp. 1–41). Sudbury, MA: Jones and Bartlett.

Leininger, M. M. (2006b). Ethnonursing research method and enablers. In M. M. Leininger & M. R. McFarland (Eds.), *Culture care diversity and universality: A worldwide nursing theory* (2nd ed., pp. 42–81). Sudbury, MA: Jones and Bartlett.

Leininger, M. M. (2011). Leininger's reflection on the ongoing father protective care research. *Online Journal of Cultural Competence in Nursing and Healthcare, 1*(2), 1–13.

Wenger, A. F. (1991). The culture care theory and the Old Order Amish. In M. M. Leininger (Ed.), *Culture care diversity and universality: A theory of nursing* (1st ed., pp. 362–363). New York, NY: National League for Nursing Press.

Zoucha, R. D. (1998). The experiences of Mexican Americans receiving professional nursing care: An ethnonursing study. *Journal of Transcultural Nursing, 9*(2), 34–44.

Chapter 6

Folk Care Beliefs and Practices of Traditional Lebanese and Syrian Muslims in the Midwestern United States

Hiba B. Wehbe-Alamah

> *The ultimate goal of a professional nurse-scientist and human-ist is to discover, know, and creatively use culturally based care knowledge with its fullest meanings, expressions, symbols, and functions for healing, and to promote or maintain wellbeing (or health) with people of diverse cultures of the world.*
>
> (Leininger, 2006b, p. 43)

INTRODUCTION

In a world that is increasingly characterized by cultural diversity and con-sumers who demand, expect, and are entitled to provision of culturally congruent care, healthcare providers are faced with a plethora of familiar and unfamiliar folk (generic or emic) care beliefs and practices. Culturally competent registered nurses, nurse practitioners, and other healthcare pro-fessionals assess, understand, and incorporate different folk care beliefs and practices into their professional plans of care. Leininger has long main-tained that integration of both professional (etic) and generic (folk or emic) caring systems is necessary to provide culturally congruent care (Leininger, 1995, 2002).

Muslims worldwide include approximately 1.6 to 2.1 billion people or nearly one-fifth of the world's total population; the exact number of Muslims in the United States is unknown but is estimated at 2 to 7 million (Grossman, 2011; Johnson, 2011; Mughees, 2006; Religious Population Worldwide, n.d.). This number is projected to double over the next two decades, according to the Pew Forum on Religious and Public Life (2011). Therefore, healthcare providers need to be prepared to care for Muslim patients, including those of Lebanese and Syrian heritage, in a culturally sensitive and meaningful way. To do so, they need to be aware of their folk care beliefs and practices to maintain and/or preserve, accommodate and/or negotiate, or restructure and/or repattern those beliefs as an integral part of their professional plan of care.

PURPOSE, GOAL, AND DOMAIN OF INQUIRY

Two ethnonursing studies conceptualized within Leininger's culture care theory were conducted with Lebanese and Syrian informants, respectively. The domain of inquiry was the generic and professional care meanings, beliefs, and practices related to health, wellbeing, and illness of Lebanese and Syrian Muslims living in several urban communities in the Midwestern United States. The purpose of these studies was to discover, describe, and analyze the influences of worldview, cultural context, technological, religious, political, educational, and economic factors on the traditional Lebanese and Syrian Muslims' generic and professional care meanings, beliefs, and practices. The goal of these studies was to provide nurses and other healthcare professionals with knowledge that can be used for cultural care decisions and actions that facilitate the provision of culturally congruent care for Lebanese and Syrian Muslims living in urban communities in the Midwestern United States (Wehbe-Alamah, 2005, 2006, 2011).

ETHNOHISTORY

In the United States, Arab Americans are found in all 50 states with one-third concentrated in the states of California, Michigan, and New York. Los Angeles, Detroit, New York, Chicago, and Washington, D.C., are the cities with the largest Arab American populations. In the state of Michigan, more than 80% of Arab Americans reside in Macomb, Oakland, and Wayne counties and one-third of the residents in the city of Dearborn claim Arabic heritage. Thirty-four percent of Arab American immigrants in the United States can trace their heritage back to Lebanese and/or Syrian origins (Arab American Institute, n.d., 2011).

Until they gained their independence from the French in 1946, Lebanon and Syria were part of what was then known as *The Levant* or Greater Syria. The first documented Syrian Lebanese family in the United States was that of Professor Joseph Arbeely, who arrived in 1878 with his wife, six sons, and a niece (Bennett, 2000). Early Lebanese/Syrian immigrants to the United States were predominately Christians who were leaving their country to escape Ottoman Turkish rule. The second wave of Lebanese and Syrian immigration took place around the late 1960s which coincided with the relaxation of U.S. immigration laws and the outbreak of the Lebanese civil war; the majority of these immigrants were Muslims (Connelly et al., 1999; Dehler, 2009). Subsequent increased immigration rates coincided with peaks of political violence in either country.

Early Lebanese and Syrian immigrants were self-employed and highly valued education (Dehler, 2009). The majority of the later Lebanese immigrants who came to the United States were medical doctors and engineers (Labaki, 1992, as cited in Fatfat, 1998). The reasons most frequently cited for leaving Lebanon were education, followed by political motivations (government instability), social factors (lack of physical security in Lebanon), and economic reasons. Factors influencing Lebanese immigrants to stay in the United States were primarily economic followed (in descending order) by educational, political, and social considerations. Female Lebanese immigrants differed slightly from males in that their reported most important reasons for leaving Lebanon were social (following a relative to the United States) and educational in nature, and their most important reasons for staying in the United States were educational, followed by economic and social reasons (Fatfat, 1998).

With the ongoing turmoil in the Middle East, and specifically in Syria, political violence has already caused more than 2 million documented Syrian refugees to flee from their country, 52% of whom are children under the age of 17. An additional 4.25 million are displaced within Syria (UNHCR, 2013). Factors behind the displacement of Syrians both within Syria and to other countries include civil war, bombing, mass destruction of cities and homes, political persecution and instability, rape and other forms of sexual violence, assaults on human dignity, and violations of human rights (United Nations News Centre, 2012). It is expected that the number of displaced and fleeing Syrians will continue to increase leading to another egress of immigrants from that country.

RESEARCH QUESTIONS

The following questions guided the two research studies discussed in this chapter:

1. What are the traditional generic (folk) and professional care beliefs, expressions, and practices related to health and illness of Lebanese and Syrian Muslims?
2. In what ways do worldview, cultural context, and social structure dimensions, such as technological, religious, political, educational, and economical factors, influence the Lebanese and Syrian Muslims' generic (folk) care beliefs, expressions, and practices?
3. In what ways can Leininger's three care modes of nursing decisions and actions facilitate the provision of culturally congruent nursing care for Lebanese and Syrian Muslims?

THEORETICAL FRAMEWORK

The theoretical framework used for the two studies to be discussed was Leininger's Theory of Culture Care Diversity and Universality (CCT), which holds that *care* is the essence and unifying focus of nursing (Leininger, 1991). The purpose of the theory is to guide the discovery, documentation, and interpretation of human culture care diversities and similarities as influenced by worldview, social structure, language, and environmental context, and to discover new knowledge which would enable nurses to provide culturally meaningful and beneficial care practices (Leininger, 1988, 1991, 1995, 1996, 1997a, 2006a). The goal of the theory is to provide culturally competent nursing care for health and wellbeing for people (Leininger, 1995, 1996, 1997a, 2006a).

Cultural diversities and universalities about human care exist among and within all cultures worldwide, and the discovery of cultural knowledge can be used to guide nursing care decisions and actions which will be beneficial to clients' health and wellbeing (Leininger, 2002). When cultural care values, beliefs, expressions, and practices of people from diverse or similar cultures are discovered and used in appropriate, sensitive, and meaningful ways, culturally congruent and therapeutic care occurs (Leininger, 2006a). The CCT has been credited with the discovery and establishment of a broad transcultural knowledge base that has led to, and will continue to contribute to, the transformation of nursing education, clinical practice, research, administration, and consultation (Leininger, 1994, 1996, 1997b). In addition, the theory has played an important role in the formulation of the Standards for Transcultural Nursing (Leuning, Swiggum, Barmore, Wiegert, & McCullough-Zander, 2002).

METHOD

Leininger's qualitative ethnonursing research method was ideal for conducting these two studies, as it fit well with the culture care theory and with their identified goals and purposes. Ethnonursing research is an open discovery and naturalistic people-centered method developed by Leininger (1991) with the goal of teasing out complex and largely unknown people's emic (local) viewpoints about nursing dimensions such as human care, wellbeing, health, and environmental influencers (Leininger, 2006a, 2006b). Leininger (1991) stated that a major reason for establishing this method was her interest in discovering the differences and similarities between folk (generic) care and professional nursing care among different cultures.

The two studies under discussion took place in several urban Midwestern communities over the period of 4 years in locations identified as comfortable by informants, such as homes, mosques, offices, Middle Eastern restaurants, and other places of the informants' choosing. Collectively, 17 *key* informants (7 Lebanese and 10 Syrians) and 31 *general* informants (11 Lebanese and 20 Syrians) were interviewed for these two studies. Informants were recruited with the assistance of community gatekeepers and using the Snowball method. All informants met the following recruitment criteria: 18 years of age or older; born to Lebanese or Syrian parents in any country in the world with relocation to the United States *or* born in the United States to Lebanese or Syrian parents; currently living in the United States; stated cultural identity as Lebanese or Syrian Muslim; knowledgeable about the domain of inquiry; and willing to participate in the study.

Key informants were considered to be more knowledgeable than general informants about the domain under study and were interviewed on two different occasions. Informants ranged between the ages of 18 and 79 years. The interviews, which were conducted in either the English or Arabic language, lasted anywhere from 45 minutes to 1.5 hours, and incorporated semi-structured questions derived from an adaptation of Leininger's Open-Ended Inquiry Guide and the Sunrise Enabler, which was translated into Arabic for these studies (see the appendix at the end of this chapter). The use of Leininger's Stranger-to-Trusted Friend Enabler and Observation–Participation–Reflection Enabler helped toward establishing trust between the researcher and the informants; developing the researcher's sensitivity for the informants' verbal and visual clues; and maintain the researcher's objectivity during data collection and analysis.

Institutional Review Board approval was secured and a written consent was obtained from each informant for participation in the studies and/or for audio-recording of the interviews. A written explanation of each study and consent form in either the English or Arabic language (depending on the informant's individual preference) was read, explained, and given to each informant for signature. Informants were also given the option to either sign their name or leave a mark on the consent form that was meaningful to them, such as an X, to preserve confidentiality. In addition to the semi-structured open-ended inquiry guide and the face-to-face audio-taped interviews used in this study, data were collected through field notes, observation, daily journals, photographing of material objects, and videotaping with preservation of anonymity.

All audiotapes were returned to Syrian informants following data transcription, as is congruent with the traditional Syrian Muslim culture and religion and per the informants' request. Lebanese informants entrusted the researcher with the destruction of the tapes. Rigorous data analysis was conducted through the use of Leininger's Phases of Ethnonursing Analysis for Qualitative Data and a software program for qualitative data analysis known as QSR NUD*IST 4 (an earlier version of the NViVO software). Leininger's (2006b) ethnonursing research evaluation criteria of credibility, confirmability, meaning-in-context, recurrent patterning, saturation, and transferability were used throughout the data analysis process (Wehbe-Alamah, 2006, 2008b, 2011).

FINDINGS AND DISCUSSION

Nine themes that address the research questions were discovered in the two studies. These themes, along with their associated patterns, descriptors, discussions, and transcultural care decisions and actions, as well as other selected findings from these studies, were previously published (Wehbe-Alamah, 2006, 2008a, 2008b, 2011). Therefore, in the following paragraphs, discussion is focused on the traditional Lebanese and Syrian Muslim folk care beliefs and practices relating to health and illness, magic and the evil eye, caregiving, health maintenance and promotion, illness prevention, illness treatment and cure, death and dying, and alternative treatments. In addition, the relationship between folk care beliefs and practices and Lebanese and Syrian worldviews, cultural contexts, and social structures is explained.

Traditional Lebanese and Syrian Muslims

Worldview

The worldview of traditional Lebanese and Syrian Muslims is embedded in both *Islamic* and *cultural* beliefs and practices. Religion controls every aspect of the life for traditional Muslims, including their folk care beliefs and practices. By comparison, the worldview of liberal and nontraditional Lebanese informants was not found to be deeply rooted in Islamic beliefs and practices. However, in most Lebanese and Syrian houses or offices visited during the research interviews, numerous religious artifacts were observed on walls or shelves.

Most traditional Lebanese and Syrian Muslims view life as a test from God and religion as the focus of life. A common belief is that humans are transit passengers in this lifetime who will go to heaven or hell in the afterlife depending on the way they lived their life while on earth. God tests people, and because life is not permanent, one should do good deeds to be eligible to go to heaven. As a result, one must live his or her life with this idea in mind and attempt to do as many good deeds as possible and to behave in a righteous way whenever conducting business, taking care of housework, or engaging in any other regular daily activity.

This belief was clearly illustrated by a Syrian physician informant, who maintained that Islam guides his daily activities, his worldview, his work, and his relationships with people. He added that he feels it is his religious duty and obligation to tell his patients to abstain from performing unnecessary procedures, regardless of personal financial benefit, for such money gained would be considered unlawful or *haram*. A Lebanese informant shared a verse from the Qur'an that also supports this view (Surat 29, Al-'Ankabut, verse 58):

> But those who believe and work deeds of righteousness, to them shall
> We give a Home in Heaven, lofty mansions beneath which flow rivers,
> to dwell therein for aye; an excellent reward for those who do (good)!
> (Ali, 1983, p. 1045)

Given that the teachings of Islam encourage people to take care of themselves, family members, relatives, friends, neighbors, and strangers, traditional Lebanese and Syrian Muslims are more likely to engage in caring activities that are congruent with or fulfill religious teachings. For example, they will rarely place their elderly parents in nursing homes because God said in Surat 17 (Al-Israa) verses 23–24:

> Thy Lord hath decreed that ye worship none but Him, and that ye be
> kind to parents. Whether one or both of them attain old age in thy life,
> say not to them a word of contempt, nor repel them, but address them
> in terms of honor. And, out of kindness, lower to them the wing of
> humility, and say: "My Lord! Bestow on them thy Mercy even as they
> cherished me in childhood. (Ali, 1983, pp. 700–701)

A Syrian informant shared that taking good care of elderly parents or relatives is a source of pride, a cultural expectation, and a religious obligation.

One has to keep in mind that not all Muslims are equally religious or apply religion in the same way. As mentioned earlier, some of the research informants were extremely liberal whereas others were particularly traditional. However, it is safe to say that the folk care practices of traditional Lebanese and Syrian Muslims are largely influenced by their worldview.

Cultural and Social Structure Effects on Folk Care Beliefs and Practices

Lebanese and Syrian cultures emphasize generosity, hospitality, and solidarity. Historically, Arabs have been known for their generosity and hospitality; the Lebanese and Syrian people are no exception. Every time the researcher interviewed an informant in his or her own home, she was offered a beverage and dessert. The beverage most commonly offered was Turkish coffee in Lebanese households and hot tea in Syrian homes. As for desserts, the researcher was offered different kinds of delicious Syrian pastries brought back from summer trips to the homeland. Lebanese informants offered baklava, cakes, and sweets, and/or insisted on having brunch (which often included a traditional salad known as *tabbouleh*) with the researcher at the end of an interview.

Traditional Lebanese and Syrian men and women consider themselves *equal* but not *identical*. From a cultural point of view, women are traditionally seen in the role of caregiver, and some men consider the act of providing physical care to the sick to be a shameful and feminine practice. A Lebanese informant reported, "To some men, it is a shame or something shameful for a man to do housework or physical work with the ill—that is, for those who follow culture." Typically, the woman is in charge of the physical and emotional care of the sick, the home, and the children; the man is responsible for the financial care. Today, men are being seen more and more in the role of caregiver. This is partly due to the absence of extended family members in the surrounding geographical area, acknowledgment of the working woman as a productive family member (following the example of the Prophet), and acculturation. This finding was supported by a Lebanese informant, who shared:

> Yeah, he will [husband will help], I don't know, because I don't have any relatives here, anyone to help . . . like when I'm sick, he cooks, he washes dishes [chuckle], he do everything, he gives the kids baths, he takes them to bed, you know, 'cause I don't have anybody . . .

Taking care of others and performing folk care practices are reflections of concern for the wellbeing of others. Strong family and community ties characterize both Lebanese and Syrian Muslim societies. Nuclear and extended family members, as well as friends and neighbors, often participate in the healthcare process and also provide emotional, spiritual, and financial support when needed. Visiting the sick and the family of the recently deceased is a folk caring practice and a cultural duty that reflects solidarity. Other folk care practices include helping with cooking, housework, child care, and sometimes the bills, as well as praying to God for a painless and quick recovery. Neglecting this caring cultural and religious duty could lead to alienation and destruction of cultural and/or family ties. As one Lebanese informant shared:

> When you know someone is sick or in the hospital, it is custom that you visit, if the family does not visit in the hospital, you're upset with them, so the true friend will be revealed.

One common traditional Syrian cultural practice is that of segregating men and women during social events such as weddings and dinners. The researcher was invited to a wedding party thrown by a traditional Syrian Muslim family. Two ballrooms were rented in the same hotel: One was reserved for women and the other for men. The researcher had a difficult time recognizing some of the informants she had already interviewed, as they were dressed up, had removed their head scarves, and applied makeup. It was as if the women had undergone a metamorphosis. Most Syrian informants maintained that separating men and women for social events was religious in origin, although some disagreed with this interpretation and insisted that this practice was more cultural than religious. However, all informants agreed that not all Syrian Muslims participate in this custom and that the more religious or traditional tended to adhere to this custom.

Greeting others in the form of shaking hands, hugging, and/or kissing is another custom that has both cultural and religious implications. In general, traditional Lebanese and Syrian Muslims tend to avoid shaking hands and hugging or kissing members of the opposite sex. The majority of informants stated that they shake hands and hug only with members of their same gender or close relatives. A male Syrian informant stated that he does shake hands with women who do not understand his religion so as not to offend them. Most informants agreed that not all Lebanese or Syrian Muslims strictly adhere to this practice and that some will shake hands with members of the opposite gender. A cultural cue that indicates a person's unwillingness to shake hands is raising the right hand and placing it flat on the upper chest over the heart. Some might gently tap their hand to their chest to bring the other person's attention to the placement of their hand. This action is similar to the way a hand is placed when pledging allegiance to the American flag.

Another cultural practice for traditional Syrian Muslims is the wearing of a coat or *jilbab* over clothes. A *jilbab* was described as a coat without a lining that is designed to look more like a dress than a coat and allows for modesty and freedom of movement. Only a few of the interviewed veiled Lebanese female informants wore a *jilbab* or coat over their clothing when in public; however, the majority of interviewed Syrian female informants did report wearing the traditional *jilbab* throughout the year. Several male informants maintained that modesty in dress is important for men as well as for women. While dressing conservatively was considered to be mandated through religion, the wearing of a coat or *jilbab* on top of clothes was considered to be a cultural practice by most informants. One should not assume, however, that this is how all Syrian or Lebanese Muslim women dress either in their native country or in the United States. Several informants clarified that many Muslim women do not wear head scarves or dress conservatively, and many Muslim women who do wear a head scarf do not necessarily wear coats or *jilbabs* on top of their everyday clothes. Nevertheless, all informants agreed that preserving modesty is an important cultural value and practice for traditional Muslim women and men.

The majority of Lebanese and Syrian informants maintained that they try to stay in touch with their culture through visits to their home country, speaking Arabic at home and with their children, watching Arabic TV, and cooking Middle Eastern food. Maintaining close ties with relatives and Lebanese or Syrian friends and following a lifestyle that is representative of the native culture are other ways Muslims attempt to instill their cultural beliefs and practices into their children. A Syrian informant shared that he instills his cultural values in his offspring through speaking only Arabic at home with them. Another informant said that he engages in the cultural practice of kissing the right hand of his parents and grandparents when greeting them as a means of conveying his respect and obedience. With advanced technology, most Lebanese and Syrians stay in touch with their cultural ties and relatives overseas through use of computer software and/or mobile applications such as Skype, Viber, Line, Tango, Vonage, Talkatone, MagicJack, Facebook, Bobsled, or WhatsApp.

Folk Care Beliefs and Practices Related to Health and Illness

Health was viewed by many Lebanese and Syrian informants as the absence of illness and as a blessing from God. Some informants associated health with happiness, strength, and living a good life. Health was found to have spiritual, physical, and emotional/psychological dimensions and involved the wellbeing of the body, mind, and soul. One Syrian informant reported that "... health has a wide spectrum that incorporates physical, emotional, and psychological aspects" and that a person needs to have a "... healthy body, mind, and soul to be considered free of illness."

Health was also considered as a requirement of, as well as a contribution to, one's faith. One Syrian informant maintained that health was a prerequisite to caring. She explained, "One needs to be in good health in order to be able to care for oneself and for others." Many Lebanese and Syrian Muslims believe that they must keep their bodies in a healthy state in order to be able to practice the requirements of their faith such as prayer, fasting, and caring for the sick. A Syrian informant maintained that health is strengthened by the application of religion. He described that drifting away from his religion is detrimental to his spiritual health and wellbeing whereas getting closer to God lifts his spirits and improves his spiritual and emotional wellbeing and, consequently, his mental and physical health.

Numerous interpretations were given to illness. Illness was associated with being weak and nonproductive. Some informants viewed illness as a time for self-reflection on their lives and shortcomings. Other informants looked at illness as a physiologic or a religious wake-up call. A Syrian informant maintained that illness is the body's way of telling one to slow down and rest. Another informant held that "Illness can be God's way of reminding you that you forgot about Him, and that it is time to address Him through prayers, because He wants to hear from you."

Many Lebanese and Syrian informants considered illness as God's will and an act of fate that may not be prevented in some cases. True believers are ones who do not question God's existence or decision when they get sick and remain patient throughout their illness in order to pass God's test and get rewarded by Him. A Lebanese informant shared:

> If someone gets sick, if something happens to someone, they will say this is God's will . . . for example, if this bacteria enters someone's body, if the Lord of the Universe wills to cure this person, he will cure without a doctor.

Illness was also viewed as a blessing in disguise. Illnesses are believed to erase sins which will lessen the torture (if any) experienced in the afterlife. As a result, by inflicting illnesses, it is believed that God is not only showing a sign of His love but is also rewarding people and elevating them in the hereafter. Many Lebanese and Syrian informants explained that this belief is what helps them endure an illness in a hopeful and optimistic manner, especially given that such an attitude will contribute to having their sins erased. A Lebanese informant declared:

> . . . if God let things [illnesses] happen to someone, it means that God
> loves him, as they say: if *Rab El 'Alameen* [Lord of the Universe] tortures
> someone in this life, he will get less torture in Hereafter.

Several Lebanese and Syrian informants maintained that their belief in fate does not mean that sick people should not seek treatment, especially given that God says in the Qur'an that He has created a cure for every illness. As a result, sick people are encouraged to seek medical and professional treatment for their illnesses. This finding was supported by the following statement from a Lebanese informant: "God also said that he sent the sickness and the cure. For example, if you are sick in your heart, treatment is found in the legs; you can take an artery from the legs." Some Lebanese and Syrian informants held that in addition to seeking treatment, ill people should pray to God to heal them anyway because He is the ultimate healer and not the physicians. A Syrian informant explained that the proof is that doctors themselves sometimes tell a patient that they did all they could and "the rest is in God's hands."

Some informants maintained that illness was a natural occurrence linked to biologic or physiologic origins. The most common example given was that illnesses could happen from shaking hands with somebody who has a cold. A Lebanese informant stated, ". . . other things that cause illness, is bacteria that was sent by the Lord of the Universe."

Folk Care Beliefs and Practices Related to Magic and the Evil Eye

Magic and the evil eye or *saybit ein/ain* were mentioned by both Lebanese and Syrian informants as phenomena that contribute to the development of sudden or unexplainable illnesses. A Lebanese informant stated:

> Many people had the evil eye; they even die from it. They discovered
> that there is nothing wrong with that person; there is nothing but the
> evil eye. It happens spontaneously.

Most informants maintained that they believe in magic and the evil eye because they are mentioned in their holy book and in several of the Prophet's *ahadeeth* (sayings). The majority of informants stated that although they believe in these phenomena, they do not live their lives in fear or expectation of harm. A Syrian informant said that she does not believe that someone will just come out and put her "under a spell." Another informant said that people should not go to extremes and interpret any bad thing that happens to them as the product of the evil eye.

The most vulnerable to the evil eye were reported to be good-looking people. Individuals who show off their fortune to others can also be affected by the evil eye. Several informants held that the evil eye tends to happen mostly to beautiful infants or children when they dress up and look very nice. The evil eye was reported to be the result of love, admiration, jealousy, or envy, which sometimes can be unintentional. Many informants shared that a mother may give the evil eye to her own children. A Lebanese informant shared:

> Even the parent can give it [evil eye] to their children. It is not because they hate the person; because they love him so much, they will give him the evil eye. Some people, because of jealousy, they might give it to the other person . . .

A few Syrian informants reported that there are scientific explanations for the evil eye effect. They reported that the human eye emits gamma radiation, which can be powerful enough to cause harm, and added that the blue color can absorb this radiation and render it harmless. One informant said that when a person feels envious, his or her body discharges an electrical current that can cause the evil eye and further explained that knocking on wood can diffuse this electrical charge and prevent the evil eye.

Many informants shared with the researcher personal encounters with the evil eye. One story involved a Syrian husband who was dressed up in a suit and was ready to leave the house when a female visitor commented to the wife that her husband was too tall and handsome. The informant reported that the second the visitor finished her sentence, her husband collapsed and had to be taken to a hospital. A Lebanese informant shared the following:

> I once had a gathering of ladies at my house and had a big brand-new tall crystal vase on my kitchen island with red roses in it. One of the guests looked at it and said: "How beautiful!" The vase cracked instantly and separated into two pieces!

The majority of informants said that the evil eye and magic can be prevented or treated by mentioning God's name or reading special chapters from the Qur'an known as *Al-Muawwathat* (The Exorcists). Many informants reported that the evil eye as well as magic can also be prevented by saying religious expressions and by eating seven dates from Medina (a city in Saudi Arabia where the Prophet lived for a long time and where he is buried) every morning. Religious expressions designed to prevent the evil eye include *Mashaallah* (What God wills) or *Subhanallah* (Glory be to Allah). A Lebanese informant reported:

> When I see something beautiful, I always say: "*Mashaallah, Subhanallah*" [What God wills, Glory to Allah], that will save the person from getting hit by the *Ain* uh, I know a lot of people like this say that about my child. Let's say you have a beautiful child, they say: "Oh, how beautiful

he is," and then before they say anything I say in my heart, you know, "*Mashaallah, Bismillah*" [In the name of God], so that always when you keep God's words in your mouth nothing can happen to you.

A Syrian informant relayed that the messenger taught his followers a supplication that words off the evil eye and harm. The supplication called *Dua' Al Tahseen* (Supplication of Protection) goes as follows:

اللهم اني أعوذ بكلمات الله التامة من شر كل شيطان و هامة و من شر كل عين لامة

Allahumma ennee aouthou bekalemaatellahe ttamah min sharre koulle shay-tanin wa hammah wa min sharre koulle aynin laamah

Oh God, I seek refuge in God's complete words from the evil of all devils and beasts and from the evil of the evil eye.

The informant explained that her sister said this *dua'* to her daughter, who later got poked in the eye with a pencil. When the mother took the daughter to a Saudi Arabian doctor (the family lived in Saudi Arabia at the time), he asked her if she was saying a *dua'* for her daughter, and said that there could be no other explanation why the eye was not lost.

In addition to reciting *The Muawwathat*, the evil eye can be treated by going to a *sheikh* (Muslim religious scholar/leader) who typically will do some read-ings from the Qur'an. A few Syrian informants reported that the evil eye may also be treated by collecting the water from a bath taken by the person who had caused the evil eye and pouring it on the person afflicted by it.

There were mixed beliefs in relation to use of blue beads to prevent the evil eye. Many informants reported that they do not believe that blue beads can prevent the evil eye and stated that this is an incorrect or outdated belief. Nevertheless, some informants did say that they believe that wearing blue beads can attract the gamma rays produced by the eye, which would divert the rays from the original target. A Syrian informant said that pin-ning gold emblems or blue beads on a baby's clothes detracts attention from the baby itself, thereby preventing the evil eye. A Lebanese informant maintained:

Envy or the evil eye might hit when something is very beautiful. It could be a kid; if this kid got sick, they assume he was attacked by the evil eye. That is why most Muslims dress their newborns with the *Kharza Zarka* [blue bead] until a certain young age.

Another Lebanese informant shared an opposing view:

You can wear *Ayat Al Kursee* [readings from the Qur'an], you could wear *Allah Akbar*, but *Al Kharza Al Zarka* [blue bead] is against Islam at all, because *Kharza Zarka* is not going to do anything for you. It's just a piece of thing with a color, that's it. It has nothing to do with the *Ain*, or anything. You can wear the Qur'an, . . . you know, Allah is the one who watches you all the time, Allah is the one who is around you all the time, not the *Kharza Zarka*. *Kharza Zarka* is just a thing.

A few Lebanese and Syrian informants shared with the researcher that some people will avoid pronouncing the name of certain illnesses or conditions such as "cancer" and will refer to it instead as "the disease that cannot be named" as a way of protecting themselves from being afflicted by the same condition. A Lebanese informant stated:

Yes, some people ask about someone's illness, they say, "*B'eed min haun,*" which is like "[keep it] far from here"; it is the disease that cannot be named. People are afraid of mentioning its name, they know it by that label . . . Because they are afraid the disease will happen to them.

Folk Caregiving Beliefs and Practices

The vast majority of informants maintained that caregiving in a Muslim community is the responsibility of the family and community members. It was very common to hear an informant describing instances where she was taken care of by her husband, children, and community friends. Typically, both men and women provide physical and emotional support to their families, relatives, and friends. Men tend to provide emotional care through actions more than words, whereas women tend to be more expressive and outspoken. Several informants explained that the man is supposed to be a pillar of strength and support. One informant said that men in the Syrian culture are supposed to be strong providers of support. Another informant held that men do not show sadness but instead encourage others to be tough.

Husbands tend to care for their wives by taking them to the doctor or hospital, purchasing and/or administering medicine, cooking healthy meals, helping with child care, cleaning around the house, and/or asking their wives to rest and not worry about housework. Some husbands hire housekeepers or cleaning ladies to help out their wives around the house instead of personally doing the chores. A Syrian informant described that her husband exhibits caring by paying for someone to help her clean the house. Another informant described how her husband cooks soup for her when she gets the flu. She added that she appreciates his help despite the fact that he creates a lot of messes while helping her. She also shared that sometimes he orders food from restaurants so she can rest in bed and not have to worry about feeding the family.

Husbands will also take care of their wives by being present for them and making themselves available for them and for the children. Many female informants reported that their spouses took time off from their work to take care of them when they were very ill or when they gave birth to their children. One informant related that when she gets sick, her husband checks on her, sits by her to keep her company, covers her with a blanket, and strokes her hair. A Syrian male informant added that he attempts to lift his wife's spirits by "bringing her flowers and helping out around the house" as much as he can. The majority of informants affirmed that the caregiving role of men is a source of pride as opposed to shame. One male informant said that in other cultures men might consider engaging in physical acts of caring as a shameful thing to do, but added that this is not the case for the vast majority of Syrian people. Lebanese informants explained that absence of extended family members being present forces husbands to help their wives when they are sick and in all aspects of life.

Traditionally, both Syrian and Lebanese men are in charge of financial care. Husbands are responsible for their family's medical expenses whether or not the wife is employed outside the home. Brothers and fathers are financially responsible for all expenses of an unmarried sister or daughter. Sons bear the religious, cultural, and moral obligation of caring for the financial, physical, and emotional needs of their retired or elderly parents. A Syrian informant maintained that he is not only responsible for the financial and emotional stability of his immediate family but that he is also accountable for his parents. He explained that when his father retires, he and his brothers will take over the financial expenses of their parents. He added that if his parents get to the point where they can no longer live independently and require someone to care for them, he will have to either bring them to the United States or move back to Syria to care for them. He explained that one of the ways he currently provides for his parents' emotional needs is through weekly international calls that enable his mother and father to hear his voice and the voices of his wife and children.

The majority of informants agreed that when the husband gets sick, it is usually the wife who provides physical and emotional care. Typically, the wife will give her husband or any other ill family member medicine and/or some home remedies. She will attempt to keep the children quiet so that the sick husband or family member can rest. A Syrian informant said that his wife provides him with a good environment when he gets sick, makes sure their children do not disturb him, and cooks special foods for him such as chicken soup. He added that women customarily express more emotional care than men. In addition, women care for children by providing them with nutritious foods, by maintaining a clean house, and by being available for them at all times to address any problems they might have.

As far as children were concerned, it was discovered that they show care to parents and other family members by keeping quiet, helping around the house, and refraining from arguments. According to a Syrian informant, children show care by hugging and kissing and checking on the sick relative. Another informant said that children show tenderness and emotion and inquire if the sick person needs any help. A different informant related that when she is sick, the children clean the house, stay quiet, and give her lots of hugs. A male informant stated that children try to lift the spirit of a sick individual and avoid mentioning negative things around the ill person. He related that when he was a child, he used to visit his sick grandfather, be kind to him, and do little things here and there to make him feel better and more comfortable. A Lebanese informant shared that when she is sick or tired, her son offers to massage her feet.

Visiting the sick person is extremely important in Lebanese and Syrian society. In addition to being identified as a way of caring, visitation is considered a cultural expectation, a religious obligation, and a source of blessing. A Syrian informant said that visitors usually bring flowers or chocolates with them when visiting an ill person. Another informant shared that the Prophet is reported to have said that God rewards people who visit the sick by erasing a sin for every step they take to reach the house or the hospital where the ailing person is staying. She added that the angels pray for the people who visit the ill and that individuals who visit a sick person should ask the ill person to pray for them, as the prayers of the ailing are usually answered by God.

Another informant described how she went to a hospital to visit a Syrian family who was involved in a car accident. She maintained that when she entered the room, she thought a party was going on because of the large number of people who were there. She described how nurses were looking at them and at one another in amazement as if they did not know what to do. Several informants told the researcher that it is not uncommon for Syrians living in the United States to travel to Syria to visit and spend time with a sick parent, especially if the ill individual has a serious or terminal illness. A Lebanese informant stated, "When someone is sick, your duty is to go and visit. If you don't, you may no longer be considered a friend."

Presence and prayer are two other expectations or roles of relatives and friends. A Syrian informant said that the best thing one can do for his brother is *dua'* (prayer/supplication). Another informant added that when her friend went to the hospital for surgery, she sat by her side, read the Qur'an, and prayed for her. Friends and relatives are expected to lend a caring hand when needed. Typically relatives will offer to physically and emotionally care for a sick woman and her children. The children are seldom sent to day care, as a relative or a friend will usually offer to babysit or care for children until the sick person recovers. The researcher observed that whenever a Syrian woman got sick or delivered a baby, other women developed a schedule and took turns in cooking, delivering healthy food, and/or cleaning her house.

Lebanese and Syrian Muslims associate caring with safeguarding and protecting people's honor and pride while caring for them. A Syrian informant explained that the local community included many people who might not be able to afford to buy medicine. These people tend to hide this fact so as not to appear like or be treated as beggars. He added that when he finds out about these people, he and his close friends offer private monetary contributions to assist these families in buying the needed medicine. Several Lebanese informants made similar comments.

Folk Health Maintenance/Promotion and Illness Prevention Beliefs, Expressions, and Practices

The majority of Lebanese and Syrian Muslim informants maintained that most of the care actions they engage in to maintain or improve their health and to prevent illness are derived from their cultural tradition and/or religious beliefs and the recommendations of the Prophet. In addition, many informants reported engaging in scientifically based care practices to maintain their health and prevent illness. Lebanese and Syrian Muslims believe that they can maintain and promote their health by eating a healthy diet, eating in moderation, exercising, fasting, praying, reading the Qur'an, drinking holy water known as *Maa Zamzam*, and maintaining cleanliness of their body and physical environment. Observing Islamic manners of eating *Adab Al Taam* as taught by Prophet Muhammad, doing good deeds, abstaining from smoking, and abstaining from the foods, drinks, and actions that are prohibited by God are other examples of ways traditional Lebanese and Syrian Muslims use to keep healthy.

Illness prevention is very important to both Lebanese and Syrian Muslims. There is a famous saying in both Lebanon and Syria that was cited by several informants from both cultures: "*Dirham Wekaya khayron Min Kintare 'elaj*" or "An ounce of prevention is better than a ton of cure." Health maintenance and promotion are closely related to illness prevention. Many of the informants stated that most of what they do to stay healthy is the same thing they do to prevent illness as well as the evil eye. It was also not rare for informants to state that they abstain from doing certain things that are harmful to their health because of clear instructions provided by their religion. For example, by staying away from pork products, they eliminate the possibility of developing trichinosis; by staying away from alcohol, they avoid alcohol-related health problems and motor-vehicle accidents; and by wrapping the *zennar* or cotton belt/belly wrap around the bellies of newborns until they are 4 or 5 months old, they help prevent stomach cramps and gas/colic problems. Wearing blue beads and emblems with readings from the Qur'an, using *bakhour* (incense), and wearing *hijabs* chase away evil spirits and the evil eye. Including a lot of lemon and garlic in the diet and staying away from ill individuals are other ways of preventing illnesses. The following are specific examples provided by Lebanese and Syrian informants.

Consuming Healthy Food in Moderation The vast majority of informants maintained that they cook Middle Eastern food in their homes, which they described as healthy because it contains a lot of olive oil and fresh vegetables. Many informants shared that they stay away from fast foods. Other informants reported that they abstain from eating a lot of meat in their diet, which they watch very carefully. A Syrian informant maintained that the Prophet recommended that people eat in moderation. As a result, her people try not to fill their stomachs when they eat. Another informant said that Syrian people include dried fruits such as apricots in their diet to maintain regular bowel movements and to prevent constipation. A Lebanese informant stated:

> I try to avoid fatty foods, cut much on junk food especially [for] my kids. We have low-fat milk, we use vegetable oil instead of butter, we avoid fries. I don't allow my kids to eat fast food except occasionally. We eat too much vegetables and fruits.

Consuming foods rich in lemon juice and garlic is also believed to maintain health and prevent illness. A Lebanese informant said:

> . . . citrus is very good for anything to be taken in advance; we should add lemon and garlic as much as we can to food. Garlic is like antibiotic; this use is to make antibiotics, to kill the bacteria. Lemon is very important to the body; it will prevent many things, any disease.

One informant said that the messenger of God recommended that people eat *Habbet el Barakeh*, known as the Blessed Seed or Black Seed (**Figure 6-1**), in the morning an herb which is supposed to boost the immune system and prevent illnesses. He also recommended that people eat honey in the morning for the same reason. Some informants told the researcher that they mix honey with warm water and drink it in the morning. A Syrian informant explained that her 76-year-old father takes two teaspoons of honey mixed with two teaspoons of Black Seed every morning. She maintained that her father, who looks younger than her own husband, is physically fit and

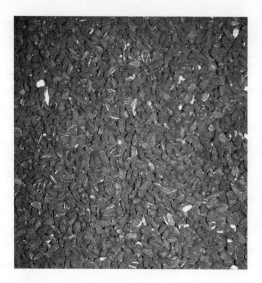

Figure 6-1 Black seeds
© Hiba Wehbe-Alamah, 2012.

has good mental health, and attributes his condition to his daily morning intake of this mixture.

Fasting   Abstaining from eating and drinking from dawn to sunset is a religious requirement during the month of Ramadan for practicing Muslims all around the world. Some informants mentioned that the Prophet also recommended fasting on Mondays and Thursdays as well as on the 13th, 14th, and 15th days of every lunar month when the moon is full. It is believed that fasting rests the stomach, helps decrease weight, and improves spiritual and mental health. A Lebanese informant stated:

> It [fasting] is very healthy, helps lose weight, and reduces fat and cholesterol in blood. It has health and psychological benefits. It is good for a human being to bear starvation and to know how other people suffered from it.

Eating Seven A'jwa Dates in the Morning   This is another tradition of the Prophet. Many informants reported that they eat dates when they break their fast, following the example of their Messenger. Several informants reported that the Prophet advised people to eat seven A'jwa dates (a type of date) from the city of Medina every morning to ward off different illnesses. According to a Syrian informant, the Prophet said that eating dates in the recommended way protects individuals from magic, poison, the *Juzam* (infection of the skin that leaves scars on the face), and the *Ta'oun* (plague).

Exercising Many informants reported that exercise is good for the body. A Syrian informant held that exercise is very important because a strong believer is more beloved to God than a weak believer. Another informant reported that he tries to exercise as much as he can by going to the park and staying active. Several informants shared that although they believe that exercise is good for one's health, they do not feel that they are exercising enough. A Syrian informant explained that he tries to exercise through sports and going up and down the stairs instead of using elevators, but admitted that he does not do that often. A Lebanese informant stated, "To keep well and remain healthy . . . I do sports."

Abstaining from Alcohol, Drugs, Smoking, Pork Products, Premarital Sexual Relations, and Other Actions Prohibited by God All informants maintained that they abstain from drinking alcohol and blood, taking mind-altering drugs, eating the meat of dead animals, and consuming any pork products such as ham, pepperoni, lard, sausage, gelatin, and bacon because of their religion, which forbids these actions as they are believed to be harmful to health. A Lebanese informant said:

> Regarding to health, anything that was prohibited by the *Rabb El Alameen* [Lord of the Universe], I stay away from it, because if it wasn't harmful, the Lord won't prohibit it.

Several Lebanese and Syrian informants maintained that pork is not good because it contains a parasite that can cause illness (trichinosis) and complained of the fact that U.S. hospitals serve Jello and use medications that contain pork-derived gelatin. There was a consensus among informants that smoking is harmful to health, although many Lebanese informants reported that smoking cigarettes as well as the *argheeleh* (also known as *hubbly bubbly* or water pipe; **Figure 6-2**) is becoming increasingly popular among Lebanese youth. A Lebanese informant stated, "To stay healthy we do not smoke or drink . . . in Lebanon, there is no pollution or smoking awareness." Some informants considered smoking to be forbidden by religion whereas others disagreed. A Syrian informant held that taking care of one's body and mind is a religious obligation and therefore one should not intentionally harm the body by smoking or doing any of the harmful actions outlined previously. Several Syrian informants maintained that practicing Muslims in general avoid sexual relations outside of marriage, adultery, and homosexuality, which are prohibited by their religion, to

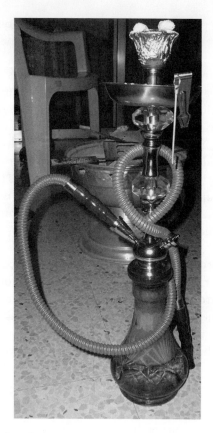

Figure 6-2 Argheeleh in Lebanon
© Hiba Wehbe-Alamah, 2012.

protect themselves from contracting illnesses such as sexually transmitted infections (STIs) and HIV/AIDS.

Waking up and Going to Bed Early   Many Syrian informants reported that the Prophet recommended that people go to bed early and wake up early. One informant held that the Prophet said, *"La Samara Ba'adal Isha"* (no chatting after evening prayer), and that going to bed early gives one strength and energy in the morning. She added that the best and most beneficial sleep children can get is during the first third of the night. Another informant said that he tries to finish his studying as early as possible and that if he does not have a reason to stay awake, he does not. Going to bed and waking up early is believed to promote one's health and energy.

Maintaining a Clean Body and Environment   Many Lebanese and Syrian informants maintained that cleanliness is part of the Muslim religion which encourages people to live in a clean environment and have hygienic bodies. Lebanese and Syrian Muslims value cleanliness from religious, cultural, and social perspectives. It is not customary for guests to call ahead and announce their intention to come and visit; for this reason, houses should be clean and ready at all times to receive guests. A Lebanese informant explained:

> We have to keep our houses clean because we can have visitors at any time. Back home, women spring clean their houses every day—well, it is almost like spring cleaning, they don't have to do their windows every day, but everything else, yes.

In addition, cleanliness of the body is a prerequisite for prayer and is often portrayed in the act of *wudu'*, which precedes prayer up to five times per day. For example, a Syrian informant quoted a popular Arabic saying: *Annazafatou Minal Iman* (cleanliness is from faith). She added that prayer is not accepted by God unless it is performed in a clean place by a clean person wearing clean garments. Another informant held that washing hands before eating is recommended by the Prophet, as is using the toothbrush and *siwak* (tree stick used for cleaning teeth). He went on to describe how making *wudu'* or ablution up to five times per day before prayer is another healthy practice that maintains health and keeps illness away by getting rid of germs. In addition, the researcher observed the presence of a watering can in the bathrooms of several informants. The watering can was used to clean the private area after each bathroom use.

Staying Warm During Cold Weather and Keeping Distance from Ill People   A few Lebanese and Syrian informants reported that staying warm during cold weather keeps them healthy and prevents them from catching colds. A Syrian informant shared that she and her baby will stay inside the house when it is too cold outside. Another informant stated that she will make sure her family is well covered before they leave the house during the winter season. A Lebanese informant described the following practice: "Sometimes to stay away from the ill person, not to get very close to him. Not in all kinds of illnesses—in case of colds, for example." Another said: "To prevent kids from getting sick, we keep them at home if it is cold outside. We don't give them ice cream in cold weather."

Boosting Immunity with Fruit Cocktails, Herbal and Green Teas, and Vitamin and Mineral Supplements   Several informants reported taking vitamin and mineral supplements to maintain or improve their health. A Syrian informant shared that she took her mother to Wal-Mart when she came to visit from overseas and bought her gelatin-free calcium supplements for her bones. Another informant reported that she and her husband prepare fresh carrot or fruit cocktails for their children and drink green tea because of its antioxidant properties, which boost the immune system. Another informant shared that on a daily basis her mother steeps a pot of tea consisting of a mixture of herbs including sage, fennel, anise, and ginger. She tried this tea herself and felt that it gave her energy and boosted her immunity. Two informants stated that some Syrians drink raw eggs with milk in the morning to get good nutrition and energy but maintained that this was now an almost extinct practice. A Lebanese informant stated:

> Fresh carrot, lemonade, and orange juice are very popular in Lebanon. We drink carrot juice to improve vision and lemonade and orange juice to prevent colds and boost our energy and immune system.

Maintaining Annual and Routine Medical Checkups and Staying Up-to-Date with Vaccinations   Several Lebanese and Syrian informants relayed that they make sure their children are up-to-date with their required vaccinations. A Syrian informant shared that she took the Hepatitis A and Hepatitis B vaccines before going on a trip to Syria. Another informant indicated that she updates her tetanus shot every 10 years. A Lebanese informant stated, "We also believe in immunizations to prevent serious diseases like polio. All of my kids have had their immunizations."

Some informants reported that another way of maintaining one's health is through regular annual physical examinations. A Syrian informant maintained that she sees an obstetrician on an annual basis and takes her children to the dentist every 6 months for a checkup and teeth cleaning.

Applying the *Zennar* to Prevent Hernias and/or Colic   Both Lebanese and Syrian informants reported using a wide, thin cotton belt called a *zennar* by wrapping it around a newborn's abdomen to prevent hernias or colic. A Syrian informant reported that the *zennar* is one of many other items that are typically provided for a first-time pregnant woman. She explained that she had received one from her mother but that she had never used it. A Lebanese informant stated:

> I used the belt for all my children. A lot of people use it. Children move a lot and they uncover, which might cause stomachache or gases. This belt will protect his stomach. I don't know, I learned this from my mother and my grandmother . . .

Saying Different Supplications, Reading the Qur'an, and Praying Lebanese and Syrian Muslims view praying as a form of mental and physical exercise that strengthens the body, improves the spiritual state, and allows for mental relaxation. A Lebanese informant shared:

> ... praying by itself is like exercise; we have to bend and kneel and touch the ground several times a day. Also, praying helps people to be on a certain schedule and mentally it is good for them ...

In addition, both Lebanese and Syrian informants reported use of supplication as a means of protection and to ward off harm and illnesses. A Syrian informant maintained that she says *Bismillah allathi la yadurrou maa'smihi shay'* (In the name of God with whom nothing can cause harm with the mention of His name) to protect herself from food poisoning or if she feels worried or suspicious about something she is about to consume, such as sushi. Another informant reported that she says the different supplications taught by the Prophet for use in various situations. For example, when riding a car, she says a *dua'* that is supposed to protect her while using any form of transportation; she says another supplication before going to bed. She added that she feels that the prayers are helping her stay safe from harm. Several informants stated that reading certain verses from the Qur'an, such as *Al-Muawwathat* (which have a protective function), plays a role in preventing harm, promotes mental relaxation and psychological comfort, and thus preserves health. A Lebanese informant stated:

> There is something in me, is that when I get upset I read in the Qur'an, I feel very relaxed, if I cry, I read in the Qur'an, I feel that the Qur'an gives me relaxation. I do not know why, the Lord of the Universe only knows.

A Syrian informant maintained that "memorization and recitation of Qur'an improve memory and retard Alzheimer's disease."

Drinking Holy *Zamzam* Water Lebanese and Syrian Muslims believe that drinking *Zamzam* water (**Figures 6-3** and **6-4**), also referred to as *Mayet Zamzam or Maa Zamzam*, will keep them in good health, prevent illnesses, and even cure diseases. *Zamzam* water was described as a special kind of water that people who make a pilgrimage to *Makkah* (also known as Mecca) usually bring back home with them. It is considered holy and blessed. A Syrian informant declared:

> Prophet Muhammad, peace be upon him, said: *"Maa Zamzam bema shouriba lah,"* which kind of means that if you make a wish when you drink it, your wish comes true. Many people drink it and wish for health or wish to be cured from their illness.

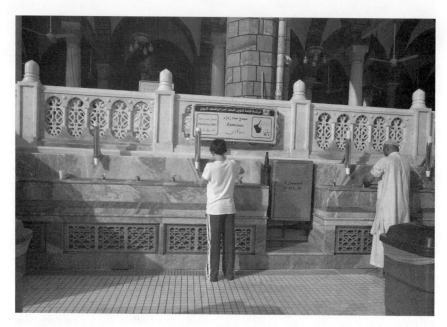

Figure 6-3 Zamzam Holy Water fountain, Makkah, Saudi Arabia.
© Hiba Wehbe-Alamah, 2012.

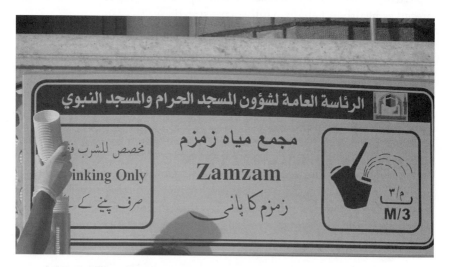

Figure 6-4 Sign for Zamzam Holy Water fountain, Makkah, Saudi Arabia.
© Hiba Wehbe-Alamah, 2012.

A Lebanese informant stated:

> *Maa Zamzam* is very, very good water to drink and wash with, 'cause the story of *Mayet Zamzam* is very, very touching story, from *Sayyedena Ismaeel*; he's the one who God gave him this water. This water has special taste; it doesn't have any kind of bacteria in it at all, so it's very healthy water, . . . it is blessed water.

Observing *Adab Al Taam* (Etiquette of Food/Eating) Lebanese informants associated Muslim etiquette regarding the consumption of food as taught by Prophet Muhammad with maintenance of good health and prevention of illness. Such etiquette includes (but is not limited to) abstaining from eating hot foods, examining water before drinking it, chewing food slowly, eating only when hungry, and avoiding getting full. A Lebanese informant explained:

> There's a way in our religion too. We call it *"Adab Al Taam"* so the way we eat well, first we don't eat food very hot, we do not blow on it, this is from the behaviors, we don't eat too much, we learned bout eating uh, . . . we do not eat a lot of fat foods, we could eat meat, but we eat a lot of vegetables, which is very healthy for the person . . .

Preventing Future Hair Loss with Early and Frequent Haircuts Lebanese informants reported resorting to frequent haircuts as a means of strengthening hair and preventing future or early hair loss. An informant shared:

> We cut our baby's hair bald or very short to make it grow strong and thick, I cut my daughter's hair bald three times already. This way when she is older, she will always have strong hair and she will not lose it early.

Syrian informants reported shaving newborns' hair bald at one week of age following the example of Prophet Muhammad, but did not relate the custom to strengthening hair or prevention of future hair loss.

Folk Illness Treatment Beliefs, Expressions, and Practices

The majority of both Lebanese and Syrian informants affirmed that they used their folk healing practices or home remedies either as a first-line treatment or in conjunction with professional management such as medications. A few Syrian informants admitted that they tend toward antibiotic use at the first sign of a cold or cough because they can easily obtain medication samples from physician friends. Some informants shared that they occasionally self-diagnose and use leftover medications from previous minor illnesses such as colds. Other informants relayed that they feel that antibiotics are overused and expressed their dislike at consuming them unless their use was declared necessary by a primary care provider.

In the following paragraphs, several folk cure practices that were discovered when conducting these two studies are described. It is important to note that not every interviewed informant knew about or practiced all of the discovered rituals and/or practices. Some informants even depicted treatment procedures that are now rarely practiced and some illustrated techniques used by other members of their culture.

Treatment for Hair Loss   Lebanese informants reported treating hair loss with homemade shampoos of a Lebanese wine known as *Arak, Hinneh* (henna), or eggs with olive oil. A Lebanese informant stated:

> We put *Arak* on our hair to strengthen it when we notice that it is starting to fall or shed; we put *Hinneh* for the same reason. We use eggs and olive oil, too.

Syrian informants reported using olive oil as a shampoo that is applied on the hair for one hour prior to taking a bath. They explained that this is supposed to render the hair silky and stimulate its growth.

Treatment for the Common Cold, Cough, Stomachache, Gas, and Sore Throat   Both Lebanese and Syrian informants reported using herbal teas to treat the common cold, stomachaches, gas, and sore throats. *Zhourat* (tisane) is a mixture of herbs that is boiled to make a tea that is used for multiple purposes including throat pain, cough, cold, flu, constipation, and stomachache. *Naa'naa'* (mint tea) is used to treat colds, coughs, stomachache, the flu, diarrhea, and gas. *Baboonej* (chamomile tea) is used for stomachaches, colds, coughs, the flu, and colic. It is also believed to be calming and soothing to the nerves and is occasionally given to soothe cranky babies. Sage is boiled with regular tea to treat stomachache. *Matta* (mate tea) is used as a diuretic and a digestive aid. *Yansoon* (anise) is used to treat colic and stomachache; it is also used for insomnia and as a sleep aid for cranky babies. *Kammoon* (cumin) was reported as the ideal treatment for gas, stomachache, and colic; several Syrian and Lebanese informants affirmed that they used it and obtained successful results. *Maleeseh* (an herb from the same family as mint) is boiled and used for colds and the flu. A tea made from fennel, sage, anise, and ginger is believed to have diuretic effects. A Syrian informant stated that it worked for her and decreased the swelling around her ankles. Another Syrian informant said that she heard of an herb called *Zoofa* that is used to help people urinate but that she had never tried it herself. Another informant reported that insomnia used to be treated with a tea from a plant known as *Khashkhash* (corn poppy). She stated that Syrians stopped using this herbal tea because it was discovered that it contained a narcotic (opium). Insomnia is now more commonly treated with warm milk. Warm milk is also mixed with honey to relieve sore throats. Lebanese informants also reported using hot water bottles to treat stomachache and salt-and-water or plant-based gargles to treat sore throats. Other similar Lebanese home remedies are illustrated in the following statements:

> For a cold, it is good to boil black figs like tea, drain it and drink it, or you can mix a teaspoon of honey with two teaspoons vinegar in a glass of water, which is good for colds, blood and arthritis . . . we use *Khoubayzeh* (mallow plant) for throat pain, gargle with *Khoubayzeh* and half a teaspoon of baking soda, it will get rid of the infection . . . and *Maward* (rose water), *Mazahr* (orange blossom water) and *Ayzakan* (a plant) are used for stomachaches.

Home-made humidifiers were described by Syrian informants as an excellent treatment for colds and chest or head congestion. An informant described the practice as follows:

> One puts a large pot of water on the stove to boil, then puts the pot on a low table and sits in front of it with a towel over his head so that the steam from the pot is trapped between the pot and the face of the person.

Finally, Lebanese informants reported using "*Serej Al Taheeneh*" (the oil on top of the sesame paste) to treat cough:

> I know that if a person is coughing too much, my mother used to take the *Taheeneh* sesame oil, she used to get oil from the *Taheeneh*, and drink it, then they won't cough anymore.

Treatment for Fever   Lebanese informants reported treating fever by immersing the body (of infants or children) in a cold to tepid bath and by using ice packs. A Lebanese informant stated, "If my son has fever, I try to put ice packs, ice towels; I try to break the fever down; I try putting him in the bathtub . . ." A mixture of isopropyl alcohol, vinegar, and olive oil is used by some Lebanese to bring down elevated body temperature:

> If someone has high fever, they can use vinegar, alcohol, and olive oil to help spread it on the body, take off the person's clothes, and apply the mixture all over the body; the fever will go down better than using suppository.

Another Lebanese informant reported the following almost extinct practice:

> To treat an infant with fever, bring a rectangular piece of *Amr Eddine* [dry apricot sheet], make a hole in the middle of it as big as the infant's navel, wipe it with vinegar and dry mint [the sheet], put it on the infant's belly, and put the *zennar* over it. It will absorb the fever from the baby and when you remove it, you will see that the baby's belly is orange in color just like the color of *Amr Eddine*.

A few Syrian informants mentioned the use of cold-water compresses to reduce fever. One informant related that cold wet compresses are typically placed on the forehead.

Treatment for Head Lice   Both Lebanese and Syrian informants reported that some members of their culture may apply kerosene to the hair to treat head lice. Syrian informants explained that this practice is becoming rare and is being replaced with shampoos that can be purchased from pharmacies. Some Lebanese informants described this practice as more efficient than shampoos:

> For *Seebain* (head lice), we treat with *Kaz* (kerosene). I think it is better than the medicine nowadays. Even olive oil, but *Kaz* is better.

Treatment for Migraine Headache   Older Syrian informants described the use of *mandeel* to treat headache but explained that this procedure is extremely rare these days. A *mandeel* was portrayed as a big handkerchief that is made out of heavy cotton and is triangular in shape. It is wrapped tightly around the head, and a knot is formed over the migraine site, where a big key is placed. The technique consists of applying pressure to the migraine site to relieve the headache.

Treatment for Ringworm   Older Lebanese informants described the use of garlic and banana root to treat ringworm. One recounted:

> *Taalabeh* [ringworm] is treated with a piece from the banana root called "*Ermieh*." You squeeze it on the ringworm; it has a watery substance in it which forms bubbles when put on the ringworm. It heals it in days.

Another stated:

> . . . *Taalabeh*, as soon as you see it, rub it with garlic before it spreads, it will heal before you go to the doctor instead of [the doctor] telling [the patient to] come after a week, this will freeze [the ringworm] and heal it. I did that for my granddaughter . . . it worked.

Treatment for Minor Bleeding   Ground coffee was reported by several Lebanese and Syrian informants as an excellent way for stopping minor bleeding. A Syrian informant explained that a lot of ground Turkish coffee is placed over the bleeding area and that something in the coffee causes coagulation which causes the bleeding to stop. A Lebanese informant reported: "For minor cuts and bleeding, I wash the cut and put coffee to stop the bleeding. It works."

Treatment for Low Blood Pressure   Syrian informants reported using a cold beverage derived from licorice root to treat fainting episodes associated with low blood pressure and to increase dangerously low blood pressure levels. One informant said that licorice increases blood pressure and, therefore, is very good for people with low blood pressure who tend to faint a lot and for people with ulcers. The researcher observed several informants as well as other Syrian Muslim women drink a cold beverage made from licorice at the end of a fasting day during the month of Ramadan.

Treatment for Bee Stings   Garlic was reported by both Lebanese and Syrian informants as a very good management tool for bee stings. A Syrian informant described that when a person gets a bee sting, the skin should first be squeezed to let the stinger out. The skin should next be rubbed with a peeled garlic clove. This treatment is supposed to prevent infection and provide pain relief. A Lebanese informant explained: "For bee stings, we rub the affected area with garlic, which is used as antibiotic."

Treatment for First-Degree Burns   Lebanese informants reported using toothpaste, aloe, and yogurt to treat superficial burns. One informant said, "I used to apply toothpaste, but when I came here, I learned about the aloe herb and I used it since then for burns, pains, or anything. . ." Syrian informants reported successfully using toothpaste to treat minor burns. An older Syrian informant shared that she uses slices of a ripe red tomato to treat skin burns.

Treatment for Constipation and Diarrhea   Lebanese informants reported using molasses, olive oil, honey, anise, *Khoubayzeh* (Mallow plant used as a laxative), and pine seeds to treat constipation. A Lebanese informant explained how pine seeds are used:

> I used it for my first child [infant]. You insert a pine seed in the baby's bottom, also a tiny piece of soap, because it slips, and that makes the baby go.

Lebanese informants also reported using tea, yogurt, rice water, and boiled potatoes to treat diarrhea: "For diarrhea we boil rice and drink its water, or we eat boiled potatoes . . . drink dark, dark tea . . . and eat some yogurt on bread . . ."

On the other hand, Syrians reported using dried apricots and prune juice to treat constipation. A Syrian informant shared her personal experience with prune juice and how it had worked for her in the past. Another popular home remedy for Syrians is the ingestion of boiled potatoes and yogurt to treat diarrhea. A Syrian informant stated that she gives her children Pepto-Bismol and regular black tea, a combination that so far has worked very well for her. Another informant added that 7-Up is great for the dehydration associated with diarrhea as well as for nausea. Some Syrian informants stated that they feed their constipated family members fruits and salads to loosen their bowels if they are constipated. An older Syrian informant shared that she used to drink soup or warm goat milk whenever she got constipated.

Treatment for Vaginal Infections   Both Lebanese and Syrian informants described folk practices that they described as becoming rare when it comes to treating vaginal infections. Syrian informants relayed the use of two herbs called *Hoummaydah* and *Hasheeshat al Zujaj*, which are usually boiled with 1 kilogram (2.2 pounds) of barley and lots of water. The herbs are then separated from the water, and the water is poured into a tub or a big bucket. The affected woman would sit in that water and clean her private area with it; she would sit in it twice a day for three days. Lebanese informants relayed a similar, but almost extinct practice using *Khoubayzeh* (Mallow plant): "If the woman has vaginal infection, she can make douche with boiled *Khoubayzeh*; it is the best treatment ever for infections."

Treatment for Anemia   Raw liver is believed by both Lebanese and Syrians to be rich in iron and, therefore, is thought to be an excellent food for a person who is anemic or has iron deficiency. It is also often prescribed for pregnant women. Ingestion of raw liver is common in Lebanon. Unlike Lebanese informants, some Syrian informants described this practice as on its way to extinction. Some informants shared that raw meat is also part of a very popular dish called *Kibbeh Nayyeh* that is consumed by both Lebanese and Syrians. A Syrian informant reported that she feels guilty when she eats it but she still eats it anyway because she loves the taste. She added that she has tried a vegetarian imitation dish that tastes the same and plans to use it as a permanent replacement. Lebanese informants also described consumption of lentils and spinach as a means of treating anemia.

Treatment for Male Impotence   Lebanese informants reported boiling *Zallouah*, also known as *Zallouh* (*Ferulis harmonis*) tea, as a treatment for sexual impotency or to boost men's sexual performance. These informants maintained that *Zallouah* is considered the equivalent of modern-day Viagra. A Lebanese informant shared:

> There is a plant called *Zallou'a* in the mountains of Lebanon . . . they interviewed the persons who found this plant and which they have been using for a long time; they said it's a lot better than Viagra or it could be in the same rank with it.

Treatment for Pain and Mosquito Bites   Lebanese informants reported using vinegar to treat mosquito bites. An informant explained, "If you get a mosquito bite, put vinegar on it right away—it stops the itching and makes it heal quickly." Lotions known as *Abu Shanab* or *Abu Fais* (which smells like Vick's Vapo-Rub) as well as pain patches known as *Lazka* are used to treat pain associated with arthritic nerves. An informant shared:

> *Abu Shanab* is lotion like Vicks—has a terrible smell but it is very good for the nerves for people suffering from arthritis. There is also *Lazka*. My grandmother used to put *Laskat* on the back, to release *Wahm*, absorb infection. They used it in villages; it was very effective.

Homemade patches were reported as a treatment for back pain:

> For back pain or any kind of muscle pain, bring a *Khameh* [piece of dry cloth], dip it in *Arak*, bring some *Bakhour*, crush it and sprinkle it on that wet cloth like a *Lazka*.

Treatment with Cupping   *Hujamah* or cupping was declared by many Syrian informants as an old home remedy that dates back to the time of the Prophet and is currently experiencing a comeback. Cupping consists of lighting a piece of paper and putting it inside a glass cup (**Figure 6-5**); the cup is then placed on the back. As soon as the glass is placed on the back, a vacuum seal is created, resulting in a suction that causes the person's bad blood to accumulate under the skin. The suction seal is broken when the lighted paper in the glass is consumed. The process is repeated three times, at the end of which the skin over the bad blood is cut with a sterilized blade. Another

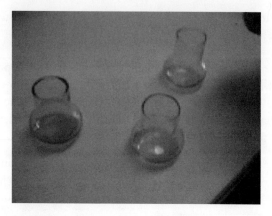

Figure 6-5 Hujamah cups
© Hiba Wehbe-Alamah, 2012.

cup is placed over the small cut and a paper is again lit inside it. The newly created suction draws out the *bad blood*, which is then collected in the cup.

A Syrian informant, who had taken lessons in cupping in Syria, explained that this practice is recommended as a treatment for diabetes and hypertension and is usually done once a year during the springtime, early in the morning and on an empty stomach. According to her, cupping was extremely popular about 50 years ago in Syria and people are now going back to it because of its long-lasting effects, despite the fact that it leaves bruises on the back for a month. The informant shared that cupping lowered her blood sugar by 100 points after one session and decreased her systolic blood pressure from 150 mm Hg to 130 mm Hg. The systolic blood pressure of the informant's mother went down from 180 mm Hg to 120 mm Hg after two treatments.

Lebanese informants also reported using cupping to treat back pain and inflammation, but they referred to it as *Kasset El Hawa*.

Treatment with Arabic Kohl The application of Arabic kohl to newborns' eyes was described by Syrian informants as a controversial practice designed to protect the eyes of the newborn from infection and to make the eyes larger and thus more attractive. One informant said that the old Arabic kohl used to contain lead, which is harmful to babies, but the new Arabic kohl does not have lead in it. She added that Arabic kohl contains mercury, which is a good thing to put on the eyes of newborns to prevent infection. Nowadays hospitals apply their own medications to the eyes of newborns, she noted, so people tend to use Arabic kohl more to make the eyes of their infants bigger (which is a mark of beauty for Syrians).

Alternative Treatment Options Used by Lebanese and Syrian Muslims

Lebanese and Syrian informants shared the existence of alternative care and healing systems to prevent or seek cure from certain illnesses. Syrian Muslims with no health insurance or low income reported seeking medical advice and medication samples from physician friends and family members who work in the healthcare field. One informant related that her physician husband tells the people who call him on the telephone for a diagnosis or treatment that he has to see them before making any recommendations. Another Syrian informant shared that some people have strong *dua'* (prayer supplication), meaning that their *dua'* usually comes true. Such people are therefore approached by ill individuals and their relatives and are asked to pray for the healing of the sick.

Lebanese and Syrian informants maintained that it is common to ask a person who is traveling to the holy land of Makkah in Saudi Arabia to perform the pilgrimage (*Hajj;* **Figure 6-6**) or mini-pilgrimage (*Umrah*) to pray for the healing of a sick person. When a man performs *Hajj*, he becomes

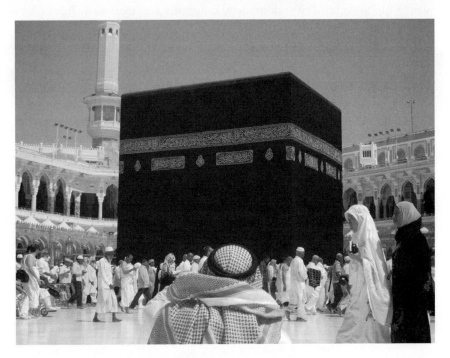

Figure 6-6 Holy Kaaba in Makkah, Saudi Arabia, where Muslims from all around the world congregate to perform Hajj or Umrah.
© Hiba Wehbe-Alamah, 2012.

known as a *Hajj*; a woman who has performed the pilgrimage is known as a *Hajjeh*. An older *Hajjeh* is often sought for her wisdom, experiences in life, folk practices handed down from generation to generation, and her status as a *Hajjeh* for medical advice, blessings, and prayer supplications.

Lebanese and Syrian informants also reported that a Muslim *Sheikh* is often sought for counseling and/or asked to pray for a sick person. The *Sheikh* is a Muslim religious leader and scholar. He is most often sought to help cure or pray for someone affected by the evil eye, chronic illnesses, or states of mind believed to have been caused by evil spirits, *Jinn*, or *Kateebeh* (a form of black magic). A Lebanese informant shared:

> They [people] told me I had the evil eye, and it was true, I felt changes, I went to the doctor and had X-rays. There was nothing wrong. They referred me to the *Sheikh*, he told me that I had the evil eye for bad things. He gave me a paper with verses from the Qur'an, he warned not to open, he told me to soak it in warm water and stir then drink the water. I tried it and it worked . . .

In Syria and Lebanon, people who cannot afford to see a physician or who want a quick fix tend to seek medical diagnosis and treatment from pharmacists. A Syrian physician informant reported that she saw a pharmacist dispense the wrong treatment to a customer after delivering an incorrect diagnosis solely based on the customer's description of symptoms. Most pharmacists in Lebanon are licensed. However, a pharmacist can hire a relative or any layperson to help him run the pharmacy. In addition, some pharmacies do not require their customers to have a prescription from a physician to purchase certain medications such as antibiotics. As a result, some Lebanese people who cannot afford a visit to the doctor ask the pharmacist (or anyone running the pharmacy at the time of visit) to recommend a medication to treat their symptoms. A Lebanese informant reported:

> Yes, it is true that they [pharmacy owners] will hire a relative to help in the pharmacy. In Lebanon, some pharmacies will sell medications without a prescription, but some pharmacies will only sell you if you have prescriptions. People, let's say a mother with a lot of kids, if her kid is coughing or has diarrhea, and she knows what medications he needs, she will not go to the doctor because she wants to save money, so she will go to the pharmacist and tell him give me this medication, or she will tell him give me a medication for diarrhea for my child. Here in America, you have to have a prescription even in Lebanese pharmacies.

In addition to the folk practices described previously, Lebanese informants reported engaging in polypharmacy and sharing medications from friends and family when seeking cure for illnesses. A Lebanese informant shared:

> I went to the pilgrimage, *Hajj*, had fever over there, I took medicine from a lot of people, a lot of people told me: "Here, take this it works for me, my doctor prescribed it for me, try it." I came back home, find that my liver and my kidneys were not working from all the medicines I was taking. From now, I tell everybody this is no good, very bad to take other people's medications. A lot of people do this.

A few Lebanese informants reported that in some remote villages, there is often a shortage or absence of licensed physicians or professional health-care providers. To accommodate the health needs of the residents in these areas, some lay persons move to a big city, seek work in a hospital or an office, learn some basic medical or nursing skills such as inserting IVs and giving injections, and then return to their villages and become the "doctor" in that area. They often rely on their experiences, memory, medical books, and consultations with licensed physicians or pharmacists when delivering care. A Lebanese informant stated:

> We had a man in our village, he was smart, he got sick and stayed at the American Hospital, accompanied the doctors and stayed with them, he learned many things from them. He went back to the village, he started giving shots. I can't tell you how smart he was, finally, he had a stethoscope, and starting testing patients, there was snow and the roads are blocked, you can't leave the village. He used to call over the phone. For example, my husband when he was single, he had typhoid fever and bronchitis, . . . He diagnosed the two diseases, he called the doctor in Zahle and described symptoms, . . . the doctor told that what he was doing was right. . . . He treated him and saved him from the two disease. I also had fever from drinking from *Abu-Ali River* in Tripoli, he treated me, I was in a very bad condition. . . . I had my children by a midwife, she used to treat us for everything . . .

It is important to note that not every single Lebanese or Syrian Muslim necessarily holds all of the beliefs shared in this chapter. Variations exist even within the same family unit. Therefore, conducting cultural assessments is important to avoid generalizations that may turn into stereotypical assumptions.

Discoveries for Culture-Specific Care

Leininger (2006a) held that nurses (as well as other healthcare providers) can creatively bridge professional and generic/folk care beliefs and practices and deliver meaningful and helpful care to their clients through the use of the three nursing care modes of decisions and actions in the provision of culturally congruent care.

Culture Care Preservation and/or Maintenance

This mode refers to professional decisions or actions that assist, support, facilitate, or enable cultures to "retain, preserve, or maintain beneficial care beliefs and values or to face handicaps and death" (Leininger, 2006a, p. 8). Accordingly, a healthcare provider interested in preserving and/or maintaining the culture care beliefs and practices of Lebanese or Syrian Muslims may engage in any of the following actions:

- Acquire some basic holding knowledge related to traditional folk care beliefs and practices, worldviews, and cultural and social structure beliefs, practices, and expressions of Lebanese and Syrian Muslim cultures.
- Accept gestures reflecting the hospitality of Lebanese and Syrians within the healthcare system, such as chocolate, candy, or baklava and other Middle Eastern sweets.
- Understand that Lebanese and Syrian men and women consider themselves equal but not identical. Their roles are reflective of this belief. Healthcare providers are encouraged to refrain from imposing their own values on their patients.
- Observe transcultural communication principles respectful of Lebanese and Syrian beliefs related to eye contact, personal space, and touch.
- Inform clients and family members of the location of an interfaith chapel and/or provide a copy of the Qur'an (holy book for Muslims; **Figure 6-7**) when appropriate.
- Refrain from effusive or passionate admiration of newborns—an action associated with unintentional infliction of evil eye according to some folk beliefs.
- Evaluate herbal and other folk care practices reported by clients and support use of ones that are considered safe.

Culture Care Accommodation and/or Negotiation

This mode refers to professional decisions or actions that assist, accommodate, facilitate, or enable cultures to "adapt to or negotiate with others for culturally congruent, safe, and effective care for their health, wellbeing, or to deal with illness or dying" (Leininger, 2006a, p. 8). Accordingly, a healthcare provider interested in accommodating and/or negotiating the culture care

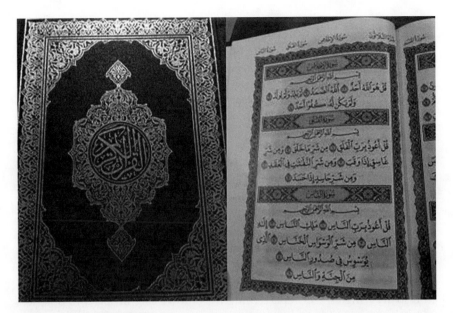

Figure 6-7 Left: Muslim Holy Book (Qur'an). Right: The Muawwathat verses (the exorcists).
© Hiba Wehbe-Alamah, 2012.

beliefs and practices of Lebanese or Syrian Muslims may engage in any of the following actions:

- Utilize transcultural professional interpreters when caring for nonbilingual Lebanese or Syrian patients to ensure effective communication.
- Provide physical space or accommodations for a relative to spend the night with a hospitalized patient or for a large number of visitors during the daytime. Alternatively, negotiate the number of visitors with the client and/or family.
- Accommodate dietary needs and/or restrictions by providing *halal*, vegetarian, or seafood menu options and by prescribing or dispensing gelatin/pork/alcohol-free medications.
- Accommodate the need for privacy, modesty, and a same-gender healthcare provider when needed. Provide a chaperone when unable to accommodate the request for a same-gender healthcare provider.
- Negotiate (with clients and administration) use of cell phones or tablets with Wi-Fi to allow hospitalized patients to stay in touch (via Skype or similar programs) with long-distance or overseas family

members—an important cultural belief and practice for members of Lebanese and Syrian cultures.

- Assist clients with performance of ablution. Provide a water container for use in the bathroom. Arrange for a clean and private space for prayer rituals. Position the bed in the northeast direction if the client is unable to get out of bed for prayer.
- Accommodate hospitalized or outpatient fasting patients by switching medication regimens from daytime to nighttime administration. Negotiate with hospital dietary service for a meal prior to sunrise for hospitalized patients.

Culture Care Repatterning and/or Restructuring

This mode refers to professional decisions or actions that assist, support, facilitate, or enable cultures to "reorder, change, modify, or restructure their lifeways and institutions for better healthcare patterns, practices, or outcomes" (Leininger, 2006a, p. 8). Accordingly, a healthcare provider interested in restructuring and/or repatterning the culture care beliefs and practices of Lebanese or Syrian Muslims may engage in any of the following actions:

- Discourage use of polypharmacy, medication sharing, and reliance on nonprofessional self-claimed lay doctors. Provide resources for free or affordable healthcare services.
- Educate clients about the harmful ramifications of using kerosene to treat head lice (flammability; irritation to skin, eyes, and respiratory system; and potential fatal aspiration; Tesoro Corporation, 2012) and herbal douching to treat vaginal yeast infections. Provide access to or education about healthier alternatives.
- Repattern use of *argheeleh* by educating clients about the effect of smoking tobacco via water pipe and the effects on the pulmonary and other systems involved. Provide smoking cessation kits adapted for use of *argheeleh*.
- Educate clients about herbal–drug interactions following an individualized assessment of herbal folk practices reported by the client.
- Educate clients about development of antibiotic resistance and discourage use of antibiotics without professional prescriptions.
- Restructure consumption of raw liver and meat by educating clients about possible repercussions for ingesting uncooked meats which could be contaminated with bacteria or parasites such as *Salmonella, Escherichia coli,* and *Listeria* (Centers for Disease Control and Prevention [CDC], 2012).

- Educate clients about the harmful effects of lead and provide resources for lead-free kohl alternatives.
- Encourage clients who use cupping to rely solely on the services of professional healthcare providers with formal academic training.

Healthcare providers who incorporate folk care beliefs and practices and Leininger's culture care modes of decisions and actions into their professional plans of care deliver culturally sensitive, meaningful, and beneficial care to the people they serve. In addition, they contribute to increased patient satisfaction, establishment of trust, and commitment to participation in and adherence to professional plans of care.

CONCLUSION

Different cultures present with a plethora of folk care beliefs and practices. Knowledge of these folk care beliefs and practices is essential for maintenance and promotion of health and wellbeing. People of diverse cultural backgrounds are entitled to professional care that is sensitive to and respectful of their cultural beliefs, needs, and prohibitions. Professional healthcare providers have the moral and ethical obligation to provide the best possible care to their clients. Such care must be inclusive of both professional and generic/folk care beliefs and practices. In this chapter, the worldview of traditional Lebanese and Syrian Muslims, as well as their folk care beliefs and practices related to health and illness, health maintenance and promotion, illness prevention and treatment, death and dying, and alternative treatments, were shared. In addition, the relationship and effects of folk care beliefs and practices on Lebanese and Syrian worldview, cultural context, and social structure were explained. Readers are encouraged to consider the presented findings as holding knowledge and to conduct individualized cultural assessments when caring for members of these or other similar cultural groups to avoid generalizations and stereotyping and to provide culturally congruent care that is tailored to the cultural beliefs and needs of the people they serve.

DEDICATION

This chapter is dedicated to Lebanese and Syrian immigrants residing in the United States and across the world, and to educators, students, and current/ future primary care providers who are passionate about providing culturally congruent care to those whom they serve.

DISCUSSION QUESTIONS

1. Why should healthcare professionals develop plans of care that are inclusive of folk care beliefs and practices?
2. Why should healthcare professionals become aware of folk care beliefs and practices?
3. What are some important cultural and social folk care beliefs and practices of Lebanese and Syrian Muslims? Why?
4. List three Lebanese and Syrian folk care beliefs and practices that healthcare providers can/should accommodate and/or negotiate when caring for these cultural groups.
5. List three Lebanese and Syrian folk care beliefs and practices that healthcare providers can/should repattern and/or restructure when caring for these cultural groups.

APPENDIX 6-A: LEININGER'S SUNRISE ENABLER IN ARABIC

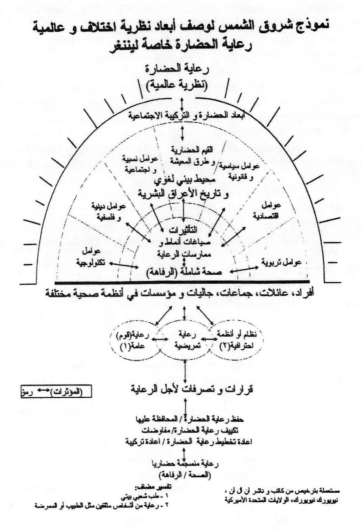

Appendix 6-A Leininger's Sunrise Enabler translated into Arabic.
Modified with permission from © M. Leininger 2004, by Wehbe-Alamah.

REFERENCES

Ali, A. Y. (1983). *The holy Qur'an*. Maryland: Amana Corp.

Arab American Institute. (n.d.). Demographics. http://www.aaiusa.org/pages/demographics/

Arab American Institute. (2011). Michigan. http://aai.3cdn.net/961a14b93140d532a5_yym6iyilb.pdf

Bennett, S. H. (2000). Lebanese or Syrian ancestry—immigration. http://www.genealogytoday.com/family/syrian/part3.html

Centers for Disease Control and Prevention (CDC). (2012). Food safety. http://www.cdc.gov/foodsafety/specific-foods.html

Connelly, M., Hammad, A., Hassoun, R., Kysia, R., & Rabah, R. (1999). *Guide to Arab culture: Health care delivery to the Arab American community*. Dearborn, MI: ACCESS Community Health Center.

Dehler, T. (2009). Genealogy: Syrian, Lebanese immigrants arrived in U.S. in 1870s. http://tribstar.com/history/x1896315608/Genealogy-Syrian-Lebanese-immigrants-arrived-in-U-S-in-1870s

Fatfat, M. (1998). *The migration of Lebanese professionals to the United States: Why they left Lebanon and why they are staying in the United States*. Doctoral dissertation. Available from ProQuest Dissertations and Theses database (UMI No. 9837494).

Grossman, C. L. (2011). *Number of U.S. Muslims to double*. http://usatoday30.usatoday.com/news/religion/2011-01-27-1Amuslim27_ST_N.htm

Johnson, T. (2011). Muslims in the United States. Council of Foreign Relations, Campaign 2012. http://www.cfr.org/united-states/muslims-united-states/p25927

Leininger, M. M. (1988). Leininger's theory of nursing: Culture care diversity and universality. *Nursing Science Quarterly, 2*(4), 152–160.

Leininger, M. M. (1991). *Culture care diversity and universality: Theory of nursing*. New York, NY: National League for Nursing.

Leininger, M. M. (1994). *Transcultural nursing: Concepts, theories, & practices*. Columbus, OH: Greyden Press.

Leininger, M. M. (1995). Overview of Leininger's culture care theory. In *Transcultural nursing: Concepts, theories, research, & practice* (2nd ed., pp. 93–114). New York, NY: McGraw-Hill.

Leininger, M. M. (1996). Culture care theory, research, and practice. *Nursing Science Quarterly, 9*(2), 71–78.

Leininger, M. M. (1997a). Overview of the theory of culture care with the ethnonursing research method. *Journal of Transcultural Nursing, 8*(2), 32–52.

Leininger, M. M. (1997b). Transcultural Nursing Research to Transform Nursing Education and Practice: 40 Years. *Image: Journal of Nursing Scholarship, 29*(4), 341–347.

Leininger, M. M. (2002). The theory of culture care and the ethnonursing research method. In M. M. Leininger & M. R. McFarland (Eds.), *Transcultural nursing: Concepts, theories, research, & practice* (3rd ed., pp. 71–98). New York, NY: McGraw-Hill Medical.

Leininger, M. M. (2006a). Culture care diversity and universality theory and evolution of the ethnonursing research method. In M. M. Leininger & M. R. McFarland (Eds.), *Culture care diversity and universality: A worldwide nursing theory* (2nd ed., pp. 1–42). Sudbury, MA: Jones and Bartlett.

Leininger, M. M. (2006b). Ethnonursing research method and enablers. In M. M. Leininger & M. R. McFarland (Eds.), *Culture care diversity and universality: A worldwide nursing theory* (2nd ed., pp. 43–82). Sudbury, MA: Jones and Bartlett.

Leuning, C. J., Swiggum, P. D., Barmore Wiegert, H. M., & McCullough-Zander, K. (2002). Proposed Standards for Transcultural Nursing. *Journal of Transcultural Nursing, 13*(1), 40–46.

Mughees, A. (2006). Better caring for Muslim patients. *World of Irish Nursing & Midwifery, 14*(7), 24–25.

Pew Forum on Religion and Public Life. (2011). The future of the global Muslim population projections for 2010–2030. http://www.pewforum.org/The-Future-of-the-Global-Muslim-Population.aspx

Religious Population Worldwide. (n.d.). World religious population in 2011/2012. http://www.religiouspopulation.com/World/

Tesoro Corporation. (2012). Safety data sheet: Kerosene. http://www.tsocorp.com /stellent/groups/corpcomm/documents/tsocorp_documents/msdskerosene .pdf

UNHCR—The UN Refugee Agency. (2013). Number of Syrian refugees tops 2 million mark with more on the way, 3 September, 2013. http://www.unhcr .org/522495669.html http://data.unhcr.org/syrianrefugees/download .php?id=1631

United Nations News Centre. (2012). Magnitude of human rights violations in Syria has dramatically increased—UN panel. http://www.un.org/apps/news /story.asp?NewsID=42909#

Wehbe-Alamah, H. (2005). *Generic and professional health care beliefs, expressions and practices of Syrian Muslims living in the Midwestern United States*. Doctoral dissertation. Available from ProQuest Dissertations and Theses database (UMI No. 3197399).

Wehbe-Alamah, H. (2006). Generic care of Lebanese Muslims in the Midwestern United States. In M. L. Leininger & M. R. McFarland (Eds.), *Culture care diversity and universality theory and ethnonursing research method* (2nd ed., pp. 307–325). Sudbury, MA: Jones and Bartlett.

Wehbe-Alamah, H. (2008a). Bridging generic and professional care practices for Muslim patients through the use of Leininger's culture care modes. *Contemporary Nurse, 28*(1–2), 83–97.

Wehbe-Alamah, H. (2008b). *Culture care of Syrian Muslims in the Midwestern USA: The generic and professional health care beliefs, expressions, and practices of Syrian Muslims and implications to practice*. Saarbrucken, Germany: VDM Verlag Dr. Muller.

Wehbe-Alamah, H. (2011). The use of culture care theory with Syrian Muslims in the Midwestern United States. *Online Journal of Cultural Competence in Nursing and Healthcare, 1*(3), 1–12.

Chapter 7

Transcultural Midwifery: Culture Care for Mauritian Immigrant Childbearing Families Living in New South Wales, Australia

Lynette Mary Raymond
Akram Omeri

INTRODUCTION

Australia is a country of many diverse cultural and linguistic societies, with its people drawn from more than 200 of the world's nations and speaking more than 80 languages (Commonwealth of Australia, 2001, 2008). Because it is a nation of immigrants, the Australian government has made a commitment to increasing positive immigration and healthcare policies and maintaining Australia's Multiculturalism with an obligation toward meeting the diverse cultural and linguistic healthcare needs of all Australians (Bottomley & Lepervanche, 1990; Commonwealth of Australia, 1999, 2003, 2008; Idrus, 1988; Jupp, 1990). The principles upon which Australia's multiculturalism policy is based include the importance of valuing differences; ensuring access and equity; and utilising the cultural knowledge and skill contributions of people from different backgrounds, experiences, and perspectives so as to generate new ideas and ways of doing things in all sectors of society. Accordingly, it is a policy intended for all Australians, not just for those people from non-English-speaking backgrounds (Commonwealth of Australia, 2003, 2008).

BACKGROUND

Maternity care service providers in New South Wales (NSW), Australia, include a variety of healthcare workers such as midwives; obstetricians; mothercraft nurses; registered nurses (working in the specialty areas of family planning/fertility, neonatal intensive care, baby health, and women's health); obstetric ethnic liaison officers; enrolled nurses; and allied maternity staff such as physiotherapists, childbirth educators, antenatal and postnatal instructors, dieticians, and paediatricians. However, registered midwives comprise the largest number of maternity care service providers in NSW. In 2003, there were 76,190 nurses registered in NSW; 19,201 were listed as authorised to also practise midwifery (New South Wales Nurses' Registration Board, 2001). Mothercraft nurses have qualifications in childhood development and their role and function include care for the postnatal mother and her newborn until 5 years of age. Since 2010, mothercraft nurses in Australia have been granted general registration as enrolled nurses with the conditions that they may practise only in the area of mothercraft nursing and that they are not eligible to administer and monitor medications in the work environment.

The Australian College of Midwives Incorporated (ACMI) asserts midwifery as a "profession in its own right," with midwives best positioned to provide holistic, appropriate, and cost-effective professional maternity care to women, babies, and their families (ACMI, 2002a, p. 2). In recognition of the differences between the two professions (not all midwives are nurses), the Nurses Act of 1991 was amended by the Australian federal government in 2003 and legislated as the Nurses and Midwives Act 1991 (Brodie, 2003). Approval of direct-entry Bachelor of Midwifery courses commenced soon afterward. As of July 2012, 27 universities across Australia offered undergraduate and/or postgraduate courses in midwifery. In addition to the undergraduate Bachelor of Midwifery, other courses on offer included a double degree with a Bachelor of Nursing and Bachelor of Midwifery; Conversion and Honours study pathways were also available. Post-Graduate Diploma, Master's, and Doctor of Midwifery degrees were also on offer at many Australian universities.

CULTURAL AND LINGUISTIC DIVERSITY AMONG NSW CHILDBEARING FAMILIES

In 1996, there were 86,429 births to 85,302 women in New South Wales; by 1999, this figure was little changed with approximately 27% of births occurring to women who were born overseas. Approximately 20% of these women were from non-English-speaking backgrounds, a proportion that remained relatively stable until 2002 (Australian Institute of Health and Welfare, 2001; NSW Department of Health, 1998, 2001, 2002a). During the period 2002–2009, the number of births from mothers who were born overseas had increased to nearly 32% (NSW Department of Health, 2009, 2010; NSW Ministry of Health, 2011). The importance of recognising and addressing cultural and linguistic diversity issues by maternity care service providers has become increasingly evident during the late twentieth and early twenty-first centuries (Barclay & Jones, 1996; NSW Department of Health, 2002b).

The Mauritian immigrant community represents one of the many diverse cultural and linguistic groups giving birth in NSW. The health and wellbeing of the Mauritian mother and baby throughout the childbearing experience and the relationship with their immigrant family members' cultural beliefs, values, meanings, and patterns of care was a central focus of the research study discussed in this chapter. Both in the past and at present, Mauritian-born mothers giving birth in NSW have been collated under the group classification of *Other*, *Middle East*, or *Africa*. Also, only those countries of birth from which 100 or more women have given birth in the preceding year are itemised in the annual midwives' data collection report (NSW Ministry of Health, 2011). Analyses by the Epidemiology Unit of the University of NSW revealed that 360 Mauritian-born women gave birth in NSW during the 4-year period from 1994 to 1997 (Bauman & Mohsin, 1999).

PURPOSE AND DOMAIN OF INQUIRY

The purpose of this ethnonursing research study was to discover, describe, and analyse the cultural beliefs, values, care meanings, decisions, and actions as expressed by Mauritian immigrant childbearing families living in New South Wales. Leininger's Theory of Culture Care Diversity and Universality, the qualitative ethnonursing research method, and selected theory ethnonursing enablers guided this study. The domain of inquiry (DOI) focused on the culture care expressions and the behaviour patterns and lifeways of Mauritian immigrant childbearing families toward maintaining health and wellbeing during pregnancy, childbirth, and puerperium.

ETHNOHISTORY (*HISTOIRE ETHNIQUES DE L'AMBIANCE*)

Holding knowledge of an individual's ethnohistory, language, sociocultural, and environmental contexts provided valuable background information about the informants' homeland. This cultural heritage information was used to facilitate the researchers' understanding and accurate interpretation of the differing and similar beliefs, values, and behaviour patterns as expressed by the Mauritian people who participated in this study.

Geographical Location

Mauritius is a small, weathered volcanic island measuring approximately 1,969 square kilometres (760 square miles) in area, situated in the South west Indian Ocean located approximately 5,800 kilometres (3,625 miles) from Perth on the west coast of Australia and 1,100 kilometres (690 miles) from the east coast of Madagascar (located in the Indian Ocean off the west coast of Africa). The island has a humid monsoon tropical climate, with a mean seasonal temperature varying between 16 and 29 degrees Centigrade (approximately 61 to 84 degrees Fahrenheit) throughout the calendar year (Government of Mauritius Central Statistics Office [GMCSO], 2001b). The capital of the island is Port Louis, a bustling colonial-style centre of administration and commerce, servicing both domestic and international trades. Notwithstanding the island's geographical proximity to Africa, Eriksen (1998, p. 11) points out that "... Mauritius cannot be considered an African country proper ... [As] it has been built from scratch since 1715 and has in most respects much more in common with West Indian islands than with any African society of comparable scale."

The People of Mauritius

Mauritius has no indigenous population, but rather has an ethnically diverse group of people due to the pattern of recurrent possession and dispossession, colonisation, and the importation of slaves and indentured labourers throughout the past 300 years (Duyker, 1986, 1988; Eriksen, 1988, 1998). The Republic of Mauritius has a growing population; the nearly 1.06 million inhabitants identified from the 1990 population census grew to almost 1.2 million by 2000, an approximate annual increase of 1.1% during this 10-year period (GMCSO, 2001a; Republic of Mauritius, 2003). The age distribution of the Mauritian population in the year 2000 was as follows: 15 years of age or younger, 25.7%; 15 to 59 years, 65.4%; 60 to

64 years, 2.8%; and 65 years of age and older, 6.1% (GMCSO, 2001a). These figures highlight the large proportions of Mauritians who were young adults and of childbearing age; seeking travel or immigration opportunities to live, work, and/or study in another country was common among this age group (Australian Bureau of Statistics, 1997).

Ethnicity (*Ethnicité*)

In the year 2000, the population of Mauritius comprised a distinctive blend of races, diverse cultures, ethnic identities, religions, and languages (GMCSO, 2001c). The cultural and sociobiological heritages of the people consisted predominantly of European, African, Indian, and Chinese origins that through interethnic marriage resulted in a multicultural society where various ethnic identities with similar and diverse beliefs and cultural practises live harmoniously. The standard postwar official four-ethnic-group classifications identified in the 2000 population census of Mauritius included Hindu (51.8%), Muslim of Asian-Indian origin (16.6%), General Créole Population of African origin (28.4%), and a small Chinese/Sino-Mauritian settlement of people (3.2%). Within each of these four major ethnic groups, further subethnic categorisations were made based on a variety of cultural, racial, ethnic, class, and religious distinctions (Eriksen, 1998; GMCSO, 2001a, 2001c).

The General Population category was comprised of 2% Franco-Mauritian and a much larger subcategory of Créole. According to Eriksen (1998), the Créole people are usually described as being Christian (of whom the majority are Catholic) and of African or mixed African-European, African-Indian, and/or African-Chinese descent. "Ethnicity [in Mauritius] has proved to be the most powerful unifying principle both cognitively and socially, that is deeper than class membership and more relevant in everyday life than nationality" (p. 98).

In addition to the constructs of Leininger's (1991, 2002b) Theory of Culture Care Diversity and Universality, *ethnicity* was also discovered as a significant influencing social structure factor embedded in the dimensions of cultural values, beliefs, and practices for Mauritians living in NSW. The ethnic (General Créole Population) identity of the Mauritian informants covertly influenced their culture patterns of care, as was discovered within the context of the domain of inquiry. Informants identifying as a member of the General Créole Population held religious beliefs based on the principles of Christianity; collaborative family and social relationships were also highly valued as were the values of education, knowledge, and skill acquisition (formal and informal). These values provided both an impetus and the means for gaining social and economic mobility which the informants believed enhanced health and wellbeing and improved the lifeways for childbearing women and their unborn/newborn infants.

Language (*Langage*)

The official Mauritius Census data from 1990 and 2000 reported the population was multilingual, with English, French, and Créole (Kreole/Patois) being the main languages spoken. Additional smaller numbers of people were reported as being fluent in Hindi, Chinese, or 1 of 10 other languages spoken on the island (Eriksen, 1998; GMCSO, 2001a).

After the country gained independence and became a member of the British Commonwealth, English was declared the official national language on the island of Mauritius; it has remained such since the advent of British rule. English is used in all official government documents, in academia, for conducting global business, and to a limited extent in the mass media. Both English and French are taught in primary and secondary schools. Eriksen (1998) identified that many Mauritians are also fluent French speakers, most of whom acquired their French literacy as a first-spoken language. Créole is an unofficial national language of Mauritius that is often spoken at home, in the marketplace, and at other less formal social occasions. Créole is a French-lexicon language primarily associated with the Créole ethnic group dating back to the slave–master and slave–slave contexts of the early 18th century. It is the slave-development history of the Créole language that has in many ways contributed to preventing it from being declared the official language of Mauritius (Eriksen, 1998; Lenoir, 1985; Singh, Swaney, & Strauss, 1999; Willcox, 1999).

Family, Kinship, and Social Factors (*Famille, Parenté, et Facteurs Sociaux*)

Eriksen (1998, p. 15) suggested that, unlike other nations, the "... social construction of persons in Mauritius is based on ethnicity." Ethnicity is viewed as a dominant structural dimension that influences the development of social relationships, beliefs, and values among the Mauritian people. Other, less dominant influencing structural dimensions that were also identified as the "basis of many [Mauritian] social networks" included interethnic marriages (i.e., marriage between individuals with differing ethnic identities), gender, class, age, individualism, region, locality, and globalisation (p. 103). Ethnographic descriptions of family and kinship systems in postcolonial Mauritius have been described in general as "... male dominated and highly dependent on ethnic membership" (p. 60). Nevertheless, of all the ethnic groups on the island of Mauritius, Créole women have maintained the highest degree of personal freedom and have had the greatest number of women representatives participating in public life and political activitism.

Marriage is confined to the private life domain, with all major political parties taking a neutral position on the issue of interethnic marriages. Notwithstanding these differences, outside of the marriage relationship interethnic relationships do commonly exist between women in social and workplace settings, transcending ethnic boundaries and differences in both these social contexts (Eriksen, 1998).

Culture (*Culture*)

The relationship between "ethnicity and culture is complicated" in Mauritius and highly dependent on context (Eriksen, 1998, p. 25). Competing cultural systems are sustained and reproduced through the process of socialisation. They are largely defined by interethnic relations in diverse social contexts that contribute to the maintenance of both shared culture and diverse ethnic identities. Eriksen (1998) referred to culture ". . . as the ways in which one can conceivably lead one's life." With respect to Mauritian society, he explained:

> Culturally specific knowledge may include knowing when to speak French instead of *Créole*, how to vote, for whom and why, understanding why a *Séga* song is funny, knowing how and when to get into and out of debt. . . [Knowing the] implicit rules for the cultural expression of spontaneity: The display of emotions, cursing, laughter, shrugging and nearly all forms of body movements. . . It is inscribed in the bodies of the carriers. (p. 23)

The duality of culture in this context refers not so much to the distinction between identity (sameness) and difference, but rather to the communication of sameness and difference. Eriksen (1998) stated that, ". . . societies and cultures are open systems" whose boundaries are likely to shift according to each individual's (emic) perspective and as such, the integrated relationship between culture and diverse ethnicity must be first understood if one is to understand the Mauritian people as a whole (p. 27).

Worldview (*Vue de Monde*)

Some anthropological studies undertaken on the island of Mauritius have attempted to convey the worldview of the Mauritian people as a whole.

Eriksen (1998) described the underlying ". . . current spirit of Mauritian society as one of *compromise*" [italics added] (p. 6). Sussman (1981) discovered that regardless of their ethnic and religious differences, the Mauritian peoples' outlook on life encompassed the unifying belief that ". . . illnesses of God are phenomena that exist and are part of the natural order of the universe as God created it" (p. 253). Both Sussman's (1981) and Eriksen's (1998) anthropological study findings described the elements contained in the worldview of the Mauritian people, but also explored how they see themselves in relation to the world around them. Elements of unity and compromise and the belief that what happens to the individual is the direct result of God's will were identified as key beliefs and values underlying the worldview of the Mauritian people.

The discovery of the informant's worldview or outlook on life was important to understanding the embedded and covert cultural values, meanings, and patterns of care for Mauritian immigrants. These discoveries were aided by the use of the ethnonursing qualitative research method and enablers. Like many other cultures, the Mauritian immigrants residing in NSW are not a homogenous group; nevertheless, more commonalities than differences were discovered among the informants. However, some differences existed among informants and informant experiences with professional maternity care practises.

Based on a review of the literature and this study's findings, the Mauritian immigrants' worldview or outlook on life can best be described as being comprised of several dominant characteristics common to all key and general informants. The dominant characteristic of the Mauritian immigrants was that they were a family-oriented people who valued reciprocity and collaborative, mutually supportive relationships. Through prayer, the informants maintained openness to God's will, which in turn influenced their decision making and acceptance of consequences beyond their control. Education and lifelong learning were highly valued as was taking responsibility for one's own learning and self-care. The informants believed in living an active, balanced lifestyle, and together they enjoyed the present and anticipated life experiences and aspirations associated with being pregnant, giving birth, parenting, and grandparenting. These worldview discoveries were congruent with findings from previous studies conducted by Sussman (1981) and Ericksen (1988, 1997, 1998).

The following descriptors explain and support the informants' worldview or outlook on life with regard to the significant life event of childbearing. The openness to God's will through prayer was a recurrent pattern found embedded within all five themes and the supporting culture care patterns of the study. A summation of those beliefs and patterns was reflected in the following comments made by one key informant:

> I believe there is a balance. God does not cause bad things to happen. I have a say in which direction my life goes. We need to work with things that happen to us, as with many things we do not have control over. However, like my choice to have a Caesar [caesarean section] rather than a normal delivery, that was my decision and if something went wrong that is the chance I was willing to take. I wanted some control in the birth outcome; that is why I chose to go that way. God is still with me when I make those choices, whether they turn out for the good, or the bad, but I had some say in the decision.

All key and general informants placed great value on the acquisition of knowledge and skills, with learning viewed as a lifelong process, a value discovered to be innately driven by a strong sense of responsibility toward self and self-care. The informants believed neither professional nor folk (generic) knowledge possessed all the answers and were proud to be participating in this study and contributing in some small way to further the development of professional knowledge and maternity care practice. A summation of these discoveries is reflected in the following informant comments. One mother said:

> I believe people are to a large extent masters of their own fate and need to take a larger portion of responsibility for their own health outcomes. The system is only in a small way responsible for positive health outcomes.

Another stated:

> The combination of the long visits and traveling over several months [visiting her sick baby] started to take its toll. I could feel I was starting to get run down with a loss of sleep and was not eating well. I was having too many take-away foods. I had to take charge of that, so I made sure I had an afternoon nap and started eating more nutritious meals that I was eating previously when I was pregnant. I also really wanted to maintain the breastfeeding, so I had to do something before my supply reduced too much. I started eating again more rice and lentils and the Mauritian diet I was use[d] to eat[ing] that also included lots of green vegetables. . . I felt much better if I did that. I could also emotionally cope much more with all the stress and constant changes in our baby's condition. When I had that afternoon nap my breastmilk supply also increased.

Religions and Philosophies (*Religions et Philosophies*)

Since Mauritian independence in 1968, religion has not been politicised and the approach to religious diversity has reflected the symbolic focus and values underlying Mauritian nationalism: *Unity in diversity*. Issues pertaining to the various religious belief systems remain in the private domain and are not a topic for interethnic or public discourse. This approach to religious diversity among Mauritians has allowed for the ". . . shared cultural notion of difference" to be reproduced and contributes to the achievement and maintenance of compromise and peace among the people of Mauritius (Eriksen, 1998, p. 90).

The population census of Mauritius in 1990 and 2000 reported approximately 90 different religions in a population of just over 1 million (GMCSO, 2001a). The numerous Hindu temples, Islamic mosques, Buddhist pagodas, and Catholic and other Christian churches scattered throughout the island were evidence of the diverse religions and belief systems that could be found on Mauritius. Mauritians in general related pragmatically to their own and others' religious beliefs and practises. The diverse religious groups and their places of worship harmoniously coexisted. The Mauritian people were described as a nation that respected one another's differences and honoured celebrations associated with the various religions, whether performed in private or religious settings (Eriksen, 1988, 1998; GMCSO, 2001a, 2001b; Mountain & Proust, 1995; Singh et al., 1999; Willcox, 1999). The influence of the Catholic Church is reflected in the 1996 Australian Bureau of Statistics (1997) census figures which show that 82.8% of Mauritian immigrants living in NSW were affiliated with the Catholic Church (see the appendix at the end of this chapter). For the remainder of the Mauritian immigrant population, affiliations with other religions were reported to include other Christian denominations, Hinduism, Islam, Buddhism, and other non-Christian religions as well as some without any known or clearly stated religious affiliation.

Political and Legal Systems (*Systèmes Politiques et Légaux*)

The Republic of Mauritius is a sovereign democratic nation state within the British Commonwealth and has been described as one of the few stable democracies in the postcolonial world today. Mauritius has a long tradition of a stable multiparty parliamentary democracy that has experienced several peaceful changes of government since its independence in 1968. The symbolic slogan *Unity in Diversity* adopted by the government of Mauritius is representative of the principles underlying the political system on the island (Republic of Mauritius, 2003; Sussman, 1981).

Economy and Natural Resources (*Économie et Ressources Naturelles*)

Mauritius was colonised by the Dutch (1598), French (1710), and British (1810–1968), with each colonial power capitalising on and being in part responsible for the extermination of some of the island's best natural resources. These natural resources have included the island's geographic and strategic location as a maritime base; its pleasant climate and fertile volcanic soil; the readily available sources of food and seafood; and the now-extinct dodo (a flightless, goose-like bird). During their occupation, the Dutch introduced sugar cane, tea, and Javanese deer farming practises to the island. Despite the country's diminished economic assets, Mauritius remained relatively unscathed by World Wars I and II. Damage to the economy during this period was the result of natural disasters such as cyclones and malaria epidemics rather than the worldwide slump in the monetary value of sugar (Eriksen, 1988, 1998; GMCSO, 2001b).

The Mauritian economy has evolved and diversified from being dependent on the sugar cane industry in the 1970s toward becoming a modern economy based on manufacturing (textiles and knitted garments), sugar, tourism, tea, fishing, salt, and coral quarries. Evidence of the growth in the economy is demonstrated by the very high levels of private home ownership which increased from 98.6% in 1990 to 99.1% by 2000 (GMCSO, 2001b). The lack of employment mobility and career opportunities on the island contributed to the large numbers of Créoles who emigrated to other Commonwealth nation-states.

Education and Employment (*Éducation et Emploi*)

Since 1976, primary and secondary education on the island of Mauritius has been offered free to all residents, resulting in a high literacy rate. Despite this, the Mauritian 2000 census indicated only a small proportion (4.4:100) of males and females continued their education with either postsecondary, technical, and/or university-level courses. These figures are not congruent with the Australian 1997 census figures which indicated that approximately 50% of Mauritian immigrants living in NSW had attained a postschool qualification. Bunwaree (2001) stated that the education system and official policy of *equality of opportunity* in Mauritius was not a working reality, as the policies masked the powerful factors of "... class, gender, and ethnic inequality" (p. 257).

Health and Generic (Folk) Care (*Santé et Soins Génériques/Traditionnels*)

A review of the literature revealed that throughout history, Mauritian people have utilised a wide variety of professional medical practises, folk care treatments, and healing resources as they were introduced by each new government or wave of immigrants. The people accessed diverse healing resources in order to maintain and preserve health (*santé*) and wellbeing (*bien être*) and to assist with the healing processes in response to illness (*maladie*) and disease (Kalla, 1995; Ministry of Health, 1990; Republic of Mauritius, 2003).

Medical anthropologist Sussman (1981) investigated the relationship between diverse medical traditions and health-seeking behaviours among the diverse ethnic groups of Mauritius. Her findings revealed that a plural medical belief system provided a "... unitary conceptual system that promoted the maintenance of several ideologically diverse therapeutic traditions" (p. 247). These diverse therapeutic traditions were found to include a wide variety of both secular and religious healers reflecting the polyethnic, religious, and cultural diversity that existed on the island. The types of healing resources available included biomedicine healthcare services (government medical services, sugar estate dispensaries, private physicians and clinics, nurses, and pharmacists); homeopathic, Chinese, and Ayurvedic medicine; professional and folk herbalists; specialised secular healers; a sorcerer; and religious temples, shrines, and specialists (Hindu maraz; Sai Baba Temple Tamil poussari; Muslim *miadee*, Buddhist sisters; Christian priests, ministers, charismatic groups, healing churches, and a healing shrine dedicated to the missionary Saint Père Laval) (pp. 248–252).

Sussman's (1981) findings indicated that when sick, Mauritians initially obtained advice from family and friends. Once the illness was identified and the healing resource decided upon, in the majority of cases the individual sought treatment from practitioners who treated "illnesses of God," with biomedical treatment usually being the first choice. Other factors found to influence choice of treatment included pragmatic reasoning, such as the economic resources available to the person; the convenience of the geographic location; religious preferences; past knowledge of the therapists' services; and the practitioner's ability to treat particular symptoms and illnesses. Mauritians were found to place greater "... emphasis upon treatment results and techniques than upon understanding the cause of the illness and the ideological foundations of the therapeutic techniques themselves" (Sussman, 1981, pp. 255–256). Following the initial phase of treatment, if cure or a reduction of symptoms was not obtained, Mauritians continued (in *most* instances) to seek a cure from another therapeutic source or (in *some* instances) accepted their illness as chronic and incurable, believing that God may have willed it (pp. 255–256). Medical pluralism continues to be accepted by the majority of polyethnic, multicultural, and socially heterogeneous Mauritians (Sussman, 1981).

Healthcare and Technology Services (*Soins De Santé et Services De Technologie*)

By the year 2000, Mauritius had a total of eight government-run regional (principal) and district hospitals, one psychiatric hospital, and six specialty clinics (ear, nose, and throat; ophthalmology; respiratory; cardiac; and dermatology). The available hospital and clinic beds were reported to total 3,819 (excluding private clinics, cots for newborns, and outpatient beds). Of these hospital beds, 388 were allocated to obstetrics, 199 to gynaecology, and 333 to paediatric services which included incubators and cots for newborns requiring special care. In addition, there were many family planning clinics, community health centres, vaccination centres, area health centres, medi-clinics, family health centres, dental health clinics, private nursing homes, a chest clinic, sugar estate dispensaries, a mobile dispensary, and a social hygiene clinic. These do not include a number of private healthcare facilities also located on the island (Republic of Mauritius, 2003).

A variety of medical and paramedical staff were employed by both the Ministry of Health and private practise clinics. The 2000 census data on selected workforce statistics revealed 2,748 qualified nurses and midwives; 569 student nurses; 663 registered doctors (417 in private practise); 146 dentists (99 in private practise); and 295 pharmacists (all but 17 in private practise). In addition to these professional health workers, the Ministry of Health employs smaller numbers of physiotherapists; occupational therapists; speech therapists; medical laboratory technicians; radiographers; inspectors; social workers; dispensers; and engineers, in addition to larger numbers of assistants and students for each specialty profession (Republic of Mauritius, 2003).

Mauritian childbearing women were found to utilise technology and healthcare services for both themselves and their babies as made available by the Ministry of Health. One indicator of this was the high levels of usage and adherence in regard to the expanded immunisation program introduced in the mid-1990s. By the year 2000, 12,913 pregnant women had attended vaccination clinics for their first dose of tetanus toxoid immunisation.

There was also a major shift from domiciliary confinements with a midwife toward hospitalised childbirths, with 18.5% home births in 1991 but reduced to zero by 1998; during that period, medical maternity care interventions also increased (Republic of Mauritius, 2003).

Overseas published information on pregnancy care, childbirth, and baby care were widely used by Mauritian women experiencing the life-changing event of childbearing. Popular literary resources from the United States include books such as *What to Expect When You're Expecting* (Murkoff, Eisenberg, & Hathaway, 2002) and *Dr. Spock's Baby and Childcare* (Spock & Parker, 1998); the French book *J'attends un Enfant* (Pernoud, 2003); and the British book *Conception, Pregnancy, and Birth* (Stoppard, 2002) were purchased and recommended by women and maternity care health professionals throughout the island. British, French, and South African pregnancy and baby care magazines such as *Neuf Mois*, *Parents*, *Pregnancy & Birth*, and *Living and Loving* were also readily available.

Information brochures and posters depicting images of healthcare advice during the childbearing period have been jointly published by the Ministry of Health and Quality of Life (*Ministère de la Santé et Qualité de la Vie*) together with the United Nations International Children's Emergency Fund (UNICEF) for display at hospital clinics, health centres, and family planning centres. The information contained in the posters and brochures convey childbearing healthcare messages in French. The general message conveyed in the posters and brochures encourages all expectant mothers to be well prepared and to seek medical care from the beginning of their pregnancy to ensure the best possible birth outcomes for both mother and baby (*une grossesse bien prepare, plus de chances d'avoir un bébé en bonne santé*). Other messages in these childbearing healthcare posters included the importance of attending a healthcare clinic on a regular basis; the need for regular balanced and nutritional meals; the importance of breastfeeding; the need to monitor safe levels of weight gain; rest; avoiding harmful substances such as medications, alcohol, and cigarettes; the need for family members to assist with work in the home; vaccinations; family planning; and the importance for the mother to prepare for labour, delivery, and baby.

Maternal and Child Health 1990–2000 (*Santé Maternelle et Infantile 1990–2000*)

During the year 2000, 19,398 live births and 263 stillbirths were registered in Mauritius. Of this number, 16,962 (86.3%) delivered in hospitals, with 11,484 (67%) delivered by a nurse–midwife and/or midwife and 5,478 (32%) delivered by doctors (Republic of Mauritius, 2003). The remaining 2,436 births were attended by nurse–midwives, midwives, and doctors working at private clinics. Domiciliary visits are also undertaken by the nurse–midwife and/or midwife when providing antenatal and postnatal care, with only a small number of home births during the years between 1990 and 1998. Since 1999, midwives or nurse–midwives in Mauritius have attended no home births. The largest number of live births were to women between 20 and 29 years and a smaller but significant number to women aged 30 to 34 years (Republic of Mauritius, 2003).

During the year 2000, antenatal examinations carried out at clinics by a nurse–midwife and/or midwife numbered 15,963 for first attendances and 61,174 for subsequent visits, with an additional 17, 226 antenatal and postnatal domiciliary visits undertaken by a nurse–midwife during that same period. By comparison, Mauritian doctors during the same period provided antenatal examinations for 14,615 first attendances and 38,442 subsequent visits. No domiciliary care was reported as being provided by the Mauritian doctors, although additional postnatal examinations were performed by doctors at the clinics (Republic of Mauritius, 2003).

The infant mortality rate is an accurate indicator of the health (*santé*) profile of a specific cultural group and/or a nation's people. During the period 1945–1968, the infant mortality rate in Mauritius averaged 58 infant deaths per 1,000 live births; the highest level—81.3 infants per 1,000 live births—was recorded during the period 1951–1955. By 1981, the infant mortality rate had dropped to 27.4 infant deaths per 1,000 live births, attributed in part to the eradication of malaria on Mauritius and the implementation of an immunisation program during that same period (Choolun, 1985). Between 1990 and 2000, the infant mortality rate was reduced from 19.9 deaths per 1,000 births to 15.8 deaths per 1,000 births; and the perinatal mortality rate was reduced by approximately 7% per 1,000 births during this same period due in part to expansion of the existing immunisation program (Republic of Mauritius, 2003).

Neither male nor female circumcision (*circoncire et exciser*) is routinely practised on the island of Mauritius, except when medically indicated. No statistical figures could be located regarding the exact number of circumcisions undertaken on the island. Since 1957, both government (*Mauritius Family Planning Association*) and private (*Action Familiale*) family planning services have been active on the island of Mauritius and continue to be widely used (Jones, 1989; Ministry of Health & Quality of Health, 2001). Family planning methods such as oral contraceptives, barrier or intrauterine devices, hormonal injections, and the sympto-thermal method (temperature rhythm method) are available and commonly used by men and women during their childbearing years (Republic of Mauritius, 2003).

Nurse and Midwifery Education Programs (*Programmes d'Éducation des Infirmières et des Sages-femmes*)

Generalist nurse and midwifery education programs prior to and since independence had been offered at Mauritian government teaching hospitals and clinics but no nursing programs were available through the University of Mauritius. Educational preparation of nurses and midwives in Mauritius was undertaken at the School of Nursing Victoria Hospital in Candos, a major teaching hospital on the island. The School of Nursing at Victoria Hospital had more than 500 student nurses and midwives enrolled in its programs, with maternal and child care as integral components of the curricular and clinical student experiences (Republic of Mauritius, 2003).

There were two educational pathways to become a registered midwife in Mauritius. Midwifery programs could be undertaken either as a 3-year direct-entry undergraduate program or as a 1-year post-graduate program after completion of a 3-year general nursing course with at least 1 year of postgraduation clinical work-based experience. Satisfactory completion of either program-track met the Mauritian government standard requirements for registration as a midwife or nurse–midwife. Both the direct-entry and nurse-to-midwifery undergraduate programs were 3 years in duration, with the curriculum for both closely based on the U.K. hospital system. A small number of practising midwives had obtained their midwifery certification overseas in places such as the United Kingdom, South Africa, and France. All registered midwives and nurse–midwives in Mauritius were female, reflecting the Mauritian cultural belief that labour and childbirth are women's business except for treatment interventions by male obstetricians and other physicians. Whilst labour and childbirth were perceived as a female domain in Mauritius, Hurloll pointed out that these views are gradually changing; many of the private clinics involve the husband in the antenatal, labour, and delivery phases of childbirth (Mr. Khee Alee Hurloll, Senior Nurse Educator, Mauritius, personal communication, April 24, 2003). The choice to include the father in the birth experience at the private clinic did result in an out-of-pocket expense that the majority of families could not afford.

Morbidity and Mortality 1945–2000 (*Morbidité et Mortalité 1945–2000*)

The poor socioeconomic and health status of the Mauritian people prior to their 1968 independence was reflected in high morbidity and mortality rates, with diseases such as cholera, malaria, and plague then found to be the major causes of illness and death. However, since independence the adult morbidity and mortality rates have markedly improved, with the major causes of illness and death now showing characteristics similar to those of other developed countries (Kalla, 1995). By 2000, the life expectancy at birth for males had increased from 65.6 years in 1990 to 67.1 years and for females from 73.4 to 74.6 years (Bah, 1994; GMCSO, 2001a; Ministry of Health and Quality of Life, 2001; Republic of Mauritius, 2003).

Customary Food and Infant Feeding Practises (*Nourriture Coutumière et Pratiques d'Alimentation Infantile*)

The customary food practises of the Mauritian people reflected the multi-ethnic influences, tropical climate, and rich volcanic soil of the island. With the exception of recently introduced processed Western foods, Mauritius has become increasingly self-sustaining, with tropical fruits, vegetables, dairy products, oils, grains, pulses [legumes and beans], nuts, spices, herbs, sugar cane, seafood, and meat farmed and readily available throughout the many markets located on the island. A diet of rice, pulses, and vegetables served with either meats or fish and accompanied by salad, spices (curries), chutneys, or other condiments was found to be the overall staple diet of the Mauritian people.

Dietary practises during childbearing have been discussed in several well-known British, French, and U.S. pregnancy care, childbirth, and baby care books readily available and popular on the island of Mauritius; these are discussed further in the healthcare technology section of this chapter. Despite the lack of culture-specific literature promoting breastfeeding, health professionals and lay women have always encouraged breastfeeding during the first year of the baby's life for its nutritional, immunoprotective, and family planning purposes (Republic of Mauritius, 2003).

In 1991, the Mauritius Contraceptive Prevalence Survey (CPS) included a special module on infant feeding patterns in Mauritius. Grummer-Strawn, Kalasopatan, Sungkur, and Friedman (1996) found in their study that the incidence of breastfeeding had fallen from 86% in 1985 to 72% by 1991; however, the duration of breastfeeding remained constant throughout this period at 13.6 months.

Immigration History of Mauritian People in Australia (*Histoire de l'Immigration du Peuple Mauricien en Australie*)

From a historical perspective, shipping and other registry records indicate Mauritians have had links with Australia for several centuries. Beginning with Abel Tasman in 1642, Mauritius was an important Indian Ocean base utilised by the French and British as a stopover prior to exploration of the Australian coast, with trade beginning as early as 1802. It was during this period that Mauritius was captured by the British from the French. Following British colonisation, approximately 60 Mauritian slaves were transported as convicts to New South Wales and Van Dieman's Land (Duyker, 1986, 1988).

At the time of the Australian Federation's formation, there were reported to be 740 Mauritian immigrants in Australia comprised of merchants, mariners, and other free immigrants who had relocated there in search of gold during the 1800s. During the latter part of the 19th century, Mauritian cane farmers and chemists also made significant contributions to the development of Australia's sugar industry. The next major Mauritian wave of free migration to Australia occurred during the period following the 1968 Declaration of Independence of Mauritius from the British. These increased numbers during this period were largely due to fear surrounding the worsening economic situation in Mauritius, desire for further educational and career opportunities, and the final abolition of the White Australia Policy which had dominated immigration selection criteria during the first half of the 20th century (Bottomley & Lepervanche, 1990; Browne, 1991; Duyker, 1986, 1988; Hage & Couch, 1999).

The Australian Bureau of Statistics (ABS, 1997) reported the 1981 Mauritian immigrant population in NSW numbered approximately 3,218 persons. By 1991, the number of persons born in Mauritius and residing in NSW increased to 5,556 persons (ABS, 1997). This growth was largely due to a shift in immigration policy criteria and objectives, with the focus changing from *assimilation* to *multiculturalism* by the 1980s. In 1996, the ABS (1997) Census of Population and Housing recorded 17,064 Mauritian immigrants Australia-wide, with the majority of change occurring in Victoria, New South Wales (5,606), Western Australia, and Queensland, respectively, and only a few residing in South Australia, Tasmania, the Northern Territory, and the Australian Capital Territory. The small number of persons emigrating from Mauritius during this time has been attributed in part to the changed immigration policies and criteria in Australia, which made the immigration process extremely difficult. In comparison, between 1981 and 1991, the Mauritian immigrant population increased by 2,338 persons, but from 1991 to 1996 the recorded increase was only 50 persons.

REVIEW OF LITERATURE

Mauritian Immigrant Studies

A review of the literature revealed no previous transcultural nursing or transcultural midwifery studies involving either the Mauritian people or Mauritian immigrants that could be located in Australia or overseas.

Similarly, no research studies investigating the culture care meanings and patterns of health and wellbeing, as expressed by Mauritian women or Mauritian immigrant childbearing women and their families, were identified. However, other research studies investigating either medical, social, and/or cultural issues relating to the Mauritian people were located and when relevant were used for the ethnohistory section of this chapter.

Culture Care Studies of Childbearing Women

A number of studies investigating other culture-specific care patterns and issues related to the domain of childbearing were examined and found to utilise a variety of research methodologies. Qualitative research methods such as ethnography, ethnonursing, phenomenology, grounded theory, and multimethods were most commonly used to investigate the cultural aspects of childbearing. Examples of *ethnography* studies included early works by Carrington (1978); Clark (1978); Kay (1982a, 1982b); Mead & Newton (1967); and Oakley (1980); and later works by Browner and Sergeant (1990); Callister (1998); Hughes, Deery, and Lovatt (2002); Kendall (1992); Rossiter (1998); and Stainton, Solaiman, and Strahle (2002). *Ethnonursing* studies were completed by Berry (1999); Bohay (1991); Finn (1995); Higgins (2000); Horn (1990); Lamp (2002); Morgan (1996); and Nahas and Amasheh (1999). To a lesser extent, qualitative research methods such as phenomenology (Callister, Semenic, & Foster, 1999; Finn, 1995); grounded theory (Sawyer, 1999); and mixed methods (Kim-Godwin, 2003; Mercer & Stainton, 1984) were also identified as being used to conduct investigations into culture care. Quantitative methods were found to be utilised far less frequently; however, at the time of this study there was an increasing trend toward using multimethods or mixed methodology that included quantitative methods in combination with qualitative approaches, such as work by Homer (2000); Martinez-Schallmoser, Talleen, and MacMulleen (2003); Pincombe (1992); Riordan and Gill-Hopple (2001); and Weber (1996).

Culture Care for Childbearing Women

Previous research studies that investigated culture-specific care practises for childbearing women have been conducted with both Western and non-Western cultural groups. In summary, the dominant cultural care themes identified by previous research studies included traditional folk beliefs; involvement and support by immediate and extended family members (a role often held by females and to a lesser extent by males); respect; presence of significant other; significance and normality of the childbearing experience; breastfeeding and eating well; observing the principles of hot and cold;

avoidance of sexual intercourse during puerperium; a trusting relationship; touch; encouragement; empowerment; first spoken language valued; continuation of gender roles and female support persons; belief that professional, folk, and complementary therapies perceived as beneficial and having their place; co-participatory care as desired; professionals needing to anticipate the needs of mother and baby; spiritual dimensions as important; avoidance of evil spirits; and avoidance of washing hair and full-immersion bathing.

The findings from the review revealed that transcultural care modes of decisions and actions supported the preservation and maintenance of traditional cultural care patterns as important for maintaining the health and wellbeing of the mother and baby during the childbearing period. These findings were consistent with Lauderdale's (2003) comment that "few cultural customs related to pregnancy are dangerous; although they might cause a woman to limit her activity and her exposure to some aspects of life, they are rarely harmful to herself or her fetus" (p. 101). The research studies conceptualised within Leininger's theory substantiated the suitability of the culture care theory, enablers, and ethnonursing method to discover diverse and similar culture care meanings, decisions, and actions as patterns of health and wellbeing for diverse cultural groups experiencing the significant life-changing event of childbearing within a variety of professional maternity clinical and sociocultural contexts.

THEORETICAL FRAMEWORK

This study used the Theory of Culture Care Diversity and Universality as the framework to discover the culture care meanings of health and wellbeing for Mauritian immigrant childbearing families living in New South Wales, Australia (Leininger, 1991). The researcher's formal education in the disciplines of anthropology, sociology, nursing, and midwifery was the basis for choosing the culture care theory (CCT) to guide the study in addition to previous research studies that had used both the theory and the ethnonursing method to explore the relationship between culture care for mothers and babies and their health and wellbeing. Discovered culture care knowledge from the research findings was intended to contribute to the body of transcultural knowledge and culturally congruent nursing practises for specific cultural groups.

Several select ethnonursing enablers were used to guide the research study data collection and analysis process. Leininger's (2002c) Sunrise Enabler was primarily used as a cognitive map to examine the major assumptions (tenets) of the culture care theory in relation to the research study domain of inquiry. The Sunrise Enabler guided the explication and interpretation of emic data related to the diverse cultural and social structural dimensions that were assumed to influence childbearing care behaviours and health outcomes among Mauritian immigrants participating in the study. The enabler was translated from English into French for the benefit of the informants (see the appendix at the end of this chapter).

Other enablers utilised to enhance the discovery and analysis of the emic data included the ethnonursing Observation–Participation–Reflection (OPR) Enabler, Stranger-to-Trusted Friend Enabler, and Leininger's Acculturation Healthcare Assessment Guide for Cultural Patterns Traditional and Nontraditional Lifeways, along with two specific domain of inquiry enablers (DOI) that were primarily developed and used by the researcher to explicate culture care phenomena from a holistic emic perspective (Leininger, 2002c).

RESEARCH QUESTIONS

The following research questions guided this study's interviews with participants:

1. What is the meaning of care for Mauritian immigrant childbearing families living in New South Wales, Australia?
2. How do worldview, cultural and social structure dimensions, environmental context, language, and ethnohistory influence and strengthen the culture care expressions, meanings, and patterns of care for the Mauritian immigrant childbearing woman and her baby during pregnancy, childbirth, and the puerperium?
3. What are the beliefs, values, and culture-specific care patterns Mauritian immigrant childbearing family members express toward self or another during pregnancy, childbirth, and puerperium in order to preserve, maintain, and/or improve the health and wellbeing and to prevent illness for the mother and unborn/newborn baby?

ORIENTATIONAL DEFINITIONS

The following adapted orientational definitions were used as nondefinitive guides to discover, interpret, and evaluate emic data from interviews and observations with Mauritian immigrant key and general informants (Leininger, 1991, 2002c):

- Culture care (*soins de culture*): Refers to those supportive or facilitative care behaviours specific to the Mauritian immigrant (*General Créole Population*) that assist childbearing families to preserve and maintain the health and wellbeing of the mother and her baby during pregnancy, childbirth, and puerperium (adapted from Leininger, 1991, 2002c, p. 83).

- Professional care (*soins professionels*): Refers to the attributes (knowledge, skills, and attitudes) formally taught, learned, and offered by maternity service providers to Mauritian immigrant childbearing families within a clinical and/or familiar environmental context (adapted from Leininger, 1991, p. 48).

- Folk (generic) care (*soins [génériques] traditionnels*): Refers to the traditional and nontraditional knowledge, skills, and attitudes culturally learned and transmitted to the Mauritian immigrant childbearing woman and her baby by other immediate and extended family members or significant others within familiar environmental or maternity service clinical contexts (derived from Leininger, 1991, p. 48; 2002c, p. 61).

- Worldview (*vue de monde*): Refers to the way the Mauritian people tend to view the world and universe and their place in it to form a picture or outlook about their life and the world around them (adapted from Leininger, 1991, 2002c, p. 83).

- Cultural and social structure dimensions (*dimensions de la structure culturelle et sociale*): Refers to the past and present dynamic, holistic, and interrelated influences of religion and spirituality; kinship (gender and ethnicity); political (and legal); economic; educational; technology; philosophy; language; and ethnohistorical factors about the beliefs, values, and patterns of care for the Mauritian immigrant *General Créole Population* within an environmental context (adapted from Leininger, 2002c , p. 48).

- Environmental context (*contexte environnemental*): Refers to the totality of an environment (physical, geographic, and sociocultural) within which the childbearing processes are experienced that give interpretative meanings to guide human expressions and decisions with reference to the promotion of health and wellbeing during the childbearing period (adapted from Leininger, 1991, 2002c).

- Political factors (*facteurs politique*): Refers to the dynamic dimensions of power—social relationships, choice, decision making, economics, and politics—in relation to the personal, professional, and state alliances of an individual (adapted from Leininger, 1991, p. 48).

- Health (*santé*): Refers to a holistic, balanced, dynamic state of physical, mental, social, and spiritual wellbeing that is culturally constituted, defined, valued, and practised by the Mauritian immigrant childbearing woman and her family, and that enables them to function in their daily lives (adapted from Leininger, 2002c, p. 84).

- Transcultural midwifery: Refers to a sub-area of study and practise within the discipline of midwifery that focuses on comparative holistic culture care and healthcare patterns for childbearing women and their babies with the goal of providing culturally congruent, safe, sensitive, and competent maternity care for culturally and linguistically diverse childbearing women and their families (adapted from Leininger, 1991, 2002c, p. 84).

- Culturally competent midwifery care: Refers to the explicit use of culturally-based care and health knowledge that is congruent with the general lifeways and needs of the Mauritian immigrant childbearing woman and her family in order to achieve a beneficial and meaningful state of health and wellbeing, or to cope with illness or death (adapted from Leininger, 1991, 2002c, p. 84).

- Transcultural competence standards for midwives: Refers to a continual and dynamic process whereby a combination of personal and professional attributes—knowledge, skills, beliefs, values, and attitudes—result in the delivery of culturally congruent, safe, and sensitive maternity care (adapted from Leininger, 2002c).

- Ethnicity (*ethnicité*): Refers to relationships between groups whose members consider themselves distinctive in terms of their social identity, sense of belonging, culture, history, symbolism (language), ideologies, political alliances, and myths of common origins (adapted from Eriksen, 1997, pp. 35–36).

- Mauritian immigrant: Refers to a female or male adult person who has immigrated to Australia and identifies their country of birth as Mauritius and perceives their ethnicity as being part of the *General Créole Population* of Mauritius (GMCSO, 2001b).

ASSUMPTIVE PREMISES OF THE RESEARCH

The following assumptive premises underpinning the Theory of Culture Care Diversity and Universality were modified and used as a guide by the researcher to systematically discover culture care meanings of health and wellbeing for Mauritian immigrant childbearing families living in New South Wales, Australia. The assumptive premises included:

- Culturally-based care for Mauritian immigrants is essential for health and wellbeing, growth, and survival, especially during the significant life-changing event of childbearing (adapted from Leininger, 2002c, p. 79).

- Culture care beliefs, values, meanings, and behaviour patterns are influenced by and embedded in the Mauritian immigrant woman's worldview and the cultural and social structural dimensions of kinship (including gender and ethnicity); religion (or spirituality); political (and legal); educational; economic; generic; folk and professional care; technology; language; ethnohistory; and environmental contexts (adapted from Leininger, 2002c, p. 79).

- Culture care diversities (differences) and universalities (commonalities) exist among and between the Mauritian immigrant childbearing woman, her family, and professional (adapted from Leininger, 2002c, p. 79).

METHOD

The ethnonursing method was used to investigate the culture care meanings of health and wellbeing for Mauritian immigrant childbearing families living in New South Wales, Australia (Leininger, 1991, 2002c) and enabled the researcher, through an open inquiry discovery approach, to inductively explore in a naturalistic way the informants' differing and similar cultural beliefs, values, meanings, and patterns of care. The naturalistic settings for observing and interviewing both the key and general informants were contexts familiar to and chosen by them, such as own place of residence or the workplace. One informant chose to meet at the researcher's home as a matter of convenience; another two key informants were interviewed in the researcher's work office. The familiar contexts for the interviews provided the informants with an environment that was conducive to sharing, memory recall, and reflective thought processes of past and current childbearing events.

Data Collection Procedure

The study was conducted between the years 1999 and 2003 in the state of New South Wales, Australia. The major data-gathering activities involved the use of audiotaped, semi-structured, and open-ended interviews based on questions contained in the Childbearing Culture Care Practises of Mauritian Immigrants domain of inquiry guide developed for the study. As the informant interviews and observations unfolded, many answers to the researcher's questions were naturally revealed as the informants told their stories, without direct questioning (Leininger, 2002c, p. 82). The interviews also focused on the informants' time focus, human activity, social relationships, spiritual connectedness, and their perceived relationship with their environment (Hall, 1959; Ibrahim, 1985; Kluckholn & Strodtbeck, 1961; Sue & Sue, 1990).

Human Subject Considerations

This study was undertaken in consultation with informants from the Mauritian immigrant community living in New South Wales, Australia. The consultation process included a preliminary visit with key Mauritian immigrant group members personally known to the researcher with the purpose of seeking permission to undertake the study. The University of Sydney's Human Ethics Committee granted ethics approval to conduct the study in May 1999; thereafter, invitation and consent to participate in the study were gained from the informants. At the time of the first interview, each informant was provided with a detailed information letter about the study and a consent form to read and sign. Both documents were written in French and English for the benefit of the informant. Each informant retained a copy of the signed consent form; the researcher collected a duplicate copy that was retained for contact information and ethical purposes. Key and general informants were assured that participation was without obligation and that they could decline to answer any question or withdraw from the study at any time without prejudice. The informants were further reassured that the data collected from the interviews would be presented in such a way that anonymity and confidentiality would be preserved.

Selection of Informants

For the purpose of the study discussed, only those Mauritian immigrants who were originally from the island of Mauritius that identified as being part of the General Population (Créole) ethnic identity were invited to participate as study informants because this ethnic group comprised the largest number of immigrants to migrate to Australia since 1968 and were the main Mauritian ethnic group personally associated with the researcher in Australia since 1974.

Purposive and Snowball selection methods were used to select and invite prospective 15 key informants and 27 general informants to participate in the study. The informants included both female and male Mauritian immigrants with multilingual knowledge, skills, and commands of the English, French, and Créole languages, which significantly aided their effective communication with the researcher and enabled a better mutual understanding and interpretation of the informants' beliefs, values, and meanings of care about childbearing families. Spradley (1979) stated that language is an important cultural "symbolic expression" and means for humans to construct and understand the world around them. Leininger (2002c) also noted that language needs to be understood in relation to the ". . . cultural and social structural dimensions of kinship [gender and ethnicity] and social factors; cultural values, beliefs and lifeways; educational, political, legal, economic and religious factors; together with the ethnohistorical and environmental context of cultures" (p. 79).

Together, these influences have provided meaning-in-context for language guidelines in culturally congruent communication processes, interpretations, and patterns of care. Accurate identification of care terms along with their semantic and heuristic meanings was aided by consultation with all key and general informants in conjunction with a Mauritian immigrant interpreter and translator accredited by the National Accreditation Authority for Translators and Interpreters (NAATI) for the purposes of comparing and confirming the informants' views with the researcher's personal (etic) interpretations of the emic data. Professional support was provided in the form of an interpreter; however, all informants participating in this study identified themselves as being multilingual with high levels of both written and spoken French, Créole, and English language proficiency. All interviews were conducted in English with only occasional words (idioms and clichés) or phrases translated by the informants for the benefit of the researcher.

Furthermore, the selection criteria required that all informants were either currently pregnant or had been pregnant and given birth in Australia since migration; and/or had given birth in Mauritius; and/or socialised with a Mauritian relative or friend who was either currently pregnant or had been pregnant and given birth in Australia since migration.

DATA ANALYSIS AND EVALUATIVE CRITERIA

The analysis of the data was an ongoing process relying heavily on Leininger's (2002c) *Four Phases Ethnonursing Qualitative Data Analysis Guide*. The guide provided the researcher with a systematic, credible, consistent, and accurate means by which the analysis could be undertaken and universal and diverse themes identified.

Phase I involved collecting, describing, documenting, and coding of raw data from key and general informant interviews (emic data) together with the researcher's reflective observations and viewpoints (etic data). On completion of each interview and observation period, the researcher electronically transcribed the audiotaped recordings and journal field memos.

The completed transcriptions were then transported into The Ethnograph V5.07 (Qualis Research Associates, 1998) qualitative computer analysis software database program. The computer program was found to be congruent with the ethnonursing method and phases of data analysis, as it aided the recording and organisation of voluminous quantities of raw data. Further formatting included the organisation and coding of data with both parent and child codes together with the researcher's (etic) observations and reflections of the event from which cultural inferences were later generated and analysed.

The second phase of analysis involved the identification and categorisation of descriptors and components for similarities and differences as related to the domain of inquiry. In keeping with the phases of analysis guide, additional descriptions of interview settings and contexts and field journal memos were also included. During the third and fourth phases of analysis, the trustworthiness of the data was evaluated further for credibility, confirmability, meaning-in-context, recurrent patterning, saturation (redundancy), and transferability of the study findings.

Credibility refers to the truth-value, trustworthiness, accuracy, dependability, and believability of data findings. In order to improve credibility, several measures were undertaken to ensure a high degree of rigour was achieved and to limit researcher bias. *Confirmability* or verifiability of data findings was achieved by seeking feedback from both key and general informants in relation to the formulation of themes and interpretation of emic data about culture care meanings, expressions, and patterns of care for Mauritian immigrant childbearing women and their families.

The criterion of *recurrent patterning* refers to human events, experiences, or lifeways that reflect a tendency to recur in designated sequences or patterns over time. *Saturation* refers to having taken in all that can be known or understood about the phenomenon under study. *Redundancy* is a term closely related to saturation, with similar, repeated, or duplicated data discovered in relation to the informants' ideas, meanings, descriptions, and other human expressions. Based on these criteria, the number of key and general informants obtained by the researcher was determined by the saturation level and richness of the data generated from the interviews. The researcher sought no further informants once the degree of repetition and confirmation of previously collected data became redundant and no new insights or revelations, meanings, and descriptions were being observed and/or presented at interview.

The final criterion of *transferability* refers to the feasibility of whether the findings will have similar meaning, relevance, or significance in other similar situations or contexts. Transferability of data findings differs from the term *generalisability* often associated with quantitative methodologies in that transferability of findings from one cultural group to other similar cultural groups is only undertaken with full cognisance of contextual factors taken into consideration (Leininger, 2002c, p. 88). Further information on the ethnonursing method and accompanying four phases of ethnonursing data analysis guide can be viewed in earlier chapters in this text.

FINDINGS WITH DISCUSSION

Five dominant themes depicting the universal cultural meanings and patterns of care were discovered: Care as extended family and friendship support (*soins comme soutien de la famille élargie et l'amitié*); self-care as responsibility (*soin de soi comme responsabilité*); care as best professional and/or folk practises (*soins comme les meilleures pratiques professionelles et/ou traditionnelles*); care as enabling and empowerment (*soins comme rendre capable et habile*); and care as maintenance of a hygienic and supportive environment (*soins commele maintien d'un environnement hygiénique et supportif*). Differences were discovered to exist among the informants' culture care patterns and the professional care practises experienced by them.

Each of the five themes identified what *care* means for Mauritian immigrants and how care is expressed through decisions and actions during the various phases of childbearing. Examples of descriptors and other emic raw data and patterns derived from the study interviews and observations are presented to substantiate the dominant universal culture care themes and subsequent transcultural care modes of decisions and actions developed for culture-specific clinical midwifery care.

Universal Theme 1: Care as Extended Family and Friendship Support (*Soutien de la Famille Élargie et par Amitié*)

Extended family and friendship support was discovered and confirmed by all informants as a significant and highly valued expression of culture care. Mauritian immigrants believed in a direct link between the health and wellbeing of the childbearing mother and her baby and the provision of extended family and friendship support during the childbearing period. This support was described by the informants as collaborative and interdependent with the greatest emphasis placed on support during the puerperium and during periods of illness. Immediate and extended family members and friends included, but were not exclusive to, parents, siblings, grandparents, in-laws, cousins, aunts, uncles, and friends. Five recurrent culture care patterns identified by the researcher substantiated this universal theme: *Collaborative and interdependent relationships; offer of support; assistance with domestic duties; presence;* and *advocacy.*

Care Pattern 1a: Collaborative and Interdependent Relationships (Les Relations Collaboratives et Interdependents)

The traditional folk care pattern of family and friendship support throughout the childbearing period has been successfully continued within the Australian context because of the Mauritian immigrant kinship system together with their social and cultural lifeways of collaboration and interdependency. This interconnectedness and comfort of knowing that the significant life event of childbearing was not being experienced alone brought with it a strong sense of health and wellbeing for the Mauritian immigrant mother and her family. As one key informant shared:

> It is different here. I did not know the neighbours that well and you hardly see one another. In Mauritius, you are much closer to the neighbours. They look out for you. If they cook a meal and some is left over, they would bring some of it to you. Everyone keeps much more to himself or herself here in Australia. . . It makes it difficult to cope with everyday activities. It is very different to what it is like in Mauritius. . . . Our neighbours [in Mauritius] were involved in everything, our birthdays and parties everything. . . We had a very good support network. Which here [in Australia] you do not have that. . . That is why here in Australia, the Mauritian people like to maintain a network and so we can support one another in situations like that. Like, for instance, when I had my second child, I started to worry how I was going to manage to take my daughter to school, but I need not have worried because a Mauritian friend of mine rang and said, "I have been thinking about how I can help out with dropping your daughter off at school and this is what we could arrange if it suits you." I did not even have to worry about it and if I had been in her position, I would have done the same.

Additional accounts of collaborative support by extended family, friends, and hired domestic help are exemplified by the following comment from one general informant:

> The help I received from my mother, sisters, husband, and maids did not undermine my role as a mother; it was just the opposite. They supported me in such a way that I had more energy to care for the baby while the others did all the household chores. I coped better mentally and physically because I was able to get enough sleep and rest, as well as nutritious food and did not have to worry about anything else.

These excerpts highlight the value informants placed on collaboration, interdependency, reciprocity, and networking as means of sustaining relationships at a significant time in life when family and friendship support was needed most. This pattern of care supports the theoretical assumptive premise that the cultural and social structural dimension of kinship is needed for preserving and maintaining holistic health and wellbeing.

Care Pattern 1b: Offer of Support (Offre de Soutien)

Anticipating the needs of the childbearing family and offering support rather than waiting for it to be requested was a recurrent cultural care pattern for the Mauritian people participating in this study. Informants expressed the desire for maternity care health professionals such as doctors or midwives and family and friends to anticipate the needs of the childbearing family. Offering their support or services at the time the need arose, rather than waiting for a request by either the mother or another member of the family, was identified as caring. This pattern of culture care is reflected in the following comment:

> There is no way I would have not been there to be with my sister. I did not have to wait until she asked me to help or to visit. I just offered and then get in and help. That is the way we still do things in Mauritius.

In addition, another informant said that:

> With my first baby, my husband took time off while she was very sick in the hospital and for the six weeks after we had brought her back home a few months later. My mother also stayed with us at home during the first week with both my children, and then she and my sisters would visit regularly after that.

The most common types of care offered by family, friends, and hired help included domestic duties such as cooking, cleaning, washing, presence, prayer, and advocacy, and to a lesser extent baby care.

Care Pattern 1c: Assistance with Domestic Duties (Aide pour les Travaux Ménagers)

Support from family and extended members and friends with domestic duties significantly contributed to the health and wellbeing of the mother and unborn/newborn baby. Performing domestic duties was found to be the form of support most often provided during the postpartum period and during periods of illness whilst pregnant. Traditionally, childbearing support in Mauritius included care provided by extended family members, friends, and employed staff such as maids who were hired to undertake domestic duties such as cooking, cleaning, and washing for the mother and, to a lesser extent, care of the newborn baby. During the puerperium period, the hired domestic help contributed toward making life for the new mother and her family easier and more restful. As one general informant commented, "We were treated like princesses following the birth of the baby." Another said, "We did not have to lift a finger; we were treated like a queen." One key informant stated that the cleaning support provided ". . . more time to spend with my baby." Trust was a key factor in determining whether the support was perceived to be positive and to enhance health and wellbeing. As one general informant concurred:

> I had maids help me with the chores around the house just like the other women, but there was something different about the support your mother, sisters, and husband gave you. I trusted them more with the baby and the advice they gave. I know my family had my interest and the baby's interest at heart, more so than the maids would have.

Supportive care in the form of assistance with domestic duties such as cooking, washing, and cleaning continues to be a valued and frequently expressed pattern of support in both Australia and Mauritius. Instead of obtaining hired domestic help, the support role for household maintenance has become more heavily weighted toward the childbearing family's mother, husband, sister, in-laws, and other extended family members and friends. As one key informant stated:

> My husband would come home from work and cook for me, because I could not stand the smell of cooking. It used to make me sick, so I would look after the baby instead. . . My sister-in-law helped me with the first three babies as well. She lived with us at that time. She helped with the cooking, cleaning, and washing and with the other children. When I had the second and third baby, my mother stayed with us.

Care Pattern 1d: Presence (La Présence)

Knowing that at least one family member or friend she trusted was present with the expectant mother during labour, childbirth, and the postpartum period was believed to contribute to the mother's health and wellbeing. The cultural pattern of presence was important to all the informants. One informant stated:

> He was not too keen to go into the theatres for the caesarean section, but I said to him, "You are not going to let me go through this on my own; you have to be there." I needed him to be someone who could act on my behalf and be my voice in relation to choices about me and for

the baby, as I was pretty tired from the long labour and the pethidine [meperidine hydrochloride or Demerol] they had given me previously. I also wanted him to share the special moment with me; he, like me, just did not think it would turn out like this. So, it was really for both those reasons that I wanted him there.

Another said, "My husband really wanted to be there and when he was born, you should have seen the smile on his face."

Care Pattern 1e: Advocacy (L'intercession)

Knowing that at least one trusted family member could speak, pray, and/or act as an advocate on behalf of the mother during labour, childbirth, and the postpartum period was believed to contribute to the health and wellbeing of the childbearing family. One informant stated:

> When you are in such a vulnerable position and if the pressure continued and your husband was not there, you may have given in just to get them off your back. Rather than do something you did not want to do in the first place. . . I must say I admire the support my husband gave when I was having the children. If I was he, I do not know whether I would have been as capable or as good at support as he was. He constantly reassured me, acted and asked on my behalf, and protected me from unnecessary worry or pain when possible. I told him recently how grateful I was to him for that.

Another informant commented:

> They even would not call the doctor until I was ready to have the baby. So, Mum finally said to the nurse, they have to call the doctor to come and see me. Then the nurse called the doctor. . . . Whatever the nurse was telling me, I did not believe her [referring to the nurse–midwife]. I always asked Mum again afterwards.

Informants shared their views on the advocacy role that God and prayers to God played in maintaining the health and wellbeing of the mother and unborn/newborn throughout the childbearing period. Prayers requesting the maintenance and/or restoration of health were offered on behalf of the childbearing family, by the mother herself, and by other immediate and extended family members. One informant commented, "I remember they prayed with me to have peace. It was as if a whole weight had been lifted off my shoulders. I was no longer sad and much more relaxed when feeding." Another stated, ". . . It is important to support the new mother with prayers and by bringing around extra food so she does not have to cook." Yet another mother offered:

> I did pray to God to help make everything alright. I do think God has something to do with what happens to us, but I do not think He does that without us caring for our baby or ourselves. As we cannot do what we want and think, He will fix everything. I have my responsibility in addition to God's help.

Together these patterns of care support and confirm the assumptive theoretical premise that culturally-based care for Mauritian immigrants was essential for health and wellbeing, growth, and survival especially during the significant life-changing event of childbearing. Summarised in the following comment made by one general informant:

> My family have been my greatest support from the time I found out I was pregnant. My husband, Mum, mother-in-law, cousins, and aunties have all been involved during the pregnancy, birth, and with the care of the baby. . . My mother-in-law also comes and helps me with the cooking, washing, and holding the baby if I need to rest. We learn from each other the way. . . I learn what she used to do with her babies and I show her what I have found works. . . Supporting each other like that . . . is a cultural thing. It is something we do in our everyday life.

The discoveries revealed that differences existed between folk and professional maternity care practises. Past maternity care practises in Australia disallowed the presence of a woman's husband, mother, or any other significant other during labour and childbirth; this was perceived by informants as contributing to additional unnecessary stress and emotional upset. One key informant remembered:

> I would have liked him to be there for both of the births. But in those days it was not that common and it was only just starting to happen where they had the husband present at the birth. But we had talked about it and I had always said I wanted him to be there, but it never happened.

Another informant recalled:

> When I gave birth in Australia, my husband was not allowed to be in the room until after the baby was born. . . It was even more difficult [for me] because I knew no one and my husband was not allowed in to be with me. It was just terrible; it made me really scared. I had no one to talk on my behalf if something had gone wrong—thank God, nothing did.

Several informants interpreted this denial as a means by which health professionals could maintain power and avoid professional accountability for their actions. One male informant suggested, ". . .it could be a power thing, as they could avoid being more accountable and responsible if people were not there to witness their behaviour or question them or their care."

Universal Theme 2: Self-Care as Responsibility (*Soin de soi Comme Responsabilité*)

Care means self-care responsibility. Taking responsibility for one's own health and wellbeing was discovered by the researcher and confirmed by all informants as an important value and expression of cultural folk care. The mother was believed to be the person largely responsible for maintaining her own health and the health and wellbeing of her unborn/newborn baby. Eight recurrent culture care patterns identified by the researcher substantiated this theme: *Maintaining a balanced healthy lifestyle; knowledge and skill acquisition; avoidance of harmful substances, experiences, and practises; keeping active, exercising, and working hard; eating nutritional foods; rest and sleep; breastfeeding; and prayer and acceptance of God's will.*

Care Pattern 2a: Maintaining a Balanced Healthy Lifestyle (Maintenir un Mode de Vie Sain et Équilibré)

The self-care culture pattern of maintaining a balanced healthy lifestyle was reflected in the following excerpts made by two key informants. One mother said:

> I perceive we are meant to coexist in harmony with nature and things happen if it is God's will. He is in control. God exists but people are to a certain extent responsible for their own destiny and are responsible for their own health. The system is only in a small way responsible for positive health outcomes.

Another stated:

> I believe health is achieved through maintaining a balanced lifestyle. I drink plenty of water, and taking long walks has also helped. I also eat a lot of fruit and vegetables. When I was pregnant and [later] breastfeeding, I was conscious that I needed to eat more foods that had calcium and iron, such as vegetables and milk. I avoided foods that were too spicy and my Mum said cabbage and red beans. However, I ate plenty of things like lentils. Health is having a holistic approach to my life. . . I do believe you need to nurture each part of self. Wholeness includes my relationship with God, as well as a balanced diet and knowledge.

Both these descriptors highlight the collaborative approach that informants maintained with others and God in order to achieve self-care, rather than as an independent activity.

Care Pattern 2b: Knowledge and Skill Acquisition (L'acquisition de Connaissances et de Compétences)

The recurrent culture care pattern of knowledge and skill acquisition about childbearing and childrearing was highly valued by the Mauritian informants. One key informant expressed, "...My prime reason for wanting to migrate here was to be able to study at university." Another stated, "We both [referring to her husband] think an education is so important, as it can influence your decisions regarding maintaining your health. It does help you make the best decisions I think for the baby and me." Yet another commented:

> Education is of great significance to most Mauritian people and for me also. I am not sure why that is, but it has been that way ever since I can remember. In fact, furthering our educational opportunities is one of the major reasons for migrating to Australia. Knowledge and choice in the decision-making process are of great value to me. The more knowledge I have, I think it improves the outcome of my health.

Educational resources described by the informants included sharing of knowledge and skills between immediate and extended family members and friends; reading books; and asking questions of the midwife, nurse, obstetrician, and/or paediatrician. For a small number of informants, knowledge was acquired through attendance at antenatal classes delivered by maternity care professionals in NSW. Acquiring knowledge and skills was achieved by accessing a diverse number of resources. One key informant said:

> I read the pregnancy care book put out by the government and Sheila Kitzinger's book...I liked her work... and the pregnancy care book that my friends had passed on to me once they found out I was pregnant... My obstetrician gave me information when I went for my visits, and two of my sisters, although younger than me, had already had children and they gave me some information... my learning was basically from books.

The major reasons given for nonattendance at antenatal classes in Australia included being content with being self-educated; tiredness; unsuitable antenatal class time schedules; inadequate number of classes offered throughout the suburban Sydney region; the restrictive rule of attendance only in the latter 10 weeks of pregnancy; the expectant mother's self-confidence with previous childbirth experience; and preexisting folk knowledge and skills. One informant said:

> They [midwives] did provide these [antenatal] classes, but I did not go because I did not have time and I was working. I read a lot of books on

pregnancy and childbirth; they were called *Ma grossesse* and *J'attends un enfant* both by Laurence Pernoud. These books are in French and are available in Mauritius.

These exemplars show how the acculturation process of an individual living in a new country inevitably adopts some of the host culture's lifeways, whilst at the same time retaining some of traditional values and folk care practices.

Care Pattern 2c: *Avoidance of Harmful Substances, Experiences, and Practises (*Éviter les Substances, Expériences, et Pratiques Nuisibles)

Through the acquisition of knowledge and skills informants in this study were aware of the many harmful substances, experiences, and practises that needed to be avoided during the childbearing period in order to preserve and maintain the health and wellbeing of the mother and unborn/newborn baby. All informants described cigarette smoking and taking alcohol and other illicit drugs as harmful substances to both the expectant mother and unborn/newborn baby. None of the female informants stated that they knowingly consumed any harmful substances once they were planning pregnancy, confirmed pregnant, or during pregnancy. Similarly, harmful substances, experiences, and practises were avoided during labour, childbirth, and the puerperium; whilst breastfeeding; or in the presence of the baby and/or expectant mother.

One general informant commented:

> When I was pregnant, I was aware I had to avoid substances that could harm the baby and me. I knew that smoking and alcohol were not good for you, and we ate more green vegetables. I also remember taking folic acid and iron tablets that the clinic gave me when I went to visit the midwife during my pregnancy.

Several informants described the fear, stress, and worry experienced when they were unable to avoid what they believed were harmful substances, experiences, and practises. The following story depicts the culture shock and fear informants experienced when they were unable to avoid what they believed was a harmful substance. One informant shared:

> With the first pregnancy, I had a miscarriage, and then I fell pregnant again after that, but I ended up having a problem with my foot, so I went to the doctor. . . He gave me a very strong medication and he said to me, "Lucky you came to see me, because if you had waited one day later, we may have had to amputate your foot!" He said be very careful and not to fall pregnant whilst on that medication because you could lose your baby. . . . Then during the month I was taking the medication,

I did not have my period and I thought it was because I was taking the medication, that maybe it was changing my cycle a bit. Then I went to get a test, and they said to me "You are pregnant" and I was really frightened, really frightened. Once again I said to the Lord, "If you want me to have this baby and for the baby to be healthy, please help the baby and me." I did not do it on purpose and yet He might say she has to pay the consequences.

Another informant said:

After I had my first baby here in Australia, I was shocked. Because the nurse just took me in the shower with all the tubes from the drip things, and she was helping me to have a shower and I thought I was just going to die after everything I had heard about not washing [by full immersion] for 40 days. I was brought up like that, you know. I did not even have a shower—just a hand wash until after my period—and I thought to myself I should not be doing this and washing my hair just after I have had a baby. But after the shower, I realised I was still alive and nothing happened... I do not know if I told her that, but she said "That is alright, you will be alright, do not worry."

Healthcare policies and practises change over time, as new research evidence becomes available to those practitioners who provide maternity care. The study findings indicated neither male nor female circumcision has ever been culturally or professionally supported or valued as a best practise in Mauritius. The Mauritian people participating in this study believed it is a Western practise that is totally unnecessary, unhealthy, and culturally incongruent with their beliefs, values, and lifeways. A common response to the question "Was your baby circumcised?" was met with a universal reply of "Oh no, no, definitely not" or "... No, he is not circumcised; the men are not circumcised in Mauritius." One key informant talked about the disempowering pressure that maternity care health professionals placed on a mother to enforce their culturally incongruent policies and practises:

No, no. I chose not to. But had my first baby been a boy, it may have been different, because there was a lot of pressure at that time to do it to boys. They may have pushed me into doing it, because it seemed to me to be the done thing at that time. By the time my boy was born, things had changed and there were very few who promoted it... for us Mauritians, the dads are not done anyway.

These discoveries revealed the power and influence that maternity care health professionals can have over the mother's existing belief systems and the cultural imposition a professional maternity care provider can cause through his or her own ignorance, bias, blindness, or inappropriate abuse of authoritative power.

In contrast, some informants expressed a high level of trust in professional maternity care providers' opinions, knowledge, and expertise as expressed by one general informant who commented, ". . . they must know what is best for the mother and baby, as that is their area of expertise." However, one young general informant questioned the high levels of trust and compliance by informants with professional maternity care treatments, stating, ". . .I was surprised at the high level of trust placed on the maternity care professionals' judgements and opinions by my cousin who has recently given birth."

Care Pattern 2d: Keeping Active, Exercising, and Working Hard (Être Actif, Faire de l'Exercice, et Travailler Dur)

The culture care pattern of keeping active, exercising, and working hard was highly valued by all informants. The Mauritian immigrant mothers maintained an active lifestyle during normal pregnancies and rested when experiencing illness, a non-normal pregnancy, or when regaining her strength post birth. The informants believed physical activity maintained health and wellbeing for both the mother and her unborn/newborn baby. One key informant commented, ". . .I had morning sickness, but it was not severe. I was able to work for nearly eight months."

Another said:

> I worked up until the day I had both babies. I also did aqua-aerobics during my pregnancy and lots of walking—nothing too aggressive, though. I probably did more than I did prior to my pregnancy. . . I tended to also cope better and had more energy if I had a power nap in the afternoon, especially when I was pregnant with my second child, as my first was only two at the time and very active. . .

Various culture care pattern responses to experiences of illness or complications during pregnancy, childbirth, and postpartum in relation to activity, exercise, and work were identified in this study. Regarding a diagnosis of postnatal depression, one key informant said, ". . .Exercise works for me when I feel a bit low. Power walking is really helpful." Another stated:

> I felt better until the seventh month when I started to have contractions because I use to travel a long way to work. . . the obstetrician told me to stop, so I had to stop work. Then I had to stay in bed until I had the baby, as it was too early to have a baby. I stayed in bed up until I was eight and half months. My mother came from Mauritius to help me.

*Care Pattern 2e: Eating Nutritional Foods (***Consommer des Aliments Nutritifs***)*

All the informants were extremely knowledgeable about the need for consuming nutritious foods and fluids during the childbearing period. The experience of both illness and wellness and the desire to prevent illness for both the mother and baby were major influences on the eating habits of the childbearing women participating in this study. High-protein pulses such as lentils, green and other vegetables, fish, poultry, fruit, grain (rice and oats), and smaller amounts of dairy products were identified as both traditional and contemporary foods currently consumed by Mauritian immigrant childbearing women living in NSW. As one key informant described:

> I had fish three times a week. I remember my Mum also saying to eat more lentils, greens, rice, and other legumes—things I normally eat anyway. . . also was more conscious of eating foods rich in iron and more fibre.

Mauritian women throughout the childbearing period consumed foods based on their nutritional value as well as personal tolerances, cravings, likes, and dislikes. Two informants shared:

> [First] I remember I could not stand the smell of fried food. . . I would have taken less greasy foods, but otherwise the normal Mauritian foods. Lots of greens, green vegetables, we tend to eat a lot of greens. Rice and lentils. . . Friends would say, "Have a piece of dried toast or apple before you get up in the morning or out of bed." Sometimes they helped and sometimes nothing. . . .

> [Second] I tended to follow what many Mauritian mothers tended to say. Eat a lot of porridge, because we believe oats helps you to get milk. . . I would avoid black lentils like split peas and broad beans that cause more wind. They also talk about chicken soup to help build your strength and increase your milk supply.

Another mother commented:

> I think I still had the chillies the first three months and then I stopped taking the chillies. For the morning sickness, I would mainly have dried foods. . . I found for me each time I had lentils the baby had problems. . . some people said do not eat cabbage or chili; others said eat lots of green vegetables, but I ended up eating what I wanted.

During periods of illness, changes to dietary choices were made. As one mother said, "I had gestational diabetes during all three pregnancies. . . I was diet controlled, but I had to be careful as to what I ate. . . I was not trying to increase my milk supply; I ate it for my strength."

Care Pattern 2f: Rest and Sleep (Repos et Sommeil)

All key and general informants valued the contribution rest and sleep provided in aiding the health and wellbeing of the mother and baby during pregnancy and the puerperium. Immediate and extended family and friendship support sustained the culture care pattern of rest and sleep during the postpartum period and during periods of illness. For example, husbands and other family members encouraged and promoted rest and sleep of the new mother whilst other family members or hired help attended to routine domestic duties. This pattern of care was reflected in a comment made by one general male informant whilst observed speaking with his wife several days post delivery: ". . .it does not matter if she [newborn baby] doesn't have a bath every day. . . you are still breathless from the haemorrhage, so take it easy and we can bathe her tomorrow." Another informant commented, ". . .I tended to also cope better and had more energy if I had a power nap in the afternoon, especially when I was pregnant with my second child."

Care Pattern 2g: Breastfeeding (Allaitement au Sein)

All the informants valued and believed breastfeeding was in the best interest of the health and wellbeing for both the mother and the newborn, whether or not they actually commenced breastfeeding; started and discontinued breastfeeding because of problems associated with feeding; and/or continued to breastfeed following discharge from hospital. One informant stated, "I breastfed all my children for more than one year, as it was the best nutrition you could give to your baby and you were able to bond to your baby more easily because of closeness as well." Another said, ". . .For nearly one year, I ended up feeding her. She was healthier for it." Many participants in this study breastfed their babies for extended periods. One key informant commented:

> I breastfed all my children. I fed my first child until she was four years old, the next child till she was three, my boy until he was two, and this baby who is now two. Sometimes I give it to her just to keep her quiet. But other people cannot handle it all the time, but I don't care. Sometimes she wants a drink, other times she just mucks around.

Informants were not only aware of the nutritional value of breastmilk for the newborn baby, but also the passive immunity properties of breastmilk. One key informant shared:

> I do believe I played a significant role in the maintenance of my health during pregnancy and the health of my baby. That is why I felt so strongly about expressing my breastmilk for all those weeks when my baby was unable to suck, so my baby would have the best there was to offer and would recover quicker. . . I also wanted to feel like I was more actively involved. The expressing of breastmilk helped in that respect, as I knew it helped with her immunity to fight the infection she had.

In addition, another said of her child, "Initially he was okay, then on day three he developed jaundice [*jaunisse*] and they put him under phototherapy lights. I was able to continue to breastfeed him, though." One of the mothers who had experienced breastfeeding difficulties commented:

> I breastfed all three babies, but they were all painful. So, I did not feed them for long at all. Two to three weeks, I was in pain all the time. And when the baby started to cry for her feed, I would cry in anticipation of the pain. It was not an enjoyable experience. So, I changed to the bottle. . . My Mum did try to tell me all that it will get better and that it was the best food for the baby, but I could not cope with all the pain.

The contraceptive benefits of fully breastfeeding a newborn baby for the first six months of life were widely known by all key and general informants. One key informant explained, ". . .I don't use contraceptives, but I breastfed for very long periods; I breastfed all of my children for two to three years." The acquired knowledge regarding the benefits of breastfeeding was found to be derived from resources such as their female family members (mother, sister, sister-in-law, and mother-in-law) and friends, in addition to pregnancy and baby care books and, to a lesser extent, advice received from their midwife, nurse, and/or obstetrician. The childbearing women were aware of which foods improved their lactation production and which foods were best avoided, passing on this traditional folk knowledge to other female friends and relatives.

Unlike breastfeeding, the informants viewed the topic of contraception and fertility as private and more commonly discussed between the husband and wife. The informants shared with the researcher how the couple during the postnatal period sought out additional information about family planning and fertility issues from pregnancy and baby care books, their doctor, pharmacist, and/or midwife. However, in the majority of circumstances, this was done on a one-to-one basis and not as a group activity. In addition to breastfeeding, Mauritian immigrant couples practised other natural family planning methods, such as the temperature and mucous method and barrier methods (condoms, spermicidal creams, and sponges) as preferred choices and natural means of avoiding and spacing pregnancy. Two key informants stated that they were hoping their husbands would have a vasectomy in the near future; one other key informant and one general informant stated they had been taking the contraceptive pill to avoid pregnancy. Another informant shared that she had used injectable hormones as a long-term method to prevent pregnancy, whilst two other informants stated that they had each used the surgical procedure of therapeutic abortion on one occasion each.

Care Pattern 2h: Prayer and Acceptance of God's Will (La Prière et l'Acceptation de la Volonté de Dieu)

The informants' religious and spiritual beliefs, values, and patterns of care were embedded within the five dominant culture care themes. The mother and the immediate and extended family members used the culture care pattern of prayer together with other culture care patterns to achieve health and wellbeing outcomes or to accept God's will in the case of illness and death. All informants shared their views on how God and prayers contributed to the health and wellbeing of the mother and unborn/newborn baby. One informant commented:

> I think God played a big part in it. I think that because you have a relationship with God, it helps you worry less about the future, whether the baby is going to be born okay and healthy. These are the things that cross the mother's mind now and then. Even with the girls and my boy, every one of them you were hoping and praying that they would be okay. You can trust in God, although what happens, happens; but if you know he is in control, you can trust Him that everything will be okay and if something does go wrong, He will be there to comfort you.

The theme of self-care responsibility was substantiated by the recurrent culture care patterns of maintenance of a balanced healthy lifestyle; knowledge and skill acquisition; avoidance of harmful substances, experiences, and practises; keeping active; exercising and working hard; eating nutritional foods; rest and sleep; breastfeeding; prayer; and acceptance of God's will.

Universal Theme 3: Care as Best Professional and/or Folk Practises (*Soins Comme les Meilleures Pratiques Professionelles et/ou Traditionnelles*)

All key and general informants valued best professional and folk practises and believed both forms of care contributed toward the health and wellbeing of the mother and unborn/newborn baby. The four culture care patterns for best professional and folk practises included *respect for diverse knowledge and skill expertise*; *utilising best professional maternity practises*; *utilising best technology*; and *utilising best folk (traditional and nontraditional) practises*. The following care pattern descriptors substantiated this universal theme.

Care Pattern 3a: Respect for Diverse Knowledge and Skill Expertise (Respect Pour les Diverses Connaissances et Expertises de Compétences)

All key and general informants believed that no one maternity care provider had the ability or resources to meet all the needs of the childbearing family, and in particular those of the mother and unborn/newborn baby. The informants valued a collaborative approach by professional maternity care providers and wanted them to work in partnership with mothers and their family and to not disregard the benefits of folk care practises. One woman stated:

> I was raised a Catholic, so we did call a priest in to anoint her. All our families were in the adjoining room attached to the neonatal intensive care unit at the . . . hospital praying with their rosary beads for her recovery. It was at that point we knew she was gravely ill. As much as I do believe God plays a part in allowing life to continue, I also believe it was the expertise of the doctors and nurses and the technology that saved her life. . . . We tried everything in the hope that something would work. . . . My husband and I . . . purchased three healing crystals each. They were supposedly capable of projecting different strengths. We clung to those crystals the whole time she was in hospital. . . Both my husband and I were willing to try anything that would help.

Another said:

> I believe both medical technologies and traditional or folk treatments to be advantageous during pregnancy, childbirth, and following delivery. They need to be relied on equally, as both forms of treatment and as a preventative measure. I think it is [to] important not to quickly push aside alternative traditional forms of treatment, such as heat packs or thyme infusions, for example, [which] were of great assistance when I was in pain.

A variety of professional and folk care was sought when a family needed maternity healthcare services; however, doctors (general practitioners and obstetricians), followed by midwives, were usually the initial person consulted for diagnosis of pregnancy and non-normal illness experienced by either the mother or her unborn/newborn baby. One informant stated, "I saw a midwife with all of my children and it was fine. All of the midwives were female who cared for me." Other diverse professional and folk care opinions and treatments were sought and utilised by informants for what they described as normal physiological or psychological changes. Another informant stated:

> The doctor delivered my first baby, because I was in labour for a long time; but with the next two, they came so quickly that the midwives delivered them. . . I found the midwives very competent and they did their job in some ways better than the doctors did, and you know the aftercare in the hospital was also very good. . . I think it was in their approach—they appeared to know what they were doing, they were knowledgeable, and they shared information with me.

The economic status of the childbearing family was believed to not directly influence the type of care provided for either the mother or her unborn/newborn baby within the Australian maternity clinical healthcare context. Informants remarked that there were minimal differences between the public and private maternity care services offered to childbearing families. One informant noted, ". . .being a private patient just meant more bills, not necessarily better care in my situation." Another informant said:

> I was really surprised because I had been told public hospitals were not the best and I have private healthcare cover and people had given me some warning that they are not very caring and do not give you much attention. . . I was very happy with the care that I had received. . . I found that they were there all the time, explaining what the procedures were, and they sat down with my husband and I and explained everything to us both . . . I kept telling everyone I was very pleased.

Care Pattern 3b: Utilising Best Professional Maternity Practises (Emploi des Meilleures Pratiques Professionnelles)

All informants willingly utilised best professional maternity care practises and viewed diagnostic technology as important. As one general informant commented, "I think all people in all cultures want the best care available; this is not unique to Mauritians. I want to know what is happening to my baby and me so I can make the best decision possible." Another key informant stated:

> Sometimes you do not have any choice and you do what the doctors recommend. I trust them to offer the best treatment possible, as I am not a nurse or a doctor. What I know is from books and what my Mum and friends have told me.

Best practise included the continuation of congruent care within diverse clinical and community contexts. As one key informant stated:

> They gave him my breastmilk in a tube until he was able to start sucking by himself. . . I actually went home soon after that and used to come in to visit him while he was recovering and I would bring in my expressed milk. I ended up breastfeeding him for about eight months.

Further recurrent patterns found to support the theme of best professional practise included *genuine care by doctors, midwives, and nurses; anticipation of the needs of the mother;* and *acknowledgement of the diverse range of normality among childbearing women and their babies.* The following descriptors depicted these best practise characteristics. One informant stated:

> I would like to see midwives and doctors acknowledge the normality of the fact that not all mothers necessarily instantly have love and/or want to dote on their babies. . . I just needed someone to say it was okay and you just have to give it time. . . I am sure that [their denial] contributed to my emotional response as well.

Another informant said:

> She was small, but my husband always argues about that, saying that they incorrectly compare the petite size of Mauritian babies with larger-boned white Australians. It is wrong because in Mauritius she would have been a normal-size baby. . . Some babies her weight they put in special care, but for her they said she is fine. A woman had had a 10-pound baby and it looked huge next to my little one, like a beached whale, and mine was wiggling and turning.

Best professional practise included the ability of the health professional to anticipate the needs of the mother and offer the best care available, rather than wait for it to be requested by either the mother or another member of the childbearing family. One informant said, "I did want to know what happened to it [placenta] and I wanted to have a look for my own interest, but I did not feel right asking them to see it and they did not offer." Another said, "Each time I went to visit my son, they would bring and take the meals away again untouched. . . The maternity ward was a long way from the children's hospital and I could never get back in time."

Healthcare policies and practises change over time as new research evidence becomes available to practitioners who deliver maternity care. However, not all changes are perceived by consumers as being conducive to positive healthcare outcomes. One key informant commented:

> With the boy, on the other hand, he was with me constantly and I had
> to do most of the care. So in the hospital, he was even sleeping in a cot
> next to my bed with me at night so I could not sleep easily. . . I know
> what they are trying to do to get the mother to spend more time with
> the baby to bond, but at the same time it does not give you a break and
> able to rest more to recover more quickly.

These descriptors demonstrate how a lack of culture care knowledge can result
in cultural conflict, cultural imposition, cultural stress, and cultural pain.

Care Pattern 3c: Utilising Best Technology (Emploi de la Meilleure Technologie)

It was important to all informants that they could access the best technologies available to the childbearing mother and her baby. The technology utilised by informants included blood tests; monitoring of a mother's blood pressure, urine, and weight; hospitalisation; and surgical procedures such as caesarean section, dilatation and curettage, tubal ligation, and vasectomy. In addition, diagnostic procedures such as ultrasound, foetal monitoring, and newborn screening tests such as those currently used for testing blood or hearing were identified as acceptable practises to all informants. Additional technologies utilised included intravenous therapy, blood transfusions, and administration of medications such as antibiotics, contraceptives, syntocinon (oxytocin), vitamin K, and immunisations. One informant stated, ". . .the ultrasound proved that the baby was growing normally"; a second said, ". . .at four months it became so severe—the nausea and vomiting—that I was admitted to hospital and given intravenous fluids to correct the imbalance in my blood and system." Another reported:

> There was no question at all that I was going to be giving birth straight
> away, so they put a drip in and gave me some medication to try and
> delay the labour while the baby's lungs matured enough for her to
> breathe. . . they just kept saying your baby is very sick, she is very sick. . .
> I do not blame them for how they went about the whole thing, because
> they were just trying to do their best and they did not really know what
> was going on. All they knew was she was very sick.

Another informant commented:

> I kept bleeding quite heavily with bright blood and then on the ninth
> day I haemorrhaged. I was passing large clots. They had to take me to
> theatre to remove a piece of retained placenta. I was okay after that. I
> came close to having a blood transfusion, but in the end, I did not have
> one and I had had enough of hospitals and just wanted to go home.

Referring to the loss of her baby, one female informant stated:

> We had lost our first baby at four to five months' pregnancy, and he saved my life by taking me to the hospital to get treatment. If it was not for what he did, I would not have been alive today. Thank God, he did not listen to me. My Mum saw the baby in the toilet at home, but not the placenta.

The universal acceptance and usage of technology by both key and general informants was discovered to be not completely without question. The informants were consciously aware of the many risks associated with new and existing technologies and the various maternity-related medical and surgical treatment modalities available. One informant stated, "I wanted to know what was happening and what the effects of treatments had on my baby and me in advance." The same informant went on to say, "I did not want to have the epidural. I did not like the thought of someone sticking a needle in your back. I hate pain, but I hate even more thinking of losing control, like paralysing your legs." Another informant highlighted the ambivalence experienced toward professional treatment modalities by stating, "I was able to breastfeed, but I had to give it away when I took the tablets [antidepressants]. That was really tough because she was breastfeeding really well."

The desire to maintain control over their own body's functions during the phases of labour and childbirth contributed to the ambivalence experienced by informants toward professional treatment modalities. For both older and younger Mauritian immigrants, concern was raised about maternity practises that medicalised the childbearing experience. Eight informants stated that they preferred to reserve professional maternity care treatment modalities such as hospitalisation or other midwifery, nursing, medical, and surgical procedures for only non-normal childbearing and illness episodes. One mother commented, "I don't like it when they cut you." Another said, "When we came here to Australia, we were surprised when my children had to go to hospital to have their babies. We only went to hospital if something was wrong. Not if everything was normal." Another younger informant commented:

> They gave me an enema and shaved me in those days. It was shocking, really shocking. How could they do this to us. . . What happened afterwards was even worse, but at that stage, you were in their care and you had to do what the nurses and doctors wanted you to do. It was shocking. How degrading. I remember I went to the shower because I had been sick; I was vomiting, so when I was in there I was going both ends. It was so horrible and it was just awful.

Despite the expression of ambivalence toward technology and professional treatment modalities, the study informants indicated they universally trusted that health professionals knew what they were doing. The informants trusted the doctors, midwives, and nurses to only provide treatments or undertake diagnostic tests that were in the best interests of both the mother and the baby. This pattern of care is conveyed in the following descriptors which highlighted the high level of trust all informants placed in the professional maternity care staff and their choice of practises. One mother said, "I know there are risks with all of these, like when I had the epidural in my back for the Caesar [caesarean section]. I guess, though, I am prepared to take the risk, trusting that they know what to [do]." Another commented, "During pregnancy, you have to be careful not to take anything that would harm the baby, but I trust that they [doctors, midwives, and nurses] would not intentionally do that [harm]." In contrast, one general informant stated, "I was surprised at the high level of trust placed on the maternity care professionals' judgements and opinions, as I found with my Mauritian cousin who recently gave birth."

Care Pattern 3d: Utilising Best Folk (Traditional and Nontraditional) Practises (Emploi des Meilleures [Traditionelles et Non-traditionelles] Pratiques)

The Mauritian informants' universally valued best folk traditional and nontraditional patterns of care in addition to best professional maternity care services. Choosing the best care available from a variety of folk and professional care practises is common among many cultural groups during a significant life event such as childbearing (Lauderdale, 2003). Traditional and nontraditional best folk practises used by the informants included the use of herbs; massage therapy; rest, activity, and exercise; eating nutritional foods, breastfeeding, and drinking adequate quantities of water; heat foments; natural family planning and contraceptive barrier methods; prayer; and family and friendship support. Both key and general informants commented on the benefits of using folk (generic) treatments in accord with professional maternity care practises. One informant stated:

> It was really beautiful I just stayed in the spa. It really relieved the pain. . . every time I felt uncomfortable I went into the spa, it was really nice. . . I wanted to deliver in the spa, but the doctor said it would be safer because of the cord to deliver on the bed. I really did not want to get out of the comfortable spa. . . But he had been so good to me, I didn't mind compromising; and so, I let the staff and my husband put me on the bed to deliver. When it was at this point, my Mum had to go

because she was very disturbed. She could not cope with watching me in the spa, because in Mauritius when your waters have broken you are not supposed to immerse yourself in hot water until after the uterus has healed and the cervix reclosed to prevent infection. But I would have been happy to deliver in the bath. It was so comfortable it was far better than the pethidine.

Another stated:

When we wanted to have children, I read all about the natural products and herbal treatments; I wanted to have only these kinds of things. I was really healthy. Eating lots of foods like brown rice, lentils, and fruit.

Another key informant raised concerns about the efficacy of narcotic use with regard to pain experienced during labour and delivery:

I remember saying, "You have to get pain when you have a baby." In Mauritius, they do not try to get rid of the pain; they say you have to have it. Not like here in Australia, when they give you something for the pain if you want it. . . I know that in the Bible I have read that God has said that for a woman to get a baby, she must have pain. It is true, isn't it? Every woman who gets a baby has to go through that pain. All the women, everywhere—women got pain. Even if they gave you something for the pain, you still feel the pain. God meant for you to have pain. You cannot take that away. I had an injection for the pain during the birth of my second, but it did not take away all the pain. It was still there.

Universal Theme 4: Care as Enabling and Empowerment (*Soin Comme Rendre Capable et Habile*)

All key and general study informants believed care meant enabling and empowering the childbearing woman. Four major culture care patterns were discovered to support this theme: *Knowledge and skill acquisition*; *open and honest communication*; *involvement in decision-making care processes*; and *choice.* These patterns of care provided the mother with the means, power, and/or ability to maintain her own health and wellbeing and that of her unborn/newborn baby.

Care Pattern 4a: Knowledge and skill acquisition (L'Acquisition de Connaissances et de Compétences)

Knowledge and skill acquisition was highly valued among all informants and believed to enable and empower the childbearing woman. The *approaches* by which the mother acquired knowledge and skills were found to be just as important as the knowledge and skills themselves. Several informants expressed concern about professional care practises that disempowered the mother and the potential impact on the health and wellbeing of the mother and baby. Patterns of care discovered to enhance knowledge and skill acquisition included *patience, reassurance,* and *encouragement by maternity care providers.* One key informant expressed her view:

> There was one midwife in particular, though, that was really helpful. I am not really sure what was so different between her and the others, but I think it had to do with how she kept reassuring me of my own capabilities. She helped me maintain my confidence in my ability . . . and the care I was giving to my baby. I found it comforting. The presence of that kind of supportive person is just so important when you are a new mum or dad. All the questions I asked did not seem to bother her in the slightest. She was happy to give me all the information I wanted. I had read heaps of information throughout my pregnancy, so it was reassuring to be able to discuss it with her.

Shared traditional and nontraditional folk knowledge and skills by family members and friends were found to empower the women with their mother-crafting skills. Knowledge and skills offered in an encouraging manner instilled confidence in the mother's ability to care for her own baby. As one mother stated:

> A cousin of mine kept encouraging me to stick to breastfeeding and do not give up because it is best for you and the baby. It was because of what she said that I persisted and kept on trying. About a fortnight later, she was sucking by herself and I did not [need to] use the shield.

All informants viewed pregnancy as normal, with the experience of *some morning sickness* included in their definition of normality. One informant stated, ". . .all my pregnancies were okay. I just had morning sickness like everybody has." The normalisation of the childbearing experience by maternity care providers, family members, and friends was an enabling and empowering pattern of care, as reflected in the following statement:

> When I experienced the baby blues on my return home from hospital about seven days later, I started to get worried. I started to fret over silly things, like how I was going to care for her in seven years' time when she is going to go to school and I just cried all the time for no reason. I thought about things I have never thought about before. It all came flooding in. It was not until I talked to some other young Mauritian mums who had said it was normal that I suddenly snapped out of it and stopped spiralling down into what appeared to be a big black hole.

Some mothers said they cried when they looked at a bucket of soiled nappies they had to wash. I was not that bad. From the time I realised it was normal to be somewhat sad after you have a baby, I got back on my feet and life went on as normal. I just needed someone to say it was okay to be sad—that was enough for me. It was weird I know, but I just freaked out. . . That was all I needed to get going. I thought I could cope. It gave me the confidence and the hope that I was not having a nervous breakdown.

Care Pattern 4b: Open and Honest Communication (Communication Ouverte et Honnête)

For all informants participating in this study, open and honest communication was a valued and expected pattern of care and was found to enable and empower the childbearing family to cope better with unexpected illness, change, and/or loss experienced by the mother or unborn/newborn baby. One informant stated, "We trusted their judgment and we appreciated their open and honest communication right from the beginning, when they had told us she most likely would not survive." Another informant shared, "No matter how bad the news, we want the doctors and midwives to be open and honest with us. We want to share in the final decision-making. . . [we] needed to know exactly what was happening and be involved."

In contrast, disempowering patterns of professional care included closed communication styles, dishonesty, isolation, control, and lack of collaboration between the mother and maternity care providers. One informant stated, "So many different people attended to me and so there was a lack of consistent care with people that knew me. . . People did not seem to know what was going on they did not communicate with each other." Another informant stated, ". . .the nurse wanted me to lie. I wasn't going to tell the doctor something that was not true." Yet another stated:

> My husband and I were so upset when that professor dropped that bad news on us and then left without discussing the treatment or delivery options further with us. I felt powerless in that situation. It was just terrible. . . I was left alone for very long periods not knowing what was happening. . . They never took the initiative to communicate what was happening with my baby son or me.

Still another shared, "What was even worse, I remember they tied my legs up in the stirrups. I remember that was horrible. I am a very private person and to me it was just exposing myself."

All but two informants believed their command of English did not warrant the services of an official interpreter when seeking explanations for professional maternity care or diagnostic results. One informant commented:

> We learn and speak English in Mauritius. For the first one, though, my sister-in-law came with me to every visit and she interpreted for me if they spoke too fast. By the time I went into labour and visited the clinic during the second pregnancy, my English was good enough to understand what they were saying and the explanations they gave to me. So, I do not mind them speaking English to me.

Conversely, one key informant shared the initial difficulties she and her husband experienced immediately following their arrival in Australia: "If people speak slowly and clearly, I usually understand them. Like you, you are easy to understand. You do not speak too fast like some other Australians."

Recent immigration was not identified as an accurate indicator of English language proficiency and/or the need for interpreter services when receiving professional maternity care advice or treatments. Instead, the determining factors contributing to a Mauritian immigrant's level of understanding and command of the English language were largely influenced by the individual's age at the time of migration, level of education attainment prior to immigration, and number of years spent working in Mauritius prior to arrival in Australia.

Mauritian informants use their right hand to shake another person's hand when meeting or greeting for the first time or in a formal or professional context such as a healthcare setting. However, unlike many other Australians, the Mauritian people greet people known to them with a kiss repeated twice or three times on both cheeks especially among familiar people and within familiar contexts such as at home or social gatherings. They use the family name of a person when being introduced until an invitation to use their first name is given—a social pattern commonly practised by most Australians (Commonwealth of Australia, 2003, p. 20).

Care Pattern 4c: Involvement in Decision-Making Care Processes (Participation à la Prise de Décision des Processus de Soins)

Informants expressed the desire to be collaboratively involved in the clinical decision-making process with professional maternity care providers. One key informant stated:

> I had made this agreement with my doctor very early on in the pregnancy that when the pain arises that I did not want to have to put up with the pain, just like when I go to the dentist I do not want to

have fillings done without pain relief given first. However, I think they [midwives] only gave me Panadol [acetaminophen] or Panadine [acetaminophen with codeine] when I was in labour, because I got the distinct impression that the midwives thought I was putting on an act and that I could not have been in labour, as they thought I was still only three centimetres dilated. And I remember holding the bed handbars and I was using the bars to help breathe and control the pain.

About the pain experienced and practises used to relieve pain during labour and childbirth, one informant commented:

I think for the first time I really wanted to experience what it was like to be in pain and if I am strong enough to go through with the pain and to see how much I can cope. So, they gave me the gas mask when I was finding it hard to cope with the pain. I did not have an epidural or whatever, and after the birth, it felt good to know that I had coped.

Another key informant raised the issue about the timing of discussions:

I was prepared to have some pain from what I had read, but at no time did I think it was bad enough to have morphine. The pethidine was all that I needed and I knew about. I started to feel like this lamb that was going to the slaughterhouse. It was not the right time to offer something new. I could not make a decision. I wanted to work with what I already knew.

Care Pattern 4d: Choice (Choix)

The study findings showed that choice was highly valued and contributed to the enabling and empowerment of the mother. All informants viewed choice as an important value and expression of care. One key informant commented, "I want to have choice and I want to be fully informed of any treatment or care decision that is going on that could impact on my family and me." Another said, "I want to choose what kind of treatment they do to the baby and me, but at the same time I trusted their professional judgment and usually accept what they recommend." An additional informant stated, "I prefer they ask me and explain why it is necessary, but I want to make the final decision." From another perspective one informant shared:

I think differently about it now compared to when I was younger. Now I think I am the one who makes the choices and God is there to give me the strength to get through life and its experiences. I used to think He caused things, but I do not think like that anymore. I am much more at peace with myself since I made that decision to trust He will be there no matter what happens.

For some informants, their strong desire for choice was based on painful past childbearing experiences. One informant stated:

I was traumatised by that experience. When I fell pregnant with my third child, I just cried. I thought that I am going to die; I am not going through that again. It was so painful [referring to the episiotomy]. So, when I saw my doctor for my third child I said to him, "I am not going to have a normal delivery. . . . I want a caesarean section."

From a comparative perspective, some informants viewed lack of choice as a disempowering, noncaring practise and was a major cause of emotional upset among Mauritian immigrant childbearing women. One informant stated, ". . .unless they offer you alternative choices, you really have no choice and have to go along with what they ask or suggest you do." Another said, "I looked at him and said that 'I do not want to take it,' but the doctor there, the [doctor] there, did not offer other options." Another informant recalled:

Everyone says, "Do not do this" and "Do not eat that." Everyone that spoke to you made some comment about what you should and should not do or eat. Eventually I just ate what I wanted. . . I remember the nurse coming into the room and saying, "You are breastfeeding, aren't you?" I said, "Yes." "Well, you cannot eat that," she said. I looked at her and I was going to say, "I do not care," but then she said, "Listen, you eat everything you want. You will soon find out what is suitable for you and what is not." I think that was the best thing she could have told me. You will find out what is right for you because what is upsetting for some people's babies is not upsetting for others.

Childbearing experiences that left the mother feeling disempowered with regard to her personal choices often resulted in the childbearing women finding other ways of achieving their goals. An example of a behavioural response to feeling disempowered is exemplified by the following comment:

I was smarter with the second one because a trusted friend gave me the advice not to go to the hospital too early—that way you will not have the doctors poking you and hurting your abdomen. I waited until the waters had broken and the pains were coming frequently. When I got to the hospital, my baby was born 30 minutes later. The midwife delivered my baby and none of the doctors were there to poke me. I did not have any tear with the second baby. She is the one I breastfed for two years or so.

Universal Theme 5: Care as Maintenance of a Hygienic and Supportive Environment (*Soin Comme le Maintien d'un Environnement Hygiénique et Supportif*)

Care means the provision of a hygienic and supportive environment for the mother and her newborn baby. These findings supported the culture care patterns of *avoidance of harmful environments, privacy,* and *cleanliness,* expressed by all key and general informants as substantiated by the following descriptors.

Care Pattern 5a: Avoidance of Harmful Environments (*Éviter les Environnements Destructifs*)

The provision of a safe and comfortable environment included the monitoring of light, temperature, and noise levels by professional maternity care providers, family members, and friends in hospital and home contexts. A typical definition of a safe environment (*la securité milieu*) for the mother and newborn baby is reflected in the etic description by the researcher of one key informant's home that was visited 2 weeks following the birth of her first child:

> The house was small, quiet, and extremely clean, with everything appearing to have its place. The baby's room was warm and sunny, with a bassinette, cot, and toys all arranged in the room. In the lounge [living] room, there was one specific recliner chair set up with tables surrounding it [to make] access[ing them] easier whilst the mother was feeding. The baby was dressed in contemporary baby clothes suitable for the temperature of the room.

Informant descriptions of what they believed constituted a safe and comfortable environment included the following statements. One informant commented, "...when I come to visit, I am always conscious of the need to be quieter if the baby is sleeping or my sister is resting." Another said, "...a lot of people have offered us second-hand baby things; however, we have turned them down because I think with a first baby it is nice to have new things." Yet another said, "...the baby was always kept safe and under the watchful eye of the maid or my mother if I was sleeping." Still another shared:

> Sometimes the maids would also pull the curtains to dim the light so that I could sleep and rest more comfortably. They helped me with this for many weeks. I literally did nothing but care for the baby. It was wonderful.

Care Pattern 5b: Privacy (**Intimité**)

Privacy was discovered to contribute to the health and wellbeing of the newborn baby as expressed by a significant number of female informants.

Privacy for Mauritian immigrant mothers meant having an environmental space to one's self during the delivery of care, control over noise levels, and a choice of topics acceptable for public discussion. Topics related to illness, family planning, and fertility were discovered to be viewed as private and having the potential to increase levels of stress if discussed in a public space. Informants had a preference for one-on-one teaching activities, as opposed to large group activities with people they did not know or trust. As one informant stated, "After I had breakfast, I asked if I could have a private room because I did not want to be with other ladies and their crying babies." Another commented on the topic of family planning by stating, "...that is such private information, but thinking about it we will probably use condoms considering I had difficulty falling pregnant with this baby. I will make a decision when I go back to visit the doctor." Another said, "All I wanted was a room by myself because seeing all the other bigger, healthier-looking babies made me feel a little depressed."

Care Pattern 5c: Cleanliness (Propreté)

All key and general informants discussed the importance of a clean environment for maintaining the health and wellbeing of the mother and newborn baby and for preventing illness. One informant described that "...traditionally, the maids were responsible for keeping everything clean, such as nappies and clothes, as well as helping the midwife when she delivered the baby and washed me afterwards." In modern Australia, immediate and extended family and friends of the childbearing family continue to play a major role in the maintenance of a clean and safe environment for both the mother and newborn baby during and following the birth of the baby. The type of support offered allowed the mother to have more energy to care for herself and the newborn thereby maintaining her confidence in her own mother-crafting skills. One informant shared, "Since my grandchild has arrived, I have helped my daughter-in-law with all the general household chores. I try to work in with what she wants, as it is her home." Another commented, "They were also pretty clean at the clinic. . . I did not want to get an infection. It was a private clinic, so it had to be clean. There is a certain level of standard you have to keep." From a different perspective, one mother offered a word of advice to maternity care providers:

> The Mauritian people are extremely house proud and therefore it takes much more effort to have a stranger come to your home and offer you support than it does for your own mother and other family members to come and visit and provide or offer their support following the birth of your baby. The midwives and other healthcare workers need to realise that.

The study findings indicated that traditional personal hygiene practises for women post delivery have changed very little over the years because older mothers and women have shared their knowledge and skills with younger Mauritian women who have immigrated to Australia. The cultural practise of passing on knowledge and skills intergenerationally is reflected in the following descriptors. One informant stated:

> After my delivery I had a shower straight away, but my Mum warned me not to wash my hair. . . It is because in Mauritius they say it has something to do with the blood loss and staying warm, not cold. They also say only drink warm or hot water, never cold water, after you have had a baby. You need to do this for at least one week.

Another commented:

> I had a shower, but it was not a full shower, not my head, more just the lower part of my body and I did not stay in bed. I was up walking around the house. With my second baby, however, it was different. I could not walk. It hurt too much. I was in pain. I had pain everywhere; even when I breastfed, I was in pain.

Another key informant's comment demonstrated how acculturation and access to new knowledge can change a person's beliefs and patterns of care.

Summation of Findings

The co-participatory or collaborative expressions of care embedded within the five dominant themes—*care as extended family and friendship; self-care as responsibility; care as best professional and/or folk practises; care as enabling and empowerment;* and *care as maintenance of a hygienic and supportive environment*—together with their supportive culture care patterns highlight the interrelationship of the cultural and social structural dimensions and their powerful influences perceived by the informants as culturally safe, congruent, and sensitive care.

The assumptive theoretical premise of the study—that culture care is essential for the health and wellbeing of the mother and baby, and for foetal development and a healthy birth—supported the literature review findings by Berry (1999); Bohay (1991); Callister (1998); Callister, Semenic, and Foster (1999); Finn (1995); Higgins (2000); Horn (1990); Kendall (1992); Kim-Godwin (2003); Lamp (2002); Morgan (1996); Nahas and Amasheh (1999); Rossiter (1998); Sawyer (1999); and Stainton, Solaiman, and Strahle (2002). The emic data descriptors revealed that the culture-specific care patterns were influenced by a person's worldview, ethnohistory, language, and the environmental context within which care took place. The culture care patterns of *avoidance of harmful environments, privacy,* and *cleanliness* contributed to the health and wellbeing of the mother and her newborn baby. These patterns of care substantiated the assumptive premise that culturally-based care for Mauritian immigrants is essential for health and wellbeing and the prevention of illness especially during the significant life-changing event of childbearing.

In unison, the patterns of culture care supported the assumptive premise of the study that the informants' worldview and accompanying cultural and social structural dimensions of kinship (gender and ethnicity), religion and spirituality, education, politics (including legal), and economics influenced the health and wellbeing outcomes for mothers and babies in a diverse range of environmental contexts.

The folk (traditional and nontraditional) dietary patterns practised by the Mauritian immigrants supported the major feature of the theory and study assumption that differences and similarities do exist between individuals belonging to a particular cultural group and that the cultural ". . .learned and shared beliefs, values, and lifeways of a designated or particular group are transmitted inter-generationally [in order to continue to] influence one's thinking and action modes" (Leininger, 2002a, p. 9). These culture care pattern discoveries supported the premise that both folk and professional care practises were utilised concurrently. The choice of treatment modality was highly dependent on what was believed by the mother to be the best care option at that time.

In addition, the study discoveries and patterns of care descriptors for theme five supported the interactional phenomenon of the theory: Immigrant individuals, families or community groups living in a new country not only gain new knowledge and skills intergenerationally but also often adopt many of the ". . .values, behaviours, norms, and lifeways" (Leininger, 2002b, p. 56) of the host culture through the process of acculturation.

DISCOVERIES FOR CULTURE-SPECIFIC CLINICAL MIDWIFERY CARE

Consistent with the Theory of Culture Care Diversity and Universality, three culture-specific clinical midwifery care decision and action modes were developed from the study findings and dominant themes. Leininger's three nursing care modes of decision and action are culture care preservation and/or maintenance; culture care accommodation and/or negotiation; and culture care repatterning and/or restructuring. The primary aim of the care modes of decision and action is to preserve and maintain existing culture-specific patterns of care. The culture-specific care knowledge discovered to sustain the health and wellbeing of the Mauritian immigrant childbearing woman and her unborn/newborn baby is intended to serve as a guide for midwives to maintain, accommodate, and repattern practise in order to provide culturally congruent, safe, and competent midwifery care.

Culture Care Preservation and/or Maintenance

The themes and supportive pattern descriptors revealed how health and wellbeing for the Mauritian immigrant childbearing family are closely interrelated with their beliefs, values, meanings, and patterns of care. Culture-specific folk care meant *extended family and friendship support; self-care responsibility; best professional and folk (traditional and nontraditional) practises; enabling and empowerment of self and others; and maintenance of a hygienic and supportive environment.* All informants confirmed their desire to maintain these culture care patterns. The dominant theme of extended family and friendship support was shown to be sustained by the culture care patterns of *collaborative and interdependent relationships* that included reciprocity and acceptance of God's will; *offers of support; assistance with domestic duties; presence;* and *advocacy.* The interconnectedness and comfort of knowing that the significant life event of childbearing was not experienced alone brought with it a strong sense of health and wellbeing for the Mauritian immigrant mother and her family.

From a comparative perspective, the core competency standards of practise for midwives in Australia focus on holistic, individualised woman-centred care within their family and community of significant others (ACMI, 1998, 2002a; New South Wales Nurses' Registration Board, 2001). The competency standards of midwifery practise are, in broad terms, congruent with culture-specific folk care for Mauritian immigrants. Even so, it must be kept in mind that the successful transferability of the culture care patterns to midwifery practise is not automatic. Key factors contributing to the success of culture-specific patterns of folk care relied heavily on well-established trust relationships developed over many years between the mother and her immediate and extended family members and friends. Reciprocity, equality, and a high level of privacy also accompanied those same trust relationships.

The professional relationship between maternity care providers and the mother and her baby takes place during the antenatal, intrapartal, and postnatal periods. The childbearing mother and her family seek out best professional therapeutic treatment modalities and folk care during this period. Unlike professional practise relationships, folk care practises involve established trust relationships between the mother and her family and friends. These trust relationships are often intergenerational and exist for the duration of the mother's and baby's lifetime. Midwifery-led models of care are not readily available at all NSW maternity care service facilities, although other models of shared obstetric and maternity care services are available to childbearing women. However, modern midwifery-led models of care provide continuity of care and offer opportunities for the development of a trusting relationship between the childbearing woman and her midwife (Homer, Brodie, & Leap, 2008).

Because the midwife's involvement with the mother and baby is short term the immediate and extended family members and friends with whom the mother has already developed a trusted relationship are better positioned to perform folk care. Conversely, midwives are in a prime position to support and encourage the continuation of culture-specific folk care alongside their own professional practises. This dual approach is thus more likely to contribute toward the preservation and maintenance of health and wellbeing for childbearing women and their babies.

The study findings showed that Mauritian immigrant childbearing families placed great value on the enabling and empowering culture care patterns of *knowledge and skill acquisition; open and honest communication; choice;* and *involvement in decision-making care processes.* The midwifery profession recognises the "right" and importance of women having ". . .choice, control and continuity of care throughout their experience of childbirth" (ACMI, 2002a, pp.1–2). In addition to these professional core values, the core competency standards also expect midwives to practise a co-participatory, individualised, woman-centred, problem-solving approach to their maternity care. Professional midwifery care includes assessment, planning, implementation, monitoring, and evaluation. It is expected of the midwife that the mother and her family will be central to these care processes and involved in clinical decision making throughout their childbearing experience. Likewise, the culture care pattern of open and honest communication is an expected professional behaviour reflected in the competencies and code of ethics for midwives, as are the principles of adult teaching and learning with regard to knowledge acquisition about childbearing care issues. These enabling and empowering culturally congruent midwifery competency standards of practise contribute in a positive way to the preservation and maintenance of health and wellbeing for Mauritian immigrant childbearing families and can prevent cultural conflict, imposition, stresses, and pain.

The Australian College of Midwives Incorporated (2002a) states, "It is the responsibility of the midwife to maintain high standards of health care within the community through continued education and research" (p. 1). The discovery of the culture care pattern of *self-care responsibility* highlighted the congruency between the Mauritian immigrants' well-established health-promoting patterns of care and the midwifery competency standards of practise relating to health education and promotion (ACMI, 1998, 2002a; New South Wales Nurses' Registration Board, 2001). Through the self-monitoring, health-promoting care decision and action patterns of *maintaining a balanced healthy lifestyle; knowledge and skill acquisition; avoidance of harmful substances, experiences, and practises; keeping active, exercising, and working hard; eating nutritional foods; rest and sleep; breastfeeding;* and *religious and spiritual practises,* the Mauritian immigrant mother was discovered to preserve and/or maintain her own health and wellbeing as well as that of her unborn/newborn baby.

Embedded in the culture-specific patterns of care were the informants' religious beliefs and practises. Religious (Christian) and spiritual beliefs and practises such as prayer were important to the Mauritian people, especially during the significant life-changing event of childbearing and even more so during periods of illness. However, other than showing respect for an individual's religious belief system, the informants viewed professional involvement by midwives in this aspect of their lives as unwarranted, because of the private nature of those beliefs and their personal relationship with God. The practise behaviour of showing respect for an individual's religious belief system is congruent with the competency standards for midwives as well as their philosophy and code of ethics (ACMI, 1998, 2001, 2002a, 2002b; New South Wales Nurses' Registration Board, 2001). The study findings indicated that maternity care services provided by midwives were more similar than different when compared to those culture patterns of care practised by Mauritian immigrant childbearing families.

Culture Care Accommodation and/or Negotiation

Culture-specific patterns of care practised by Mauritian immigrant childbearing families were discovered to enhance the health and wellbeing of the mother and her unborn/newborn baby. Despite the commonalities (universalities) found to exist among and between informants' patterns of care and the competency standards guiding maternity practises, the study findings indicated that disparities (differences) also existed. Therefore, the transcultural care mode of accommodation and/or negotiation has greater significance for providers of maternity care services than it does for the

Mauritian immigrant mothers as recipients of their care. Both past and present competency standards require midwives to work collaboratively with the childbearing mother and her family with the goal of developing an individualised plan of care. However, standardised practises were the approaches more commonly experienced by the informants, including restrictions and differences associated with hospital routines and visiting schedules; the ward layout and sleeping arrangements; group antenatal and postnatal education sessions; and medical and midwifery interventions that medicalised the childbearing experience including such procedures as the use of stirrups, episiotomies, and epidurals. In combination with these professional practises, some Mauritian immigrant mothers also included the transference of personal beliefs, values, and attitudes by individual staff members onto the mother, especially in relation to what the mother could or could not eat when breastfeeding; personal hygiene practises; and baby care—practises that were perceived as culturally imposing and/or culturally incongruent with Mauritian folk (generic) care.

Informant suggestions for overcoming these practise differences included greater flexibility in hospital accommodations with separate rest and sleeping arrangements; self-directed dietary and hygiene practises; the need for privacy from strangers; and for quietness in the clinical environment. These suggestions were found to be especially relevant during the postnatal period. When sleeping in a room that accommodated more than one new mother and her baby, adequate rest and sleep were reduced and choices were limited for involving and receiving support from extended family members and friends. While the informants acknowledged that changes to existing maternity care infrastructures, practises, and room arrangements were not always achievable or economically viable, it was suggested that consideration of these factors be addressed in the short- and long-term strategic planning of maternity care services or facilities.

The discovery of the informants' respect for and utilisation of diverse professional and folk knowledge and skill expertise reflected the informants' belief that maternity care providers such as midwives and doctors, or any other allied health professionals, cannot solely meet the whole needs of the childbearing family. The informants valued the input from professional maternity care providers, as well as the traditional and non-traditional folk care offered by extended family and friends. High levels of trust, together with the expectation that maternity care professionals such as midwives would provide and offer best practises, accompanied the informants' respect for midwifery and other maternity care knowledge and skill expertise. The Mauritian immigrants' pluralistic approaches to and respect for the diverse range of therapeutic maternity care treatment modalities available are congruent with the competency standards for midwives (ACMI, 1998, 2002a) and are reflected in the growing number of midwives who are incorporating a diverse range of evidenced-based traditional and complementary treatment modalities (such as herbal medicine) in their practises (Belew, 1999; McCabe, 2001; Nanayakkara, 2001; Nice, Coghlan, & Birmingham, 2000). However, despite the professional recognition of the need for midwifery practises and education to be predominantly evidenced based (ACMI, 1998, 2001, 2002a, 2002b), the informants suggested midwives need to show consideration for the health benefits and contributions of non-scientific-research-based folk (traditional and nontraditional) care expertise, knowledge, and practises.

The multilingual (English, French, and Créole) skills of the Mauritian informants in the majority of cases did not require the services of an accredited French healthcare translator or interpreter. However, because of the diverse levels of English language proficiency found among Mauritian cultural groups and the obstetric healthcare terminology frequently used by professionals, it is suggested that interpreter services be offered during the cultural assessment phase to accommodate diverse communication needs and to prevent unnecessary misunderstandings.

Culture Care Repatterning and/or Restructuring

Transcultural care decisions and actions of repatterning and/or restructuring have significance for the providers of maternity care services. Mauritian immigrants suggested there is a need for maternity practises to acknowledge the diverse range of normality (both physically and psychologically) that exists among and between childbearing women and their babies. Informants raised the issue that the existing maternity and baby percentile measurement scales were ethno-specific and therefore did not accurately reflect the physical and genetic characteristics of the Mauritian people, whom they argued are on average more petite in size and stature than the average Australian. The informants believed that development of a diverse range of culture-specific percentile measurement scales would contribute to the normalisation of the physical attributes of the Mauritian infants and their maternal experience. Research into the redevelopment and/or repatterning of current maternity care assessment practises would minimise psychological stresses experienced by Mauritians when cultural differences among mothers and babies are identified and referred to as abnormal.

Maternity care practises that adopted a collaborative or group approach to parental education in the absence of having first developed a trusting relationship were less likely to be successful in terms of participation than when offered individually by the midwife whom the childbearing family members knew and trusted. According to the study findings, group activities were more likely to be economically viable and reflective of many NSW antenatal and postnatal maternity care education sessions on offer. Collaboration with groups of strangers to discuss family planning issues was a teaching approach that informants viewed as culturally incongruent with their folk care. Group activities did not afford the same level of privacy or create the trusting environment that the informants believed could be achieved with the use of individualised care. The informants preferred maternity care that could be provided by a midwife on a one-on-one basis. Accessibility of midwifery-led models of care for Mauritian immigrant childbearing families could improve the cultural congruency of some culturally incongruent maternity or obstetric care practises.

CONCLUSION

Childbearing is a significant life event in any culture. Folk (generic) care knowledge and skills specific to each cultural group are essential to transcultural midwifery practise within a diverse range of clinical or community healthcare contexts. One universal finding from this study was that culture-specific folk care for Mauritian immigrant childbearing families was important for the health and wellbeing of the mother and unborn/newborn baby. All 15 key informants and 27 general informants viewed childbearing as a significant, normal, and joyful life event that the woman was not expected to experience alone. Each of the five themes exemplified what care and caring meant for Mauritian immigrants and how care was expressed through the nursing care modes of decision and action during the various phases of childbearing. These patterns of care supported and confirmed the assumptive premise that culturally-based care for Mauritian immigrants was essential for health and wellbeing and for growth and survival, especially during the significant life-changing event of childbearing.

Culture care beliefs, values, meanings, and patterns were influenced by and embedded in the Mauritian immigrants' worldview, together with the cultural and social structural dimensions of kinship (gender and ethnicity); religion (and spirituality); politics; technology; education; economics; language; ethnohistory; and environmental context. The study findings were evaluated for trustworthiness according to the criteria of credibility, confirmability, meaning-in-context, recurrent patterning, saturation, and transferability. The discoveries substantiated the fittingness of the Theory of Culture Care Diversity and Universality, the qualitative ethnonursing research method, and selected enablers to discover and interpret culture-specific care for the discipline and practise of midwifery for Mauritians in the Australian environmental context.

Based on these discoveries, three transcultural midwifery nursing care modes of decision and actions were developed. Their overall aim was to preserve and/or maintain existing Mauritian culture-specific folk care. Recommendations for accommodation and/or negotiation and repatterning and/or restructuring professional midwifery care practises were also made. Culturally congruent and beneficial care for the Mauritian immigrant childbearing woman and her baby can occur only when the cultural values, lifeways, expressions, and patterns of care are known and explicitly used for the delivery of competent, safe, sensitive, and meaningful transcultural clinical midwifery care.

DEDICATION

This chapter is dedicated to the Australian Mauritian community. The authors also wish to acknowledge the New South Wales Nurses Registration Board and the Royal College of Nursing, Australia for their financial support during the final year of this doctoral study.

DISCUSSION QUESTIONS

1. Based on the findings in this study, discuss the efficacy of the ethnonursing research method and accompanying enablers for their fittingness to discover culture-specific clinical midwifery care.
2. Discuss the advantages and disadvantages of utilising folk or generic-based knowledge and skills to contribute to the development of professional maternity care practise knowledge.
3. Using Leininger's Sunrise Enabler as a guide, identify the cultural and structural dimensions addressed in the antenatal clinical assessment forms, birth plans, and postnatal clinical pathways of your local maternity care service.
4. Discuss how a midwife could use the five dominant themes discovered in this study to assist with the development of culturally safe and congruent antenatal and postnatal education courses in nursing education and in primary care practise, health clinic, or hospital care settings.

APPENDIX 7-A

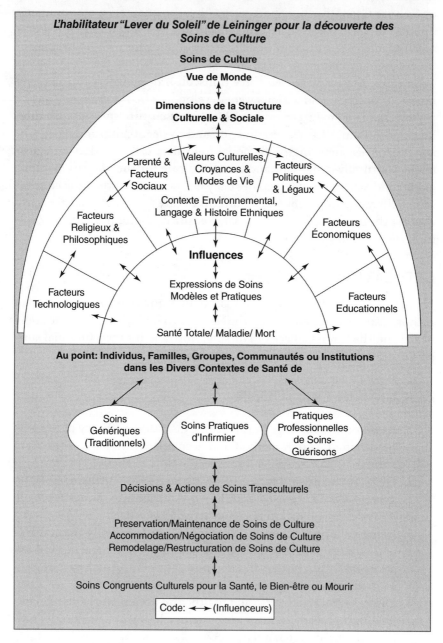

L'habilitateur "Lever du Soleil" de Leininger pour la découverte des Soins de Culture

Soins de Culture

Vue de Monde

Dimensions de la Structure Culturelle & Sociale

Parenté & Facteurs Sociaux

Valeurs Culturelles, Croyances & Modes de Vie

Facteurs Politiques & Légaux

Contexte Environnemental, Langage & Histoire Ethniques

Facteurs Religieux & Philosophiques

Facteurs Économiques

Influences

Expressions de Soins Modèles et Pratiques

Facteurs Technologiques

Facteurs Educationnels

Santé Totale/ Maladie/ Mort

Au point: Individus, Familles, Groupes, Communautés ou Institutions dans les Divers Contextes de Santé de

Soins Génériques (Traditionnels)

Soins Pratiques d'Infirmier

Pratiques Professionnelles de Soins-Guérisons

Décisions & Actions de Soins Transculturels

Preservation/Maintenance de Soins de Culture
Accommodation/Négociation de Soins de Culture
Remodelage/Restructuration de Soins de Culture

Soins Congruents Culturels pour la Santé, le Bien-être ou Mourir

Code: ←→ (Influenceurs)

Appendix 7-A Leininger's Sunrise Enabler translated into French.
Modified with permission from © M. Leininger 2004, by G. S. Raymond.

REFERENCES

Australian Bureau of Statistics. (1997). *1996 census of population and housing for Mauritius.* Sydney, Australia: Author.

Australian College of Midwives Incorporated (ACMI). (1998). *ACMI competency standards for midwives.* Canberra, Australia: Author.

Australian College of Midwives Incorporated (ACMI). (2001). Code of ethics. http://www.acmi.org.au/shared/docs/codeofethics.htm

Australian College of Midwives Incorporated (ACMI). (2002a). ACMI competency standards for midwives. http://www.acmi.org.au/shared/docs/competency.htm

Australian College of Midwives Incorporated (ACMI). (2002b). ACMI philosophy and position statements. http://www.acmi.org.au/shared/docs/position_statements_intro.htm

Australian Institute of Health and Welfare National Perinatal Statistics Unit. (2001). *Australia's mothers and babies 1998* [Rep. No. 10)]. Sydney, Australia: Author.

Bah, S. M. (1994). Influence of cause-of-death structure on age patterns of mortality in Mauritius. *Social Biology, 41*(3–4), 212–228.

Barclay, L., & Jones, L. (1996). *Midwifery: Trends and practice in Australia.* Melbourne, Australia: Churchill Livingstone.

Bauman, A., & Moshsin, M. (1999). *Midwives data collection: Analysis by Mauritian status 1994–1997* (Unpublished). Liverpool, NSW, Australia: NSW Health Department Epidemiology Unit.

Belew, C. (1999). Herbs and the childbearing women: Guidelines for midwives. *Journal of Nurse–Midwifery, 44*(3), 231–252.

Berry, A. (1999). Mexican American women's expressions of the meaning of culturally congruent prenatal care. *Journal of Transcultural Nursing, 10*(3), 203–212.

Bohay, I. (1991). Culture care meanings and experiences of pregnancy and childbirth for Ukrainians. In M. Leininger (Ed.), *Culture care diversity and universality: A theory of nursing* (pp. 203–229). New York, NY: National League for Nursing Press.

Bottomley, G., & Lepervanche, M. (1990). The social context of immigrant health and illness. In J. Reid & P. Trompf (Eds.), *The health of immigrant Australia: A social perspective* (pp. 36–76). Sydney, Australia: Harcourt Brace Jovanovich.

Brodie, P. (2003). Nurses and midwives act in NSW: We did it! *Midwifery Matters, 21*(4), 29.

Browne, E. (1991). Australia's immigration context. In B. Ferguson & E. Browne (Eds.), *Health care and immigrants: A guide for the helping professions* (pp. 46–66). Artarmon, NSW, Australia: MacLennan & Petty.

Browner, C. H., & Sargent, C. F. (1990). Anthropology and studies of human reproduction. In T. M. Johnson & C. F. Sargent (Eds.), *Medical anthropology: A handbook of theory and method* (pp. 215–229). New York, NY: Greenwood Press.

Bunwaree, S. (2001). The marginal in the miracle: Human capital in Mauritius [Electronic version]. *International Journal of Educational Development, 21*(3), 257–271.

Callister, L. C. (1998). Culturally competent care of women and newborns: Knowledge, attitude, and skills. *Journal of Obstetric, Gynecologic, and Neonatal Nursing, 30*(2), 209–215.

Callister, L. C., Semenic, S., & Foster, J. C. (1999). Cultural and spiritual meanings of childbirth: Orthodox Jewish and Mormon women. *Journal of Holistic Nursing, 17*(3), 280–295.

Carrington, B. W. (1978). The Afro-American. In A. L. Clark (Ed.), *Culture, childbearing health professionals* (pp. 34–52). Philadelphia, PA: F. A. Davis.

Choolun, R. (1985). Infant mortality and socio-economic development in Mauritius. *Journal of Tropical Pediatrics, 31*(3), 174–176.

Clark, A. L. (1978). *Culture, childbearing and health professionals.* Philadelphia, PA: F. A. Davis.

Commonwealth of Australia. (1999). *Australian multiculturalism for a new century: Towards inclusive.* Canberra, ACT, Australia: National Multicultural Advisory Council.

Commonwealth of Australia. (2001). *Australian migration, settlement website.* Canberra, ACT, Australia: Department of Immigration and Multicultural and Indigenous Affairs. http://www.immi.gov.au

Commonwealth of Australia. (2003). Multicultural Australia: United in diversity. Updating the 1999 new agenda for multicultural Australia: Strategic directions for 2003–06. http://www.immi.gov.au/media/fact-sheets/06evolution.htm

Commonwealth of Australia. (2008). A new lease of life for multicultural Australia. http://www.minister.immi.gov.au/parlsec/media/media-releases/2008/lf08004.htm

Duyker, E. (1986). *Mauritian Heritage: An anthology of the Lionnet, Commins and related families.* Victoria: Australian Mauritian Research Group.

Duyker, E. (1988). *Of the star and the key: Mauritius, Mauritians and Australia.* Sylvania, NSW, Australia: Australian Research Group.

Ericksen, T. H. (1988). *Communicating cultural difference and identity: Ethnicity and nationalism in Mauritius.* Oxford, UK: Berg.

Ericksen, T. H. (1997). Ethnicity, race and nation. In M. Guibernau & J. Rex (Eds.), *The ethnicity reader: Nationalism, multiculturalism and migration* (pp. 33–42). Cambridge, UK: Polity Press.

Ericksen, T. H. (1998). *Common denominators: Ethnicity, nation building and compromise in Mauritius.* Oxford, UK: Berg.

Finn, J. (1995). Leininger's model for discoveries at the Farm and midwifery services to the Amish. *Journal of Transcultural Nursing, 7*(1), 28–35.

Government of Mauritius Central Statistics Office (GMCSO). (2001a). Central Statistics Office. The National Computer Board (Mauritius). http://ncb.intnet.mu/cso/index.htm

Government of Mauritius Central Statistics Office (GMCSO). (2001b). Constitution. The National Computer Board (Mauritius). http://ncb.intnet.mu/govt/constitu.htm

Government of Mauritius Central Statistics Office (GMCSO). (2001c). History of Mauritius. The National Computer Board (Mauritius). http://ncb.intnet.mu/govt/history.htm

Grummer-Strawn, L. M., Kalasopatan, S., Sungkur, J., & Friedman, J. (1996). Infant feeding patterns on Mauritius Island, 1991. *Social Science and Medicine, 43*(12), 1697–1702.

Hage, G., & Couch, R. (1999). *The future of Australian multiculturalism: Reflections on the twentieth anniversary of Jean Martin's "The Jean Martin's—The migrant presence."* Sydney, Australia: Research Institution for Humanities and Social Sciences, University of Sydney.

Hall, E. T. (1959). *The silent language.* Sioux City, IA: Doubleday Books. [Anchor Books reprint in 1973 by publisher arrangement.]

Higgins, B. (2000). Puerto Rican cultural beliefs: Influence on infant feeding practices in western New York. *Journal of Transcultural Nursing, 11*(1), 19–30.

Homer, C. (2000). Incorporating cultural diversity in randomized controlled trials in midwifery. *Midwifery, 16*(4), 252–259.

Homer, C., Brodie., & Leap, N. (2008). *Midwifery continuity of care: A practical guide.* Sydney, Australia: Churchill Livingstone Elsevier.

Horn, B. (1990). Cultural concepts and postpartal care. *Journal of Transcultural Nursing, 2*(1), 48–51. [Reprinted by permission from [1981] *Nursing and Health Care, 2*(3), 516–517; 526–527.]

Hughes, D., Deery, R., & Lovatt, A. (2002). A critical ethnographic approach to facilitating cultural shift in midwifery. *Midwifery, 18*(1), 43–52.

Ibrahim, F. A. (1985). Effective cross-cultural counselling and psychotherapy: A framework. *The Counselling Psychologist, 13*, 626–638.

Idrus, L. (1988). Transcultural nursing in Australia: Response to a changing population base. *Recent Advances in Nursing, 20*, 81–91.

Jones, H. (1989). Fertility decline in Mauritius: The role of Malthusian population pressure. *Geoforum, 20*(3), 315–327.

Jupp, J. (1990). Two hundred years of immigration. In J. Reid & P. Trompf (Eds.), *The health of immigrant Australia: A social perspective* (pp. 1–38). Sydney, Australia: Harcourt Brace Jovanovich.

Kalla, A. (1995). Health transition in Mauritius: Characteristics and trends. *Health and Place, 1*(4), 227–234.

Kay, M. A. (Ed.). (1982a). *Anthropology of human birth.* Philadelphia, PA: F. A. Davis.

Kay, M. A. (Ed.). (1982b). Writing an ethnography of birth. In M. A. Kay (Ed.), *Anthropology of human birth* (pp. 1–24). Philadelphia, PA: F. A. Davis.

Kendall, K. (1992). Maternal and childcare in an Iranian village. *Journal of Transcultural Nursing, 4*(1), 29–36.

Kim-Godwin, Y. S. (2003). Postpartum beliefs and practices among non-Western cultures. *MCN: The American Journal of Maternal/Child Nursing, 28*(2), 74–78.

Kluckholn, F. R., & Strodtbeck, F. L. (1961). *Variations in value orientations.* Evanston, IL: Row, Patterson & Co.

Lamp, J. (2002). Finnish women in birth: Culture care meanings and practices. In M. M. Leininger & M. R. McFarland (Eds.), *Transcultural nursing: Concepts, theories, research & practices* (3rd ed., pp. 403–414). New York, NY: McGraw-Hill.

Lauderdale, J. (2003). Transcultural perspectives in childbearing. In M. Andrews & J. Boyle (Eds.), *Transcultural concepts in nursing care* (4th ed., pp. 95–131). Philadelphia, PA: Lippincott Williams & Wilkins.

Leininger, M. M. (1991). *Culture care diversity and universality: A theory of nursing.* New York, NY: National League of Nursing.

Leininger, M. M. (2002a). Transcultural nursing and globalization of health care: Importance, focus, and historical aspects. In M. M. Leininger & M. R. McFarland (Eds.), *Transcultural nursing: Concepts, theories, research, & practice* (3rd ed., pp. 3–43). New York, NY: McGraw-Hill.

Leininger, M. M. (2002b). Essential transcultural nursing care concepts, principles, examples and policy statements. In M. M. Leininger & M. R. McFarland (Eds.), *Transcultural nursing: Concepts, theories, research, & practice* (3rd ed., pp. 45–69). New York, NY: McGraw-Hill.

Leininger, M. M. (2002c). Part I: The theory of culture care and the ethnonursing research method. In M. M. Leininger & M. R. McFarland (Eds.), *Transcultural nursing: Concepts, theories, research, & practice* (3rd ed., pp. 71–116). New York, NY: McGraw-Hill.

Lenoir, P. (1985). *Mauritius: Isle de France en mer Indienne.* Port Louis, Mauritius: Isle de France.

Martinez-Schallmoser, L., Talleen, S., & MacMulleen, N. J. (2003). The effect of social support and acculturation on post-partum depression in Mexican American women. *Journal of Transcultural Nursing, 14*(4), 329–328.

McCabe, P. (2001). *Complementary therapies in nursing and midwifery.* Melbourne, Australia: Ausmed.

Mead, M., & Newton, N. (1967). Cultural patterning of perinatal behaviour. In S. A. Richardson & A. F. Guttamacher (Eds.), *Childbearing: Its social and psychological aspects* (pp. 142–244). Baltimore, MD: Williams and Wilkins.

Mercer, R. T., & Stainton, M. C. (1984). Perceptions of birth experience: A cross cultural comparison. *Health Care for Women International, 5*(1–3), 29–47.

Ministry of Health. (1990). *Mauritius report of the Ministry of Health 1982–1988, 2.* Port Louis, Mauritius: Silvio M. Empeigne, Government Printer.

Ministry of Health and Quality of Life. (2001). *Family planning and demographic yearbook 2000.* Port Louis, Mauritius: Ministry of Health and Quality of Life. http://www.health.gov.mu

Morgan, M. (1996). Prenatal care of African American women in selected USA urban and rural cultural contexts. *Journal of Transcultural Nursing, 7*(2), 3–9.

Mountain, A., & Proust, A. (1995). *This is Mauritius.* London, UK: New Holland.

Murkoff, H., Eisenberg, A., & Hathaway, S. (2002). *What to expect when you're expecting.* (3rd ed.). New York, NY: Workman.

Nahas, V., & Amasheh, N. (1999). Culture care meanings and experiences of post-partum depression among Jordanian Australian women: A transcultural study. *Journal of Transcultural Nursing, 10*(1), 37–45.

Nanayakkara, S. (2001). Complementary therapies in midwifery practice. In P. McCabe (Ed.), *Complementary therapies in nursing and midwifery* (pp. 291–303). Melbourne, Australia: Ausmed.

New South Wales Department of Health. (1998). *New South Wales mothers and babies 1996.* Sydney, Australia: Author.

New South Wales Department of Health. (2001, January). *New South Wales mothers and babies 1999* [Rep. No. S-4, Volume 13]. North Sydney, NSW, Australia:

Centre for Epidemiology and Research, NSW Department of Health. http://www.health.nsw.gov.au/public-health/mdcMDCRep01.pdf

New South Wales Department of Health. (2002, December). *New South Wales mothers and babies 2001* [Rep. No. 1]. North Sydney, NSW, Australia: NSW Department of Health.

New South Wales Department of Health. (2002b). *Women's health outcomes framework* [Rep. No. SHPN: (PH) 010171]. Gladesville, NSW, Australia: Better Health Centre Publications Warehouse.

New South Wales Department of Health. (2009). *New South Wales mothers and babies 2006.* Sydney, Australia: Centre for Epidemiology and Research, NSW Department of Health.

New South Wales Department of Health. (2010). *New South Wales mothers and babies 2008.* Sydney, Australia: Centre for Epidemiology and Research, NSW Department of Health.

New South Wales Ministry of Health. (2011). *New South Wales mothers and babies 2009.* Sydney, Australia: Centre for Epidemiology and Research, NSW Ministry of Health.

New South Wales Nurses' Registration Board. (2001). Statistics: Registered nurses, certified midwives and enrolled nurses. *NRB Board of Works,* 8.

Nice, F., Coghlan, R. J., & Birmingham, B. T. (2000). Herbals and breastfeeding: Which herbals are safe to take while breastfeeding? *Birth Issues, 9*(3), 77–84.

Oakley, A. (1980). *Women confined: Towards a sociology of childbirth.* New York, NY: Schocken Books.

Pernoud, L. (Ed.). (2003). *J'attends un enfant [I am waiting for my baby]* (3rd ed.). Paris, France: Horay.

Pincombe, J. (1992). Transcultural approaches to midwifery care. *Australian College of Midwives Incorporated, 5*(2), 11–14.

Qualis Research Associates. (1998). *The Ethnograph (Version 5.7)* [Computer software]. Thousand Oaks, CA: Scolari, Sage Publications Software. http://www.scolari.com

Republic of Mauritius. (2003). *2000 Ministry of Health and Quality of Life island of Mauritius health statistics annual report of the principal medical statistician.* Port Louis, Mauritius: Ministry of Health & Quality of Life. Retrieved from http://mih.gov.mu/English/Pages/Info%20Gateway%20-%20Natural%20Health%20Info/Annual-Health-Statistics—2000-.aspx

Riordan, J., & Gill-Hopple, K. (2001). Breastfeeding care in multicultural populations. *Journal of Obstetric, Gynecologic, and Neonatal Nursing, 30*(2), 216–223.

Rossiter, J. C. (1998). Promoting breast feeding: The perceptions of Vietnamese mothers in Sydney, Australia. *Journal of Advanced Nursing, 28*(3), 598–605.

Sawyer, L. (1999). Engaged mothering: The transition to motherhood for a group of African American women. *Journal of Transcultural Nursing, 10*(1), 14–21.

Singh, S., Swaney, D., & Strauss, R. (1999). *Mauritius, Reunion and Seychelles* (3rd ed.). Hawthorne, Victoria, Australia: Lonely Planet.

Spock, B., & Parker, S. (1998). *Dr. Spock's baby and child care* (7th ed.). New York, NY: Pocket Books.

Spradley, J. P. (1979). *The ethnographic interview.* Fort Worth, TX: Harcourt Brace Jovanovich College Publications.

Stainton, M. C., Solaiman, S., & Strahle, A. (2002). Providing culturally sensitive health services in partnership with childbearing Bangladeshi women. *Nursing Matters, 29,* 12.

Stoppard, M. (2002). *Baby and child health care.* London, UK: Dorling Kindersley.

Sue, D. W., & Sue, S. (1990). *Counselling for the culturally different: Theory and practice* (2nd ed.). New York, NY: John Wiley.

Sussman, L. (1981). Unity in diversity in a polyethnic society: The maintenance of medical pluralism on Mauritius. *Sociology, Science, and Medicine, 15B,* 247–260.

Weber, S. (1996). Cultural aspects of pain in childbearing women. *Gynecology and Neonatal Nursing, 25*(1), 67–72.

Willcox, R. (1999). *Mauritius, Reunion and Seychelles: A travel survival kit* (2nd ed.). Hawthorn, Victoria, Australia: Lonely Planet.

Chapter 8

An Examination of Subculture as a Theoretical Social Construct Through an Ethnonursing Study of Urban African American Adolescent Gang Members

Edith J. Morris

> *Problems of adjustment [to societal values] to which the delinquent subculture is a response are determined, in part, by those very values which respectable society holds most sacred.*
>
> (Cohen, 1955, p. 137)

INTRODUCTION

Purpose

The purpose of this chapter is to explore the concept of a subculture through a study of African American adolescent gang members. In an ethnonursing study conceptualized using the Theory of Culture Care Diversity and Universality (Leininger, 1991), this author found that a gang subculture exists within the African American culture, and its intended function is to improve the lifeways of poor African Americans in an urban context (Morris, 2004). The practices of the subculture had roots in the African American culture, but deviated in some beliefs, values, and lifeways. The gang subculture was identified through characteristics discovered from the study and included the use of a specific and unique language spoken within the gang; an illegal economy consisting of drug and weapon sales; specific types and colors of clothing to identify gang members; and violent activities. These characteristics are consistent with Leininger's (2002a) definition of a subculture as well as the anthropological definitions by Haviland, Prins, McBride, and Walrath (2011) and the sociological definitions by Becker (1963); Brake (2003); Cohen (1955); Fine and Kleinman (1979); and Herzog, Mitchell, and Soccio (1999).

Subculture Background

Subcultures exist within many cultures and may even transcend cultural lines, yet the concept of a subculture is often either ill defined based on the anthropological definition or so broadly defined as to make it difficult to distinguish a culture from a subculture. Haviland, Prins, McBride, and Walrath (2011) defined subculture as ". . . a distinctive set of ideas, values, and behavior patterns by which a group within a larger society operates, while still sharing common standards with the larger society" (p. 30). This seminal textbook offered ethnic groups as examples of subcultures, noting that they are distinguishable from the dominant culture by shared ancestry, language, customs, and traditional beliefs and values, yet share some commonalities with the dominant culture. In particular, Haviland et al. identified the Amish people in the United States as an example of an ethnic subculture of the American dominant culture. Herein begins confusion over what is and what is not a subculture.

If the Amish are a subculture of the American culture, then would not all ethnic cultures in the United States be subcultures of the American culture? Following this line of thought, African Americans, Latinos, Asians, and Euro Americans would also be examples of subcultures within the American culture. It would seem to follow, then, that American culture is indeed a "melting pot" and, therefore, a new and separate culture overriding all distinct ethnic groups within the United States. The final result of this definition is that diversity is not held in as high esteem as is generally espoused. Thus this author suggests that ethnic groups do not fit the traditional definition of a subculture, but rather are an overriding culture from which groups emerge who remain part of said overriding culture, yet have some significant and distinct differences from it. This definition allows for honoring the diversity found within ethnic groups, yet clearly defines *subculture* as a group within an overriding or dominant ethnic culture.

This author would like to go a step further and define a subculture as a group within an overriding ethnic culture that subscribes to many of the lifeways, practices, values, and beliefs of that culture, but differs in some distinct ways that are expressed through daily lifeways, beliefs, and values. Haviland et al. (2011) suggested that subcultures may exist in distinct groups within an overriding culture, and within these distinct groups may exist a complex organizational culture. This definition would indicate that one must first define the culture before describing subcultures that are within that culture. It would further indicate that *culture* is a loosely defined term—and hence *subculture* is even more loosely defined. Nanda and Warms (2011) share a similar definition of a subculture, stating that it is a term ". . . used to designate groups within a single society that share norms and values significantly different from those of the dominant culture" (p. 84). The term *subculture* was coined by the Chicago School of Sociology in the 1940s and was defined as loosely associated social groups organized around shared interests and practices (Herzog et al., 1999). It would appear by these definitions that both culture and subculture are loosely defined. In this author's opinion, defining culture loosely and subculture even more loosely may lead to difficulty in conducting research studies, thereby leading to less rigorous cultural healthcare research.

The term *subculture* was first used to describe adolescent groups who pulled away from mainstream culture (society) because of their inability to fit into the societal norms of the overriding culture. This subculture offered an alternative set of values and norms where adolescent boys were able to fulfill the expectations of the subculture and experience some measure of success (Cohen, 1955; Thrasher, 1963). Frederic Thrasher (1927, 1963), a University of Chicago sociologist, first studied these gangs (groups) systematically in a 50-year longitudinal study. Later, Cohen's (1955) work on delinquent boys further solidified the concept of a delinquent subculture. Becker (1963) later hypothesized that the idea of a subculture could be used to describe many groups who could not fit into their ethnic culture.

Another current sociological definition of subculture includes elements common to the group which include identifying as a group; commitment to the rules, values, and norms by the members of the group; consistent behaviors that establish the distinctiveness of the group; and autonomy from the overriding societal culture (Herzog et al., 1999). Brake (2003) used a more recent sociological definition of subculture that emphasized interrelationships, where subordinate groups interact with the overriding culture to mediate contradictions that arise from the larger social context to form alternative meaning systems and modes of expression (lifestyles). In other words, the interaction between the societal cultural norms and the alternative societal norms defined by the group forms the subculture.

Dr. Madeleine Leininger, world-renowned nursing theorist and innovative author of books and articles on the Theory of Culture Care Diversity and Universality and the ethnonursing research method (Leininger, 1978, 1991, 2002b), defined a subculture as "closely related to culture, but refers to subgroups who deviate in certain ways from a dominant culture in values, beliefs, norms, moral codes, and ways of living with some distinctive features that characterize their unique lifeways" (Leininger, 2002a, p. 47). As a nurse with a PhD in anthropology, Leininger developed her theory using *culture* from anthropology and *care* from nursing to conceptualize her theory of culture care. This theory was borne out of her dissertation study with the Gadsup of Papua, New Guinea. Since its inception, her Theory of Culture Care Diversity and Universality has been widely used throughout the world to study various cultures (Leininger, 1994). As a doctoral student of Dr. Leininger, this author was cautioned about conducting a study of a subculture, as such groups were difficult to define and ascertaining whether subsequent findings related to the subculture or the culture would be difficult. Hence, this researcher studied African Americans with adolescent gang members as the key participants. Care constructs discovered in this study were compared to previously discovered care constructs from earlier African American culture care ethnonursing studies. The care constructs discovered by this researcher were examined for their congruence and closeness of alignment with characteristics of gang subculture. These new constructs were not found in other African American studies reviewed.

DOMAIN OF INQUIRY AND THEORETICAL FRAMEWORK

The domain of inquiry for this culture care study was the expressions, meanings, and cultural lifeways of selected African American adolescent gang members and their daily and nightly experiences within their environmental context. The Theory of Culture Care Diversity and Universality with the ethnonursing research method was used to study and explicate the domain, which led to the discovery of largely unknown ontologic and epistemic transcultural nursing knowledge (Leininger, 1991, pp. 22, 24).

ETHNOHISTORICAL CHARACTERISTICS OF GANGS

As a way of defining an adolescent gang subculture, an ethnohistory of youth was explored in selected cultures worldwide. Characteristics of subcultures were described in relation to the overriding cultures to which these gang members belonged. The essence of each subculture was found embedded in the social structure factors of the dominant culture. The specific characteristics of each subculture were teased out to define that subculture within the culture of a dominant ethnic group (Leininger, 1991, 2002a). Transcultural studies of gangs revealed that cultures with no social rites of passage for adolescents experienced increased numbers of gangs and gang activity (Bloch & Niederhoffer, 1958). Historical, technological, and economic factors are cited as prolonging the adolescent period and adding pressure and tension to the youths' quest to achieve adult status.

In Europe, gang activity has been reported since the 14th and 15th centuries; the Muns, Hectors, Bugles, and Dead Boys were reported in London during this time. France and Germany reported gang activity into the 18th century (Covey, Menard, & Franzese, 1992; Hay, Linebaugh, & Rule, 1975; Pearson, 1983). Gangs are present in most industrialized and post-industrialized cultures worldwide (Balme, 1985; Boyle, 2010; Glaser, 1992; Goddard, 1992; Kulik, 1993; Leininger, 1994; Nibbring & Nand, 1992; Sheldon, Tracy, & Brown, 2003).

Goddard (1992) reported that the gang phenomenon in Papua, New Guinea, had been ". . . contextualized by observers in the high rate of unemployment and relative poverty which has accompanied urbanization" (p. 20). Goddard (1992) and Kulik (1993), both anthropologists, suggested that criminal gangs in Papua, New Guinea, were a result of a precapitalist behavior integrated into a capitalist environment. Although there was fear and concern with the increased gang activity, it seems to have been tolerated. In fact, a gang known as the Rascals has reported by Kulik (1993) as receiving

> . . . great support among the villagers because the villagers see them as surrounded by an aura of adventure, education, and power. Villagers believe that Rascals are fighting a kind of protracted guerrilla war against corrupt politicians, greedy businessmen and obstructionist missionaries. (p. 9)

Leininger (1994b), when revisiting Papua, New Guinea, in 1991, discovered and met the Rascals; her findings were similar to those of Kulik (1993). The discovery of gold and oil in that country brought new wealth, along with a dearth of entrepreneurs and research scientists. The indigenous people realized few gains from their nation's newfound wealth, and the resulting political and economic factors threatened their health and wellbeing. Leininger likened the Rascals to the "big men" of the Gadsup—the warriors who fought to maintain political, economic, and cultural rights. "The Rascals seemed to be playing a role to curtail their losses and to regain what foreigners, corrupt politicians, missionaries, businessmen, and others have or are taking away from the PNG [Papua New Guinea] people" (Leininger, 1994, p. 25).

The ethos of external political caring was nonexistent and noncaring prevailed among the Gadsup people. A major purpose of the Rascals, according to Leininger (1994a), was to regain a caring ethos in order to protect their Gadsup culture, its food and mineral resources, and to avoid exploitation by the non-Gadsup (largely European) in noncaring ways. Much of the self-esteem for the members of the Rascals was accomplished through organized street crime to acquire food, cash, and beer. The consumption of beer defines manhood for the Rascals (Nibbring & Nand, 1992). This pattern is similar to that seen with the early ethnic gangs in the United States, which fought to protect their cultural group from robbery and harm from outsiders. Hence, Leininger (1994a) and Kulik (1993) each independently discovered the Rascals and the reasons for their gang behavior.

The Totsies of South Africa is another subculture gang that seemed to be in search of a rite of passage in the midst of the process of urbanization. Although the Totsies have a clear identity in terms of race, class, generation, and gender, as Black working-class male youth they were subordinate in race, class, and generation but dominant by gender. They guarded their gender privilege carefully and asserted their masculine and sexual difference against females, who were property to be won, and once won were branded with a "Z", the mark of Zorro. The gang owned females. The attitude of Totsi men toward women in the township was similar to the attitude of the White working class toward the Black working class in South Africa (Glaser, 1992).

The Rascals and the Totsies, like American gangs, seemed to define their manhood to some degree through women. Gang rape was one activity that bonded the brotherhood of the gang. Rascals believed women were magical, and that they (Rascals of the Papua New Guinea culture) received some of their black magical powers from women (Kulik, 1993). In all three cultures, it appears women of low self-esteem who lacked self-confidence were targeted for the gang rapes (Glaser, 1992; Kulak, 1992; Orenstein, 1994). By contrast, Leininger (1978, 1994b, 1995) found that the Gadsup women of Papua, New Guinea, did not have low self-esteem or low self-confidence, but were confident and strong in self-identity and image. Moreover, manhood was achieved through male avenues and rites of identity, and not through women. The rites of passage were very strong in the Gadsup of Papua, New Guinea (Leininger, 1994b, 1995), although less structured and less strong than those of the Rascals of Papua, New Guinea (Kulik, 1993). Research conducted globally about gangs with discoveries of similar findings include studies in Belize (a Caribbean nation) (Matthei & Smith, 1998); Hong Kong (Lee, 1998); Mexico (Ferrera-Pinto, Ramos, & Mata, 1997; Glittenberg, 2008); New Zealand (Eggleston, 1997); Chinatown, Oakland, California (Mark, 1997); Guam (Schmitz & Christopher, 1997); United States [Mexican Americans (Valdez & Kaplan, 1999) and Southeast Asians

(Hunt, Joe, & Waldorf, 1997)]; Northern Ireland (Montgomery, 1997); and El Salvador (Ward, 2013).

Since 1927, gang phenomena have been studied in sociology, anthropology, and psychology; in more recent criminal justice studies, gang phenomena have also begun to take on the characteristics of subculture. Theoretically discovered empirical data from research in these disciplines seem to represent a gang subculture or a subculture with activities related to those of the gang. The findings presented herein are various researchers' conceptualizations from their cited research of the context and subculture in which gangs develop and flourish.

Gangs have also been in existence throughout the history of the United States and have functioned to serve a specific societal purpose (Sheldon et al., 2003; Thrasher, 1927). Jean Lafitte and his buccaneers and the Wild West gangs such as the Younger Gang and the James (Frank and Jesse) Gang are examples of legendary gang activity. Urban youth gangs in the United States emerged as a result of the shift from an agrarian society to an industrial capitalistic society. The growth of the urban areas with a rapidly expanding economy seemed to stimulate gang development further (Cohen, 1955; Thrasher, 1927). The Mob, Al Capone, Bonnie and Clyde, and the Ma Barker Gang were all active during the Depression years (Cohen, 1955; Miller, 1958).

Immigrants moving into urban areas during the latter nineteenth and early 20th centuries frequently encountered a racially prejudiced environment. Ethnic, religious, and cultural lines were drawn as multiple ethnic groups began to live within close proximity to one another. Businessmen and merchants of various ethnic cultures became victims of robbery and extortion from the rival ethnic groups (Sheldon, Tracy, & Brown, 1997, 2003; Taylor, 1989; Thrasher, 1927). Ethnically indigenous gangs formed to protect these businesses and merchants. They fought fiercely to protect their own ethnic enterprises—and thus began gang warfare. Protection of the ethnic group from robbers and extortionists was the major function of many of the early youth gangs formed during the post-industrialization era (Sheldon et al., 1997, 2003). America's national crime syndicate began with the Purple Gang formed in Detroit in 1920 (Taylor, 1989). The Sugar House Gang, which protected Jewish merchants, and Norman Purple and his group joined forces to form the Purple Gang (Taylor, 1989).

REVIEW OF THE LITERATURE

Thrasher (1927) studied urban gangs from 1927 until 1963 conducting a 50-year study of 1,313 gangs considered to be the classic study of urban gangs. Thrasher reported that these gangs were beyond the ordinary controls of police and other social agencies, describing members as "lawless, godless, and wild" (p. 6). The 1920s Chicago gangs were composed of immigrants, mostly Poles, Italians, and Irish, along with a smaller number of Jews, Slavs, Germans, and Swedes. Thrasher also reported that slightly more than 7% of the gangsters were African American and that stealing was their main activity (pp. 74, 130, 132).

The famous Forty-Two Gang of Chicago's West Side, known as "Little Italy," from the late 1920s is considered the worst juvenile gang ever formed in the United States. Eventually, some of the Forty-Two moved into the lower ranks of the Capone mob, a highly organized group of adult criminals. Capone gangsters were cautious of these wild, reckless, and amoral youth, believing they were too extreme for organized work (Taylor, 1989).

Cohen (1955), a sociologist from the University of Connecticut, in his classic work on delinquent boys described juvenile delinquency as a subculture. He described the "working-class" boy as one who frequently finds himself at the bottom of the status hierarchy as he tries to fit in with his middle-class peers, his middle-class teacher, and middle-class standards. If he has a problem adjusting to class standards, he then seeks a solution. He may choose the delinquent subculture of the gang or group as a vehicle to elevate his societal status. The youth chooses this alternative value system, the delinquent subculture, because he has been denied respectable status in middle-class society.

Three years later, Bloch and Niederhoffer (1958)—an anthropologist and a sociologist, respectively—together with a lieutenant from the New York Police Department studied adolescent behavior through the context of gangs. Following Cohen's (1955) lead related to nonachievement of status for the adolescent, they attributed the phenomenon of gangs and delinquency to the lack of a social rite of passage into adulthood.

Social disorganization theory developed by the Chicago School of Sociology in the 1920s and 1930s attributed decreasing sense of community as a cause of increased criminal activity and hence the formation of subcultures. Groups moving into and out of an area prohibited a sense of community from developing and caused social disorganization. The Old World norms collapsed, but there were no new effective standards to replace them. Urbanization, industrialization, and immigration were cited as key factors in social disorganization (Thrasher, 1963). Thrasher (1927) reported that the failure of social norms that direct and control institutions and the deteriorated housing, sanitation, and other substandard conditions found in slums were responsible for increased youth group activity. Gang activities were viewed as a result of uneven societal development, with social change and conflict affecting adolescent behaviors. Additional research studies by Sheldon, Tracy, and Brown (1997); Goldstein (1991); and Dukes, Martinez, and Stein (1997) have all conceptualized gangs within a social disorganization model.

Social strain theory originated with Robert Merton (1957), who borrowed the term *anomie* from the work of the 19th century French sociologist, Emile Durkheim (1915). *Anomie* refers to inconsistencies between social conditions and opportunities for growth, fulfillment, and productivity within society. According to social strain theory, the incongruity between goals and a legitimate means to achieve them leads to a deviant subculture. Hagedorn's (1997) research with Milwaukee gangs was conceptualized within social strain theory.

Cultural deviance theory proposed delinquency is a result of an attempt to conform to cultural values that are in conflict with conventional society, which then forces the formation of a delinquent subculture. Cohen (1955), Cloward and Ohlin (1960), and Miller (1969) all found in separate research studies incongruities between opportunity and social conditions that support the attainment of respectable goals. Their research was conceptualized within cultural deviance theory.

Social bond or social control theory is a theory of prevention (Hirschi, 1969). This theory suggests people are bonded to society through the validity of their beliefs and values, and because of this strong bond, one does not commit crime. The research of Travis Hirschi (1969) conceptualized gangs within this framework and defined the elements of the bond as *attachment* (to significant others); *commitment* (to ideal requirements of childhood); *involvement* (in structured time activities); and *belief* (in law and morality), thus forming a subculture in lieu of the ideal society.

Social learning theory purported that criminal and delinquent behaviors are learned through a subcultural process that is like that of any other learning process. Edward Sutherland (1947) described "differential associations" in his research, suggesting that delinquent youth learn by their association with other delinquent youth. The work of Ferrera-Pinto, Ramos, and Mata (1997), as well as that of Sutherland (1947), were conceptualized within social learning theory.

The labeling perspective (Becker, 1963) addresses the relatedness of how and why certain actions are labeled criminal; the response to the crime on the part of authorities; and the effects of these definitions and responses by officials on labeled persons. Often such labeled persons within the overriding culture form a delinquent subculture.

Critical Marxist theory (Quinney, 1970) argues that much of what is known about gang behavior, including gang-related crimes, can be understood as an attempt by an oppressed subculture to accommodate and resist the problems created by capitalist institutions. The research by Quinney (1970, 1977) and Quinney and Trevino (2001) about gangs was conceptualized within critical Marxist theory and goes on to discuss capitalistic systems and crimes of control which are the crimes committed by the oppressing group and are related to control and domination over the oppressed. These are oftentimes crimes committed by the government in an attempt to control and be dominant over people.

In summary, many current social, psychological, and anthropological theories support the concept of gang formation by adolescents who are unable to fit into the norms of society. These subcultures serve various functions including protection and maintaining a personal reputation.

> Most gang boys are driven by a need for what they call "rep." Reputation, standing, is the most important thing in their lives. They're denied it in their homes. The schools, overcrowded and understaffed, can't give it to them. So they look for it in their gangs. That explains why they fight such ferocious wars over the right to softball fields or a stolen girlfriend or a casual shove or some imaginary insult. (Bloch & Niederhoffer, 1958, p. 166)

The 1960s and 1970s are not well represented in the literature in relation to gangs. This may be due to the denial of the presence of or any significant problem with gangs (Albanese, 1994). During this time, many major metropolitan cities dissolved their gang task forces, believing the problem no longer existed (*Juvenile Justice Bulletin*, 1989). The antiwar movement, the emphasis on peace, the search for freedom, and the unrest that caused middle- and upper-class society to reexamine their core values and beliefs took attention away from urban street violence (Sheldon et al., 1997, 2003).

Focus on adolescent gangs began to increase again during the late 1980s and early 1990s once the interest in the "hippie" counterculture movement had subsided (Sheldon et al., 2003). Public fear of adolescent gangs increased exponentially during this time, as news reports highlighted violence and random killings of innocent people. These adolescent gangs soon realized that they could control others by fear and intimidation; this became their main mode of operation, which led to even greater public fear. In response to increased public cry for safety, many cities reinstated gang task forces (Boyle, 2010; Sheldon et al., 2003). Additionally, gangs from other countries began moving inside U.S. borders, further threatening public safety and projecting fear on citizens. An example is the famous Mara Salvatrucha (MS-13) gang, whose members traveled from El Salvador to Los Angeles to protect the El Salvadoran immigrants who had previously moved to the area (Ward, 2013).

The 21st century has seen governments institute multiple gang-related prevention and antiviolence programs (Sheldon et al., 2003; Ward, 2013). The major economic work of adolescent gangs remains unchanged from the late 1980s and 1990s, and includes drug and weapon sales. Gang-related research has also become more prominent, particularly in the fields of criminal justice and sociology. However, increased research and increased funding for and proliferation of prevention programs have not demonstrated a significant reduction in the number of gangs, nor their level of violence and activity within American society (Sheldon et al., 2003).

RESEARCH DESIGN

This transcultural research study was designed using the ethnonursing research method. Generally, findings from the method are reported in themes and patterns. However, sometimes findings emerge from the data that are neither a theme nor a pattern, but are additional findings important to culture care theory. In this study, four universal themes (Morris, 2012) and one diverse theme (Morris & McComish, 2012) emerged. The additional finding (and topic of this chapter) that emerged from the data was defining *subculture* within the African American culture. The finding of adolescent gangs as subcultures is significant because it helps us understand how diverse subcultures function within the structure of dominant ethnic cultures, as well as supports the anthropological definition of a subculture. It is important to understand that many groups function within a culture that are not necessarily subcultures of the overriding culture, but represent social groups that have formed based on a common bond. These social groups should not be confused with a subculture, as they do not fit the accepted parameters of a subculture as carefully defined by anthropology, sociology, and nursing.

ETHNONURSING RESEARCH QUESTIONS

The domain of inquiry (DOI) for this study was the expressions, meanings, and cultural lifeways of African American adolescent gang members and their daily and nightly experiences within their environmental context.

- What are the caring expressions, meanings, functions, interpretations, and practices of African American adolescents within the gang?
- What are the holistic social and cultural factors influencing African American adolescent gang members in the urban setting?

- What are the caring behaviors of African Americans that influence their adolescents to join gangs?
- What are the purposes of selected African American adolescent gang member expressions and practices in American society?
- What are the culture care needs of African American gang members in the urban setting?
- What are the African American gang members' emic generic care expectations and what are the etic professional care expectations of nurses?
- What nursing decisions and actions related to Leininger's three modes of care preservation and/or maintenance, accommodation and/or negotiation, and repatterning and/or restructuring are necessary to provide culturally congruent care to African American adolescent gang members that is safe and health promoting?
- Can African American gang expressions be repatterned into healthier lifeways?
- Does a gang subculture exist within the African American culture for many adolescents?

In using Leininger's culture care theory, an open discovery approach within the qualitative paradigm of the ethnonursing research method was used to guide the researcher to discover constructs of culture care. Predetermined expectations of participants were held in abeyance so as to obtain their emic views and experiences.

ORIENTATIONAL DEFINITIONS

In order to systematically study in depth the stated domain of inquiry, maintain consistency with the tenets of the theory, and follow the purposes of the investigation, the following orientational definitions were adapted from the culture care theory for the study within the ethnonursing qualitative method:

- Caring: Refers to actions and activities directed toward assisting, supporting, or enabling another individual or group with evident or anticipated needs to ameliorate or improve a human condition or lifeway, or to face death (Leininger, 1991, p. 46).
- Gangs: Refers to a group or collectivity of persons with a common identity who interact in cliques or sometimes as a whole group on a fairly regular basis and whose activities the community may view in varying degrees as legitimate, illegitimate, criminal, or some combination thereof; and who are distinguished from other youth groups

by their communal, collective, or fraternal relationships (adapted from Curry & Spergel, 1992).

- Gang subculture: Refers to a collective group of young African Americans who deviate in certain ways, particularly illegal activities including drug sales, violence, and thefts from the African American culture and the dominant culture, yet who have many attributes in common with the ethnic culture's values, beliefs, and lifeways and some characteristics of the dominant culture (adapted from Cohen, 1955; Leininger, 1995; Sheldon et al., 1997).
- Gang members: Refers to African American adolescents who are associated with an urban street gang (Morris, 2004, p. 16).
- Adolescent: Refers to a young person who may or may not have engaged in criminal behavior and is between the age of 10 and 17 years.
- Gang violence: Refers to destructive gang behaviors that may result in physical injuries, handicaps, or death to the gang member, rival gang member, or non-gang member (Morris, 2004, p. 16).
- African American adolescents: Refers to young people who identify themselves as of African American descent and living in the United States.
- Culture: Refers to the learned, shared, and transmitted values, beliefs, norms, and lifeways of African American adolescent gang members that guide their thinking, decisions, and actions in patterned ways (adapted from Leininger, 1991, p. 47).
- Cultural values: Refers to the powerful directive forces that give order and meaning to African American gang members' decisions and actions (adapted from Leininger, 1978, 1991, 1995).
- Enculturation: Refers to in-depth learning about a culture with its specific values, beliefs, and practices in order to prepare children and adults to function or to live effectively in a particular culture (Leininger, 1995).
- Socialization: Refers to the process of learning the ways of the gang subculture (adapted from Leininger, 1995; Oswalt, 1986).
- Culture care diversity: Refers to the variability and/or differences in meanings, patterns, values, lifeways, or symbols of care within or between collectivities that are related to assistive, supportive, or enabling caring expressions of gang members (Leininger, 1991, p. 47).
- Culture care universality: Refers to the common, similar, or dominant uniform care meanings, patterns, values, lifeways, or symbols of care within or between collectivities that are related to assistive, supportive, or enabling caring expressions of gang members (adapted from Leininger, 1991, p. 47).

- Generic care: Refers to learned and transmitted, indigenous, gang subculture knowledge and skills used to provide assistive, supportive, enabling, or facilitative acts toward or for another gang member or the collectivity of the gang with evident or anticipated needs, to ameliorate or improve a human lifeway or health condition, or to deal with despair and death situations (adapted from Leininger, 1991).
- Professional care system: Refers to formally taught, learned, transmitted professional care, health, illness, wellness, and related knowledge and practice skills that prevail in professional institutions usually with multidisciplinary personnel to serve customers (Leininger, 1991, p. 48).
- Health: Refers to a state of wellbeing that is culturally defined, valued, and practiced, and which reflects the ability of individuals to perform their daily role activities in culturally expressed, beneficial, and patterned lifeways (Leininger, 1991, p. 48).
- Culture care preservation and/or maintenance: Refers to those assistive, supporting, facilitative, or enabling professional actions and decisions that help African American gang members retain and/ or preserve relevant care values to help maintain wellbeing, recover from illness, prevent violence or destructive acts, or face handicaps, despair, and/or death (adapted from Leininger, 1991, p. 48).
- Culture care accommodation and/or negotiation: Refers to those assistive, supporting, facilitative, or enabling creative professional actions and decisions that help African American adolescent gang members to adapt to, or to negotiate with, others for safe, beneficial, or satisfying health and wellbeing outcomes (adapted from Leininger, 1991, p. 48).
- Culture care repatterning and/or restructuring: Refers to those assistive, supporting, facilitative, or enabling professional actions and decisions that help African American adolescent gang members to reorder, change, or greatly modify their lifeways for new, different, and beneficial health beliefs and still providing a more beneficial or healthier lifeway than before the changes were co-established with the adolescents (adapted from Leininger, 1991, p. 49).
- Cultural congruent (nursing) care: Refers to those cognitively based assistive, supportive, facilitative, or enabling acts or decisions that are tailor-made to fit with the gang member subculture, the gang, or the dominant African American cultural values, beliefs, lifeways in order to provide or support meaningful, beneficial, and satisfying health-care or wellbeing services (adapted from Leininger, 1991, p. 49).

- Culturally competent care: Refers to the use of culturally based or subculturally based knowledge that is used in sensitive, creative, and meaningful ways to fit with the general lifeways of the gang subculture and leads to beneficial and satisfying health, wellbeing, and care or to face violence, difficult situations, disabilities, or death (adapted from Leininger, 1978, 1991, 1995).
- Cultural context: Refers to the totality of shared meanings and life experiences in a particular social situation, cultural, subcultural, and physical environment that influences attitudes, thinking, and patterns of behavior (adapted from Leininger, 1995).

ASSUMPTIVE PREMISES OF THE RESEARCH

The following assumptive premises for this study were adapted from Leininger's (1991) work:

- Culture care for urban African American adolescent gang members was aimed at promoting safety, health, and wellbeing and to ameliorate the harsh lifeways on the streets.
- Culture care meanings, practices, and lifeways can be discovered within the social structure factors of the African American adolescent gang culture, along with the diversities and commonalities from the African American culture.

METHOD

Setting

The research setting centered on a charter school that enrolled children and adolescents from kindergarten age through junior high school. Traditional grade categories, such as first grade, seventh grade, and so on, were not used in this school. The building had formerly been a parochial grade school and was attached to an active Roman Catholic church. The church participated in the activities of the school through board memberships, teacher assistants, and maintenance of the building. The school was located in a poor urban area of a Midwestern city. Three housing projects were located within close proximity to the school, and many of the students came from one of these projects. The homes in the area were older, and the surrounding neighborhoods had obviously been established long ago. Students were enrolled from all over the city, but the greatest number came from the urban area immediately adjacent to the school.

The building was typical of an older school, with wide hallways and central staircases; the ground floor contained the cafeteria, gymnasium, and restrooms. Classrooms were located on the second and third floors and were large; one wall in each room had windows typical of the era in which the school was built. The adolescents' classrooms contained several round tables with four to five chairs at each table. There were many posters and wall hangings with motivational messages on them. One room was painted bright yellow, and the other a medium pink.

Initially, the researcher sat to the side of the room and observed; then later sat at the table with the students and helped with class assignments or homework. Once the researcher and the students were comfortable with one another, the individual interviews began. After the initial interview with the key participants, the researcher told them that she would be giving $25 to the class trip fund for each participant in the study. Additionally, the researcher had candy that the key participants were allowed to eat during the interview. The candy was a major incentive in the beginning for them to come to the interview. As one participant said, "You didn't even need to give us $25 for our field trip; the candy was all you needed to get us to talk to you."

Two of the key participants wanted to start a "candy business" at school where they could make money for a class trip and also have a percentage for themselves. The researcher helped them start the candy business as a class project. The students learned to keep a ledger and knew how much money was needed each week to buy more candy for the following week. The net profit was divided equally between the spring trip fund and the two key participants. The researcher also participated actively with the school and the participants through dances, parent–teacher organization (PTO) meetings, graduation, field trips, and funerals.

The researcher believes that the stories of the youth were consistent with naturalistic inquiry (Leininger, 1991; Lincoln & Guba, 1985), while a safe environment was provided for discussions with each of the key participants. Most of the interviews with key participants took place in different school rooms, but were private at the time of the interview.

General participant interviews took place in a variety of settings, as mentioned previously. While safety is always an issue in an urban environment, less vigilance was required when choosing a place to meet with general participants. Additionally, it was beneficial to be out in the community of the key participants, so the researcher could have more knowledge of the naturalistic setting of the participants.

The urban African American adolescent gang members were asked to talk about their daily lifeways, values, and beliefs about care, caring, wellbeing, and health using a form of expression that was comfortable for them. The Sunrise Enabler and the Open Inquiry Guide (described in the Data Analysis section), along with the two assumptive premises of the culture care theory, were used to guide the research and the discussion (Leininger, 1991).

Selection of Participants

General participants were asked to express the daily lifeways, values, and beliefs related to their interactions with gang members through a dialogue with the researcher. According to Leininger, in an ethnonursing study, the term *informant* is typically used instead of participants. However, there are instances where this term may not be culturally appropriate. This was the case with this study which focused on teenage gang members who had extensive experiences with the legal system. Therefore, this study's informants will be referred to as participants throughout. Upon further reflection regarding these terms, Dr. Leininger indicated she believed that using participants was much more congruent with the theory "...as it implies more active and equal participation in the study" (M. M. Leininger, personal communication, unknown date, 2004).

Key and general participants are important sources for transcultural nurse-researchers to learn about the people and their cultural care expressions, meanings, and lifeways and in order to enhance wellbeing and health by providing culturally congruent care. Key participants are the most knowledgeable about the domain of inquiry and are believed to accurately reflect norms, values, beliefs, and lifeways about the culture being studied and are generally the most interested in participating in the study (Leininger, 1991). General participants are less knowledgeable about the domain of inquiry, but have general ideas about the domain and are able to accurately give information from an etic perspective (Leininger, 1991).

Thirteen key participants—11 male and 2 female—were purposefully selected for the study to explicate the domain of inquiry: Adolescents who declared or were known urban street gang members; adolescents between 10 and 15 years of age; adolescents who were African American; adolescents interested in participating in three or four interviews; and adolescents with signed informed and voluntary consents. Most of the key participants were interviewed at an urban charter school in a Midwestern city where they were students. Some key participants lived in the community surrounding the school and were volunteer assistants with the basketball team at the school.

Twenty-eight general participants who were familiar with African American gang members, but were not part of that subculture, were purposefully selected for the study. The general participants all had contact with urban African American adolescent gang members in some manner. They included teachers, school staff, and administrators; former gang members; nurses who cared for gang members; juvenile detention staff; adolescent friends or peers of gang members; parents, foster parents, and families of gang members; and ministers of gang members. Adolescents who were non-gang members, but were from urban areas and knew and recognized gang members, also shared their viewpoints.

Data Collection

The researcher interviewed the key participants from two to five times, for a period of one to four hours per interview. The interviews in the first part of the data collection process were generally about an hour, but as the researcher moved further along the continuum from stranger to trusted friend, the interview time increased greatly in length and frequency. The interviews were generally one on one, but on some occasions, two participants came together. The last encounter with the key participants occurred near the end of the school year, when 10 of the 13 participants requested to meet together around a table to talk about their lifeways. There were a number of occasions where the participants asked if they could "rap" their story. This involved more than one participant, as one could "beat" (with two pencils on the desktop) while the other would rap. The rap interviews were not transcribed for use in this study because of difficulty in accurately transcribing the tapes. There were many impromptu interactions with the key participants (e.g., over lunch, in the hallway, in the car while taking them home from school) where there was no tape recorder running and no data were collected. The rap and the impromptu interactions were used merely to add richness to the contextual background of the study.

The general participants were interviewed once for a period of 1 to 2 hours. These interviews took place in a variety of informal settings. For example, the researcher invited a group of mothers and caregivers to a Saturday morning breakfast at a Bob Evans Restaurant for the purpose of discussing their children and gangs. Interviews took place both at the school and in the community so the researcher could gain a broad perspective on the lifeways of urban African American adolescent gang members in their naturalistic settings. Interviews took place on porches, at kitchen tables, at school functions, on the sidewalks of the neighborhood, and at churches.

Five to six hours per week were spent with individual adolescents. Leininger's (1991) Observation–Participation–Reflection Enabler was used to gain entry into the subculture of the gang. Field notes were kept from the initial entry into the setting. All formal interviews were recorded. The data collection phase ended with evidence of saturation of data (Leininger, 1991).

Human Subjects Considerations

Written consent forms were sent home with the participants and reviewed verbally with parents or custodial caregivers, either in person at the school or by telephone, and the significance of the certificate of confidentiality was described to them. Once the signed consent forms were returned, their son or daughter would be approached about participating in the study. The study purpose was explained, along with what they would be asked to talk about. Each part of the adolescent written assent was reviewed with the participants, and they signed the assent form if they chose to participate. They were informed that they could discontinue participation at any time and they could choose when they wanted to be interviewed. All interviews took place during the school day, and plans were made with teachers so that students would be taken out of class only at times specified by the teacher.

All participants were given a copy of the written consent/assent form and explanation of the study. Information about the details of the study was discussed with each participant individually and given to them in writing, and included risks and benefits of participating in the study, their right to withdraw at any time, protection from harm, and adherence to confidentiality. The certificate of confidentiality from the National Institutes of Mental Health was discussed in detail with each participant.

Each participant was told that the certificate of confidentiality gave them assurance that the information they shared would be held in confidence and reported only as group data. The researcher shared that she did not want them to report any crimes, because that was not the purpose of the research, but if they mentioned a crime incidentally during the interview, it would not be reported to law enforcement, nor could the tapes and transcriptions be subpoenaed into a court of law. Participants were also informed that the certificate of confidentiality did not cover abuse of any sort, and in the event that they reported elder or child abuse, the researcher would be required to report that particular action to authorities.

The key participants became increasingly comfortable in talking with the researcher about impactful situations that had occurred on the streets. It was difficult for the key participants to understand that at the conclusion of the data collection phase, when the certificate of confidentiality had expired, they could no longer talk with the researcher about certain criminal activities. The researcher always reminded them whenever they wanted to talk that the certificate of confidentiality had expired, and while they could still talk, they must know that any criminal activity mentioned would now have to be reported to law enforcement authorities.

DATA ANALYSIS

Leininger's (1991) *Four Phases of Data Analysis Guide* was used in analyzing the data collected during the study beginning at the data collection phase. This enabler was essential to obtain "rigorous, in-depth, and systematic analysis of ethnonursing qualitative research data and especially research findings bearing on the theory of culture care" (Leininger, 1991, p. 94). During Phase I, the raw data were collected, described, and documented with the use of a field journal, tape recorder, and computer. During Phase II, descriptors were identified and categorized. Patterns and context analyses were done simultaneously during Phase III. Finally, major themes, research findings, theoretical formulations, and recommendations were identified and presented during the fourth phase (Leininger, 1991, p. 95).

A qualitative paradigmatic inquiry requires the use of qualitative evaluation criteria so that truth in the findings can be assured. Using evaluation methods appropriate to the paradigm of the study was essential given that the purposes, goals, predicted outcomes, and philosophical underpinnings differ between qualitative and quantitative paradigms (Leininger, 1991). Leininger expanded Lincoln and Guba's (1985) criteria from four to six criteria for evaluating qualitative ethnonursing research. This set of six criteria was used to evaluate data collected in this study:

- *Credibility*, which refers to the truth of the findings, and derives largely from the emic findings throughout the observation participation and reflection phases of the study
- *Confirmability*, which refers to the repeated descriptions from key and general participants and reaffirms the researcher's observation, participation, and reflection
- *Meaning-in-context*, which refers to the significance of the findings within the emic environment of the participant
- *Recurrent patterning*, which refers to the repeated experiences and lifeways of participants designating patterns that are repeated over time
- *Saturation*, which refers to taking in all that was known or understood about the phenomena under study with no further new discoveries emerging from the data
- *Transferability*, which refers to whether the findings from the study would have similar meanings with similar environments, contexts, or circumstances

Quotations were critically analyzed to discover patterns of behavior, structural meanings, and contextual analysis. Interpretations, components, or categories of data were examined to demonstrate recurrent patterning. The researcher sought credibility, confirmability, meaning-in-context, recurrent patterning, and saturation of the data. Culture care patterns were identified from the participants' observations, recurrent participant descriptors, raw data, and field notes from the school and urban environments. Patterns were derived from field observations, descriptors, and the raw data that supported each theme.

THEMATIC FINDINGS AND SUPPORTIVE CARE PATTERNS

Four universal themes (Morris, 2012) and one diverse theme (Morris & McComish, 2012) were discovered from the data. Nineteen transcultural care patterns supported these themes (**Table 8-1**).

The *dominant* care constructs discovered in this culture care study included *respect; concern for others; being listened to and accepted; love;* and *faith in God,* which had all been reported in previous studies with African Americans (Leininger, 1991; Morgan, 2002).

The universal care constructs of *protection, surveillance, trust/confidentiality,* and *worthiness* and the diverse care construct of *hope versus despair* were new discoveries from the study that had not been found in any previous culture care studies with African Americans (Morris, 2004). It is this second set of care constructs that defined and described the African American gang subculture.

During the interviews, gang members consistently talked about the importance of watching out for each other and for family and friends (surveillance). They spoke of "having each other's backs" and the need to care for and protect their family and friends from harm (protection). Confidentiality and being able to trust caregivers were critically important to them, as they discussed not knowing whether to give full disclosure in healthcare settings about issues of health and safety. Most of the gang members spoke of feeling "unworthy" or having their "dignity" stripped from them. They were tired of always being on the bottom, so they needed to do something the best—even if that meant being the best at killing. They talked about the lack of opportunities to be able to achieve things that would make them feel worthy. Younger gang members expressed hope for a house in the suburbs with a white picket fence, having a family, getting a "good education," and "making something of themselves." Older gang members (13 years and older) demonstrated a lack of hope; their hope

Table 8-1 Transcultural Care Themes

Care Themes	Social Structures [where discovered]	Pattern 1	Pattern 2	Pattern 3	Pattern 4
Culture care for African American adolescent gang members:		African American adolescent gang members:	African American adolescent gang members:	African American adolescent gang members:	African American adolescent gang members:
Universal Theme I: Means giving and receiving respect, being listened to and accepted as a worthwhile human being, receiving recognition and guidance from adult caregivers in order to promote health and wellbeing.	Kinship and family Religious/philosophical Political/legal Social and cultural lifeways	Offer respect to adults and want to be respected in return, thereby leading to a meaningful interaction.	Believe that being present with them and being listened to as they describe their lifeways is essential for adult caregivers to guide them in making decisions to promote healthier lifeways.	Want to be accepted by nurses and other professional caregivers as they expressed remorseful feelings over their destructive lifeways.	Want recognition as a means of building self-esteem and enhancing emotional wellbeing.
Universal Theme II: Includes the importance of adult caregivers understanding that protection and surveillance are essential in order to develop safe, loyal, and trustworthy support systems to survive the tumultuous life cycle in their urban environment.	Kinship and family Economic Social and cultural lifeways	Want to be protected from making destructive life choices that may jeopardize their health and wellbeing.	Use destructive ways to survive in their urban environment and need to learn healthier ways of coping with stress associated with their urban living.	Experience stress associated with feeling concern for and worrying about others close to them, and need to learn healthier coping expressions.	Believed trusting and loyal relationships with nurses and other healthcare providers were essential in feeling safe and maintaining health in the urban environment.

Universal Theme III: Is related to spiritual-religious beliefs and practices and is a means to ameliorate harsh realities of the urban environment and promote wellbeing.	Kinship and family Religious/philosophical Social and cultural lifeways	View God as omnipotent and belief in and dependence on Him as essential to their health and wellbeing.	Practice formal rituals at sacred events, such as funerals, as a means of professing their spiritual beliefs and to grieve loss.	View religion as a social coming together of friends and family with similar beliefs about God in order to promote emotional wellbeing and build self-esteem.	Memorialize local leaders who had been killed in gang warfare and give them respected status in their neighborhood.
Universal Theme IV: Means nurses having knowledge and understanding of the emotional, cultural, physical, and environmental pain, the role of economy in urban lifeways to soften the pain, and acting on that understanding with a genuine compassion to assist them in ameliorating the pain.	Kinship and family Religious/philosophical Social and cultural lifeways	Express remorse over using illegal economic means to help others and to relieve pain associated with urban living, and want to find new ways to meet material needs.	Need to learn alternative and safe strategies for dealing with life-cycle changes related to adolescence as a means of promoting healthy emotional and social maturation.	Need to trust and confide in respected and knowledgeable nurses for guidance in order to promote emotional wellbeing and healthy lifestyles.	Need to know that they were worthy of care from professional caregivers, and that the actions of these professional caregivers are honest and sincere and aimed at improving their caring lifeways.

(continues)

Table 8-1 Transcultural Care Themes (*continued*)

Diverse Theme I:	Social and cultural lifeways of the gang	Ages 12 and under look forward to their future with anticipation of completing high school, going to college, becoming gainfully employed as a professional, and having a happy family, a nice home, and a car.	From 13 years of age and up, hold little hope for health and wellbeing including being alive long enough to finish high school, being able to go to college, having a healthy family and a decent home, car, and job.
Express diversity in meanings and beliefs related to hope for health and well-being in their future.	Age/experience		

© Edith Morris, 2004.

had diminished to the level of simply staying alive and staying out of jail (Morris, 2012; Morris & McComish, 2012).

In addition to demonstrating care constructs *atypical* of the dominant African American culture, there was precise structure to the gang subculture that functioned intentionally to improve the lifeways of poor urban-dwelling African Americans as well as to maintain the organizational integrity of the gang. Hand-signing in a gang-specific language functioned to maintain the social structure integrity of the gang and keep its members and their families safe in a turbulent environment. Drug and weapon sales brought in substantial income through an illegal underground economy where gang members could meet many material needs and desires for themselves and their families. They wore specific clothing styles and colors that identified them as members of a particular group and were recognized by and feared for their violent activities. The care constructs discovered in this ethnonursing transcultural study, along with specific social structures and cultural functions, identified the gang as a subculture of the dominant African American culture.

DISCUSSION OF GANG SUBCULTURE

Evidence of the gang as a subculture was reflected by the unique language they used throughout the interviews and other conversations between the researcher and the key participants. Words were given alternative meanings such as *cheddar* for money, *ride* for car, *crib* for home, and *hood* for neighborhood, just to name a few. Sometimes these words were to engender unity within the subculture of the urban African American adolescent gang and sometimes they were specifically gang-related terms. The following are a few descriptors that reflect some of the unique language spoken by the gang subculture:

- K-2: Like maybe my girl be needin' some *cheddar* (money).
- K-2: They be comin' in our *hood* (neighborhood) and shootin' bullets.
- K-7: Like sell stuff to other gangs to set 'em up, but then you know its turnaround time because they *silly cattin'* [deceiving] them.
- K-9: You a Blood, I'm a Crip, and the chair's a Folk. We switch. I'm a Folk, the chair's a Blood, and you a Crip. That's a *flip-flop* [changing colors]. They kill ya for doin' that.
- K-10: You break their rules, you lie to the group, you die. They call you a *donut* (dishonest person).
- K-12: The whole group goes to her *crib* (home) after the dance.

Urban African American adolescent gang members were part of a lucrative and illegal underground economy within the urban area of the city.

Illegal weapons and street drugs were sold at top market value. Through sales related to drugs and weapons, gang members were able to make significantly more money than other members of the African American culture. Material wealth gave them respect and afforded human pleasures otherwise unattainable to them. K-12 noted that the gang members chose the illegal economy as opposed to respectable jobs:

> The only reason people wanna go out and sell dope rather than work at McDonald's is they want the fast money and they ain't lookin' at the long term. They lookin' for the day rather than the future.

A major worry was getting caught and losing pocket money for the day. As K-5 stated:

> They [police] gonna get wise one day, and you gonna sell it to the wrong person, and get locked behind bars, even though you probably only get 10 days. Then you still gotta worry that they [police] took almost $3,000 outta your pocket and drugs. Now you ain't got no money or drugs to get started up again.

African American adolescent gang members wore colors and/or color combinations uniquely representative of their gang. Color was a major identifier of a gang member, and most gang members wore their colors proudly. K-2 confirmed this when he said:

> Like if we wear blue [Crips] all the time, we only care about the people that wear blue. The people that wear red [Bloods], they always care about the people that wear red. The people that wear red and green [North Side], they care about them two colors. But the people that wear red and green, they don't care about the people that wear blue.

In addition to color, there were other identifiers of gang membership, including rolling up a pant leg, shoe laces in one shoe, or one shoe tied, the other not tied, or hat turned to one special side. The particular pant leg rolled up, the shoe that contains the lace, and the side to which the hat has been turned were all signifiers of membership in a particular gang. University starter jackets have also been popular with gang members; the colors chosen are the same as the gang colors. These identifying signs of the gang subculture allowed members to be easily distinguished from the overriding African American culture.

Violent activity is another difference that separates the gang subculture from the dominant African American culture. Gang members carry guns and other weapons and use them to demand respect and to protect people, property, and drug sales territory. Owning a gun made them feel powerful over others—an attribute the dominant African American culture does not ascribe to. One female participant said:

> I beat people up. Guy, girl, it doesn't matter. Cuz that's me, that's all. I gotta tell everybody that you gonna mess with me, you gonna get beat up.

Retaliation is also a big part of the violence between gangs in the gang subculture. K-11 said:

> Like in some cases, the Crips wanna get the Bloods for killin' one of they people. Now the Bloods wanna get the Crips cuz they killed one of they people.

CONCLUSION

Understanding the unique destructive lifeways of gang subcultures is important because they exemplify the importance of culturally congruent care. Knowing and understanding the gestalt of their caring and noncaring lifeways may assist nurses to recognize the uniquely identifying behaviors exhibited by gang members. An in-depth understanding of African American urban gang subcultures is essential for nurses to collaborate with them to mutually restructure and repattern their unhealthy lifeways and to provide culturally congruent care.

DEDICATION

It is with great honor that I dedicate this chapter to the memory of Dr. Madeleine Leininger, my mentor, teacher, supporter, and friend. She not only instilled in me the importance of making new discoveries about cultures, but more importantly helped me to see cultures with new eyes.

Additionally, I would like to dedicate this chapter to the memory of my parents, John and Mildred Morris. My dad encouraged me to become a nurse from the time I was very young because he admired the profession deeply, and Mom was a constant source of support and encouragement throughout my many years in school.

ACKNOWLEDGMENTS

I wish to gratefully acknowledge the efforts of Dr. Karen Burkett, who read this chapter when it was in its infancy, with a close eye to detail, offering suggestions and ideas as well as healthy discussion about the concept of a subculture.

The research study on which this chapter is based was funded in part by the Madeleine Leininger Endowed Transcultural Nursing Dissertation Award.

DISCUSSION QUESTIONS

1. Discuss the influences of African American and other adolescent gang subcultures in urban society within the United States.
2. Discuss the influences of adolescent gang subcultures within cultures frequently encountered personally and/or professionally.
3. Discuss how your nursing care practices will be influenced by the subculture knowledge gained from this chapter.
4. Discuss the concept of a subculture as defined in this chapter. Are there other ways that you would define subculture? What criteria are important to defining a subculture? Do definitions of subculture and culture vary depending on the context of the environment? The situation?
5. As mentioned in this chapter, the term *subculture* was coined by early sociologists as a means to study adolescent groups that pulled away from mainstream culture—specifically, gangs. Do you think this was an appropriate action on their part? Do you think this action has limited or broadened the use of the term *subculture* to fit other groups within cultures?
6. Discuss differences in the term *subculture* from anthropological, sociological, and nursing/healthcare perspectives. Discuss five groups that exist in society today that can each be called a subculture and then list five that you believe are not a subculture State criteria for why you believe these groups are or are not subcultures.
7. Define and then evaluate the concept of subculture in relation to advancing nursing knowledge through research. Is understanding of subcultures important in research and advancing the science?
8. Discuss the importance or lack of importance to understanding adolescent gangs as a subculture to nursing? To health care in general? What can be learned from studies of adolescent gangs to help make communities safer and healthier?
9. Discuss similarities and differences in gang structure and function worldwide. What was present in each societal culture that caused the proliferation of gangs and, in many cases, violence? How can knowledge of gangs and gang activity lead to peace? What can societies do to bring about peace and offer hope in their communities based on this knowledge? How may gangs be used to promote health and safety?

10. How is the Theory of Culture Care Diversity and Universality useful for studying the adolescent gang subculture?

REFERENCES

Albanese, J. (1994). *Dealing with delinquency: The future of juvenile justice* (2nd ed.). Chicago, IL: Nelson-Hall.

Balme, J. F. (1985). Gangs in Novelle-Nelande. *Journal de la Socciete des Oceanistes-Paris, 41*(81), 275–278.

Becker, H. (1963). *Outsiders: Studies in the sociology of deviance.* New York, NY: Free Press.

Bloch, B. A., & Niederhoffer, A. (1958). *The gang: A study in adolescent behavior.* New York, NY: Philosophical Library.

Boyle, G. (2010). *Tattoos on the heart: The power of boundless compassion.* New York, NY: Free Press.

Brake, M. (2003). *Comparative youth culture: The sociology of youth culture and youth subcultures in America, Britain, and Canada.* New York, NY: Routledge.

Cloward, R. A., & Ohlin, L. E. (1960). *Delinquency and opportunity: A theory of delinquent gangs.* New York, NY: Free Press.

Cohen, A. K. (1955). *Delinquent boys: The culture of the gang.* New York, NY: Free Press.

Covey, C., Menard, S., & Franzese, R. (1992). *Juvenile gangs.* Springfield, IL: C. S. Thomas.

Curry, G., & Spergel, I. (1992). Gang involvement and delinquency among Hispanic and African American males. *Journal of Research in Crime and Delinquency, 29*(3), 273–291.

Dukes, R., Martinez, R., & Stein, J. (1997). Precursors and consequences of membership in youth gangs. *Youth and Society, 29*(2), 139–165.

Durkheim, E. (1915). *The elementary forms of the religious life* [translated by J. W. Swain (1965)]. New York, NY: Free Press.

Eggleston, E. (1997). Boys' talk: Exploring gender discussions with New Zealand male youth gang members. *Caribbean Journal of Criminology and Social Psychology, 2*(2), 119–214.

Ferreira-Pinto, J. B., Ramos, R. & Mata, A. (1997). Dangerous relationships: Effects of early exposure to violence in women's lives. In M. O. Loustaunau & M. Sanchez-Bane (Eds.), *Life, death, and in-between on the U.S.–Mexico border.* Westport, CT: Greenwood.

Fine, G., & Kleinman, S. (1979). Rethinking subculture: An interactionist analysis. *American Journal of Sociology, 85*(1), 1–20.

Glaser, C. (1992). Mark of Zorro: Sexuality and gender relations in the Tsotsi subculture on the Witwatersrand. *African Studies—Johannesburg, 51*(1), 47–67.

Glittenberg, J. (2008). *Violence and hope in a U.S.–Mexico border town.* Long Grove, IL: Waveland Press.

Goddard, M. (1992). Big-man, thief: The social organization of gangs in Port Moresby. *Canberra Anthropology, 15*(1), 20–34.

Goldstein, A. P. (1991). *Delinquent gangs: A psychological perspective.* Champaign, IL: Research Press.

Hagedorn, J. M. (1997). Homeboys, new jacks, and anomie. *Journal of African American Men, 3*(1), 7–28.

Haviland, W., Prins, H., McBride, B., & Walrath, D. (2011). *Cultural anthropology: The human challenge* (13th ed.). Belmont, CA: Wadsworth.

Hay, D., Linebaugh, J., & Rule, E. (1975). *Albion's fatal three: Crime and society in eighteenth century England.* New York, NY: Pantheon.

Herzog, A., Mitchell, J., & Soccio, L. (1999). Interrogating subcultures. *Invisible Culture: An Electronic Journal for Visual Studies, 2,* 1–29.

Hirschi, T. (1969). *Causes of delinquency.* Berkeley, CA: University of California Press.

Hunt, G., Joe, K., & Waldorf, D. (1997). Culture and ethnic identity among Southeast Asian gang members. *Free Inquiry in Creative Sociology, 25*(1), 9–21.

Kulik, D. (1993). Heroes from hell: Representations of "rascals" in a Papua, New Guinea village. *Anthropology Today—London, 9*(3), 9–14.

Lee, F. (1998). Teens of the night: The night drifting and subculture of young people in Hong Kong. *International Journal of Adolescent Medicine and Health, 10*(3), 227–242.

Leininger, M. M. (1978). *Transcultural nursing: Concepts theories, and practices.* New York, NY: John Wiley and Sons.

Leininger, M. M. (1991). *Culture care diversity and universality: A theory of nursing.* New York, NY: National League for Nursing Press.

Leininger, M. M. (1994a). *Transcultural nursing: Concepts, theories, and practices.* Columbus, OH: Greyden Press.

Leininger, M. M. (1994b). Gadsup of Papua New Guinea revisited: A three decade view. *Journal of Transcultural Nursing, 5*(1), 21–29.

Leininger, M. M. (1995). *Transcultural nursing: Concepts, theories, and practices.* New York, NY: McGraw-Hill.

Leininger, M. M. (2002a). Essential transcultural nursing care concepts, principles, examples, and policy statements. In M. M. Leininger & M. R. McFarland (Eds.), *Transcultural nursing: Concepts, theories, research, & practice* (3rd ed., pp. 45–98). New York, NY: McGraw-Hill.

Leininger, M. M. (2002b). Part I: The theory of culture care and the ethnonursing research method. In M. M. Leininger & M. R. McFarland (Eds.), *Transcultural nursing: Concepts, theories, research, & practice* (3rd ed., pp. 71–98). New York, NY: McGraw-Hill.

Lincoln, Y., & Guba, E. (1985). *Naturalistic inquiry.* Newbury Park, CA: Sage.

Mark, G. (1997). Oakland Chinatown's first youth gang: The Suey Sing Boys. *Free Inquiry in Creative Sociology, 25*(1), 41–50.

Matthei, L., & Smith, D. (1998). Belizean "boyz 'n the hood"? *Comparative Urban and Community Research, 6,* 270–290.

Merton, R. (1957). *Social theory and social structure.* Glencoe, IL: Free Press.

Miller, W. (1958). Lower class culture as a generating milieu of gang delinquency. *Journal of Social Issues, 14*(3), 5–19.

Miller, W. (1969). American youth gangs: Past and present. In A. Blumberg (Ed.), *Current perspectives on criminal behavior* (pp. 291–320). New York, NY: Alford A. Knopf.

Montgomery, M. (1997). The powerlessness of punishment: Angry pride and delinquent identity. *Journal of Emotional and Behavioral Problems, 6*(3), 102–166.

Morgan, M. (2002). African Americans and culture care. In M. M. Leininger & M. R. McFarland (Eds.), *Transcultural nursing: Concepts, theories, research, & practice* (3rd ed., pp. 313–324). New York, NY: McGraw-Hill.

Morris, E. J. (2004*). An ethnonursing culture care study of the meanings, expressions and lifeways experiences of selected urban African American adolescent gang members* (Doctoral dissertation). Available from ProQuest Dissertations and Theses database (UMI No. 3130357).

Morris, E. (2012). Respect, protection, faith and love: Major care constructs identified within the subculture of selected urban African American adolescent gangs. *Journal of Transcultural Nursing, 23*(3), 262–269.

Morris, E., & McComish, J. (2012). Hope and despair: Listening to the voices of urban African American adolescent gang members. *International Journal of Human Caring, 16*(4), 51–57.

Nanda, S., & Warms, R. (2011). *Cultural anthropology* (2nd ed.). Belmont, CA: Wadsworth.

Nibbring, H., & Nand, E. (1992). Rascals in paradise: Urban gangs in Papua, New Guinea. *Pacific Studies—Laie, 15*(3), 113–115.

Office of Juvenile Justice and Delinquency Prevention. (1993). *Offenders in juvenile court, 1989. Juvenile Justice Bulletin.* Washington, DC: Author.

Orenstein, P. (1994). *School girls: Young women, self-esteem, and the confidence gap.* New York, NY: Doubleday.

Oswalt, W. (1986). *Life cycles and lifeways: An introduction to cultural anthropology.* Palo Alto, CA: Mayfield.

Pearson, G. (1983). *Hooligan: A history of respectable fears.* London, UK: Palgrave Macmillan.

Quinney, R. (1970). *The social reality of crime.* Boston, MA: Little, Brown.

Quinney, R. (1977). *Class state and crime: On the theory and practice of criminal justice.* New York, NY: David McKay.

Quinney, R., & Trevino, A. J. (2001). *The social reality of crime.* New Brunswick, NJ: Transaction.

Schmitz, S., & Christopher, J. (1997). Troubles in Smurftown: Youth gangs and moral visions in Guam. *Child Welfare, 76*(3), 411–428.

Sheldon, R. G., Tracy, S. K., & Brown, W. B. (1997). *Youth gangs in American society.* Belmont, CA: Wadsworth.

Sheldon, R. G., Tracy, S. K., & Brown, W. B. (2003). *Youth gangs in American society* (3rd ed.). Belmont, CA: Wadsworth.

Sutherland, E. (1947). *Principles of criminology.* Philadelphia, PA: Lippincott.

Taylor, C. (1989). *Dangerous society.* East Lansing, MI: Michigan State University Press.

Thrasher, F. (1927). *The gang.* Chicago, IL: University of Chicago Press.

Thrasher, F. (Ed.). (1963). *The gang: A study of 1,316 gangs in Chicago.* Chicago, IL: University of Chicago Press.

Valdez, A., & Kaplan, C. (1999). Reducing selection bias in the use of focus groups to investigate hidden populations: The case of Mexican American gang members from South Texas. *Drugs and Society, 14*(1–2), 209–224.

Ward, T. (2013). *Gangsters without borders: An ethnography of a Salvadoran street gang.* New York, NY: Oxford University Press.

Chapter 9

Synopsis of Findings Discovered Within a Descriptive Metasynthesis of Doctoral Dissertations Guided by the Culture Care Theory with Use of the Ethnonursing Research Method

Marilyn R. McFarland
Hiba B. Wehbe-Alamah
Helene B. Vossos
Mary Wilson

INTRODUCTION

Conceptualized within Leininger's Culture Care Theory of Diversity and Universality and using the ethnonursing research method, the purpose of this study was to present a descriptive metasynthesis of culture care findings

Revised Reprint from the *Online Journal of Cultural Competence in Nursing and Healthcare, 1*(2), 24–39.

from 23 doctoral dissertations found in the UMI Dissertation Abstracts database (see the Doctoral Dissertations Examined in Appendix 9-A at the end of this chapter for a list of these documents). The culture care findings presented are both interpretive and explanatory and were derived from further conceptualizations of the themes and patterns discovered in the original dissertation studies. New theoretical formulations based on the culture care theory and recommendations related to nursing practice were discovered. These findings were predicted to make a significant contribution to the discipline and practice of nursing as well as the epistemic and ontologic basis of culture care knowledge and evidence-based best practices.

DOMAIN OF INQUIRY

The domain of inquiry (DOI) for this study was the culture care expressions, beliefs, and practices of diverse and similar cultures. This DOI is central to the discipline of nursing and is of major importance to the profession because it may result in theory building and theory development, as well as a higher level of abstraction of findings beyond that of the individual studies examined. The researchers predicted that contributing to the existing body of knowledge previously created using the Theory of Culture Care Diversity and Universality and the ethnonursing research method might potentially benefit healthcare policy, evidence-based practices, nursing education, and future research.

RESEARCH QUESTIONS

The researchers were keenly interested in looking at the commonalities and differences in culture care, and wanted to examine how worldview, social structure factors, and environmental context influenced culture care. The researchers also wanted to discover ways in which Leininger's three nursing care modes of action and decision could be used to facilitate the provision of culturally congruent care. The following research questions were posed by the researchers so as to provide a solid foundation upon which to fully explore the domain of inquiry:

1. What are the commonalities and differences of culture care expressions, beliefs, and practices among people of diverse and similar cultures?
2. In what ways do worldview, social structure factors, and environmental context influence culture care expressions, beliefs, and practices of people of diverse and similar cultures?

3. In what ways can Leininger's three nursing care modes of action and decision facilitate the provision of culturally congruent care for people of diverse and similar cultures?

In addition to answering these research questions, this study discovered meta-themes, meta-patterns, and meta-modes that led to the creation of the new research method of meta-ethnonursing.

PURPOSE AND GOAL OF STUDY

The purpose of this study was to describe and systematically synthesize the culture care expressions, beliefs, and practices of diverse and similar cultures. The goal of this study was to synthesize generic (also referred to as folk) and professional culture care actions and decisions that promote health, wellbeing, and beneficial lifeways for people of similar and diverse cultures. This study served as an exploration of both generic and professional care documented in the doctoral dissertations reviewed and was geared toward the overriding objective of attaining an improved understanding and appreciation of how both types of care influence culture care within and among diverse cultural groups.

RATIONALE FOR THE STUDY

The United States has historically been a place where people from all over the world have migrated, seeking a better life for themselves and their families. However, the phenomenon of cultural diversity (which makes the United States a unique country) brings with it distinct and significant challenges in the context of healthcare delivery. An inherent goal for each nurse and the profession of nursing as a discipline is to provide culturally congruent care for the diverse individuals, groups, and populations encountered and/or cared for on a daily basis.

The assumptive premises of Leininger's theory that guided this study were:

- Culture care beliefs, values, and practices are embedded in both the worldview and the cultural values of environmental contexts in urban and rural settings which influence health and wellbeing or illness outcomes (adapted from Leininger, 2006a, p. 19).
- Generic and professional care practices have been discovered for providing culturally congruent care—culture care—that influence health, wellbeing, and illness outcomes (adapted from Leininger, 2006a, p. 19).

- Social structure factors such as family and kinship, religion and spirituality, economic and cultural values, and lifeways are influencers on health, wellbeing, and illness outcomes (adapted from Leininger, 2006a, p. 19).
- Leininger's three theoretical care modes of action and decision have been discovered to help people of diverse cultures across the continuum of nursing care (adapted from Leininger, 2006a, p. 19).

Leininger (1970) stated, "Culture is the blueprint for man's way of living, and only by understanding culture can we hope to gain the fullest understanding of man as a social and cultural being" (p. vii). She challenged nurses and other healthcare professionals to view the world from a global perspective and to appreciate the complexities as well as the commonalities and differences in cultures with their concerns, beliefs, values, and lifeways. As Leininger (1978) so aptly stated, "If human beings are to survive and live in a healthy, peaceful, and meaningful world, then nurses and other healthcare providers need to understand the cultural care beliefs, values, and lifeways of people in order to provide culturally congruent and beneficial health care" (p. 3).

This was the foundation of the descriptive metasynthesis of doctoral dissertations guided by the culture care theory and using the ethnonursing research method. In addition, the methodology of developing a metasynthesis of this magnitude was founded in phenomenology, which Polit and Beck (2008) defined as both a ". . .philosophical tradition concerned with the lived experiences of humans" (p. 64) and a ". . .qualitative research tradition, with roots in philosophy and psychology, that focuses on the lived experiences of humans" (p. 761). Phenomenology is used to study and explore the meanings and interpretations of experiences of individuals or groups within the social, historical, political, or cultural contexts of their unique "life world." The intricacies of qualitative research are both ". . .descriptively sound and explicit, and interpretively rich and innovative" (p. 539).

METHODOLOGIES WITHIN THE STUDY: METASYNTHESIS AND ETHNONURSING

A nurse-researcher may wonder how metasynthesis facilitates analysis and synthesis of findings from multiple research studies. Metasynthesis is described as grand interpretive–analytical narratives produced from the synthesis or comparison of similar findings in qualitative research studies (Polit & Beck, 2008). When analyzing studies, one must compare similarities, differences, instruments, advantages, or disadvantages, and the steps required to make these comparisons. Metasynthesis is controversial and researchers are taking a closer look to determine whether it is a beneficial method for nursing research.

Metasynthesis analysis begins with reviewing the literature, followed by extracting methodological data, analyzing and interpreting data, and summarizing conclusions. The metasynthesis method has been instrumental for qualitative interpretive theory building including fleshing-out and reconceptualizing abstract concepts and putting them together again as new constructs or actions. This methodology allowed the research team to build new knowledge that served as the foundation for the discovery of new features of the metasynthesis process by utilizing raw descriptive data within the qualitative research studies. These features were then compiled into a conceptual method for data analysis.

The ethnonursing research method, created by Leininger in the late 1950s, was designed within the qualitative research paradigm to facilitate naturalistic, open discovery and interpretation of data using the culture care theory. Ethnonursing is a research method to study human cultures, specifically focusing on a particular group's belief system and practices related to nursing care and related health behaviors (Leininger, 2006b). The construct of universality in ethnonursing research refers to the commonly shared "threads" that flow through culture care studies, including social structure dimensions of human beings and groups of human beings and the care patterns, values, and lifeways for diverse and similar cultural groups (Leininger, 2002a). These dimensions provide direction for the nursing profession toward improving health outcomes, integration of evidence-based practices, and providing culturally congruent care for diverse cultural groups.

The culture care theory and the ethnonursing method were created to go hand-in-hand, and ethnonursing remains the first of two nursing research methods designed within the discipline of nursing (Leininger, 1997, 2002b). According to Leininger (2006a), "Ethnonursing is a rigorous, systematic, and *in-depth method* for studying multiple cultures and care factors within familiar environments of people and to focus on the interrelationships of care and culture to arrive at the goal of culturally congruent care services" (p. 20). Prior to Leininger's creation of the ethnonursing method, the nursing profession drew heavily from other disciplines for research methods, scales, and statistical formulas to study phenomena that were unique to nursing. Most studies were also conducted within the quantitative paradigm.

According to Leininger (2006a), qualitative research methods offer an important means to discover and describe largely embedded, covert, epistemic, and ontologic culture care knowledge and practices (pp. 18–19). In addition, the theorist postulated that culture care beliefs, values, and practices are influenced by and embedded in the worldview, social structure factors, religion, kinship, politics, economics, education, technology, and cultural values within ethnohistorical and environmental contexts (p. 19). Using the ethnonursing method, a major discovery occurred within this metasynthesis of multiple ethnonursing studies that led to the expansion of culture care knowledge, higher levels of abstraction, theory building, and ultimately the development of the meta-ethnonursing research method.

SUBSTANTIATING THE RESEARCH

Leininger (2006b) developed and refined six specific qualitative criteria to be used with the ethnonursing research method and the culture care theory: Credibility, confirmability, meaning-in-context, recurrent patterning, saturation, and transferability. They have brought increasing clarity to the evaluation of qualitative data and have established the trustworthiness of data within studies using the culture care theory.

Credibility refers to the truthfulness, accuracy, or believability of findings that have been mutually established between the researcher and the informants as accurate, believable, and credible about their personal experiences and knowledge of their own cultural phenomena (Leininger 2006b, p. 76). The metasynthesis study conducted by the researchers and described in this chapter met the criterion of credibility as all 23 doctoral dissertations examined were prepared, defended, and published by culture care experts.

Confirmability is the repeated direct and documented evidence derived largely from observed and primary informational sources (Leininger, 2006b, p. 77). Confirmability means reaffirmation of ". . .what the researcher has heard, seen, or experienced with respect to phenomena under study" (p. 77) and reflects ideas and lived experiences that have occurred within cultural groups when they are encountered in familiar and natural living contexts (p. 77). The metasynthesis study conducted by the researchers met the criterion of confirmability through an agreed-upon coding scheme contained within the ethnoscript developed by the four members of the research team. In addition, the 23 doctoral dissertations were read, reread, and reviewed in great detail multiple times throughout the progression of the study.

Meaning-in-context, the third criterion, focuses on ". . .data that has become understandable with relevant referents or meanings to the informants or people studied in different or similar environments" (Leininger, 2006b, p. 77). In the metasynthesis study, this criterion achieved through the researchers' in-depth study and selection of ethnonursing as the research method that was developed to be used with Leininger's (2006b) culture care theory.

The fourth criterion of *recurrent patterning* refers to "...repeated instances, sequences of events, experiences, or lifeways that tend to reoccur over a period of time in designated ways and contexts" (Leininger, 2006b, p. 77). The focus of this criterion is on "...the repeated experiences, expressions, events, or activities that reflect identifiable sequenced patterns of behavior over time" (p. 77) and are used to substantiate this criterion. Recurrent patterning was achieved by the metasynthesis researchers when redundancy emerged across all 23 studies through documented recurrent patterns, themes, and related descriptors as evidenced through NVivo text searches.

Saturation, the fifth criterion, refers to the processing of "taking in" occurrences or meanings from key and general informants—". . .in a very full, comprehensive, and exhaustive way *all* the information that could generally be known or understood about a certain phenomenon under study" (Leininger, 2006b, p. 77). The researcher must conduct an exhaustive exploration so as to reach a point of redundancy and repetitiveness where the researcher receives no new information which is verified with the informants (p. 77). Saturation was accomplished in the metasynthesis study when certain coding categories in the ethnoscript became exhaustive with information gleaned from all 23 studies; new information no longer emerged from across all cultural groups studied regarding worldview, cultural beliefs, generic care, professional care, social structure, and environment.

The final and sixth criterion, *transferability*, refers to ". . .whether particular findings from a qualitative study can be transferred to another similar context or situation and still preserve the particularized meanings, interpretations, and inferences" from the initial study (Leininger, 2006b, p. 77). The responsibility for determining transferability lies with the researcher; however, this is not an intended goal of any study (p. 78). In the case of the metasynthesis study, the researchers believed that the required circumstances for this criterion had been met.

DATA COLLECTION AND DATA ANALYSIS

Sampling and Analysis

The sample for the descriptive metasynthesis consisted of 23 doctoral dissertation studies that were conceptualized within the culture care theory and included using the ethnonursing research method. These dissertations were acquired from October 2007 through March 2008 through the UMI Dissertations Abstracts database which has been a central source for doctoral dissertations in North America since 1861. The dissertations were reviewed by two graduate student nurse-researchers in collaboration with qualitative researcher faculty experts.

The process of data analysis using Leininger's ethnonursing research method involved four specific phases as described in the *Four Phases of Data Analysis Enabler Guide* (Leininger, 2006b, p. 60) which was adapted for use in the metasynthesis project. With this guide, the data were processed in sequence with regular and continuous coding, processing, and analysis, with reflection by the researchers at each phase (p. 61). "At all times, research findings from the data analysis can be traced back to each phase and to the grounded data in phase one" (p. 62). Phase I involved the collection and documentation of raw data comprised by the 23 doctoral dissertations studied. Phase II included the recording, processing, and coding of raw data contained within the 23 doctoral dissertations examined. The work in this phase was facilitated by the NVivo software. Phase III was characterized by data saturation, the emergence of recurrent themes and patterns, meaning-in-context, further establishment of credibility, and confirmation of findings related to the DOI. Phase IV is considered to be the highest phase of data analysis; in the study described, it involved higher-level critical thinking with synthesis and in-depth analysis of summative data from the previous three phases. It was at this level that the researchers creatively discovered new theoretical formulations resulting in new evidence-based applications for nursing practice and recommendations for future nursing research.

Technology

The researchers used the following process to code and analyze the 23 doctoral dissertations. The raw data were coded with the Leininger–Templin–Thompson Field Research Ethnoscript (see Appendix 9-B at the end of the chapter) which ". . .reflects categories and domains from the culture care theory; additional unique codes were added as the study progressed" (McFarland, 1995, p. 74). The Ethnoscript adapted for use in this study facilitated a higher level of data analysis related to the DOI with the discovery of meta-themes and meta-patterns. As part of the qualitative data analysis process, NVivo software was used to process large volumes of data within the 23 dissertations studied. The NVivo program has distinct terminology specific to its use; in an effort to provide clarity for future discussions, a few of these basic terms are described:

- **Node**: Ideas extracted from text. For this study, the nodes are the codes within the *Leininger—Templin—Thompson Field Research Ethnoscript.*
- **Source**: Data physically stored inside the NVivo project file. For this study, the sources are the 23 doctoral dissertations.

- **Coding**: The process by which items from raw data text are linked into new constructs or complex ideas.

The researchers read and re-read of each of the 23 doctoral dissertations, coded the *Results* and *Findings* narratives, and achieved *confirmability* by confirming one another's coding and analysis. After each dissertation had been analyzed, coded, and uploaded into NVivo, the researchers noted *recurrent patterning* and eventually *data saturation*. The rich data descriptors, patterns, and themes of the descriptors were then synthesized to meta-patterns and meta-themes.

The following terms are provided to guide the reader:

- **Theme**: A central concept of cultural groups' lived care expressions such as cultural values, beliefs, lifeways, kinship, social factors, religious and philosophical factors, economic factors, and educational and technological factors influenced by environmental and ethnohistory contexts.
- **Meta**: Used in the Greek language to describe *beyond, more highly organized, in succession*, or a *transformation* (Merriam-Webster.com, 2009)
- **Meta-theme**: An overarching *idea or theme* abstracted from the diverse and similar culture care themes found within the 23 dissertations
- **Meta-mode**: An overarching *mode* abstracted from diverse and similar culture care action modes found within the 23 dissertations
- **Meta-care pattern**: An overarching *pattern* abstracted from the discovery of diverse and similar culture care patterns found within the 23 dissertations
- **Meta-ethnography**: Conceptualized theory building from the discovery from enormous amounts of diverse and similar ethnographic data
- **Meta-ethnonursing**: A higher level of abstraction of the ethnonursing research method, including meta-themes, meta-modes, and meta-patterns

METASYNTHESIS FINDINGS

For the purposes of this chapter, the findings from this meta-ethnonursing study are presented in the following order: Meta-themes followed by supporting themes; meta-patterns; care patterns; and descriptors (**Figure 9-1**). The meta-themes were as follows:

- **Meta-theme I**: Generic and professional care in health and wellbeing
- **Meta-theme II**: Social structure in health and wellbeing

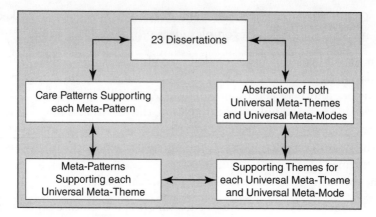

Figure 9-1 Meta-ethnonursing Process
© Marilyn R. McFarland, 2014.

- **Meta-theme III**: Culture care action and decision modes
- **Meta-theme IV**: Environmental context

Meta-themes, Themes, Meta-patterns, Care Patterns, and Descriptors

Universal Meta-theme 1: Generic and Professional Care

> Culturally congruent professional and generic care for diverse and similar cultures influence health, wellbeing, and illness outcomes.

This universal meta-theme was derived from the 23 dissertation research authors reporting generic and professional care experiences by diverse and similar cultures which influenced health, wellbeing, and illness outcomes.

Generic and Professional Care: Examples of Supporting Themes for Meta-theme 1

1. **Theme 1 supporting meta-theme 1**: Old Order Amish informants considered and selected from an array of healthcare options which included folk, professional, and alternative care (Wenger, 1988) [generic and professional care].
2. **Theme 2 supporting meta-theme 1**: Syrian Muslims have reported care as professional and generic care beliefs, values, and practices in Syrian and U.S. hospital contexts (Wehbe-Alamah, 2005). For example, generic care was reported as care given by an informant's husband, children, or community friends. Syrian Muslim men and

women provide physical and emotional support to their families, relatives, and friends [generic care]. Professional care was reported from nurses in hospitals [professional care].

3. **Theme 3 supporting meta-theme 1**: Professional care meanings and practices were reported as ritualized care that was built by respect, trust, and anticipatory care with education and advocacy; generic care was reported as protective care. For example, Finnish women giving birth reported generic care was in the context of comfort from family members by touch and presence (Lamp, 1998) [professional care].

Generic and Professional Care: Meta-pattern 1 Supporting Meta-theme 1

The context of generic and professional care patterns was reported as generic/family care patterns, professional care patterns, alternative care patterns, resident-to-resident /reciprocity care patterns, reciprocal care patterns, and protective care patterns which influenced the health and wellbeing of diverse and similar cultures and could be predictors of health, wellbeing, or illness.

This universal meta-pattern was derived from the 23 dissertation research authors reporting generic and professional care experience care patterns by diverse and similar cultures which influenced health, wellbeing, and illness outcomes. Generic care patterns included health and illness beliefs, values and practices, human care and caring, emic or indigenous care beliefs, human folk care/curing patterns, reciprocal care patterns, and protective care patterns. Professional care patterns included emic and etic beliefs, practices, professional staff and nursing care patterns, alternative care patterns, and emergency care/cure patterns.

Generic and Professional Care: Examples of Supporting Care Patterns for Meta-pattern 1

1. **Care pattern 1 supporting meta-pattern 1**: The Old Order Amish informants reported that family and their lifeways, values, and beliefs influenced their decisions about whether to use folk or professional care services; what generic care role expectations were; and, that care is first given directly through family presence (folk care), followed by the use of professional care (Wenger, 1988) [generic and professional care].
   - **Supporting descriptor**: ". . .100% of the informants made use of brauche [warm hands as a gift from God] and other folk care modalities, [alternative methods such as] chiropractic and

reflexology in addition to the services of professional physicians and nurses" (Old Order Amish; Wenger, 1988) [generic, alternative, and professional care].

2. **Care pattern 2 supporting meta-pattern 1**: Syrian Muslims reported husbands tend to care for their wives by taking them to the doctor or hospital, purchasing and/or administering medicine, cooking healthy meals, helping with the kids, cleaning around the house, and/or asking their wives to rest and not worry about housework (Wehbe-Alamah, 2005) [generic care].

   ▪ **Supporting descriptor**: One male Syrian informant shared that a caring nurse is unselfish and lives for others, whereas non-caring nurses look at their patients as a task that they cannot wait to be done with (Syrian Muslims living in the Midwestern United States; Wehbe-Alamah, 2005) [professional care].

3. **Care pattern 3 supporting meta-pattern 1**: Finnish women reported a care pattern by the nurse of continuous presence during childbirth (Lamp, 1998) [professional care].

   ▪ **Supporting descriptor**: "She [nurse] was there with me like family" (Finnish woman in labor; Lamp, 1998) [professional care].

Universal Meta-theme 2: Social Structure

Social structure factors including family and kinship, religion and spirituality, economics, cultural values, and lifeways are influencers on culture care that predict health and wellbeing.

This universal meta-theme was abstracted from the 23 dissertation research authors reporting social structure factors such as family, kinship, religion and spirituality, economics, and cultural values and lifeways which influenced health, wellbeing, and illness outcomes.

Social Structure: Examples of Supporting Themes for Meta-theme 2

1. **Theme 1 supporting meta-theme 2**: For Baganda women [rural Uganda, Africa] as AIDS caregivers, culture care means responsibility, love, and comfort derived from their kinship, religious, cultural beliefs, and values, as well as their generic health beliefs and those of professionals (MacNeil, 1994) [generic and professional care].

2. **Theme 2 supporting meta-theme 2**: Social structural factors of spirituality, kinship, and economics had great influence on the health and wellbeing of African American women receiving prenatal care in rural and urban United States (Morgan, 1994) [generic care].

3. **Theme 3 supporting meta-theme 2**: The chronically mentally ill in the community [urban Midwestern United States] are a subculture with shared social structure factors and specific cultural norms, values, and lifeways which differ in some respects from those of the dominant culture (George, 1998).

Social Structure: Meta-pattern 1 for Meta-theme 2

Within the context of social structure factors, family, kinship, religion, spirituality, economics, cultural values, and lifeways are influencers on culture care and can be predictors of health and wellbeing.

This universal meta-pattern was derived from the 23 dissertation research authors reporting social structure factors such as family, kinship, religion and spirituality, economics, cultural values, and cultural lifeways influenced health, wellbeing, and illness outcomes, with a few diverse care patterns also described. The dissertations examined discovered protective care, respectful care, comfort care from religion/spiritual beliefs, and folk and professional care patterns that influenced health and wellbeing.

Social Structure: Examples of Supporting Care Patterns for Meta-pattern 2

1. **Care pattern 1 supporting meta-pattern 1**: Traditional Baganda customs of children belonging to the paternal clan were weakened due to the numerous deaths from AIDS, often resulting from violence and family conflict, although the Baganda women sought care as comfort from God and within the Roman Catholic or Protestant religions, and prayed and bore suffering (MacNeil, 1994) [kinship, social, and religious factors].
   - **Supporting descriptor**: "This is hard to describe, but I care for my daughter, and I love her. She is all I have left" (Ugandan grandmother whose daughter was dying of AIDS; MacNeil, 1994) [kinship and social factors].
2. **Care pattern 2 supporting meta-pattern 1**: Spirituality enabled African American women receiving prenatal care to experience life with equanimity (Morgan, 1994) [spiritual and religious factors].
   - **Supporting descriptor**: "I just started talking to God about it . . . I try to trust in the Lord and everything will be all right" (African American woman in a prenatal care clinic; Morgan, 1994) [religion].
3. **Care pattern 3 supporting meta-pattern 1**: The mentally ill strove to move toward independence in achieving and maintaining stability in living arrangements, personal relationships, kinship, social

factors, and treatment of their mental illness, and in searching for a place to belong in society (George, 1998) [kinship and social factors].

- **Supporting descriptor**: "I think that sometimes people with mental health problems just sort of drift away or aren't part of the larger society" (mental health consumer; George, 1998) [kinship and social factors].

4. **Care pattern 4 supporting meta-pattern 1**: Financial disadvantage and bureaucracy made it difficult to obtain health care (Prince, 2005) [economic factors].

- **Supporting descriptor**: "Health means money. Most times to maintain your health you have to have money, insurance" (African American female prostitute living within the urban city; Prince, 2005) [economic factors].

5. **Care pattern 5 supporting meta-pattern 1**: Generosity and sharing were viewed as a care pattern influenced by kinship, cultural values of family, and lifeways (Farrell, 2001) [cultural values and lifeways].

- **Supporting descriptor**: "We always make sure family has what they need. We honor our children even if we don't like the things they do. We honor our elders. I experience that every day. It is nice to be an elder. I know that my people will take care of me if I need anything" (Potawatomi female elder living in a rural setting; Farrell, 2001) [cultural values and lifeways].

Universal Meta-theme 3: Action and Decision Meta-modes

Culture care action and decision modes for providing culturally congruent nursing care are essential and contribute to the health and wellbeing of similar and diverse cultures.

This universal meta-theme was derived from all 23 dissertation research authors reporting culture care action and decision modes were essential for providing culturally congruent nursing care and contributed to the health and wellbeing for similar and diverse cultures.

Action and Decision Meta-modes: Examples of Supporting Themes for Meta-theme 3

1. **Theme 1 supporting meta-theme 3:** Culture care preservation/ maintenance and nursing actions/decisions are essential for health and wellbeing within similar and diverse cultures. Culture care maintenance/preservation refers to assistive, supportive, facilitative, or enabling creative professional actions and decisions that help Baganda

women as AIDS caregivers to preserve or maintain a state of help, or to face handicap or death (MacNeil, 1994).

2. **Theme 2 supporting meta-theme 3:** Culture care negotiation/ accommodation of culture-specific nursing care actions/decisions is essential for health and wellbeing within similar and diverse cultures. For example, culture care accommodation and/or negotiation was reported to be a goal to alleviate barriers for African American working class women for prenatal care. Free transportation was available to accommodate women (Morgan, 1994).

3. **Theme 3 supporting meta-theme 3**: Culture care repatterning/ restructuring of unhealthy folk and alternative care practices did promote safe culturally congruent care for Finnish women. For example, pregnant Finnish women restructured a shorter length of time and cooler temperatures promoting a safer cultural care practice (Lamp, 1998).

Action and Decision Meta-modes: Meta-pattern 1 Supporting Meta-theme 3

The context of preservation/maintenance patterns, negotiation/accommodation patterns, [and] repatterning and/or restructuring patterns influences family; kinship; professional and generic care patterns; and, practices, beliefs, and cultural values that contribute toward culturally congruent nursing care that supports the health and wellbeing of diverse and similar cultures.

This universal meta-pattern was derived from all 23 dissertation research authors reporting culture care action and decision modes were essential for providing culturally congruent nursing care and contributed to the health and wellbeing for similar and diverse cultures.

Action and Decision Meta-modes: Examples of Supporting Care Patterns for Meta-pattern 1

1. **Care pattern 1 supporting meta-pattern 1**: During a period of serious illness such as AIDS, the nurse should be prepared to accommodate immediate family, relatives, and generic folk healer care patterns within the home as well as in the healthcare setting (MacNeil study in Uganda, 1994) [culture care preservation/maintenance].
   - **Supporting descriptor**: "My husband was polygamous. He had several other children with other women and brought these children home for me to look after. I did not like it, but I had no choice. I had to look after the family" (Uganda mother living in Africa; MacNeil, 1994) [culture care preservation/maintenance].

2. **Care pattern 2 supporting meta-pattern 1**: Morgan reported culture care negotiation involves alternative, generic, or folk healer care patterns in the prenatal care of African American women to enhance or shorten labor (Morgan study in Detroit, Michigan, and the rural South, 1994) [culture care negotiation/accommodation].
   - **Supporting descriptor**: "I prefer that they [babies] [are born] in the hospital—they know what they are doing, so babies are safe, better safe than sorry. . . .You need doctors and nurses to keep them safe, you need to protect your body" (African American woman in the hospital; Morgan, 1994) [culture care negotiation/accommodation].
3. **Care pattern 3 supporting meta-pattern 1**: Lamp (1998) reported pregnant Finnish women restructured care to shorten the length of time in their saunas and facilitated cooler temperatures for their saunas to ensure the safety of their unborn child [culture care repatterning/restructuring].
   - **Supporting descriptor**: "She was the only nurse and knows what happened, beginning to end" (stated by a laboring Finnish woman in a hospital; Lamp, 1998) [culture care repatterning/restructuring].

Universal Meta-theme 4: Environmental Context

> Care patterns, expressions, beliefs, and practices were viewed within urban and rural environmental contexts as a continuing life experience with both similar and diverse findings within urban and rural settings.

This universal meta-theme was derived from all 23 dissertation research authors reporting environmental context was viewed and influenced care patterns, expressions, beliefs, and practices within urban and rural settings and contributed to the health and wellbeing for similar and diverse cultures.

Environmental Contexts for Meta-theme 4   The environmental contexts of the 23 dissertation studies reviewed were both urban and rural. Examples of *urban* environments described within the studies included inner-city neighborhoods (Ehrmin, 1998), suburban/urban neighborhoods (Miller, 1997), city hospitals (Gates, 1988), city churches (Gelazis, 1994), retirement homes (McFarland, 1995), apartments, urban centers (George, 1998), and transition centers (Prince, 2005). Examples of *rural* environments described within the studies included rural American Midwest (Wenger, 1988), a Dominican village center (Schumacher, 2006), rural Ohio homes (Johnson, 2005), and rural medical clinics (Farrell, 2001).

Environmental Context: Examples of Supporting Themes for Meta-theme 4

1. **Theme 1 supporting meta-theme 4**: Anglo and African American residents viewed, expressed, and lived generic care to maintain their pre-admission generic lifeways and to maintain beneficial and healthy lifeways in the retirement home (McFarland, 1995) [urban].
2. **Theme 2 supporting meta-theme 4**: Culture care for African American adolescent gang members reported nurses have knowledge, understanding of emotional, cultural, physical and environmental pain, and genuine compassion to assist the gang members in ameliorating their pain influenced by family, spiritual/religious factors, and the social structure patterns and lifeways of the culture (Morris, 2004) [urban].
3. **Theme 3 supporting meta-theme 4**: Old Order Amish worldview, social structure, anticipatory care, and active participation in their care situations were expected to maintain high-context relationships within their community (Wenger, 1988) [rural].

Environmental Context: Meta-pattern 1 for Meta-theme 4

> Within the context of urban and rural environments, family, kinship, care patterns, practices, beliefs, expressions, and cultural values influenced health and wellbeing.

Urban and rural environments influenced universal community care patterns, maternal and paternal protective care patterns, organizational care patterns, institutional care patterns, apartment living care patterns, retirement home care patterns, nursing home care patterns, and professional care institution patterns. Urban environments influenced diverse inner-city care patterns, poverty care patterns, and destructive life care patterns. Adult females developed recovery care networks within their neighborhoods which created a cultural need for compassion, love, and understanding (Ehrmin, 1998). Rural environments influenced diverse community care patterns; generic and professional care patterns; and family and kinship care patterns.

Environmental Context: Examples of Supporting Care Patterns for Meta-pattern 1

1. **Care pattern 1 supporting meta-pattern 1**: Anglo American and African American retired male and female elders living in an urban nursing home and apartments were found to have retirement home care patterns, viewing day and night within their environmental

context as continuing life experiences. However, major differences [in worldview] were discovered between residents living in the apartment section and residents in the nursing home setting. Protective care, watchfulness, and a sense of extending family relationships were developed within these environments (McFarland, 1995) [urban].

- **Supporting descriptor**: "I help her here on and off the elevators. . . . You can't live here and just be concerned with individuality . . . and I have arranged for others to come and live here because I knew they needed care" (retired female elder living in an apartment setting; McFarland, 1995) [urban].

2. **Care pattern 2 supporting meta-pattern 1**: African American adolescent urban gang members used destructive lifeways to survive in their urban environment and needed to learn healthier ways of coping with stress within their urban environment (Morris, 2004) [urban].

- **Supporting descriptor**: "These young kids are going to jail for the older gang leaders and even beyond . . . highstakes drug dealers" (family member within the urban community of African American adolescent gang members; Morris, 2004) [urban].

3. **Care pattern 3 supporting meta-pattern 1**: The rural Amish participants discovered care patterns of community care included bonding by intergenerational family members; this was expressed through helping and participating in functions that brought people together (Wenger, 1988) [rural].

- **Supporting descriptor**: "Our people belong together. Caring for each other is what keeps the community together. Helping others is a time for bringing relatives together. It is a time for visiting. It is good for people to get together. It is how we care for each other and know about each other" (Amish person in a rural community; Wenger, 1988) [rural].

DISCOVERED THEORETICAL FORMULATIONS

Historically speaking, nursing as an academic profession has striven to build a body of knowledge to guide nursing practice. According to Cross (1981), "The systematic accumulation of knowledge is essential to progress in any profession. . . however, theory and practice must be constantly interactive. Theory without practice is empty and practice without theory is blind" (p. 110). The researchers discovered that the descriptive metasynthesis of doctoral dissertations guided by the culture care theory using the ethnonursing method has resulted in theory building, theory development, and a higher level of abstraction of findings beyond the themes discovered in the individual studies.

In building upon Leininger's body of work, the nurse-researchers were able to move the research forward. According to Leininger (2006b):

> The ultimate goal of a professional nurse-scientist and humanist is to discover, know and creatively use culturally-based care knowledge with its fullest meanings, expressions, symbols, and functions for healing, and to promote or maintain wellbeing (or health) with people of diverse cultures in the world. (p. 43)

The nurse-researchers discovered theoretical formulations within this study of 23 dissertation findings that had implications for nursing and future research. The study findings included culture care expressions, meanings, and practices for diverse and similar cultures having commonalities that influenced their healthcare practices and beliefs. These findings discovered from the dissertations facilitated a metasynthesis of their themes, care patterns, and care action modes. The data were voluminous, and the new theoretical formulations and definitions discovered derived from their themes became meta-themes, their care patterns became meta-patterns, and their modes became meta-modes.

In summary, the volume of data contained within the 23 dissertations provided the theoretical framework for the evolution of the new research method, *meta-ethnonursing* which allowed for the evaluation of previous discoveries through higher levels of abstraction and ultimately theory building. Through this descriptive metasynthesis, the researchers have expanded and embellished the existing body of knowledge for evidence-based applications in clinical practice, education, consultation, research, administration, and healthcare policy. Through the findings in this study, areas for future contributions through the continued development and enhancement of the culture care theory were discovered.

In recent years, there has been an increased number of ethnonursing studies guided by the culture care theory conducted within the discipline of nursing. Leininger (1991, 1995, 2002a, 2006a) was a pioneer in synthesizing findings from these studies and has shared culture care patterns, themes, values, meanings, and care constructs from her studies and the studies of her graduate students in her extensive publications. The voluminous amount of data contained in all of these dissertations provided the framework for the evolving qualitative research method of meta-ethnonursing which includes meta-themes, meta-patterns, and meta-modes and allowed for the expansion of a research method and further building of the Theory of Culture Care Diversity and Universality (the culture care theory).

SIGNIFICANCE AND IMPLICATIONS FOR THE NURSING PROFESSION

The implications for nursing discovered within the study findings include the discovery of culture care expressions, meanings, and practices within a cultural social structure context for diverse and similar cultures that have commonalities influencing their healthcare practices and beliefs. As shown in the metasynthesis study findings, diverse and similar cultural groups have expressed the desire for both generic and professional care. This is an important finding that can be used to provide culturally congruent care using Leininger's three modes of culture care action and decision. All 23 dissertation findings included discoveries related to Leininger's modes of care action and decision that were considered to be critical for providing culturally congruent care that is both safe and satisfying to cultural groups.

The use of the culture care action and decision mode *preservation and/or maintenance* is essential for preserving and maintaining the health and wellbeing of diverse and similar cultures and should be implemented in nursing practice. For example, McNeil (1994) reported that healthcare professionals promoted the maintenance of Baganda women as AIDS caregivers to preserve a state of helping, assisting, or facing of handicaps or death (p. 125).

The use of the culture care action and decision mode *negotiation and/or accommodation* is essential for negotiating away from and making accommodations about unhealthy cultural practices to facilitate the health and wellbeing of diverse and similar cultures and should be implemented in nursing practice. For example, Morgan (1994) reported healthcare professionals negotiated and facilitated free transportation for African American working-class women enabling them to take advantage of prenatal care (p. 254). This action lessened healthcare barriers and accommodated to improve maternal care patterns toward more favorable health outcomes.

The use of the culture care action and decision mode *repatterning and/or restructuring* is essential for minimizing or eliminating unhealthy folk and alternative healthcare practices to promote safe and culturally congruent care for diverse and similar cultures and should be implemented in nursing practice. An example of this is found in Lamp's (1998) study which reported healthcare professionals facilitated Finnish pregnant women in restructuring their sauna practices for shorter lengths of time and at cooler temperatures in an effort to promote safer maternal culture care (p. 195).

The use of Leininger's culture care action and decision meta-modes is an important contribution with strong implications for nursing practice. The modes guide the practice of culturally congruent nursing care that contributes to the promotion of the health and wellbeing of diverse and similar cultures. In addition to nursing care, nursing research will be positively affected by the metasynthesis discovery of diverse and similar cultural healthcare practices, beliefs, and expressions from the 23 doctoral dissertations. It is imperative that more cultural groups be studied to further develop the existing body of knowledge to support and expand the construct of culturally congruent care within the nursing profession.

Implications of this study for nursing include theory building, theory development, and a higher level of abstraction of findings beyond the themes from individual studies. The outcomes of this metasynthesis study have added nursing knowledge as an evidence base for practice, education, consultation, research, and administration (including policy making) toward the provision of culturally congruent nursing care locally, nationally, and globally.

CONCLUSION

Culture care represents the synthesis of two major constructs: *culture* from anthropology and *care* from nursing. These constructs guided the researchers in their endeavor to discover, explain, and account for health, wellbeing, care expressions, and other human conditions. Culture care expressions, meanings, patterns, processes, and structural forms are diverse, but many commonalities exist among and between cultures. Culture care values, beliefs, and practices are influenced by and embedded in their worldview, social structure factors, ethnohistorical, and environmental contexts. Every culture has generic and professional care practices yet to be discovered and used for culturally congruent care nursing care (Leininger, 1991, 2006a, 2006b).

The researchers discovered that this descriptive metasynthesis resulted in theory building and a higher level of abstraction of findings beyond the themes from the 23 original doctoral dissertations that were guided by the culture care theory using the ethnonursing method. The ethnonursing qualitative metasynthesis process resulted in the discovery of meta-themes, meta-patterns, and meta-modes that have contributed to the discipline and practice of nursing for providing culturally congruent nursing care. The new discovery of meta-themes, meta-patterns, and meta-modes has provided the expanded framework for the meta-ethnonursing research method and the future study of diverse and similar cultures for the continued and expanded provision of culturally congruent care.

This research blazed a trail for future meta-ethnonursing research studies and opened opportunities for further discoveries of culturally congruent care practices, beliefs, meanings, expressions, and patterns essential for the health and wellbeing of diverse and similar cultures. As Leininger (1988) wrote, "The purpose of the theory is to describe, account for, interpret, and predict cultural congruent care in order to attain the ultimate goal of the theory; namely to provide quality care to clients of diverse cultures that is congruent, satisfying, and beneficial to them" (p. 155).

DISCUSSION QUESTIONS

1. What are the commonalities and differences of culture care expressions, beliefs, and practices among people of diverse and similar cultures?
2. In what ways do worldview, social structure factors, and environmental context influence culture care expressions, beliefs, and practices of people of diverse and similar cultures?
3. In what ways can Leininger's three nursing care modes of action and decision facilitate the provision of culturally congruent care for people of diverse and similar cultures?
4. What is a metasynthesis?
5. What is a meta-care pattern?
6. Which cultures can benefit from the culture care decision and action modes?

APPENDIX 9-A: DOCTORAL DISSERTATIONS EXAMINED

Berry, A. B. (1996). *Culture care expressions, meanings and experiences of pregnant Mexican American women within Leininger's culture care theory.* Doctoral dissertation. Available from ProQuest Dissertations and Theses database (UMI No. 9628875).

Ehrmin, J. T. H. (1998). *Culture care: Meanings and expressions of African American women residing in an inner city transitional home for substance abuse.* Doctoral dissertation. Available from ProQuest Dissertations and Theses database (UMI No. 9915650).

Farrell, L. S. (2001). *Cultural care: Meanings and expressions of caring and non-caring of the Potawatomi who have experienced family violence.* Doctoral dissertation. Available from ProQuest Dissertations and Theses database (UMI No. 3010083).

Fox-Hill, E. J. (1999). *The experiences of persons with AIDS living–dying in a nursing home.* Doctoral dissertation. Available from ProQuest Dissertations and Theses database (UMI No. 9935492).

Gates, M. (1988). *Care and cure meanings, experiences and orientations of persons who are dying in hospital and hospice settings.* Doctoral dissertation. Available from ProQuest Dissertations and Theses database (UMI No.8910325).

Gelazis, R. (1994). *Humor, care and well-being of Lithuanian Americans: An ethnonursing study using Leininger's theory of culture care diversity and universality.* Doctoral dissertation. Available from ProQuest Dissertations and Theses database (UMI No. 9423710).

George, T. B. (1998). *Meanings, expressions, and experiences of care of chronically mentally ill in a day treatment center using Leininger's culture care theory.* Doctoral dissertation. Available from ProQuest Dissertations and Theses database (UMI No. 9915656).

Higgins, B. (1995). *Puerto-Rican cultural beliefs: Influence on infant feeding practices in western New York.* Doctoral dissertation. Available from ProQuest Dissertations and Theses database (UMI No. 9604699).

Johnson, C. A. (2005). *Understanding the culture care practices of rural immigrant Mexican women.* Doctoral dissertation. Available from ProQuest Dissertations and Theses database (UMI No. 3175853).

Kelsey, B. M. (2005). *Culture care values, beliefs, and practices of Mexican American migrant farm workers related to health promoting behaviors.* Doctoral dissertation. Available from ProQuest Dissertations and Theses database (UMI No. 3166257).

Lamp, J. K. (1998). *Generic and professional culture care meanings and practices of Finnish women in birth within Leininger's theory of culture care diversity and universality.* Doctoral dissertation. Available from ProQuest Dissertations and Theses database (UMI No. 9915688).

Luna, L. (1989). *Care and cultural context of Lebanese Muslims in an urban US community: An ethnographic and ethnonursing study conceptualized within Leininger's theory.* Doctoral dissertation. Available from ProQuest Dissertations and Theses database (UMI No. 9022423).

MacNeil, J. M. (1994). *Culture care: Meanings, patterns and expressions for Baganda women as AIDS caregivers within Leininger's theory.* Doctoral dissertation. Available from ProQuest Dissertations and Theses database (UMI No. 9519922).

McFarland, M. R. (1995). *Cultural care of Anglo and African American elderly residents within the environmental context of a long-term care institution.* Doctoral dissertation. Available from ProQuest Dissertations and Theses database (UMI No. 9530568).

Miller, J. E. (1997). *Politics and care: A study of Czech Americans within Leininger's theory of culture care diversity and universality.* Doctoral dissertation. Available from ProQuest Dissertations and Theses database (UMI No. 9725851).

Morgan, M. A. (1994). *Prenatal care of African American women in selected USA urban and rural cultural contexts conceptualized within Leininger's cultural care theory.* Doctoral dissertation. Available from ProQuest Dissertations and Theses database (UMI No. 9519936).

Morris, E. J. (2004). *An ethnonursing culture care study of the meanings, expressions and lifeways experiences of selected urban African American adolescent gang members.* Doctoral dissertation. Available from ProQuest Dissertations and Theses database (UMI No. 3130357).

Prince, L. M. (2005). *Culture care and resilience in minority women residing in a transitional home recovering from prostitution.* Doctoral dissertation. Available from ProQuest Dissertations and Theses database (UMI No. 3174259).

Rosenbaum, J. N. (1990). *Cultural care, cultural health, and grief phenomena related to older Greek Canadian widow within Leininger's theory of culture care.* Doctoral dissertation. Available from ProQuest Dissertations and Theses database (UMI No. 9118922).

Schumacher, G. C. (2006). *Culture care meaning, beliefs and practices of rural Dominicans in a rural village of the Dominican Republic: An ethnonursing study conceptualized within the culture care theory.* Doctoral dissertation. Available from ProQuest Dissertations and Theses database (UMI No. 3217484).

Wehbe-Alamah, H. (2005). *Generic and professional health care beliefs, expressions and practices of Syrian Muslims living in the Midwestern United States.* Doctoral dissertation. Available from ProQuest Dissertations and Theses database (UMI No. 3197399).

Wekselman, K. (1999). *The culture of natural childbirth.* Doctoral dissertation. Available from ProQuest Dissertations and Theses database (UMI No. 9936027).

Wenger, A. F. Z. (1988). *The phenomenon of care in a high context culture: The Old Order Amish.* Doctoral dissertation. Available from ProQuest Dissertations and Theses database (UMI No. 8910384).

APPENDIX 9-B: CODING DATA SYSTEM FOR THE LEININGER–TEMPLIN–THOMPSON FIELD RESEARCH ETHNOSCRIPT META-ETHNONURSING/ METASYNTHESIS

Categories and Domains of Information (Includes observations, interviews, interpretive material, and non-material data)

Category I: General Cultural Domains of Inquiry

Code Description

*Italics indicates codes created specifically for this study.

1. Worldview
2. Cultural–social lifeways and activities (typical day/night)
3. Ethnohistorical (includes chrono-data, acculturation, cultural contracts, etc.)
4. Environmental contexts (i.e., physical, ecological, cultural, social)
5. Linguistic terms and meanings
6. Cultural foods related to care, health, illness, and environment
7. Material and nonmaterial culture (includes symbols and meanings)
8. Ethnodemographics (numerical facts, dates, population size, and other numerical data)
9. *Racism, prejudice, race**

Category II: Domain of Cultural and Social Structural Data

(Includes Normative Values, Patterns, Function, and Conflict)

10. Cultural values, beliefs, norms
11. Economic factors
12. Educational factors
13. Kinship (family ties, social network, social relationships, etc.)
14. Political and legal factors
15. Religious, philosophical, and ethical values and beliefs
16. Technological factors
17. Interpersonal relationships (individual groups or institutions)
18. *Recreation* *

Category III: Care, Cure, Health (Wellbeing), and Illness of Folk and Professional Lifeways

19. Folk (includes popular health and illness beliefs, values, and practices)
20. Professional health
21. Human care/caring and nursing (general beliefs, values, and practices)
22. Folk care/caring (emic or indigenous beliefs, values, and lifeways)
23. Professional care/caring (etic beliefs, values, lifeways)
24. Professional nursing care/caring (etic and emic) lifeways (congruence and conflict areas)
25. Noncare/caring beliefs, values, and practices
26. Human cure/curing (general ideas, beliefs, values, and practices)
27. Folk cure/curing (emic beliefs and practices)
28. Professional cure/curing (emic and etic perspectives)
29. Alternative (new) or emergency care/cure systems
30. *Caring for others (resident to resident)* *
31. *Reciprocal care* *
32. *Self-care* *

Category IV: Health and Social Service Institutions

(Administrative Norms, Beliefs, and Practices with Meanings-in-Context)

33. Cultural–social norms, beliefs, values, and contexts
34. Political–legal aspects
35. Economic aspects

36. Technological factors
37. Environmental factors
38. Educational factors (formal and informal)
39. Social organization or structural features
40. Decision and action patterns
41. Interdisciplinary norms, values, and collaborative practices with medicine, social work, nursing, auxiliary staff, etc.
42. Nursing specialties and features
43. Non-nursing specialties and features
44. Ethical/moral aspects
45. *Religious aspects**

Category V: Life Cycles and Intergenerational Patterns

(Includes Ceremonies and Rituals)

46. Lifecycle male and female socialization and enculturation
47. Infancy and early childhood
48. Adolescence or transitions to adulthood
49. Middlescence
50. Advanced years
51. Cultural lifecycle values, beliefs, and practices
52. Cultural lifecycle conflicts and congruence areas (i.e., intergenerational; independence versus dependence)
53. Special subculture
54. Life passages (i.e., birth, marriage, death)
55. *Additional life passages in retirement home (nursing home to apartment, apartment to nursing home, entering home)**
56. *Acculturation, assimilation, adjustment to retirement home**

Category VI: Methodological and Other Research Features of the Study

57. Specific methods of techniques used
58. Key informants
59. General informants
60. Enabling tools or instruments used
61. Problem areas, concerns, or conflicts
62. Strengths, favorable and unanticipated outcomes of researcher and informants (i.e., subjective data and questions)
63. Unusual incidents, interpretations, and questions, etc.
64. Factors facilitating or hindering the study (i.e., time, staff, money)

65. Emic data
66. Etic data
67. Dialogue by interviewer
68. Dialogue by someone other than informant or interviewer
69. Additional contextual data (including nonverbal symbols, total view, environmental features, etc.)
70. Informed consent factors

Category VII: Study Findings

71. *Themes**
72. *Patterns**
73. *Descriptors**

Category VIII: Culture Care Modes

74. *Preservation and/or maintenance**
75. *Accommodation and/or negotiation**
76. *Repatterning and/or restructuring**

REFERENCES

Cross, P. (1981). *Adults as learners.* Washington, DC: Jossey-Bass (John Wiley & Sons).

Ehrmin, J. T. H. (1998). *Culture care: Meanings and expressions of African American women residing in an inner city transitional home for substance abuse.* Doctoral dissertation. Available from ProQuest Dissertations and Theses database (UMI No. 9915650).

Farrell, L. S. (2001). *Cultural care: Meanings and expressions of caring and non-caring of the Potawatomi who have experienced family violence.* Doctoral dissertation. Available from ProQuest Dissertations and Theses database (UMI No. 3010083).

Gates, M. (1988). *Care and cure meanings, experiences and orientations of persons who are dying in hospital and hospice settings.* Doctoral dissertation. Available from ProQuest Dissertations and Theses database (UMI No.8910325).

Gelazis, R. (1993). *Humor, care and well-being of Lithuanian Americans: An ethnonursing study using Leininger's theory of culture care diversity and universality.* Doctoral dissertation. Available from ProQuest Dissertations and Theses database (UMI No. 9423710).

George, T. B. (1998). *Meanings, expressions, and experiences of care of chronically mentally ill in a day treatment center using Leininger's culture care theory.* Doctoral dissertation. Available from ProQuest Dissertations and Theses database (UMI No. 9915656).

Johnson, C. A. (2005). *Understanding the culture care practices of rural immigrant Mexican women.* Doctoral dissertation. Available from ProQuest Dissertations and Theses database (UMI No. 3175853).

Lamp, J. K. (1998). *Generic and professional culture care meanings and practices of Finnish women in birth within Leininger's theory of culture care diversity and universality.* Doctoral dissertation. Available from ProQuest Dissertations and Theses database (UMI No. 9915688).

Leininger, M. M. (1970). *Nursing and anthropology: Two worlds to blend.* New York, NY: John Wiley & Sons.

Leininger, M. M. (1978). *Transcultural nursing: Concepts, theories, & practices.* New York, NY: John Wiley & Sons. (Reprinted Columbus, OH: Greyden Press, 1994.)

Leininger, M. M. (1988). Leininger's theory of nursing: Cultural care diversity and universality. *Nursing Science Quarterly, 1*(4), 152–160. doi: 10.1177/089431848800100408

Leininger, M. M. (1991). *Culture care diversity and universality: A theory of nursing.* New York, NY: National League for Nursing.

Leininger, M. M. (1995). *Transcultural nursing: Concepts, theories, research, & practices* (2nd ed.). New York, NY: McGraw-Hill.

Leininger, M. M. (1997). Classic article: Overview of the theory of culture care with the ethnonursing research method. *Journal of Transcultural Nursing, 8*(2), 32–52. doi: 10.1177/104365969700800205

Leininger, M. M. (2002a). Transcultural nursing and globalization of health care: Importance, focus, and historical aspects. In M. M. Leininger & M. R. McFarland (Eds.), *Transcultural nursing: Concepts, theories, research, & practice* (3rd ed., pp. 3–43). New York, NY: McGraw-Hill.

Leininger, M. M. (2002b). Part I: The theory of culture care and the ethnonursing research method. In M. M. Leininger & M. R. McFarland (Eds.), *Transcultural nursing: Concepts, theories, research, & practice* (3rd ed., pp. 71–116). New York, NY: McGraw-Hill.

Leininger, M. M. (2006a). Culture care diversity and universality theory and evolution of the ethnonursing method. In M. M. Leininger & M. R. McFarland (Eds.), *Culture care diversity and universality: A worldwide nursing theory* (2nd ed., pp. 1–41). Sudbury, MA: Jones and Bartlett.

Leininger, M. M. (2006b). Ethnonursing research method and enablers. In M. M. Leininger & M. R. McFarland (Eds.), *Culture care diversity and universality: A worldwide nursing theory* (2nd ed., pp. 42–81). Sudbury, MA: Jones and Bartlett.

MacNeil, J. M. (1994). *Culture care: Meanings, patterns and expressions for Baganda women as AIDS caregivers within Leininger's theory.* Doctoral dissertation. Available from ProQuest Dissertations and Theses database (UMI No. 9519922).

McFarland, M. R. (1995). *Cultural care of Anglo and African American elderly residents within the environmental context of a long-term care institution.* Doctoral dissertation. Available from ProQuest Dissertations and Theses database (UMI No. 9530568).

Merriam-Webster.com. (2009). Meta [definition]. Retrieved from http://www.merriam-webster.com/

Miller, J. E. (1997). *Politics and care: A study of Czech Americans within Leininger's theory of culture care diversity and universality.* Doctoral dissertation. Available from ProQuest Dissertations and Theses database (UMI No. 9725851).

Morgan, M. A. (1994). *Prenatal care of African American women in selected USA urban and rural cultural contexts conceptualized within Leininger's cultural care theory.* Doctoral dissertation. Available from ProQuest Dissertations and Theses database (UMI No. 9519936).

Morris, E. J. (2004). *An ethnonursing culture care study of the meanings, expressions and lifeways experiences of selected urban African American adolescent gang members.* Doctoral dissertation. Available from ProQuest Dissertations and Theses database (UMI No. 3130357).

Polit, D. F., & Beck, C. T. (2008). *Nursing research: Generating and assessing evidence for nursing practice* (8th ed., pp. 665–690). Philadelphia, PA: Lippincott Williams & Wilkins.

Prince, L. M. (2005). *Culture care and resilience in minority women residing in a transitional home recovering from prostitution.* Doctoral dissertation. Available from ProQuest Dissertations and Theses database (UMI No. 3174259).

Schumacher, G. C. (2006). *Culture care meaning, beliefs and practices of rural Dominicans in a rural village of the Dominican Republic: An ethnonursing study conceptualized within the culture care theory.* Doctoral dissertation. Available from ProQuest Dissertations and Theses database (UMI No. 3217484).

Wehbe-Alamah, H. (2005). *Generic and professional health care beliefs, expressions and practices of Syrian Muslims living in the Midwestern United States.* Doctoral dissertation. Available from ProQuest Dissertations and Theses database (UMI No. 3197399).

Wenger, A. F. Z. (1988). *The phenomenon of care in a high context culture: The Old Order Amish. Doctoral dissertation.* Available from ProQuest Dissertations and Theses database (UMI No. 8910384).

Chapter 10

Application of the Three Modes of Culture Care Decisions and Actions in Advanced Practice Primary Care

Marilyn K. Eipperle

Leininger's three theoretical modes of culture care [decisions and actions] offer new, creative, and different therapeutic ways to help people of diverse cultures . . . and were predicted to provide ways to give culturally congruent, safe, and meaningful health care to cultures.

(Leininger, 2006a, pp. 18, 19)

The nurse practitioner needs to be able to sensitively and competently integrate culture care into contextual routines, clinical ways, and approaches to primary care practice through role modeling, policy making, procedural performance and performance evaluation, and the use of the advance practice nursing process. By using Leininger's Sunrise Enabler and the three care modes to guide nursing actions and decisions. . . the nurse practitioner would be able to provide culturally congruent, safe, meaningful, and beneficial care to clients in primary care contexts.

(McFarland & Eipperle, 2008, p. 49)*

---

*McFarland, M. R., & Eipperle, M. K. (2008). *Contemporary Nurse, 28*(1–2), 48–63.

INTRODUCTION

The three modes of culture care decisions and actions were postulated by Leininger (1995a, 1995b, 1996, 1997, 2002c, 2006a) as a tenet of the Theory of Culture Care Diversity and Universality. "*Tenets* are the positions one holds or are [the] givens that the theorist uses with a theory" (Leininger, 2006a, p. 17). The three modes of culture care decisions and actions are culture care preservation and/or maintenance; culture care accommodation and/or negotiation; and culture care repatterning and/or restructuring (Leininger, 2006a).

The modes have been reviewed and presented within the individual and unique contexts of other chapters in this text. In this chapter, the discussion focuses on application of the modes in the context of advanced practice nursing in primary care settings and examines their appropriate foci, differentiation, and interpretation from both the client/emic and professional/etic perspectives with explication and clarification of overlapping areas in their application. Further consideration will be given to what the modes are and how they relate to the applied constructs of *care, caring, culturally congruent care*, and *cultural competence*.

PURPOSE/RATIONALE

The purpose of this chapter is to provide the reader with an in-depth overview of the three modes of culture care decisions and actions so as to explicate their meanings, intentions, and applications in primary care practice settings by advanced practice nurse practitioners. Making the modes explicit will facilitate their appropriate use by transculturally prepared nurse practitioners in the collaborative [client/provider coparticipative] provision of culture-specific, culturally congruent care that is meaningful and beneficial to individuals, families, communities, institutions, and organizations. Understanding what the modes are and how they are applied in practice will assist nurse practitioners to provide care in an accepting and acceptable manner that supports diverse cultural worldviews, lifeways, beliefs, practices, and expressions and to avoid cultural imposition through ethnocentric care decisions and actions that incur pain, harm, or negative outcomes.

ETHNOHISTORY OF NURSE PRACTITIONERS AND THEIR CARE/CARING

Advanced practice nursing began when the role of nurse practitioner was created by Dr. Loretta Ford (a nurse) and Dr. Henry Silver (a physician), who developed the first nurse practitioner program at the University of Colorado in 1965 (American Association of Nurse Practitioners [AANP], 2013a). Other programs soon followed and by 1973 more than 65 nurse practitioner programs existed in the United States (AANP, 2013a). As early as 1972, the Burlington Study (Spitzer et al., 1974) presented quantitative data demonstrating that "...a nurse practitioner can provide first-contact primary clinical care as safely and effectively, with as much satisfaction to patients, as a family physician ... [and] without a reduction in quality" (p. 255).

A case study entitled *Nurse Practitioners, Physician Assistants, and Certified Nurse-Midwives: A Policy Analysis* was conducted in response to a request from the Senate Committee on Appropriations and released in 1986 by the Office of Technology Assessment (OTA). The study evaluated the contributions of nurse practitioners (in addition to those of certified nurse–midwives and physician assistants) toward meeting healthcare needs in the United States and was considered to be the most comprehensive study on the subject then undertaken. In a comparative explication about the art of care and caring, the report stated, "...the medical model may be less suitable for measuring the interpersonal quality or art of care, which is more characteristic of care provided by nurse practitioners, physician assistants, and certified nurse midwives. ... Indeed, health promotion, teaching, and counseling [as care] are the essence of nursing education and are also stressed in the curricula for training nurse practitioners (NPs) and certified nurse–midwives (CNMs)" (p. 17).

The 1986 OTA study included an extensive review of the then extant literature of comparison physician versus nurse practitioner care (as well as individual) studies and concluded "...NPs appear to have better communication, counseling, and interviewing skills than physicians" (Congress of the United States, OTA, 1986, p. 19). Nurse practitioners were found to demonstrate more thorough history interviewing and documentation, physical assessment, client teaching, and follow-up care; provide greater depth of discussion; give more advice on child health, prevention, and wellness; and offer more caring therapeutic listening and support (p. 19).

The National Organization of Nurse Practitioner Faculties (NONPF) first issued its *Core Competencies for Nurse Practitioner Education* in 1990; its most current document (2012) recognizes as a core competency the ability of the nurse practitioner [candidate] to facilitate "...the development of healthcare systems that address the needs of culturally diverse populations, providers, and other stakeholders." Credentialing bodies for nurse practitioner national certification to practice also recognize cultural competence as a core value. The American Association of Colleges of Nursing (AACN) cites culture as a key element among its *Essentials for Practice* in its documents for both Doctor of Nursing Practice (2006) and master's-prepared (2011) nurse practitioners. Cultural competence has also been assessed as a core examination element by the American Academy of Nurse Practitioners (AANP, 2013b). Thus, cultural knowledge or cultural competence has been established as part of the national standardization for the scope and standards of practice for all nurse practitioners in the United States.

THEORETICAL FRAMEWORK

As a consequence of her experiences with culturally diverse children in a psychiatric hospital and her 2-year research study with the Gadsup people in Papua New Guinea (1966), Leininger was inspired to develop the Theory of Culture Care Diversity and Universality in the 1960s to help nurses provide culturally congruent care. "There was no one person or philosophic school of thought or ideology per se that directly influenced my thinking. I developed the theory by working on the potential interrelationships of culture and care through creative thinking, and by philosophizing from my past professional nursing experiences and anthropological insights" (Leininger, 1991b, p. 20).

The Sunrise Enabler and the tenets of the theory gave structure to the constructs, premises, and definitions by which nurses and other healthcare professionals could apply the theory in practice. "Transcultural nursing had already been conceived as a comparative field of study and practice, but it needed a theoretical and research base to explain and predict nursing as a discipline and to guide nursing practice. . . . I was interested further in explicating culture care from a humanistic viewpoint" (Leininger, 1991b, p. 29). The Sunrise Enabler is used as a cognitive map to guide advanced practice nurses in their understanding of the cultural influences upon generic and professional care expressions and patterns of the people and ". . .often leads to [the] discovery of embedded, backstage, or deeply valued and meaningful data about human care and wellbeing" (p. 33). In viewing the Sunrise Enabler, one will note that nursing care practices (including generic and professional care) are provided to clients by means of the three culture care modes of decisions and actions for culturally congruent care for health, wellbeing, or death (2006a, p. 25). Leininger intended for the modes to be the means by which nurses applied culture care constructs in the care of diverse people from a culturally holistic perspective for culturally congruent care and beneficial outcomes—the goal of the culture care theory (Horn, 2002, p. 269; Leininger, 2002c, p. 27).

Advanced practice nurses endeavor through the three culture care modes of decisions and actions [which include client participation and education] to provide health promotion and disease prevention as well as treat acute and chronic illness. Conceptualizing advanced practice nursing as a humanistic, caring nursing science and discipline will assist people to retain their health and wellbeing and avoid illness (Leininger, 1991a).

EXPLORATORY QUESTIONS

The main foci of this chapter are to explore relevant answers to the following questions in the context of the primary care nurse practitioner role:

- What are the three culture care modes of culture care actions and decisions?
- How do the modes differ?
- How should the modes be used in primary care by advanced practice nurses?

Explorations for answers to these questions are intended to assist the reader to ultimately gain a stronger grasp of what the modes are and how to appropriately conceptualize and utilize them in primary care and other clinical settings for optimal client health outcomes through the provision of culturally congruent care.

ORIENTATIONAL DEFINITIONS

The selected orientational definitions that follow provide broad focus in relation to the three culture care modes of decisions and actions. These definitions are intended to serve as guides to permit new care discoveries in primary care for advanced practice nurses to identify and explicate inductively phenomena from people and situations and how they know, experience, and define ideas or situations about care (Leininger, 1991b, p. 46).

- **Care** (noun)/**caring** (gerund): Refers to abstract and concrete phenomena related to understanding and knowing human beings in a natural or human way as possible; being with other human beings in assisting, supporting, or enabling experiences, acts, or behaviors toward or for others with expressed, evident, or anticipated needs to ameliorate or improve a human condition or lifeway, or to face death through the application of the culture care modes of decisions and actions in primary care (adapted from Leininger, 1991b, pp. 30, 46).
- **Culture care**: Refers to subjectively and objectively learned and transmitted values, beliefs, and patterned lifeways that assist, support, or enable another individual or group to maintain their

wellbeing, health, improve their human condition or lifeway, or deal with illness, disabilities, or death in primary care decisions and actions (adapted from Leininger, 1991b, p. 47).

- **Emic**: Refers to local, indigenous, or insider's views and values about a phenomenon or experience (adapted from Leininger, 2002b, p. 84); influences care decisions and actions in primary care.

- **Etic**: Refers to outsider's or more universal views and values about a phenomenon or experience (adapted from Leininger, 2002b, p. 84); influences care decisions and actions in primary care.

- **Generic-lay-folk care/systems or caring**: Refers to culturally learned and transmitted lay, indigenous (traditional), or folk (home care) knowledge and skills used to provide assistive, supportive, enabling, and facilitative acts or phenomena toward or for another individual, family, group, community, or institution with expressed, evident, or anticipated needs to ameliorate or improve a human health condition or state of wellbeing, disability, lifeway, or to face disability or death (adapted from Leininger, 1991b, p. 38); relates directly to care decisions and actions in primary care.

- **Professional care/systems**: Refers to formally taught, learned, and transmitted professional/primary care, health, illness, wellness, and related knowledge and practice skills that prevail in professions and professional settings or institutions (often with multidisciplinary personnel) that serve consumers (adapted from Leininger, 1991b, p. 48); relates directly to care decisions and actions in primary care.

- **Health**: Refers to a state of a restorative state of being that is culturally constituted, defined, valued, and practiced and which reflects the ability of the individuals, families, groups, or communities to perform their daily role activities in culturally expressed, meaningful, beneficial, and patterned lifeways (adapted from Leininger, 1991b, p. 48; 2002b, p. 84).

- **Wellbeing**: Refers to an implied quality of life or desired state of existence; serves as a guide for decisions and actions toward desired, meaningful, and beneficial care outcomes (adapted from Leininger, 2006a, p. 11).

- **Culturally congruent care**: Refers to the explicit use of culturally-based health care and health knowledge in sensitive, creative, and meaningful ways to fit the general lifeways and needs of individuals, families, groups, communities/populations for beneficial and meaningful health and wellbeing or to face illness, disability, or death (adapted from Leininger, 2002b, p. 84); a linkage between generic care and professional care (Leininger, 1991b, p. 37) achieved through the application of the three culture care modes of decisions and actions in primary care settings.

- **Cultural competence**: Refers to the ability of advanced practice nurses in primary care settings to provide culturally congruent, safe, and beneficial care through the use of the culture care theory and application of the three culture care modes of decisions and actions (adapted from Leininger, 1991b, 2002b, 2006a).

ASSUMPTIVE PREMISES

Leininger (1991b) formulated and refined a set of assumptive premises ". . .in light of the theoretical conceptualizations, philosophical position, beliefs, and predictive theoretical hunches . . . to guide nurses in their discovery of culture care phenomena" (p. 44). The selected assumptive premises relevant to this chapter are from Leininger (1991b, pp. 44–45; 1995a, pp. 103–104; 2002b, p. 79):

- Care (caring) by the nurse practitioner in the primary care context is essential for wellbeing, health, healing, growth, survival, and to face handicaps or death.
- Culture care is the broadest holistic means to know, explain, interpret, and predict advanced practice nursing care phenomena to guide nurse practitioner practices.
- Culturally congruent or beneficial nursing care can only occur when the individual, group, family, community, or culture care values, expressions, or patterns are known and used appropriately and in meaningful ways by the advanced practice nurse with the people.

CULTURE CARE MODES OF DECISIONS AND ACTIONS

One of the major tenets of the Theory of Culture Care Diversity and Universality is that the three predicted theoretical modes for nursing decisions and actions are key factors to provide congruent, safe, and beneficial care. Culturally congruent care can be realized by co-participation of the nurse and client through the three culture care modes of decisions and actions. Leininger (1991b, 1995a, 2002b, 2006a) defined the modes as:

- Culture care preservation and/or maintenance refers to those assistive, supportive, facilitative, or enabling professional acts or decisions that help cultures to retain, preserve, or maintain beneficial care beliefs and values or to face handicaps and death.

- Culture care accommodation and/or negotiation refers to those assistive, accommodating, facilitative, or enabling creative provider care actions or decisions that help cultures adapt to or negotiate with others for culturally congruent, safe, and effective care for their health, wellbeing, or to deal with illness or dying.
- Culture care repatterning and/or restructuring refers to those assistive, supportive, facilitative, or enabling professional actions and mutual decisions that would help people to reorder, change, modify, or restructure their lifeways and institutions for better (or beneficial) healthcare patterns, practices, or outcomes.

It is the three modes that will continue as the major focus throughout the remainder of this chapter. Although greater emphasis will be placed on the use of the modes by nurse practitioners in primary care settings, the concepts and ideas that remain relevant to other nursing care settings and for use by other advanced practice and registered nurses will be presented as well. Elements of culture care predominate in the use of the modes by advanced practice nurses are *care/caring, quality of life, ethics of care, cultural competence*, and *culturally congruent care* which will be explicated further in a review of the relevant extant literature.

REVIEW OF LITERATURE

Care/Caring

Leininger (2002a) presented nursing as a humanistic and caring science with a societal mandate to serve people (pp. 46–47). Early on in her theory work, she recognized that caring in nursing had a fundamental role in promoting and preserving the health and wellbeing of society but remained on the periphery of political and economic policy decisions (Leininger, 1988, pp. 71–72). Yet she maintained her assertion that caring was a central and essential construct to nursing that should be valued by the profession and the healthcare system. "Objective analysis of motivation for caring in nursing can lean to a clearer perspective of the concept of caring as a significant universal human capacity as well as an intentioned, proficient, and professional service in nursing" (p. 72). Sherwood (1991) later lamented:

> Yet the expression of caring in nursing faces increasing challenges. The expanding applications of technology compounded by the demands of the nursing shortage have created a climate which submerges the caring ethic. . . . Rewards and incentives involve cost-effective treatment modalities and efficient use of time and personnel. But where, as Leininger (1986) pointed out, is the line item in the budget for caring? (p. 80)

These are meaningful and valid words even in the 21st century. Nurses need to take hold of their practice, their profession, and their reputation and work actively as role models in their daily practices and as change agents in their organizations, institutions, and communities to change not only the face of nursing but its perception by lay persons and healthcare professionals alike.

Leininger (1991b) believed ". . .nursing needed to transcend its primary focus on nurse-patient interactions and dyads to that of conceptualizing nursing as a caring science that could focus on families, groups, communities, total cultures, and institutions" (p. 22). This meant viewing culture care not as an integration of compartmentalized elements or perspectives but from a ". . .holistic stance to reflect human functioning and caring existence" (p. 23), [seeing] ". . .culture care from a humanistic standpoint and . . . what would constitute scientific caring in nursing" (p. 29). Leininger meant for care and caring to be literal hands-on experiences such as touching, comforting, assisting, supporting, and expressions of compassion between the nurse and the client—not simply abstractions of thought: ". . . I viewed caring as a humanistic mode of being with others, to assist them in times of need or to help them maintain their wellbeing or health" (p. 29).

Leininger (1991b) recognized that nurses used the terms *care* and *caring* interchangeably; she believed that culture care ". . .had different linguistic uses, meanings, essences, patterns, expressions, functions, and structural features in different cultures that had to be explicated . . . in relation to health and wellbeing" (p. 32). Without knowledge about these ". . .care or caring patterns . . . nursing could not become a caring profession or a legitimate nursing discipline" (p. 32). Leininger posited that the constancy, continuity, familiarity, and credibility of culture have meaning and significance because ". . .human beings are born, live, become ill, survive, experience life rituals, and die within a cultural frame of reference" (p. 37). Therefore, the social structure dimensions of the Sunrise Enabler need to be used to apply cultural knowledge in people-caring modes (p. 37).

Care and *caring* should be integral to every nursing decision or act which should also be made collaboratively or in co-participation with clients in a manner that permits ". . .the client and professional [to] use their knowledge and desires for culturally congruent care with the specific three [decision and] action modes" (Leininger, 2002b, p. 82), ". . .working together to identify, plan, implement, and evaluate each caring mode for culturally congruent care" (Leininger, 1991b, p. 44). The theorist predicted that the failure to link *generic* and *professional* care would result in the absence or lack of *culturally congruent care* which would subsequently result in cultural conflicts, cultural impositions, cultural pain, cultural stresses, and other non-caring acts or unfavorable client care outcomes (Leininger, 1991b, 1995a,

2002c, 2006a). "Care is the nurse's way of being with and helping people" and entails "...essential professional knowledge...art and skill" (Leininger, 1991b, p. 40). It is essential that clients feel comfortable and involved in the care process to "...keep health maintenance and prevention [aspects] of nursing care practices alive and important" (p. 55) to cultures.

Leininger stressed that all caring was human caring, and emphasized the importance of listening to clients, hearing their story, and obtaining clients' emic care knowledge first before presenting etic professional knowledge because "...care without a cultural, holistic perspective in practice is meaningless" (1998, p. 48). In addition, she believed that using the three culture care modes in a co-participative involvement approach essential to ultimately providing culturally congruent care that is both meaningful and beneficial to clients (2002b, p. 82).

Quality of Life

Quality of life is a holistic culturally constituted phenomenon that is "...largely an abstraction of values, beliefs, symbols, and patterned expressions" held by cultural groups and individuals (Leininger, 1994, p. 22). Understanding culture care meanings and values about quality of life in different life contexts from an emic perspective can assist nurses to explain, interpret, and predict human behavior and is valuable to guide their judgments, decisions, and actions in the provision of culturally congruent care (p. 22). Leininger's (1994) review of five cultures demonstrated wide differences among cultures in that "...what constitutes quality of life is by no means universal" (p. 28). Quality of life can be preserved, maintained, or accommodated by nurse practitioners through the collaborative or co-participative use of the three culture care modes of decisions and actions to achieve health outcomes that are both meaningful and beneficial (Leininger, 2007, p. 11). "Most importantly, the three modalities would guide practitioners away from using largely inappropriate, routine, unsafe, traditional, or destructive actions that failed to fit or to be acceptable to cultures" (p. 12).

Ethics of Care

Leininger (2006b) predicted "...many more ethical and moral issues will be identified related to culture care practices as individuals, families, and groups assert their rights to preserve their own ethical values and lifeways" (p. 393). The theorist also predicted increased research and debate on ethical and moral issues related to cultural practices and philosophies with resultant changes in political policies and healthcare guidelines. Cortis and Kendrick (2003) believed that the synergy between ethics and caring when translated into practice should reflect inclusive mores and that nurses should be able to demonstrate an awareness of care as it relates to clients who have a different cultural identity to their own (p. 77). In addition, they noted ". . .the evidence suggests that nurses are woefully unaware of care expectations held by members of minority ethnic groups. This is of central moral concern because it is difficult to talk of a *caring ethic* when research indicates that members of certain minority ethnic communities feel alienated and isolated in the health care equation" (p. 77).

Cultural Competence

Cultural competence describes *the abilities of the nurse*—not the care being provided—in regard to the provision of care for indigenous people or cultural groups. The term *cultural competence* has been mainly defined within transcultural nursing (Curren, 2006; Jeffreys, 2006). Curren (2006) presented her model of cultural competence, *Curren Cultural Competency Guide: Phases of Development to Achieve Cultural Competency* (p. 164), as a visual guide to the educational and experiential steps of a series of transcultural learning sessions she developed for a community hospital toward ". . .the provision of respectful, meaningful, and culturally competent care . . . and to assist employees to effectively manage cultural conflicts with clients" (p. 163). Curren held that the need to acquire cultural knowledge and competence may be either *internally* or *externally* driven, but that *willingness*, a developed sense of self-awareness or *recognition*, followed by *understanding* gained through learned knowledge, needed to occur.

Cultural competence has been defined by Jeffreys (2006) as a multidimensional learning process that integrates transcultural skills in the cognitive, practical, and affective dimensions that aims to achieve culturally congruent care (p. 25). This process fits with Leininger's (1995a) premise that the primary goal of the nursing profession is to serve people by providing culture-specific care through the three culture care modes of decisions and actions which the theorist deemed necessary for the provision of culturally congruent care (p. 103).

Culturally Congruent Care by Nurse Practitioners

Leininger (1996) predicted ". . .providing culturally congruent, meaningful, and responsible care would have many health promoting benefits to people . . . if used in explicit and knowing ways with clients . . . [and that] culture care had to be holistically integrated in practice to lead to client health and wellbeing" (p. 73). She further postulated that use of the culture care theory would continue to be a driving force to move nursing away from the medical model in the 21st century (p. 75). As early as 1998, Leininger applied culture care theory constructs to advanced practice nursing with the recognition that nurse practitioners were ". . .realizing the power of using explicit care modalities to heal and improve health or to help people" (p. 45). Indeed, Leininger (1990) realized the importance of ". . .giving more attention to the impact of modern health practices upon different cultural groups" (p. 52). Without knowledge of cultural norms, mainstream professional healthcare therapeutic efforts resulted in outcomes of limited help or benefit to indigenous peoples or cultural groups (Leininger, 1990, pp. 52–53).

McFarland and Eipperle (2008) discussed how the Theory of Culture Care Diversity and Universality provided an appropriate theoretical framework to guide nurse practitioners in the provision of culturally congruent care in primary care contexts (p. 48). "Given that culture care is a core competency domain for nurse practitioners, it is our view that nurse practitioners need to recognize the need, validity, and *missing component* of culture care in nursing" (p. 49). The authors asserted that the ". . .nurse practitioner needs to be able to sensitively and competently integrate culture care into contextual routines, clinical ways, and approaches to primary care practice through role modeling, policy making, procedural performance and performance evaluation, and the use of the advanced practice nursing process" (p. 49). They further predicted it was through the use of the three culture care modes of decisions and actions that nurse practitioners would be able to provide culturally congruent care to clients and achieve safe, meaningful, and beneficial care outcomes in the primary care setting (pp. 49–50).

In focusing on the emic perspective, McFarland and Eipperle (2008) stated that establishing a trusting relationship with clients to assist them in their endeavors to prevent and treat disease and move toward health and wellness was essential for clients' care and caring by the nurse practitioner (p. 50). Becoming knowledgeable about the individual or family worldview, lifeway, and caring values as well as their social structure factors will facilitate obtaining accurate clinical and nonclinical information through advanced nursing observation and assessment (p. 51). It is imperative that sensitively and respectfully obtained, accurate, culture-specific information is used to develop therapeutic regimens that will be beneficial and acceptable to the clients who will implement them (p. 51). "Integrating generic and professional care concepts into advanced practice nursing within the nurse practitioner role is essential to achieving beneficial care outcomes for the client" (p. 52).

Primary care serves as a first contact in the healthcare system for most consumers. The three culture care modes of decisions and actions are key to providing culturally congruent care by nurse practitioners in the primary care setting.

> It is most essential for the nurse practitioner to use the three modes of care and caring with respect for the client's beliefs, values, and expressions regarding health and wellbeing and to advocate for the client based on the client's worldview, and to do so in partnership with the client to ensure that safe, beneficial, and appropriate as well as culturally congruent care decisions and actions are mutually chosen. (McFarland & Eipperle, 2008, p. 51)

Leininger (2002b) stated that ". . . cultural conflicts, cultural imposition practices, cultural stresses and cultural pain reflect the lack of culture care knowledge to provide culturally congruent, responsible, safe, and sensitive care" (p. 79). Therefore, it is vital for the nurse practitioner to use the three culture care modes through the emic lens of the client as well as the etic lens of the professional (McFarland & Eipperle, 2008, p. 53).

DISCOVERIES FOR CULTURE-SPECIFIC CARE

The three culture care modes of decisions and actions are unique approaches to providing culture-specific and congruent care to individuals, families, groups, communities, organizations, and institutions. As previously mentioned, the three culture care modes of decisions and actions are:

- Culture care preservation and/or maintenance
- Culture care accommodation and/or negotiation
- Culture care repatterning and/or restructuring

Throughout many years of clinical practice and in teaching transcultural nursing to various levels of nursing learners, this author has found that the modes have been most challenging for "newcomers" to the culture care theory to understand in class and apply to practice situations. As a nurse practitioner, the reader may indeed ask: *What exactly are the modes?* This author offers that the culture care modes of decisions and actions are *emically applied clinical practices or expressions of care/caring for or with the client rather than applied to or upon the client for his/her physical, emotional, psychological, social, or spiritual care.* The ideas, plans, thoughts, values, beliefs, expressions, patterns, and most practices used in efforts to provide culturally congruent care should stem from the worldview and lifeways of the client, not from the nurse or the care setting or organization. The modes are not derived from the etic perspective of the nurse, other health professionals, or the healthcare setting or institution. The modes most definitely do not entail a "nursing plan of care" developed with the "patient at the center" that is presented to the patient and/or family/significant others for "approval" or "acceptance" as is commonly done throughout healthcare systems in the United States and elsewhere. This approach completely misses the mark regarding culturally congruent care despite the best of intentions.

Using the three modes of culture care decisions and actions is part of the advanced practice nursing process and requires active engagement in critical thinking. Appropriate client culture-specific focus and care application are essential to prevent cultural imposition or cultural pain. *Holding knowledge* [noun] of the client's culture with thoughtful and thorough attention to detail is required to fully integrate the care modes into primary care practices. Cultural assessment skills must be learned, developed, and honed to become proficient or expert in their application. This requires motivation and dedication to active learning by the nurse practitioner to be able to collaboratively engage with and advocate on behalf of one's culturally diverse clients.

In the medical model of healthcare delivery, healthcare professionals tend to begin with efforts to "change" the client and his/her care practices to fit with the protocols, policies, preferences, or preferred evidence currently extant in the care setting. In the transcultural model of care based on the Theory of Culture Care Diversity and Universality, the approach is opposite. Culturally competent nurse practitioners begin with what can be retained, endeavoring to "keep" all that is beneficial or does no harm. If indicated, they then address generic care practices that may have been identified as needing or would benefit from an approach of mutual compromise based on safety, effectiveness of outcomes, or conflicts or negative interactions with other treatments of consent. Thereafter—again, only if indicated—culturally competent nurse practitioners may need to move on to care areas needing adjustment or change based on known hazards or significant risks to safety, or serious situations that place a client in jeopardy. It is indeed much easier to evaluate which of the culture care modes was used in past or prior practice applications of the theory than to determine this while "in the act" of endeavoring to provide culturally congruent care. Nevertheless, culturally competent nurse practitioners must be cognizant about which of the three modes of culture care decisions and actions is being used. Strong critical thinking skills are needed to reflect on the rationale about which mode is chosen to ensure the provision of culturally congruent care—the challenge, mission, and goal of the theory.

In the nursing literature, only one article (Wehbe-Alamah, McFarland, Macklin, & Riggs, 2011) was found that reported a research study in a primary care setting using the Theory of Culture Care Diversity and Universality with the ethnonursing research method. In addition, both Courtney and Wolgamott (2015) and Mixer (2015) used the modes as the context to present findings or outcomes in their respective chapters of this text. Therefore, the exemplars cited in the following discussion present the use of the three culture care modes of decisions and actions in the provision of culturally congruent care across diverse healthcare settings by registered nurses as well as nurse practitioners.

Culture Care Preservation and/or Maintenance

Following Leininger's lead, culturally competent advanced practice nurses endeavor (in most circumstances) *first* to preserve and maintain client care practices, beliefs, values, and expressions. Sensitive assessment of the effectiveness, safety, and meaningfulness of generic care practices will avoid cultural imposition and cultural pain while *preserving* and respecting the client's self-determined care values, beliefs, and expressions. "It is important to first consider what people are doing right in caring for themselves and their families. Many times people are giving exquisite care in their homes or nursing homes for their children or elderly relatives and these caring actions should be maintained and supported by nurses" (M. R. McFarland, personal communication, December 18, 2013).

Further delineation of this mode reveals subtexts to its application and use. For culture care preservation and/or maintenance, *preservation* means to keep whatever care patterns and practices clients have in place for themselves such as prayer rituals, clothing items, and head covering. *Maintenance* means to support or provide care essential to the client from his/her perspective for or on behalf of the client when he/she is unable to do so—for example, religious or other dietary restrictions, death rituals, and family/kinship support patterns/practices.

Wehbe-Alamah et al. (2011) discovered that nurse practitioners in the urban primary care setting preserved and/or maintained their clients' health and wellbeing by being attentive listeners and integrating their findings into the management of clients' chronic illnesses (p. 23). Wehbe-Alamah (2008) presented appropriate culture-specific nursing and healthcare practices across all settings for Muslim clients in great detail. Other notable exemplars have described culture care preservation and/or maintenance in the *holism* beliefs, values, and practices of Hawaiian *kapuna* or elders (Davis, 2010) and the residual cultural heritage beliefs and herbal practices of African American elders in the Mississippi Delta region (Gunn & Davis, 2011), both in the home care setting. For substance-dependent African

American women who had been or were residing in a transitional home, Ehrmin (2005) stressed ". . .Family and kinship caring experiences and practices, in which the women felt cared for, listened to, understood, not judged, respected, and loved unconditionally, would need to be preserved and maintained and used as a strength to help the women improve their health and wellbeing" (p. 123). In the urban community, the protection and surveillance attributes of urban adolescent gang members were carefully explicated by Morris (2012), whereas Carr (1998) identified the close, protective involvement or *vigilance* of families caring for hospitalized relatives.

These and many other studies using the culture care theory provide strong and solid evidence of the inherent value, meaningfulness, and benefit to preserving and/or maintaining generic/folk/traditional/indigenous care practices in the provision of advanced practice nursing care that can be extrapolated for use in the primary care setting. "These modes allow for individualized approaches to care decisions and actions as well as incorporating into [advanced] nursing practice the diverse ways of knowing within cultures . . . Inherent in each of these modalities are three of the core values that underlie advanced practice nursing: respect, advocacy, and partnership" (McFarland & Eipperle, 2008, p. 51).

The nurse practitioner, staff, and practice organization have many options in the primary care setting to preserve and/or maintain clients' generic care practices. Using the Sunrise Enabler as a cognitive map, the nurse practitioner can begin by ensuring that décor is culturally appropriate and welcoming; culture-specific and language-appropriate reading, educational, and entertainment materials/media are clearly in evidence and easily accessible; content of forms and composition of staff are culturally congruent; and culture- and gender-appropriate meet-and-greet practices are well known and correctly used by each administrative and clinical staff member with special attention to needs and perceptions regarding privacy and confidentiality throughout the care process (McFarland & Eipperle, 2008, p. 53).

Nurse practitioner culture care preservation and/or maintenance practices can occur when establishing a client relationship; when co-establishing the manner of assessment to be performed; and by integrating generic care approaches when mutually developing plans of care decisions and actions with clients (McFarland & Eipperle, 2008, p. 52). The nurse practitioner can observe the client sitting in the waiting room or walking down the hall to the examination which present valuable opportunities to assess general appearance, gait, pain expressions, and signs or symptoms of potential tobacco or alcohol abuse as well as to note cultural or non-contemporary forms of dress and language use and individual means of contextualizing the reason or purpose of the healthcare visit during this introductory period of the visit (p. 57). An additional brief period of conversation with the client in the examination room will allow the nurse practitioner further time for observation while assisting the client to become more comfortable, thus enabling the nurse practitioner to obtain a more detailed and accurate health history and physical assessment.

Reflection is also a valuable part of the advanced practice nursing process. The nurse practitioner can clarify valuable information and reflect the diagnostic findings back with the client and confirm acceptability and understanding while starting the process of co-developing a plan of care with the client using culture care preservation and/or maintenance as the beginning. "Using open-ended questions, active listening techniques, and appropriate language and touch are definitive ways to demonstrate caring and facilitate client trust and sharing during the assessment process as well as throughout all phases of the [advanced practice] nursing process" (McFarland & Eipperle, 2008, p. 52). Sensitivity, flexibility, and genuine caring are essential not only to preserving and/or maintaining client's generic care practices but their continued relationship with the nurse practitioner and an active involvement in their own health and wellbeing through primary care.

Culture Care Accommodation and/or Negotiation

If, in the course of cultural or client assessment, generic care practices are identified that may need modification or adjustment to protect client safety or the effectiveness of treatments of consent, or to prevent or ameliorate care conflicts or negative interactions, then culture care accommodation and/or negotiation is the care mode used to address the situation. Here again, subtext exists. *Accommodation* means to bend, alter, change, facilitate, modify, or adjust *nursing care approaches* to meet the culture care needs of the client, such as altered medication or meal times, rearranging furniture to better meet client self-identified needs or preferences, or modifying nursing assignments based on gender. *Negotiation* is a process of discussion with the client to reach a mutually agreeable compromise regarding a generic care and/or nursing care practice that requires an element of change by both the nurse and the client, such as number or timing of visitors, use of generic remedies, or inclusion of home-prepared meals in dietary regimen when medical/illness restrictions are indicated (e.g., diabetes, postsurgical status).

In the primary care setting, Wehbe-Alamah et al. (2011) identified in their study that nurse practitioners in an urban primary care clinic were observed using the mode of culture care accommodation and/or negotiation by ". . .negotiating with participants to identify and prioritize their three most urgent concerns" (p. 24) with a plan agreed upon to address remaining concerns during a subsequent follow-up appointment. These same nurse practitioners also made themselves available to clients during off-hours via an on-call system wherein clients feeling significantly unwell or experiencing changes of condition were encouraged to contact their nurse practitioner first rather than present to the emergency room (p. 23). In using culture care accommodation and/or negotiation, sensitivity, flexibility, and respect remain essential to achieve outcomes that are both meaningful and beneficial, and to the ongoing mutuality of the nurse practitioner/client relationship.

Webhe-Alamah (2008) provided substantive, evidence-based examples of culture care accommodation and/or negotiation for Muslim clients regarding the number and frequency of visitors; providing a clean and private area for prayer; and ensuring pork- and alcohol-free diet and medications (pp. 93–94). Carr (1998) found that nurses could ". . .assist family members to negotiate and change their lifeways while experiencing transitions . . . of lifestyle and role, daily rhythm, space, and going home" (pp. 77–78) from the intensive care unit either upon discharge or death of their loved one. Schumacher (2010) described the need for nurses to show sensitivity and respect; provide presence with focused and undivided attention; and allow family involvement in the provision of physical care during visits with clients from the Dominican Republic (p. 101).

Forming collaborative relationships, permitting access to fellow gang members during emergency treatment, and listening attentively/showing respect were reported by Morris (2012) as valued accommodative care decisions and actions voiced by members of the African American adolescent gang subculture (p. 268). Hawaiian elders, however, valued having cultural foods, being heard, and receiving care that is "friendly, personal, and caring" (Davis, 2010, p. 243).

Farrell (2006) discovered that ". . .Potawatomi people need sufficient time to process information before a response can be expected" (p. 231). In addition, nurses needed to learn about and gain respect for Native American spirituality and traditional ritual or ceremonial practices for caring decisions and actions toward the provision of culturally congruent care. "Nurses and other clinicians needed to incorporate the Native American spirituality, values, and beliefs to accommodate and/or negotiate mutually acceptable changes in the Potawatomi lifeways to promote their health and wellbeing" (p. 231).

Ehrmin (2005) reported ". . .Many women talked about having felt judged by nurses and other healthcare providers" (p. 123). Her study findings supported the need for nurses to ". . .accommodate the African American women's care needs of being given time to be listened to and understood, not judged, shown respect, and loved unconditionally . . . [and] learn to *empathize with* rather than *disapprove of* and negatively judge the women based on their past or current destructive lifeways, including their violation of societal norms of abusing substances" (p. 123).

Accommodation and/or negotiation is sometimes viewed as the "gray area" in the application of the culture care modes of decisions and actions where situations or issues are less clear, more changeable, or less well-defined or identifiable by either the client or the primary care provider. The nurse practitioner may feel lost if discrete boundaries between culture care accommodation and/or negotiation and culture care preservation and/ or maintenance are not easily discernable. This is also where the co-partic-ipative mutuality of the nurse/nurse practitioner and client relationship intensifies, when areas needing accommodation are identified and/or nego-tiations for indicated adjustments take place. The client may feel vulnerable, exposed, an outsider, less powerful in an unfamiliar environment, and/or suffer from an illness or condition that diminishes strength and stamina— all of which can compromise the client's ability to fully assert his or her own beliefs or preferences. It therefore falls to the nurse practitioner to ensure that the client's voice is sought, assured, and heard in these often complex and delicate situations and that every feasible effort is made to ensure that *accommodation* occurs before *negotiation* seems necessary.

Culture Care Repatterning and/or Restructuring

Lastly, the culturally competent nurse practitioner may need move on to care areas needing adjustment or change, where culture care repatterning and/or restructuring is indicated to protect or ensure client safety and well-being. The subtext for this mode differentiates between repatterning and restructuring. *Repatterning* means doing something somewhat differently, so that the *pattern* is preserved while the *format* or *structure* is changed or made different, such as not reusing needles for acupuncture, using sterile instruments for some cultural rituals that involve cutting, or placing an impermeable glass liner in a lead-glazed cup used to administer folk remedy liquids. *Restructuring* represents a major cultural change that involves alter-ing a particular behavior or practice that is unsafe or seriously compromises health or wellbeing, such as discontinuing the cultural practice of female genital cutting/circumcision, avoiding the use of traditional herbs that con-tain toxic compounds, or stopping the folk practice of applying lead-based kohl to the eyes of newborn infants.

"This mode requires the use of both generic and professional knowl-edge and ways to fit such diverse ideas into nursing actions and goals. Care knowledge and skills should always be repatterned for the best interest of the clients" (Leininger, 1991b, p. 44). Repatterning and/or restructuring can be applied to structure of care environments, development of clinical and nonclinical routines in clinical settings and institutions, and the behavioral practices and patterns of nurse practitioners, other clinicians, and ancillary or administrative staff members. Exemplars include speaking loudly to or about clients; not assuring or being sensitive to the need for physical or informational privacy and/or confidentiality during care and noncare interfaces; and talking over and not with clients during episodes of care, among many other large and small situations where the needs of the individual have been subsumed into the mechanized clinical routines of modern Westernized health care out of a sense of justified convenience or habit. Implementing small but significant changes in habitual routines, behaviors, or environments lessens cultural stress and improves client receptivity and adherence to therapeutic plans of care; larger changes can reap greater rewards.

> Nurses should understand that it is a moral imperative to accommodate clients of diverse cultures and to avoid practicing cultural imposition that leads to cultural pain and poor outcomes. Moreover, nurses need to realize and recognize that consumers should largely guide or drive the practice. Nurses' professional etic knowledge needs to be re-examined in order to practice culturally congruent care. (Leininger, 1998, p. 48)

Matters relating to sexual practices or reproduction often require repatterning and/or restructuring, such as attempts to self-induce abortion, not practicing safer-sex methods, or continued sharing of used hypodermic needles as described by Webhe-Alamah (2008, p. 94).

Morris (2012) offered health policy and sociopolitical suggestions to help find ways that diminish violence, theft, and illegal weapon and drug sales among the African American adolescent gang subcultures of the United States as exemplars of culture care repatterning and/or restructuring (p. 268). Gunn and Davis (2011) described an indication for culture care repatterning and/or restructuring among African American elders living in the Mississippi Delta who sometimes used botanicals and other substances "...for which there is no evidence of efficacy" such as coal oil or Vicks salve, the latter of which was eaten by many (pp. 45–46). The elders also were known to ingest dirt which can harbor parasites and cause structural damage to teeth or the gastrointestinal system. Promoting "...the use of Vicks™ salve as a rub, while explaining the dangers of eating it, is an example of repatterning" (p. 46).

Lifeway repatterning and/or restructuring by forming supportive networks among women with similar backgrounds was deemed important for informants in the study by Ehrmin (2005), who stated, "...Nurses can offer these women guidance and direction through suggestions to repattern and restructure destructive lifeways to improve their health and wellbeing" (p. 124). The study by Schumacher (2010) discovered harmful lifeways among rural Dominicans with regard to male *machismo* in their spousal relationships and other uncaring actions that indicated a need for victim support systems, accountability by perpetrators, and culture-wide education regarding the negative effects of these behaviors on health and wellbeing, finding that "...Culture care repatterning and/or restructuring requires ... making changes that are deliberate and comprehensive" (p. 101). Wehbe-Alamah et al. (2011) found that underserved/underinsured urban African American clients were concerned about whether clinic funding would be continued, citing that the lack of primary care alternatives could result in reversal of achieved outcomes (reduced preventable and uncompensated hospital admissions) which seemed to indicate a need for repatterning and/or restructuring of priorities by voters and politicians (p. 24).

Mutuality, sensitivity, and respect with strong attention to cultural lifeways should remain uppermost whenever nurse practitioners initiate or engage in the process of culture care repatterning and/or restructuring of generic or folk care practices with clients (Leininger, 1991b, p. 42). The nurse practitioner (possessing extensive holding knowledge of the culture) and the client together "...creatively design a new or different care lifeway for the health or wellbeing of the client" (p. 44).

DISCUSSION

Earlier in this text, the reader will have noted that the text co-editors McFarland and Wehbe-Alamah have made some updates to the Sunrise Enabler. The revision most relevant to this author's chapter is their clarification and re-ordering of terms—i.e., calling the modes *culture care modes of decisions and actions* rather than *nursing care actions and decisions*. This change took place because various transcultural researchers had demonstrated that the three culture care modes of decisions and actions could be used effectively by multiple healthcare disciplines in various roles and/ or in diverse settings, and because culture care *decisions* are usually reached before *actions* are undertaken or implemented (H. B. Wehbe-Alamah and M. R. McFarland, personal communication, October 18, 2013). Hence, this new languaging has been used throughout this chapter (including quotations) to reflect the ongoing growth and forward movement of building the theory through ethnonursing research findings and their application in clinical practice, nursing education, and administrative/organizational endeavors.

One example of both clinical and administrative/organizational application of the three culture care modes of decisions and actions can be found in the chapter by Courtney and Wolgamott (2015). They described their Doctor of Nursing Practice Capstone Project in a primary care urban clinic where staff development education in culture care was provided toward the goal of developing their cultural competence and thereby increasing cultural assessments of clients. These authors reported that statistical evidence demonstrated increased cultural awareness with anecdotal reports of increased self-efficacy among primary care practice team members who had received cultural competency training education as well as improvement in their self-perceived levels of ". . .tolerance and compassion for diverse cultures and vulnerable populations."

In collegiate nursing education, Mixer (2011) found that ". . .fostering a community of caring within the environmental context of the college/school of nursing and university was essential for promoting faculty and student health and wellbeing and fostering the provision of culturally congruent care." A key discovery of this unique study was that among nursing educators, care was taught primarily through role modeling (Mixer, 2011) which was deemed to be an effective way to teach caring to nurses, administrators, educators, and students. Mixer also postulated that those who experience culturally congruent care may be more likely to role model and provide such care to others. The three culture care modes of decisions and actions were used by participant faculty as a means to teach cultural competence skills and to role model culturally congruent care among themselves and with nursing students.

McFarland and Eipperle (2008) provided a detailed explication of the integration of the Theory of Culture Care Diversity and Universality into the primary care practice of nurse practitioners which can be extrapolated by other advanced practice nurses in various healthcare settings. The focus of their article was the integration of emic generic care practices and perspectives into the etic professional care practices of nurse practitioners. One purpose for writing this chapter has been to further delineate how the three culture care modes of decisions and actions can be the means by which nurse practitioners integrate culturally congruent care throughout their practice settings and approaches toward changing the experience of primary care as viewed by cultures. Care and caring as core constructs of the culture care theory serve as the beginning for providing culturally congruent care. Cultural self-assessment and developing holding knowledge about frequently encountered cultural groups are the next steps toward cultural competence. St. Clair (1999) stated that cultural competence requires "...A change in mindset from viewing how clients can fit into the nurses' world and way of doing things because nurses know best (ethnocentrism) to [one of] examining how nurses may understand and fit into the patients world, [thus] changing the nurses' practice recommendations to include those beliefs, traditions, and practices that have worked for the patient (ethnorelativism)" (p. 1).

At the outset of this chapter, the intention was to answer three questions:

- What are the three culture care modes of culture care actions and decisions?
- How do the modes differ?
- How should the modes be used in primary care by advanced practice nurses?

The studies and articles cited provide strong exemplars of how cultures value and need culturally congruent care through the integration of cultural values, beliefs, patterns, expressions, practices, lifeways, and worldviews into extant professional care practices, approaches, and methods. Nurse practitioners in primary care have the means to use care and caring as the center for their curing and noncuring practices, to become culturally competent, and provide culturally congruent care to their clients using the three culture care modes of decisions and actions. Definitions of the three culture care modes of decisions and actions provided differentiations that were further explicated by delineations of their unique subtexts as well as the identification of some overlapping or gray areas in their use and application in practice. Detailed specifics for the use of the three culture care modes of decisions and actions by nurse practitioners in primary care settings were also presented.

The studies and exemplars discussed in this chapter have shown the use of the three culture care modes of decisions and actions in support of the chapter-specific assumptive premises of the culture care theory. The value and importance for integrating *care (caring)* across all aspects of practice by both the nurse practitioner in the primary care context and registered nurses across all care settings were explicated in detail. Examples supported the constructs of care/caring as essential for applying the three culture care modes of decisions and actions to provide culturally congruent care and achieve health outcomes that are both meaningful and beneficial to cultures. Having holding knowledge and being open, sensitive, and respectful are fundamental to integrate *culture care* into the holistic approach to advanced practice nursing as well as to develop cultural competence. The findings from selected ethnonursing research studies presented in this chapter reflected outcomes demonstrating that, ultimately, culturally congruent or beneficial nursing care can occur only when the individual, group, family, community, or culture care values, expressions, or patterns are known and used appropriately and in meaningful ways with the people. The basic principles of these three selected assumptive premises were extrapolated for application to advanced practice by the nurse practitioners in primary care settings.

It was startling to discover the limited number of published articles wherein the assumptive premises of the culture care theory were described; fewer still fully explicated or documented support or nonsupport for the stated assumptive premises of the study or the culture care theory (circular process). The dearth of published ethnonursing research studies in primary care settings was equally surprising to find. It is imperative for the application of theory by nurse practitioners in primary care settings for researchers to publish as well as conduct these studies to foster dissemination, evaluation, and application of their findings to build the body of culture care knowledge and practice. It is my strong recommendation that transcultural nurse researchers share their scholarly work with the broader transcultural nursing community by submitting articles for publication based not only on their dissertations, but also on their doctoral capstone/translational research projects or master's theses to ensure these valuable findings are shared and can be applied to the provision of culturally congruent care.

CONCLUSION

Care and caring are fundamental to collaborative client coparticipation in primary care. Sensitivity, respect, flexibility, and openness by the advanced practice nurse are crucial for successful application of the three culture care modes of decisions and actions as are strong critical thinking skills and attentive listening and observation throughout the clinical process. The three culture care modes of decisions and actions form a tenet of the Theory of Culture Care Diversity and Universality and serve as key elements essential to the provision of culturally congruent care by nurse practitioners in primary care settings for meaningful and beneficial outcomes for individuals, families, groups, communities, and institutions from diverse cultures.

DEDICATION

This chapter is dedicated in memory of my Mother and Best Friend, Billie J. Eipperle.

ACKNOWLEDGMENT

Appreciative acknowledgment is given to Marilyn R. McFarland and Hiba B. Wehbe-Alamah with gratitude for their patience, support, encouragement, collegiality, and humor.

DISCUSSION QUESTIONS

1. Discuss the ways in which advanced practice nurses can or should appropriately use the three culture care modes of decisions and actions in their approaches with clients and in developing an individualized plan of care.
2. Discuss ways in which your own current care approaches can be adapted by using each of the three culture care modes of decisions and actions. Be specific.
3. Discuss the critical thinking process involved in the appropriate use of the three culture care modes of decisions and actions.

REFERENCES

American Association of Colleges of Nursing (AACN). (2006, October). *The essentials of doctoral education for advanced nursing practice.* Washington, DC: Author. Retrieved from http://www.aacn.nche.edu/publications/position /DNPEssentials.pdf

American Association of Colleges of Nursing (AACN). (2011, March 21). *The essentials of doctoral education for advanced nursing practice.* Washington, DC: Author. Retrieved from http://www.aacn.nche.edu/education-resources /MastersEssentials11.pdf

American Association of Nurse Practitioners (AANP). (2013a). About AANP: Historical timeline. Retrieved from http://www.aanp.org/about-aanp /historical-timeline

American Association of Nurse Practitioners (AANP). (2013b). Testing: Knowledge areas included in the adult, adult-gerontologic, and family nurse practitioner examination. Retrieved from http://www.aanpcert.org/ptistore/control/certs /domains

Carr, J. M. (1998). Vigilance as a caring expression and Leininger's theory of cultural care diversity and universality. *Nursing Science Quarterly, 11*(2), 74–78.

Congress of the United States, Office of Technology Assessment (OTA). (1986, December). *Health technology case study #37: Nurse practitioners, physician assistants, and certified nurse-midwives: A policy analysis.* [NTIS order #PB87-177465]. Washington, DC: Author.

Cortis J. D., & Kendrick, K. (2003). Nursing ethics, caring and culture. *Nursing Ethics, 10*(1), 77–88.

Courtney, R., & Wolgamott, S. (2015). Using Leininger's theory as the building block for cultural competence and cultural assessment for a collaborative care team in a primary care setting. In M. R. McFarland & H. B. Webhe-Alamah (Eds.), *Culture care diversity and universality: A worldwide nursing theory* (3rd ed.). Burlington, MA: Jones & Bartlett Learning.

Curren, D. (2006). Clinical nursing aspects discovered with the culture care theory. In M. M. Leininger & M. R. McFarland (Eds.), *Culture care diversity and universality: A worldwide nursing theory* (2nd ed., pp. 159–180). Sudbury, MA: Jones and Bartlett.

Davis, R. (2010). Voices of Native Hawaiian *Kupuna* (elders) living with chronic illness: "Knowing who I am." *Journal of Transcultural Nursing, 21*(3), 237–245.

Ehrmin, J. T. (2005). Dimensions of culture care for substance dependent African American women. *Journal of Transcultural Nursing, 16*(2), 117–125.

Farrell, L. S. (2006). Culture care of the Potawatomi Native Americans who have experienced family violence. In M. M. Leininger & M. R. McFarland (Eds.), *Culture care diversity and universality: A worldwide nursing theory* (2nd ed., pp. 207–238). Sudbury, MA: Jones and Bartlett.

Gunn, J., & Davis, S. (2011). Beliefs, meanings, and practices of healing with botanicals re-called by elder African American women in the Mississippi Delta. *Online Journal of Cultural Care in Nursing and Healthcare, 1*(1), 37–49.

Horn, B. (2002). Urban USA transcultural care challenges with multiple cultures and culturally diverse providers. In M. M. Leininger & M. R. McFarland (Eds.), *Transcultural nursing: Concepts, theories, research, & practice* (3rd ed., pp. 263–270). New York, NY: McGraw-Hill.

Jeffreys, M. R. (2006). A model to guide cultural competence in education. In M. R. Jeffreys (Ed.), *Teaching cultural competence in nursing and healthcare* (pp. 24–38). New York, NY: Springer.

Leininger, M. M. (1966). *Convergence and divergence of human behavior: An ethno-psychological comparative study of two Gadsup villages in the Eastern Highlands of New Guinea.* Unpublished doctoral dissertation, University of Washington, Seattle, WA.

Leininger, M. M. (1988). Motivational and historical aspects of care and nursing. In M. M. Leininger (Ed.), *Care: The essence of nursing and health* (pp. 61–73). Detroit, MI: Wayne State University Press.

Leininger, M. M. (1990). The significance of cultural concepts in nursing. *Journal of Transcultural Nursing, 2*(1), 52–59.

Leininger, M. M. (1991a). Becoming aware of types of health practitioners and cultural imposition. *Journal of Transcultural Nursing, 2*(2), 32–39.

Leininger, M. M. (1991b). The theory of culture care diversity and universality. In M. M. Leininger (Ed.), *Culture care diversity and universality: A theory of nursing* (pp. 5–68). New York, NY: National League for Nursing.

Leininger, M. M. (1994). Quality of life from a transcultural nursing perspective. *Nursing Science Quarterly, 7*(1), 22–28.

Leininger, M. M. (1995a). Overview of Leininger's theory. In M. M. Leininger (Ed.), *Transcultural nursing: Concepts, theories, research, & practices* (2nd ed., pp. 93–114). New York, NY: McGraw-Hill.

Leininger, M. M. (1995b). Transcultural nursing perspectives: Basic concepts, principles, and culture care incidents. In M. M. Leininger (Ed.), *Transcultural nursing: Concepts, theories, research, & practices* (2nd ed., pp. 57–92). New York, NY: McGraw-Hill.

Leininger, M. M. (1996). Culture care theory, research, and practice. *Nursing Science Quarterly, 9*(2), 71–78.

Leininger, M. M. (1997). Classic article: Overview of the theory of culture care with the ethnonursing research method. *Journal of Transcultural Nursing, 8*(2), 32–52. doi: 10.1177/104365969700800205

Leininger, M. M. (1998). Special research report: Dominant culture care (emic) meanings and practice findings from Leininger's theory. *Journal of Transcultural Nursing, 9*(2), 45–48.

Leininger, M. M. (2002a). Essential transcultural nursing care concepts, principles, examples, and policy statements. In M. M. Leininger & M. R. McFarland (Eds.), *Transcultural nursing: Concepts, theories, research, & practice* (3rd ed., pp. 45–69). New York, NY: McGraw-Hill.

Leininger, M. M. (2002b). Part I: The theory of culture care and the ethnonursing research method. In M. M. Leininger & M. R. McFarland (Eds.), *Transcultural nursing: Concepts, theories, research, & practice* (3rd ed., pp. 71–98). New York, NY: McGraw-Hill.

Leininger, M. M. (2002c). Transcultural nursing and globalization of health care: Importance, focus, and historical aspects. In M. M. Leininger & M. R. McFarland (Eds.), *Transcultural nursing: Concepts, theories, research, & practice* (3rd ed., pp. 3–43). New York, NY: McGraw-Hill.

Leininger, M. M. (2006a). Culture care diversity and universality theory and evolution of the ethnonursing method. In M. M. Leininger & M. R. McFarland (Eds.), *Culture care diversity and universality: A worldwide nursing theory* (2nd ed., pp. 1–41). Sudbury, MA: Jones and Bartlett.

Leininger, M. M. (2006b). Envisioning the future of culture care theory. In M. M. Leininger & M. R. McFarland (Eds.), *Culture care diversity and universality: A worldwide nursing theory* (2nd ed., pp. 389–394). Sudbury, MA: Jones and Bartlett.

Leininger, M. M. (2007). Theoretical questions and concerns: Response from the theory of culture care diversity and universality perspective. *Nursing Science Quarterly, 20*(1), 9–15.

McFarland, M. R., & Eipperle, M. K. (2008). Culture care theory: A proposed practice theory guide for nurse practitioners in primary care settings. *Contemporary Nurse, 28*(1–2), 48–63.

Mixer, S. (2011). Use of the culture care theory to discover nursing faculty care expressions, patterns, and practices related to teaching culture care. *The Online Journal of Cultural Competence in Nursing and Healthcare, 1*(1), 3–14.

Mixer, S. J. (2015). Application of culture care theory in teaching cultural competence and culturally congruent care. In M. R. McFarland & H. B. Webhe-Alamah (Eds.), *Culture care diversity and universality: A worldwide nursing theory* (3rd ed.). Burlington, MA: Jones & Bartlett Learning.

Morris, E. J. (2012). Respect, protection, faith, and love: Major care constructs identified within the subculture of selected urban African American adolescent gang members. *Journal of Transcultural Nursing, 23*(3), 262–269.

National Organization of Nurse Practitioner Faculties (NONPF). (1990). *Advanced nursing practice: Nurse practitioner curriculum guidelines.* Washington, DC: Author.

National Organization of Nurse Practitioner Faculties (NONPF). (2012). *Nurse practitioner core competencies.* Washington, DC: Author.

Schumacher, G. (2010). Culture care meanings, beliefs, and practices in rural Dominican Republic. *Journal of Transcultural Nursing, 21*(2), 93–103.

Sherwood, G. (1991). Expressions of nurses' caring: The role of the compassionate healer. In D. A. Gaut & M. M. Leininger (Eds.), *Caring: The compassionate healer* (pp. 79–88). New York, NY: National League of Nursing.

Spitzer, W. O., Sackett, D. L., Sibley, J. C., Roberts, R. S., Gent, M., Kergin, D. J., . . . Wright, K. (1974). The Burlington randomized trial of the nurse practitioner. *New England Journal of Medicine, 290*(5), 251–256.

St. Clair, A. (1999). Preparing culturally competent practitioners. *Journal of Nursing Education, 38*(5), 228–234.

Wehbe-Alamah, H. (2008). Bridging generic and professional care practices for Muslim patients through use of Leininger's culture care modes. *Contemporary Nurse, 28*(1–2), 83–97.

Wehbe-Alamah, H., McFarland, M., Macklin, J., & Riggs, N. (2011). The lived experiences of African American women receiving care from nurse practitioners in an urban nurse-managed clinic. *Online Journal in Cultural Competence in Nursing and Healthcare, 1*(1), 15–26.

Chapter 11

Using Leininger's Theory as the Building Block for Cultural Competence and Cultural Assessment for a Collaborative Care Team in a Primary Care Setting

Renee Courtney
Susan Wolgamott

> *Cultural Collaborative Care approach refers to those values, meanings, and expressions by persons that reveal a desire for working together in order to attain and preserve health and wellbeing for oneself and others.*
>
> (McFarland, 2011)

INTRODUCTION

It is imperative for the health of the nation that healthcare providers recognize the need to provide culturally congruent care to patients and to be knowledgeable and skillful in the delivery of culturally congruent care to diverse populations. The researchers, as part of their Doctoral Capstone Project, wished to focus on the cultural awareness, cultural assessment, cultural competence, and documentation skills of the healthcare team in a primary care setting that strives to provide culturally collaborative care for the patients. Zaccagnini and White (2011) outlined the framework for a scholarly Doctoral Capstone Project, describing each necessary step from problem identification through evaluation (p. 458). Translational research, as utilized by the Agency for Healthcare Research and Quality (AHRQ) in its Translating Research into Practice (TRIP) program, serves as a vehicle to accelerate research being brought into practice at the bedside (White & Dudley-Brown, 2012, p. 23). Doctors of Nursing Practice (DNP) are uniquely qualified to play a dynamic role in translational research, as they are thoroughly prepared to effectively evaluate and analyze the research of discovery and "...will be key to closing the research-to-practice gap and improving health outcomes in the United States" (Vincent, Johnson, Velasquez, & Rigney, 2013, para 3).

PURPOSE OF THE TRANSLATIONAL RESEARCH PROJECT

The purpose of the described project, using the frameworks of Leininger's Theory of Culture Care Diversity and Universality and her new theoretical construct of *collaborative care,* was to facilitate and support the ongoing cultural competence education of a multidisciplinary healthcare team in an urban clinic for underserved individuals and groups. The project focused on utilizing a formal educational process as a means to expand the cultural awareness of healthcare providers and clinic staff members and to integrate cultural assessment into the documentation of each clinical encounter. The needs assessment of the clinic revealed a lack of formal cultural competence education/preparation for the clinic staff (medical assistants, nurse practitioners, and physical therapists) that impaired their ability to provide culturally congruent care. Culturally congruent care is an essential element across the healthcare continuum especially as globalization has increased the multicultural character of the United States and the world (Andrews, 2006, pp. 84–85).

The U.S. Census Bureau projects that the national population will increase by 50% from 1995 to 2050, with the majority of this growth anticipated to be among racial and ethnic minorities (Shaya & Gbarayor, 2006). The authors postulated that healthcare providers' lack of cultural awareness and experience with the customs and norms of culturally diverse patients may further aggravate the effects of health disparities and have an adverse effect on health nationwide. Consequently, healthcare providers will be challenged to provide quality care and meet the healthcare needs of a diverse and changing population.

In the 1960s, through the efforts of Dr. Madeline Leininger, nursing education programs began to recognize the importance of integrating cultural competence content foci into their nursing curricula. As the culture care theory has evolved, many practitioners have become experts in the field and have developed various models and tools that facilitate cultural awareness, cultural competence, and culturally congruent care. Although transcultural nursing education has a 50-year history, and attention to culture care has gained momentum, it is still not commonly offered either as a stand-alone course or content-focused module and no particular approach has been found to be more effective than another in educating nurses about transcultural nursing (Kardong-Edgren & Campinha-Bacote, 2008, p. 37).

Healthcare disparities in the vulnerable urban underserved population of Flint, Michigan, relate directly to their increased mortality and morbidity outcomes (U.S. Department of Health and Human Services [USDHHS], 2012a). Inadequate cultural competence education for healthcare clinical staff members coupled with an absence of cultural assessment have led to missed opportunities to really know each patient's worldview, lifeways, and culture care values, beliefs, and practices that could have led to beneficial culture care actions and decisions for optimal health and wellness outcomes (Leininger, 2006, pp. 20–21). Therefore, this translational research project was focused toward maximizing the transcultural assessment skills of healthcare clinical staff members in a primary care setting.

WORLDVIEW/SOCIAL CULTURAL STRUCTURE CONTEXT

Healthcare disparities among urban underserved populations in the United States continue to increase annually (USDHHS, 2012a). The *Healthy People 2020* goals over the past 3 decades have stressed the need for affordable and accessible healthcare (USDHHS, 2012b). Despite widespread efforts toward accomplishing this goal, "… almost one in four Americans does not have a primary care provider (PCP) or health center where they can receive regular medical services" (USDHHS, 2012a); in addition, only one in five Americans has healthcare insurance.

The staff at a large Midwestern university campus-based primary care clinic provide high-quality health care to local underserved urban populations at little or no direct patient cost. The population in the urban area surrounding the campus is comprised of a diverse mix of cultures. Cultural beliefs and values have a direct effect on the health and wellness of individuals, families, groups, and populations (USDHHS, 2005). Healthcare professionals and clinical support staff need to be culturally competent to be able to fully assess each patient's individual, and sometimes complex, healthcare needs. Assessment of a patient's cultural needs provides critical information and insight that can be valuable across the continuum of care. Educating the healthcare team to perform cultural assessments and develop a plan of care that includes consideration for the cultural care needs of clients can improve health and wellness outcomes (USDHHS, 2005).

LITERATURE REVIEW

The ability to successfully perform an adequate and appropriate cultural assessment in the primary care environment requires transcultural nursing education supported by adequate practice setting resources. The roles of the primary care nurse practitioner and the multidisciplinary healthcare team are ideally suited for identifying disparities and effecting change. Their ongoing relationships with patients are very often intimate ones that engender trust. In the length of one office visit, a cultural assessment performed by a culturally competent healthcare provider can allow for immediate mobilization of local resources or identify key social structure issues that could significantly affect patient safety or care outcomes.

Numerous education modalities to improve cultural competence can be found in the literature. For example, service learning/immersion, clinical simulation/role play, self-assessment, and lecture are approaches supported by research; creative self-assessment activities (using photos), role play/simulation, and didactic modules were utilized to educate the multidisciplinary healthcare team (Amerson, 2010; Bemker & Schreiner, 2011; Kardong-Edgren & Campinha-Bacote, 2008; Shellman, 2007; Wehbe-Alamah, 2010). Amerson (2010) and Killion (2001) both reported on the importance of using innovation to expand the cultural experience, such as photograph identification games and the compilation of reflective journals using photos to depict experiences. Shellman (2007) discussed how repeated experiences can help to increase holding knowledge thereby facilitating the progression toward cultural competence.

Kardong-Edgren and Campinha-Bacote (2008) found that no one curricular approach had better learning outcomes than another, but that the teaching approach using didactic modules appeared to elicit better clinical outcomes. At the 37th Annual Conference of the International Society of Transcultural Nursing, Bemker and Schreiner presented their study findings about enhancing multicultural perspectives in nursing education through the use of simulation. The computer-based teaching module in their project used simulation to provide education regarding cultural awareness and clinical decision making. Their findings demonstrated increased cultural competence as a direct benefit of simulated experiential teaching. Amerson (2010) and Nokes, Nickitas, Keida, and Neville (2005) both reported research findings that also supported immersion experiences as a modality that effectively increased staff confidence and cultural competence. As part of their translational research Capstone Project, the chapter authors used transculturally focused education modules taught through blended approaches and delivered via mixed media to the entire primary care urban clinic staff.

THEORETICAL FRAMEWORK

Leininger's culture care theory (CCT) is holistic and comprehensive in guiding the discovery of diverse cultural knowledge and flexible for use in teaching, research, and practice (Leininger, 2002, p. 3). The basis for the creation of the educational modules used to assist clinic providers and staff toward viewing patients as holistic beings were the CCT, the Sunrise Enabler (Appendix 11-A), and the collaborative care construct. The theory was utilized to develop materials for instruction to help the clinic staff in learning how to tease out multiple social, cultural, and environmental dimensions of patients and families for appropriate care provisions and teaching and applying the concepts.

A key point of Leininger's theory is that *care* is embedded in culture; healthcare providers are challenged to understand both *care* and *culture in order* to practice transcultural care (Leininger, 2002, p. 6). The project described focused on engaging healthcare providers in transcultural education with use of the culture care theory which served as the foundational approach to expand their cultural awareness, enable cultural assessments, and empower use of the theoretical constructs in developing and enacting their plans of care.

The Johns Hopkins Nursing Evidence-Based Practice Model (JHNEBP) was useful in translating theory and evidence into practice (Newhouse, Dearholt, Poe, Pugh, & White, 2007). The JHNEBP model was developed collaboratively with bedside nurses and nursing faculty at Johns Hopkins University. Their goal in developing the model was to demystify the process of implementing evidence-based practice (EBP) into everyday nursing practice (Melnyk & Fineout-Overholt, 2011, p. 269). In the JHNEBP model, EBP has a broad definition and utilizes a problem-solving approach to clinical decision making, integrates scientific evidence and considers internal and external forces, and then carefully applies the evidence to individual patients or populations (Newhouse et al., 2007, p. 35).

Conceptually, the JHNEBP model is supported by both research and nonresearch evidence within the nursing domains of practice, education, and research. A domain is defined as "…a field or scope of knowledge or activity" (*American Heritage Dictionary*, 2009). The components of the model that further guide evidence-based projects include developing a practice question, identifying evidence, and then translating evidence into practice—a process known as practice–evidence–translation (PET). Each of these components was developed in a stepwise approach and available tools of high utility guided staff through the critical steps (Newhouse et al., 2007, pp. 37–38); each of these tools had been independently reviewed and evaluated as positively facilitating bedside clinical decision-making (Melnyk & Fineout-Overholt, 2011, p. 271). As the JHNEBP model was provisionally tried with success with another multidisciplinary healthcare team (Newhouse et al., 2007), it was deemed an appropriate model for use with this Capstone Project.

Leininger's Theory of Culture Care Diversity and Universality was used as the framework for designing teaching modules for providing transcultural education to healthcare providers and staff members. Leininger's theory guided the project toward increasing healthcare providers' holding knowledge about cultures they commonly encounter. The culture care theory also provided a systematic approach for the delivery of culturally congruent care using the social structure dimensions and modes of care action and decision as depicted in the Sunrise Enabler. The Johns Hopkins Nursing Evidence-Based Practice Model (JHNEBP) was a practical and useful model for implementing evidence-based research into clinical practice (Newhouse et al., 2007). Combining the CCT and the JHNEBP model with a didactic module/repetitive learning educational approach linked several elements that were beneficial to the development of a pilot program for *cultural assessment* and *staff education*—the building blocks of cultural competence.

RESEARCH QUESTIONS

The project had a twofold approach encompassing two distinct objectives and is best illustrated by the formulated PICOT questions that follow. PICOT is an acronym for a format to help in developing research questions and guides the search for evidence. Each letter represents a component of the research question: P (population), I (intervention), C (comparison), O (outcome) and T (time) (Melnyk & Fineout-Overholt, 2011, p. 10).

- **First PICOT question**: Will healthcare providers and clinic staff (P) who participate in an educational transcultural nursing module (I) achieve an increase in their perceived cultural competence to provide transcultural care (O) when comparing a pre-test administered before the class with an after-class post-test (C) given at 3 months (T)?

- **Second PICOT question**: Will healthcare providers and clinic staff (P) who participate in a transcultural nursing educational module and are provided with a collection of resources to increase their cultural competence (I) increase the incidence of cultural assessment of patients (O) as evidenced by increased documentation of cultural assessments in the patient healthcare record (C) when reviewed over a 6-month period (T)?

OBJECTIVES AND GOALS

The project objectives were to increase staff cultural competence, awareness of resources, and performance of cultural assessments as depicted in the Logic Model (Appendix 11-B). Short-term goals for this project were outcomes related to increased awareness by the clinical staff members about the different cultures they routinely encounter. The long-term goals for the project were 100% staff adherence in documenting patient cultural assessments and for clinical staff members to provide meaningful and beneficial culturally congruent care. Health and wellness clinical outcomes anticipated from this project were that assessments would trigger changes that decreased health disparities for and reduced mortality and morbidity among the urban underserved primary care population.

METHOD

This project was intended to bring renewed energy to the ongoing cultural competence educational efforts for the clinical staff in an urban primary care clinic providing care to an underserved population. The clinic had a cultural diversity education program in the past but experienced significant staff turnover and restructuring over the preceding 2 years and was in need of a more comprehensive cultural competence educational program that included the entire clinic staff (administrative staff, front-office personnel, medical assistants, nurse practitioners, and physical therapists). The project proposal was welcomed and supported by the clinic administration. A careful organizational assessment was performed that included conversations with the administration, practitioners, and staff; observations of the overall patient–staff process; and review of current assessment and documentation practices. Educational approaches for the clinic staff and adaptations to charting tools were then developed as indicated based on the assessment outcomes and the established project goals and objectives. The educational modules contained components focused on cultural competence self-awareness, the culture care theory and collaborative care, cultural assessments, and practical applications.

The project was developed to include two distinct phases which were based on educational steps that had been established for the project. Phase One focused on staff education; the purpose of the translational research project and expectations of staff members were explained during this phase. Phase Two included implementation of a revised SOAPE note (Appendix 11-C) and a revised patient encounter form called a *router* (Appendix 11-D) that incorporated sufficient space for documentation of cultural assessments and culturally-based interventions. During the second phase, clinical staff members were provided with a basic list of scripted questions located on the router and on room signage (Appendix 11-E) located in patient access areas. Staff were instructed that they could choose from these questions to help them initiate cultural assessments.

Phase One included two didactic educational modules for delivery/presentation to staff members in two 55-minute sessions. Module One focused on cultural self-awareness; Module Two introduced cultural assessment guided by the Theory of Culture Care Diversity and Universality along with the theoretical construct of *collaborative care*. Modules Three and Four dealt with performing a cultural assessment and practical applications of the cultural assessment content in the context of the clinic. The modules were designed to be interactive and engage the students through participative activities and discussions as well as lectures that were supplemented by PowerPoint slides. Participative activities included an activity for exploring stereotypes and biases involving photographs and another exercise that involved discovering and sharing personal cultural beliefs. Videotaped scenarios obtained from the Office of Minority Health (USDHHS, 2010) were used to illustrate dynamic cultural assessment discussions in real-life situations.

The staff began using the revised patient encounter routing form and SOAPE note approximately 1 month after completion of the education modules. Data collection began approximately 1 month thereafter.

DATA COLLECTION

The evaluation process entailed a two-step assessment of the staff members' learning experiences in conjunction with chart reviews to determine the presence of cultural assessment documentation. Prior to beginning the first pair of learning modules, the clinic staff members were administered a pre-survey using the Transcultural Self-Efficacy Tool for the Multidisciplinary Healthcare Provider (TSET-MHP) that was created by Marianne Jeffreys (2000). Inspired by the work of Madeleine Leininger and Albert Bandura's social cognitive theory (as cited in Jeffreys, 2006), Jeffreys created a tool to measure the confidence (self-efficacy) of nurses' cultural competence (p. 40). For the Capstone Project discussed, the TSET was used to measure the effectiveness of the project interventions by determining whether an increase in self-efficacy of the clinic staff occurred from pre- to post participation in the didactic education. The clinic staff members were administered the TSET again after they had completed all of the modules and had used the content in daily practice for 5 months. This second TSET was used as a post-test to assess their perceived self-efficacy over time. In addition, after each of the two educational sessions, a post-module survey (Appendix 11-F) was conducted; this survey consisted of three open-ended questions to collect qualitative data. The questions focused on whether staff members perceived any benefit from the program and how the program content may have affected their daily practice. A face-to-face interview (Appendix 11-G) was also conducted upon completion of the project.

Eleven participants attended the first educational session: One administrator, one physical therapy intake scheduler, two physical therapists, one medical assistant, two nurse practitioners, and three front-office reception staff; another office member viewed the session at a later time via videotape. All 11 participants completed the initial TSET and the first module post-survey. Ten participants attended the second educational session, with two additional staff members viewing the videotaped session at a later time; eight participants completed the second module post-survey. At the end of the project, eight post-project TSET surveys were completed by participants. Absences, hiring, and attrition from the original group contributed to some flux in data collection numbers.

Documentation compliance was assessed by the researchers, who examined the subjective data in the SOAPE notes for evidence of cultural assessment information. The modified SOAPE note was presented to the staff during the final educational session; modifications included inserting labeled areas to record both cultural assessments and culturally-based interventions/care actions and decisions. Modifications to the patient routing form allowed for space to document patient responses to the pre-scripted cultural assessment questions. However, all notational sites and the medical decision-making areas were reviewed for the presence of cultural assessment data and/or documented interventions/care actions or decisions in the event that older versions of the chart form had been inadvertently used by the clinical staff.

HUMAN SUBJECTS CONSIDERATIONS

The university institutional review board (IRB) approval was acquired through a two-phase process congruent with the two phases of the translational research project. Informed consent was obtained from all clinical staff members prior to administration of the TSET survey and presentation of the educational modules. The study did not involve any direct patient contact by the researchers. Patient consent for chart access to review documentation for data collection was covered in the permissions clause of the patient privacy consent form signed when care was initiated with the clinic. The chart data and demographic information collected were de identified; no records were maintained outside of the clinic.

DATA ANALYSIS

Quantitative data from the two TSET surveys was collected, scored, and analyzed using the tools provided with the Toolkit. The data analysis examined survey responses in relation to the three *domains of learning* (cognitive, practical, and affective) represented in the TSET subscales. The cognitive domain rated confidence regarding knowledge of different cultural backgrounds. The practical domain rated confidence for interviewing persons from various cultural backgrounds and discussing their values and beliefs. The affective domain examined "...values, attitudes, and beliefs concerning cultural awareness, acceptance, appreciation, recognition, and advocacy" (Jeffreys & Smodlaka, 1998). Analysis of the TSET data 4 months post-intervention was consistent with pre-test results, revealing continued high levels of reported self-efficacy in the affective domain as compared to the cognitive and practical domains. The data for each domain were analyzed using an unpaired *t*-test. The limitations of this area of the data collection process include the very small number of participants and an even smaller number of participants who actually returned their TSETs.

Quantitative data were also collected from chart reviews performed on 212 medical records collected over a 4-month period starting 1 month after completion of the education modules and during concurrent implementation of the revised router and SOAPE note. Each chart was analyzed at five different data points for the documentation of cultural assessment and culturally-influenced interventions (Appendix 11-H). There was no significant difference in the consistency of cultural assessments between the medical assistants and the nurse practitioners. However, there was significant correlation between the documentation of cultural assessments by the nurse practitioners before (33.7%) and after (66.3%) the intervention. Lastly, a significant correlation was also found when charts were reviewed for documentation of culturally-influenced interventions; prior to the intervention there had only been documentation of culturally-influenced interventions 25.8% of the time whereas post-intervention consistency was 74.2%.

Qualitative data gleaned from analysis of the two post module surveys and post project interviews were encouraging and enlightening. Data from both the surveys and the interviews were small in volume and fairly simple to organize and analyze. Content analysis using the ethnonursing research method (Leininger, 2006) revealed a few major themes. The first major theme was *increased awareness*, which included awareness of differences and similarities among cultures and awareness of participants' own level of self-efficacy regarding cultural competence. The second major theme was *satisfaction/ gratification* regarding positive experiences using new knowledge and ability, and increased depth and breadth of self-perceived caring behaviors. The third major theme was *increased tolerance*, wherein participants felt less anxious and less irritated when caring for patients and families from diverse cultures. The fourth major theme was the *desire/enthusiasm to increase knowledge*. Participants expressed a desire to increase their own knowledge about cultural competence and to increase holding knowledge about different cultures.

DISCUSSION

Nearly all staff members reported an increase in cultural awareness during interviews conducted at the conclusion of the project. They expressed feeling positive and enthusiastic about their newly found awareness and increased holding knowledge about different cultures but did not report feeling confident enough to execute this new knowledge in delivering patient care. Staff who reported prior knowledge and sensitivity to different cultures reported renewed enthusiasm and a broadening of their cultural perspective. Several of the staff members reported a new sense of ownership and responsibility for cultural competence during their post project interviews. One staff person said, "…This project made me want to know more and be more." Another shared, "…I thought I was a champion for culturally congruent care until I learned how much I didn't know, and that makes me want to be a better practitioner."

Another reflection shared by several of the staff members was a sense of gratification for being able to identify disparities in access to care and feeling better able to help more people. As a significant number of the patients at the clinic are indigent or homeless, providing the scripted questions and asking staff to perform a cultural assessment gave them "…the permission and the burden to ask those questions that are difficult to ask" with this vulnerable patient population. When asked to elaborate or give examples of successful application of the concepts, the staff members shared stories about patients who had transportation concerns that prevented them from accessing the follow-up care they needed. Although the staff had limited resources to help solve the transportation problems, they felt both gratified and burdened with the challenge of finding solutions to these special needs. Prior to the educational sessions, staff found these types of questions [cultural assessment questions] difficult to ask.

Early in the project development, the clinic director had expressed a desire for validation that the project had affected the attitudes of the practitioners and staff. It was hoped that the outcomes would somehow illustrate that staff attitudes had shifted and become more focused on culturally congruent care. The translational research project design was not intended to identify this outcome due to the limited scope of a capstone project. However, the qualitative findings from the post-project interviews did reveal a shift in sympathy, compassion, and empathy as well as an important theme—tolerance. This was articulated best by one staff member, who shared, "…Every day I am more sympathetic and less biased; I am less quick to judge and I don't get irritated anymore by people from cultures I don't understand. I am comfortable asking them about their culture."

The feedback from clinic staff members revealed marked enthusiasm for the interactive educational activities in the self-awareness content and the video simulation exercise. The didactic educational format was well-received and the length of each teaching session was reported as satisfactory. All staff persons expressed a desire for more content about practical applications, including specific information about cultures and additional tools and strategies for engaging patients in dialogue about cultural needs, beliefs, values, and practices.

CONCLUSION

Initial data analysis supported the clinical significance of and positive clinical outcomes for the primary care clinic. Chart reviews revealed a significant statistical change in the documentation of cultural assessments and culturally-influenced interventions after the educational sessions and assessment form modifications were entirely completed. The outcomes data from the project provided clinic administration the desired feedback regarding improvement in the cultural awareness of the healthcare team (clinic staff and providers) as well as the benefit to clinic and staff acquired by engaging in the research process as part of their continuing journey toward cultural competence. An unintended finding from the face-to-face post-project interviews was increased feelings of *tolerance* and *compassion* for diverse cultures and vulnerable populations as reflected by the healthcare team members. Instructional manuals and video links for the videotaped educational sessions were provided to the clinic for use in training new employees and for reinforcement of cultural concepts with the regular staff. The clinic administration indicated their plan for continuing to use the materials, seeking out new information, and striving to improve the quality of culturally congruent care.

Barriers and limitations were encountered during the project. In addition to the small number of staff participants in the project, the limited level of engagement by the medical assistant hampered data generated from the revised patient encounter routing form. A second medical assistant was added midway through the project, which seemed to improve the collection of cultural assessment data. The clinic was in the process of purchasing an electronic health record but still used a paper-based system at the time of this study, which posed some inherent limitations for data collection. TSET surveys were distributed to 12 staff members and providers pre- and post- intervention/implementation, but only nine pre surveys and eight post-surveys were returned.

There are many possibilities for further study not only at this urban clinic but in other settings and locations as well. Some ideas for project expansion at the clinic include measuring staff attitude changes in greater detail; collecting more in-depth data from assessments of enrolled patients, including qualitative interview data; in-depth evaluation of the physical therapy documentation; adding a certificate of completion and/or continuing education units (CEUs) as part of the educational component; and making access to the educational videos a more streamlined process. The clinic staff expressed a strong desire for more information about different cultures; discussion has centered on creating resources in electronic/easy-access formats and/or using culturally-themed mini-learning sessions. The researchers would also like to encourage researchers from other disciplines at the university to participate in educational programs of this type.

ACKNOWLEDGMENTS

Permission was granted by Dr. Leininger for the use of the *collaborative care* content. Much gratitude is given to the tireless support and encouragement of our Capstone Project committee chairpersons Dr. Hiba Wehbe-Alamah and Dr. Marilyn McFarland. Statistician Jenny LaChance played an integral role in the statistical preparation of our data collection and study model in addition to giving tremendous support in our data analysis. Librarian Andrea Rogers-Snyr worked diligently to assist with literature searches and research. The University of Michigan Nursing Department FISCUP grant provided critical financial support to our project. The University of Michigan Frances Frazier Student Travel Scholarship contributed vital funding for the researchers to present their research outcomes at the 2012 International Transcultural Nursing Conference and at state and local professional nursing conferences.

DEDICATION

This chapter is dedicated to our families, friends, and colleagues in the DNP-2 Cohort at the University of Michigan–Flint.

APPENDIX 11-A

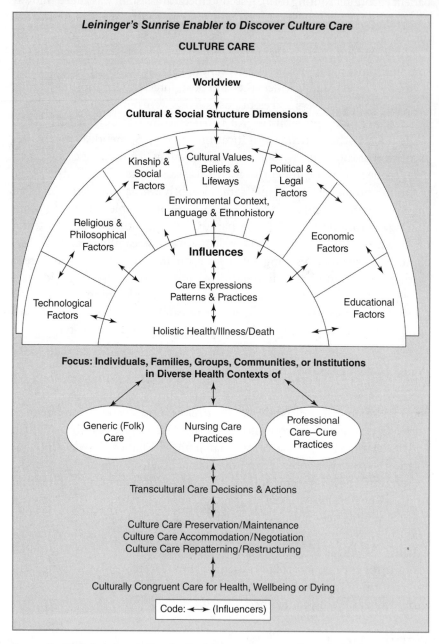

Appendix 11-A Leininger's Sunrise Enabler to Discover Culture Care
Modified with permission from © M. Leininger 2004, by M.R. McFarland and H. B. Wehbe-Alamah.

APPENDIX 11-B: LOGIC MODEL

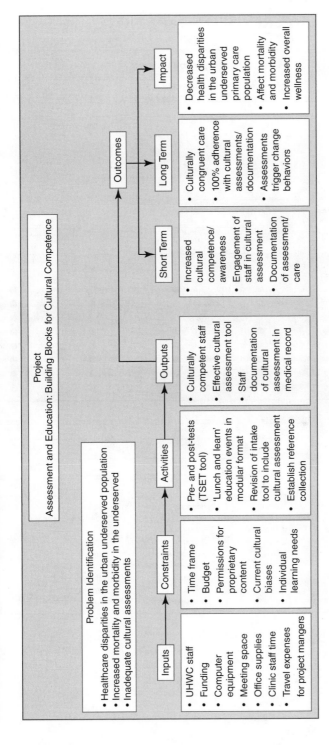

Project
Assessment and Education: Building Blocks for Cultural Competence

Problem Identification
- Healthcare disparities in the urban underserved population
- Increased mortality and morbidity in the underserved
- Inadequate cultural assessments

Inputs
- UHWC staff
- Funding
- Computer equipment
- Meeting space
- Office supplies
- Clinic staff time
- Travel expenses for project mangers

Constraints
- Time frame
- Budget
- Permissions for proprietary content
- Current cultural biases
- Individual learning needs

Activities
- Pre- and post-tests (TSET tool)
- 'Lunch and learn' education events in modular format
- Revision of intake tool to include cultural assessment
- Establish reference collection

Outputs
- Culturally competent staff
- Effective cultural assessment tool
- Staff documentation of cultural assessment in medical record

Outcomes

Short Term
- Increased cultural competence/ awareness
- Engagement of staff in cultural assessment
- Documentation of assessment/ care

Long Term
- Culturally congruent care
- 100% adherence with cultural assessments/ documentation
- Assessments trigger change behaviors

Impact
- Decreased health disparities in the urban underserved primary care population
- Affect mortality and morbidity
- Increased overall wellness

Appendix 11-B Logic Model

APPENDIX 11-C: REVISED SOAPE NOTE

Date 9/28/12   Name
                                                 DOB: Age

SUBJECTIVE

☐ Problem list reviewed and updated if indicated.   Hx

Medications

◯ No specific ROS complaints   ETOH   Smoke   LMP   ☐ Post Menopausal

☐ CV	● neg	☐ GI	● neg	☐ GU	● neg	☐ Respiratory	● neg	☐ Psych	● neg
☐ Chest Pain	● neg	☐ Abd Pain	● neg	☐ Frequency	● neg	☐ DIB	● neg	☐ Depression	● neg
☐ Syncope	● neg	☐ N/V	● neg	☐ Hem/Dysuria	● neg	☐ Cough	● neg	☐ Anxiety	● neg
☐ Edema	● neg	☐ Diarrhea	● neg	☐ Incontinence	● neg	☐ Wheeze	● neg	☐ Pain	● neg
☐ Endo/Lymph	● neg	☐ Constipation	● neg	☐ Discharge	● neg	☐ ENT	● neg	☐ Skin	● neg
☐ Fatigue	● neg	☐ Muscular	● neg	☐ Sexual	● neg	☐ Ear pain	● neg	☐ Rash	● neg
☐ Neuro	● neg	☐ Sprain/Strain	● neg	☐ Skeletal	● neg	☐ Nasal Cong	● neg	☐ Wound	● neg
☐ Neuropathy	● neg	☐ Spasm	● neg	☐ Fx/Disloc	● neg	☐ Sore Throat	● neg		● neg

ROS details

Cultural/Social

OBJECTIVE

☐ Vital signs normal   Glucose   Urine   Kg 0

HR   BP   Temp   O2 sat   RR   Ht feet   Ht in   Wt lb   BMI 0

☐ General	☐ Heart	☐ Abdomen	☐ GU	☐ Other
☐ WNL	☐ RRR, s1s2	☐ Soft, non-tender, +BS	☐ Genital exam defer	
☐ Weight gain/loss	☐ Murmur	☐ Tenderness	☐ Lesions	
☐ HEENT WNL	☐ Irregular	☐ Organomegaly	☐ Discharge	
☐ Head/face pain	☐ Lungs	☐ Musculoskeletal	☐ Skin	
☐ Eye drainage	☐ CTA	☐ ROM and function intact	☐ Intact, turgor moist	
☐ TMs/nares/pharnyx red	☐ Crackles	☐ Joint Pain	☐ Rash	
☐ Adenopathy	☐ Wheezing	☐ Edema	☐ Wound(s)	
☐ Thyroid enlarge/mass	☐ Diminished	☐ Neck or Back Pain		

Appendix 11-C Revised SOAPE note

● See dictation

9/28/12

OBJECTIVE FINDINGS

☐ No abnormal findings

ASSESSMENT/PLAN

Reviewed cultural assessment and POC requires the following culturally influenced interventions:

Labs

Rx

Education

☐ Patient stated acceptance and understanding of the treatment plan

☐ NP Student

☐

☐ FNP, BC ☐   ANP, BC

Appendix 11-C Revised SOAPE note (*continued*)

☐ Endo/Lymph ● neg	☐ Constipation ● neg	☐ Discharge ● neg	☐ **ENT** ● neg	☐ **Skin** ● neg
☐ Fatigue ● neg	☐ **Muscular** ● neg	☐ Sexual ● neg	☐ Ear pain ● neg	☐ Rash ● neg
☐ **Neuro** ● neg	☐ Sprain/Strain ● neg	☐ **Skeletal** ● neg	☐ Nasal Cong ● neg	☐ Wound ● neg
☐ Neuropathy ● neg	☐ Spasm ● neg	☐ Fx/Disloc ● neg	☐ Sore Throat ● neg	

ROS details [   ]

⟨Cultural/Social⟩ [   ]

OBJECTIVE

☐ Vital signs normal   Glucose [   ]   Urine [   ]   Kg [0]

HR [   ] BP [   ] Temp [   ] O2 sat [   ] RR [   ] Ht feet [   ] Ht in [   ] Wt lb [   ] BMI [0]

☐ **General**   ☐ **Heart**   ☐ **Abdomen**   ☐ **GU**   ☐ **Other**
  ☐ WNL   ☐ RRR, s1s2   ☐ Soft, non-tender, +BS   ☐ Genital exam defer

Appendix 11-C Revised SOAPE note (*continued*)

● See dictation

ASSESSMENT/PLAN   ☐ No abnormal findings

⟨Reviewed cultural assessment and POC requires the following culturally influenced interventions:⟩ [   ]

Labs [   ]

Rx [   ]

Education [   ]

Appendix 11-C Revised SOAPE note (*continued*)

APPENDIX 11-D: ROUTER OR PATIENT ENCOUNTER FORM

Copay collected: $_____
Not collected so due $_____
Entered in Spreadsheet Y   N

Name:	A/R + today:	
Date:	INS: A B S	
INS No.	Clinician: NP Doctor	MA
DOB:	Address:	

Phone No.	2nd phone:	HR		RR
99201	New Patient E/M Office/Outpatient Visit 10 Minutes	BP	/	HT
99202	New Patient E/M Office/Outpatient Visit 20 Minutes	Temp		WT
99203	New Patient E/M Office/Outpatient Visit 30 Minutes	Sat		Smoker Y N
99204	New Patient E/M Office/Outpatient Visit 45 Minutes	CC:		
99205	New Patient E/M Office/Outpatient Visit 60 Minutes			
99211	Established Patient E/M Office/Outpatient Visit, 5 Minutes			
99212	Established Patient E/M Office/Outpatient Visit, 10 Minutes	Allergies: Y N If Yes, list below:		
99213	Established Patient E/M Office/Outpatient Visit, 15 Minutes			
99214	Established Patient E/M Office/Outpatient Visit, 25 Minutes			
99215	Established Patient E/M Office/Outpatient Visit, 40 Minutes			

	Procedures:	Appt Time:	Cultural Assessment:
93000	Electrocardiogram, complete	Sign-in:	
94010	PFT (mod 26)	Message:	A. What transportation concerns do you have related to your healthcare?
69210	Earwash	MA Room:	
15851	Suture Removal	Stdt. Start:	
36415	Blood Draw	Stdt. End:	
	Injections:	NP Start:	B. What are your barriers or concerns that would keep you from making/keeping your appointments?
90701	DTP	NP End:	
86580	PPD	Lab. Ref:	
82607	Vitamin B12	To Front Desk:	
78272	Vitamin B12 Complex	Left Clinic:	C. What role does your spirituality or religious beliefs play in your healthcare?
90658	Flu Vaccine	Total Time:	
	Injection Type:	Stdt. Here: Y or N	
87070	Strep Culture	Stdt. Total Time Mins:	

Diagnosis:_____

Return/Remind:

____PRN____days____wk (s)____mo (s) Other____	15m	30m	60m

Referrals:_____

Laboratory:_____

Rx:_____

Appendix 11-D Router or patient encounter form

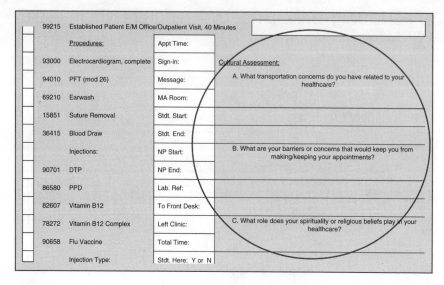

	99215	Established Patient E/M Office/Outpatient Visit, 40 Minutes		
		Procedures:	Appt Time:	
	93000	Electrocardiogram, complete	Sign-in:	Cultural Assessment:
	94010	PFT (mod 26)	Message:	A. What transportation concerns do you have related to your healthcare?
	69210	Earwash	MA Room:	
	15851	Suture Removal	Stdt. Start:	
	36415	Blood Draw	Stdt. End:	
		Injections:	NP Start:	B. What are your barriers or concerns that would keep you from making/keeping your appointments?
	90701	DTP	NP End:	
	86580	PPD	Lab. Ref:	
	82607	Vitamin B12	To Front Desk:	
	78272	Vitamin B12 Complex	Left Clinic:	C. What role does your spirituality or religious beliefs play in your healthcare?
	90658	Flu Vaccine	Total Time:	
		Injection Type:	Stdt. Here: Y or N	

Appendix 11-D Router or patient encounter form (*continued*)

APPENDIX 11-E: ROOM SIGNAGE

In an effort to better meet your needs, we would like to ask you one or more questions regarding your culture...

A   What transportation concerns do you have related to your healthcare?

B   What are your barriers or concerns that would keep you from making/keeping your appointments?

C   What role does your spiritual or religious beliefs play in your healthcare?

Assessment and Education:
Building Blocks for
Cultural Competence

Renee Courtney, MSN, RN, FNP-DC, CTN-5
Susan Wolgamott, DSN, RN, CCN, CTN-5
University of Michigan – Flint
Doctor of Nursing Practice Program

Appendix 11-E Room signage

APPENDIX 11-F: POST MODULE SURVEY

1a. What was the most helpful information you gained from participating in this educational module?
1b. Why was this information helpful to you?
2. How will the care you provide to the patients of the clinic be changed after you participated in this educational module?

APPENDIX 11-G: POST PROJECT FACE-TO-FACE INTERVIEW

1. Describe how your cultural awareness has changed after being a part of Assessment and Education: Building Blocks of Cultural Competency project.
2. Describe changes in your practice/behavior that are a result of your participation in Assessment and Education: Building Blocks of Cultural Competency project.

APPENDIX 11-H: CHART AUDIT TOOL

Presence of (non-yes/no) data on one of the cultural assessment A, B, C lines on the patient router.

Post
Data point 1

SOAPE

Cultural/Social

Presence of documentation in the cultural/social section:

1. Additional information on the assessment done by the MAs *or*
2. Additional information gleaned using the other A, B, C cultural assessment questions *or*
3. Option available to document information regarding specific culturally driven patient concerns

Pre	Post
Data point 2	Data point 3

Assessment/Plan

Presence of documentation in the assessment/plan section:

1. Utilizing the prepopulated scripting and accompanying documentation of culturally influenced interventions
2. Option to document culturally driven interventions not relating to A, B, C questions

Pre	Post
Data point 4	Data point 5

DISCUSSION QUESTIONS

1. Discuss how the Theory of Culture Care Diversity and Universality and the *collaborative care* construct can be used in your current practice environment.
2. Discuss some challenges that may be encountered when endeavoring to provide education to a multidisciplinary healthcare team.
3. Give examples of how healthcare disparities in underserved/vulnerable populations can be affected when culture is made integral to their care.
4. Describe/discuss the influences of culturally congruent care on patient–provider engagement.
5. Discuss the kinds of barriers that might be encountered when implementing a cultural competence education program with a multidisciplinary healthcare team.

REFERENCES

American Heritage Dictionary. (2009). Domain. Boston, MA: Author.

Amerson, R. (2010). The impact of service-learning on cultural competence. *Nursing Education Perspectives, 31*(1), 18–22.

Andrews, M. M. (2006). Globalization of transcultural nursing theory and research. In M. M. Leininger & M. R. McFarland (Eds.), *Culture care diversity and universality: A worldwide nursing theory* (2nd ed., pp. 83–114). Sudbury, MA: Jones and Bartlett.

Bemker, M., & Schreiner, B. (2011, October 22). *The river bends in cultural simulation: Use of simulation to enhance multicultural perspectives in nursing education.* Presentation at 37th Annual Transcultural Nursing Society Conference, Las Vegas, NV.

Jeffreys, M. (2000). Development and psychometric evaluation of the Transcultural Self-Efficacy Tool: A synthesis of findings. *Journal of Transcultural Nursing, 11*(2), 127–136.

Jeffreys, M. (2006). *Transcultural self-efficacy tool: Multidisciplinary healthcare provider.* New York, NY: Springer.

Jeffreys, M., & Smodlaka, I. (1998). Exploring the factorial composition of the Transcultural Self-Efficacy Tool. *International Journal of Nursing Studies, 35*(4), 217–225.

Kardong-Edgren, S., & Campinha-Bacote, J. (2008). Cultural competence of graduating U.S. Bachelor of Science nursing students. *Contemporary Nurse, 28*(1–2), 37–44.

Killion, C. (2001). Understanding cultural aspects of health through photography. *Nursing Outlook, 49*(1), 50–54.

Leininger, M. M. (2002). Transcultural nursing and globalization of health care: Importance, focus, and historical aspects. In M. M. Leininger & M. R. McFarland (Eds.), *Transcultural nursing: Concepts, theories, research, & practice* (3rd ed., pp. 3–43). New York, NY: McGraw-Hill.

Leininger, M. M. (2006). Culture care diversity and universality theory and evolution of the ethnonursing method. In M. M. Leininger & M. R. McFarland (Eds.), *Culture care diversity and universality: A worldwide nursing theory* (2nd ed., pp. 1–41). Sudbury, MA: Jones and Bartlett.

McFarland, M. R. (2011, October 21). *The culture care theory and a look to the future for transcultural nursing.* Keynote address presented at the 37th Annual Conference of the International Society of Transcultural Nursing, Las Vegas, NV. Text provided by M. R. McFarland.

Melnyk, B. M., & Fineout-Overholt, E. (2011). *Evidence-based practice in nursing and healthcare* (2nd ed.). Philadelphia, PA: Lippincott Williams & Wilkins.

Newhouse, R. P., Dearholt, S. L., Poe, S. S., Pugh, L. C., & White, K. M. (2007). *John Hopkins nursing evidence-based practice model and guidelines.* Indianapolis, IN: Sigma Theta Tau International.

Nokes, K., Nickitas, D., Keida, R., & Neville, S. (2005). Does service-learning increase cultural competency, critical thinking and civic engagement? *Journal of Nursing Education, 44*(2), 65–70.

Shaya, F., & Gbarayor, C. (2006). The case for cultural competence in health professions education. *American Journal of Pharmaceutical Education, 70*(6), 124.

Shellman, J. (2007). The effects of a reminiscence education program on baccalaureate nursing students' cultural self-efficacy in caring for elders. *Nurse Education Today, 27*(1), 43–51.

United States Department of Health and Human Services Healthy People 2020 20120906 Healthy People.gov U.S. Department of Health and Human Services (USDHHS), Healthy People 2020. (2012a, September 6). Leading health indicators: Access to health services. Retrieved from http://www.healthypeople .gov/2020/LHI/accessCare.aspx

United States Department of Health and Human Services Healthy People 2020 20120906 Healthy People.gov U.S. Department of Health and Human Services (USDHHS), Healthy People 2020. (2012b, September 6). Topics and objectives: Access to health services. Retrieved from http://www.healthypeople.gov/2020 /topicsobjectives2020/overview.aspx?topicid=1

U.S. Department of Health and Human Services (USDHHS), Office of Minority Health. (2005). What is cultural competency. Retrieved from http://minority-health.hhs.gov/templates/browse.aspx?lvl=2&lvlID=11

U.S. Department of Health and Human Services (USDHHS), Office of Minority Health. (2010). Culturally and linguistically appropriate services (CLAS) [Facilitator's kit]. Retrieved from https://ccnm.thinkculturalhealth.hhs.gov /GUIs/GUI_DVDorder.asp

Vincent, D., Johnson, C., Velasquez, D., & Rigney, T. (2013). DNP: Prepared nurses as practitioner-researchers: Closing the gap between research and practice. Retrieved from http://webnponline.com/articles/article_details/dnp-prepared-nurses-as-practitioner-researchers-closing-the-gap-between-res/

Wehbe-Alamah, H. (2010, March 23). *Assessing the cultural health care beliefs and practices of people from diverse cultural backgrounds and implications for clinical practice and curriculum development.* PowerPoint lecture: NUR 810 Transcultural Nursing, University of Michigan, Flint, Michigan

White, K. M., & Dudley-Brown, S. (2012). *Translation of evidence into nursing and health care practice* (pp. 23–48). New York, NY: Springer.

Zaccagnini, M. E., & White, K.W. (2011). *The doctor of nursing practice essentials: A new model for advanced practice nursing* (pp. 451–497). Sudbury, MA: Jones and Bartlett.

Chapter 12

Application of Culture Care Theory in Teaching Cultural Competence and Culturally Congruent Care

Sandra J. Mixer

> *Globalization of health care and the differences and similarities among and between human groups and cultures will continue as a growing imperative. Nurses, faculty, and mentors will act as healthcare facilitators using the culture care theory and ethnonursing research method to transform healthcare "… provide quality care services, to reduce health costs, and to promote healing."*
>
> (Leininger, 2006a, pp. 391, 393)

INTRODUCTION

Cultural diversity continues to increase among the population of the United States as well as in other countries around the globe. Every nurse in practice, education, administration, research, or consultation is professionally responsible for meeting the culture care needs of diverse and similar people worldwide (American Nurses Association [ANA], 2010; International Council of Nurses, 2012). Because people and cultures are constantly changing, nurses—regardless of their role—must engage in lifelong learning to maintain their cultural competency and their ability to provide culturally congruent care (Andrews, 2012; Institute of Medicine, 2010).

Cultural competence is described as the desire, attitude, knowledge, and skill nurses know and use to care for diverse people (California Endowment, 2003; Campinha-Bacote, 2012). Culturally congruent care (CCC) is care that recipients consider safe and beneficial. For patients, such care is satisfying and meaningful; fits with their daily lives and needs; and helps them achieve health and wellbeing or face illness, disabilities, or death (Leininger, 2006a). For faculty, providing CCC includes caring for patients and their families, students, colleagues, and themselves. In providing CCC for students, faculty may facilitate student health and success by providing professional mentoring and role modeling in didactic and clinical contexts, demonstrating respect and surveillance care, being approachable and attentive listeners, and checking in with students (Mixer, 2011). In the context of teaching culture care, faculty health and wellbeing are achieved through the caring actions of "...embracing each other's cultural similarities and differences, providing respect, and engaging in mentoring/co-mentoring" (Mixer, McFarland, Andrews, & Strang, 2013). Faculty practice self-care by attending to their nutrition, rest, exercise, emotional, and spiritual needs. Nursing administrators facilitate the health of their employees and themselves through similar caring practices. Every nurse has the ability to contribute to the health and wellbeing of those in his or her care including patients, family members, students, employees, colleagues, or self.

Teaching grounded in evidence-based best practices is essential for producing culturally competent nurses who can contribute to the health and wellbeing of all people and help reduce health disparities among underserved and vulnerable populations. The culture care theory (CCT) provides an essential framework for teaching nurses how to provide culturally congruent care. The CCT and ethnonursing research method were originally used to study the culture care needs of individuals, families, and communities. Over time, the theory and method have evolved to promote the discovery of specific care needs within the cultures of nursing administration, consultation, and education (Leininger, 2006a).

GENERATING NURSING KNOWLEDGE

Gaining nursing knowledge is a lifelong pursuit influenced by societal accountability to meet human beings' holistic needs (Barrett, 2009; Leininger, 2006a). Nursing knowledge is dynamic, is strongly influenced by context (Chinn & Kramer, 2011), and forms the foundation of contemporary and future nursing education and practice. As scholars seek to contribute to the body of nursing knowledge by developing knowledge to teach cultural competence and CCC, they are called to broaden their perspective through critical reflection, creativity, and dialogue with one another. This process compels nurses to question their assumptions and beliefs, learn to articulate their views, synthesize a variety of perspectives, and even agree to disagree with other nurses (Bond & Saucier, 2003; DeGroot, 2009).

Nursing knowledge originates from a variety of sources, including philosophical explorations, theoretical perspectives and models, research, experience, and intuition. The debate continues about which philosophical paradigms should guide nursing science. Two primary philosophical paradigms have been described in the literature: Logical positivism and constructivism. Logical positivism uses a rational, empiricist approach to observe phenomena that are scientifically verifiable by the senses. This approach, which follows reductionist thinking, is based on a rigid set of rules. Constructivism uses creative induction and interpretive analysis to construct meaning (Newman, 2009; Tinkle & Beaton, 2004). The positivist perspective focuses on gaining tangible facts deductively whereas the constructivist perspective uses an open, inductive process to facilitate the discovery of phenomena. Both positivist and constructivist paradigms provide valuable perspectives in understanding holistic human care phenomena and are foundational to nursing science and practice (Fawcett, 2009; Schultz & Meleis, 2009). Therefore, educators need to teach students both perspectives. This chapter examines the use of a constructivist approach— the culture care theory and ethnonursing research method—for discovering care practices and strategies for teaching culture care.

Figure 12-1 provides a conceptual map for generating nursing knowledge about teaching culture care using the constructivist, qualitative approaches of the culture care theory and ethnonursing research method. While this figure shows faculty as culture care teachers, the model applies to nurse educators in any context.

The conceptual map in Figure 12-1 depicts important aspects of the process of generating nursing knowledge about teaching culture care. This process is guided by the culture care theory, situated within the constructivist qualitative paradigm, and uses the processes of ethnonursing research, faculty ways of knowing and being, and praxis. Praxis is defined as "critical reflection and action to transform the world" (Chinn, 2005, p. 1). Theory, research, and practice combine to formulate teaching culture care praxis. The arrows in the conceptual map highlight the constructs' interrelatedness and interdependency, as well as their dynamic, nonlinear nature.

When teaching culture care, faculty address both epistemological and ontological perspectives. In the nursing discipline, epistemology (ways of knowing) and ontology (ways of being) are interconnected, each giving knowledge and meaning to the other (Chinn & Kramer, 2011; Silva, Sorrell,

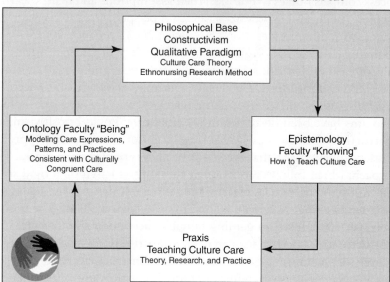

Figure 12-1 Conceptual map to generate nursing knowledge to teach culture care
© S. Mixer, 2004.

& Sorrell, 2004). For example, faculty may know the empirical, ethical, aesthetic, and personal ways of knowing (epistemology) related to teaching culture care. Faculty also may have cultural knowledge and possess effective teaching strategies for teaching culture care. Just as valuable, faculty members' way of being (ontology) also teaches culture care by role modeling through their care expressions, patterns, and practices toward patients, families, students, and colleagues. Thus a nurse's culture care knowing and being are inextricably interdependent.

A faculty member's ways of knowing and being come together to form praxis (theory, research, and practice) as he or she teaches and models culture care in class and clinical settings. Critical reflection and action are required to combine what one knows from nursing education with what one knows from participation in the daily grind—and privilege—of caring for people (Chinn, 2005; DeKeyser & Medoff-Cooper, 2009; Reed, 2009) to enable the provision of culturally congruent care.

RESEARCH SYNTHESIS

Two ethnonursing research studies guided by the culture care theory were conducted to discover care practices that enabled nursing faculty to teach cultural competentence and culturally congruent care effectively. These culture care studies with patients, families, and communities took the theory beyond research and applied it to nursing education. Extensive reviews of the literature (Mixer, 2008b) and cited study findings (Mixer, 2011; Mixer, Lasater et al., 2013; Mixer, McFarland, et al., 2013;) were previously published; the present chapter is a synthesis of these findings. While these studies were conducted in the academic setting, their findings are useful for teaching cultural competence and culturally congruent care in a variety of nursing education and practice settings.

Themes and Patterns

Forty-three nursing faculty from undergraduate and graduate nursing programs in public and private universities serving urban and rural areas across the United States participated in the combined studies. Through these studies, themes and universal and diverse patterns that contributed to teaching cultural competence and culturally congruent care were discovered (**Table 12-1**).

Table 12-1 Themes and Patterns That Contributed to Teaching Cultural Competence and Culturally Congruent Care

Themes	Universal and Diverse Patterns
Theme 1	*Universal Patterns*
Faculty teach/model culture care based on their spiritual, generic, and professional care practices.	Faculty described a spiritual foundation for their caring.
	Faculty intentionally avoided imposing their spiritual beliefs on patients/families, students, or colleagues.
	Faculty learned generic care from their families and professional care from their formal education and mentors/comentors.
	Diverse Patterns
	Some faculty described open spirituality while others expressed caring based on their religious faith.
Theme 2	*Universal Patterns*
Faculty caring for self, others, and one another is essential to promote faculty health and wellbeing in order to teach culturally competent and congruent care.	Faculty expressed respect for colleagues and students through embracing similarities and differences.
	Faculty reciprocally and collectively cared for one another.

(continues)

Table 12-1 Themes and Patterns That Contributed to Teaching Cultural Competence and Culturally Congruent Care (*continued*)

Themes	Universal and Diverse Patterns
	Faculty contributed to one another's professional growth through mentoring and co-mentoring.
	Faculty expressed a need for self-care that addressed their nutrition, sleep, exercise, and psycho-social-spiritual needs.
	Faculty described a caring environmental context within the school of nursing/University (including formal and informal leadership support) that promoted health and wellbeing.
	Diverse Pattern
	Some faculty described non-care as conflict and disrespect among faculty.
Theme 3	***Universal Patterns***
Faculty generic and professional care for nursing students is essential to promote students' health and wellbeing, cultural competence, and professional success.	Faculty showed respect for students by honoring their cultures and embracing their similarities and differences.
	Faculty provided generic care for students through expressions of kindness and concern for their health, wellbeing, and nursing school success.
	Faculty provided professional care by mentoring and modeling care and CCC for students.
	Faculty provided surveillance care by listening to students, being approachable, and checking in with students.
Theme 4	***Universal Patterns***
Faculty described universal and diverse approaches to teaching culturally competent and congruent care.	Faculty described limited culture care knowledge and effective teaching strategies to teach CCC.
	Faculty taught CCC through role modeling and mentoring in class and clinical contexts.
	Faculty designed clinical assignments to teach care for diverse persons and people in urban and rural settings.
	Faculty described limited integration of CCC throughout the curriculum. (CCC usually was taught in a module or one class session.)
	Diverse Pattern
	While a few faculty used an organizing framework to teach CCC, most taught without one.

Sources: Mixer, 2011; Mixer, Lasater, et al., 2013; Mixer, McFarland, et al., 2013.

Evidence-Based Recommendations

The data analyses for these studies led to the formulation of evidence-based recommendations for teaching cultural competence and culturally congruent care (**Table 12-2**). These recommendations were framed using the three culture care modes of decisions and actions. The first mode, *culture care preservation and/or maintenance*, refers to those supportive professional care decisions and actions that nursing faculty should maintain to facilitate teaching cultural competence and CCC. The second mode, *culture care accommodation and/or negotiation*, refers to decisions and actions that help nursing faculty negotiate new care strategies to promote student cultural competence and CCC. The third mode, *culture care repatterning and/or restructuring*, refers to decisions and actions that help nursing faculty replace noncaring practices with more beneficial ones or restructure teaching practices to improve students' cultural competence and CCC (Leininger, 2006a, p. 8.).

Table 12-2 Culture Care Decisions and Actions Modes: Recommendations for Teaching Cultural Competence and Culturally Congruent Care

Culture care preservation and/or maintenance	• Preserve faculty's spiritual foundations of caring. • Maintain generic and professional caring practices among faculty and students to promote their health and wellbeing. • Maintain diverse patient clinical assignments. • Preserve teaching CCC through role modeling and mentoring while negotiating with faculty to increase their culture care knowledge and skills.
Culture care accommodation and/or negotiation	• Accommodate faculty and students' similarities and differences. • Negotiate with faculty (and model to students) engaging in healthy self-care practices such as exercising, eating nutritiously, and getting adequate sleep. • Negotiate with faculty to integrate CCC throughout the curriculum.
Culture care repatterning and/or restructuring	• Accommodate caring faculty practices and restructure faculty conflict (noncaring behaviors). • Encourage faculty to restructure teaching CCC in class and clinical settings using an organizing framework.

Sources: Mixer, 2011; Mixer, Lasater, et al., 2013; Mixer, McFarland, et al., 2013.

Discussion of Findings

Universal and diverse findings from these faculty participants reflect the theoretical assumption that cultures share similarities and differences (Leininger, 2006a). The data supported the idea that spiritual, generic, and professional care are foundational to teaching and modeling culture care. These forms of care have been discovered in numerous CCT studies with diverse cultural groups to be foundational to *caring* (Embler, Mixer, & Gunther, in press; Wehbe-Alamah, McFarland, Macklin, & Riggs, 2011). Because "…care is the essence and the central dominant, distinct, and unifying focus of nursing" (Leininger, 2006a, p. 18) educators need to explicitly teach spiritual, generic, and professional care constructs so that students and practicing nurses can apply these foundational care actions to practice.

Fewer than one-third of faculty participants had had formal transcultural nursing or culturally-focused education (Mixer, 2011; Mixer, Lasater, et al., 2013). Among that subgroup, few had received formal education and many had only attended a workshop. These findings are congruent with the literature which reports the continued need to prepare faculty to teach transcultural nursing, cultural diversity, and cultural competence (Mixer, Lasater, et al., 2013).

While most participants lacked formal culture care training, they were able to identify and describe their generic care practices toward themselves, other faculty, students, and patients and families in the clinical setting. The importance of fostering a community of caring within the environmental context of the college/school of nursing and unversity was discovered to be essential for promoting faculty and student health and wellbeing and for fostering the provision of culturally congruent care. Care was found to be taught primarily through role modeling (Mixer, 2011; Mixer, Lasater, et al., 2013). This is an effective way to teach caring because nurses, administrators, educators, and students who experience culturally congruent care may be more likely to role model and provide such care to others. Therefore, the provision of culturally congruent care is an outcome of being taught to care (spiritually, generically, and professionally), having culturally congruent care role modeled in class and clinical contexts, and being in an environment that fosters such care. Providing, experiencing, and role modeling CCC promotes the health and wellbeing of all persons involved such as students, faculty, administrators, patients, and families.

Key Care Constructs in Nursing Education

The culture care theory guides the discovery and use of care constructs in nursing education. Care constructs, as described in the theory, are the meanings of care as articulated by individuals and cultural groups. When a nurse

Table 12-3 Care Constructs in Nursing Education

Care Constructs	Definition Within Nursing Education Context
Respect	• Honoring others for who they are and the unique contributions they make • Appreciating similarities and differences among one another.
Mentoring	• Involves sharing epistemological and ontological resources to facilitate the mentee's career success • Takes place over a sustained period and involves a faculty member making a significant impact on another's career • Frequently moves into co-mentoring
Comentoring	• A trusting, collaborative, reciprocal teaching/learning caring relationship among interprofessional colleagues working together with shared power to produce intangible and quantifiable results that mutually benefit those involved • A form of reciprocal care • Takes place over a sustained period and involves faculty members making a significant impact on one another's careers.
Self-care	• Involves healthy practices such as exercising, eating nutritiously, getting adequate sleep, and attending to one's mental, emotional, and spiritual needs
Spiritual care	• A nonjudgmental, open, caring approach that involves acknowledging people's spiritual dimensions and their need for spiritual connectedness
Reciprocal care	• Care provided by faculty to one another that involves demonstrating respect, love, forgiveness, and honoring family and work responsibilities
Collective care	• Shared caring decisions and actions that benefit all faculty members
Surveillance care	• Caring actions that involve extending oneself to monitor the health and wellbeing of another • Includes attentive listening, checking-in, being approachable, and taking opportunities to offer care

Sources: Mixer, 2008a; 2011; Mixer et al., 2012; Mixer, Lasater, et al., 2013 Mixer, McFarland, et al., 2013.

understands an individual's deeply-held care meanings, he or she is better equipped to meet that person's unique needs. **Table 12-3** lists care constructs that were found to be essential in nursing education. These definitions have been synthesized from the author's years of scholarly work in collaboration with other transcultural nurse-researchers (Mixer, 2008a; 2011; Mixer et al., 2012; Mixer, McFarland, et al., 2013; Mixer, Lasater, et al., 2013).

Understanding and employing these care constructs in nursing education are essential when working with patients, families, communities, students, fellow faculty, and other interdisciplinary colleagues. Because culture care is most often taught through role modeling and mentoring/co-mentoring, each nurse and nursing faculty should then strive to exhibit the caring behaviors comprised in these constructs during every care encounter.

TEACHING CULTURE CARE EXEMPLARS

To promote cultural competence and CCC, culture care should be integrated throughout the academic curriculum and incorporated into classroom, online, simulation, clinical, and cultural immersion assignments. To accomplish this goal, all courses should incorporate at least one objective that relates to culture care, and the environmental context and institutional culture should reflect culturally congruent practices. *Environmental context* involves the totality of the experience of teaching culture care within institutional (school of nursing and university) and clinical (hospital and community) contexts, including physical, ecological, spiritual, sociopolitical, kinship, and technological influences (adapted from Leininger, 2006a, p. 10). *Institutional culture* refers to the learned, shared, and transmitted values, symbols, beliefs, norms, and practices within the academic setting that guide the thinking, decision making, and actions of administrators, faculty, and staff (adapted from Leininger, 2006a, p. 13). Values and beliefs congruent with promoting culture care should be reflected in vision, mission, and philosophy statements; course syllabi; and university and school of nursing website content. The following exemplars provide ideas about creative ways to teach culture care in academic, community, and clinical contexts.

Exemplar 1: Transcultural Nursing Course

While transcultural nursing should be integrated throughout the curriculum, a stand-alone transcultural nursing course is the optimum format for teaching a baseline of related constructs, theoretical frameworks, and models. In this exemplar, the CCT as depicted in the Sunrise Enabler, shown earlier in this text, provides the framework for the course and assignments (Leininger, 2006a). Comprehending the broad constructs of *culture* and *care* is crucial for teaching and learning. Generic care (caring learned from one's family) and professional care (caring formally taught through education and mentors) may be combined to help students discover the roots of their own caring beliefs, patterns, and practices. This process forms the basis of providing culturally congruent and competent care for clients, community, colleagues, and self.

In a transcultural nursing course, students research and learn about a diverse array of cultural groups such as rural Appalachians; Eastern Band of Cherokee Indians; Hispanic/Mexican Americans; Arab Americans; lesbian, bisexual, gay, or transgendered (LBGT) persons; persons experiencing homelessness; and persons with disabilities. Students learn to perform cultural assessments, conduct interviews with cultural group members, and apply evidence from the literature to understand and care for diverse cultural groups.

Using the CCT approach of comparing and contrasting between and among cultures to tease out covert cultural knowledge, students gather and compare data from peer-reviewed literature and interviews with cultural group members. Next, they use the CCT culture care modes of decisions and actions to make recommendations about how to provide CCC. Students then collaborate with faculty and the simulation lab coordinator to create a relevant practice scenario. Finally, students teach their peers to provide culturally congruent care for a specific cultural group using a formal presentation and clinical simulation.

In the transcultural nursing course, honors students are given another culture care opportunity when they collaborate with nursing faculty, a philosophy professor, an institutional bioethicist, and an urban community organization to participate in an advance directive clinic for persons experiencing homelessness. Students are trained and then help individuals complete advance directives. After the clinic, students follow the same cultural group assignment described previously except that their simulation with peers involves creating advance directives with persons experiencing homelessness. In simulation debriefing, all students compare and contrast the simulated scenario with their clinical experiences in acute care settings with other cultural groups.

Exemplar 2: Community Health Course

As transcultural nursing is integrated throughout the curriculum, culture care learning is integrated in a stepwise manner into the community health course. For the major course assignment, students conduct a community assessment on a vulnerable population during a community clinical experience. The community assessment criteria mirror many other contextual cultural assessment criteria. Students examine the similarities and differences between data gathered through governmental and other sources with data generated through interviews and observations. Based on the community assessment data, students use the CCT culture care modes of decisions and actions to make recommendations that promote community health.

Community clinical assignments offer students a variety of domestic and international cultural immersion service-learning opportunities.

For example, students may work with rural Appalachians at the Redbird Mission in Kentucky; Native Americans at the Eastern Band of Cherokee Indians Health and Medical Division in North Carolina; or with diverse patient populations in Costa Rica in settings such as community clinics or at-home visits (including persons with disabilities who live in a faith-based home). The culture care theory serves as an effective guide for students and faculty in providing CCC for these diverse people. Culture care theoretical tenets and enablers, such as the Stranger-to-Trusted-Friend Enabler, have been used for many years to establish trusting relationships with community members (Leininger, 2006b). When nurse leaders and healthcare team members who are experienced with a particular cultural group and community leaders collaborate with faculty and students to create student service-learning projects, community health is promoted in a culturally congruent manner. The most significant learning outcome is that students witness firsthand how culturally congruent care benefits the health and wellbeing of persons, families, and communities in these diverse settings.

Exemplar 3: Research Practicums

Research practicums are designed to teach graduate students about use and application of the CCT, the ethnonursing research method, and culturally congruent care in a variety of teaching, research, and practice contexts. Students participate in literature reviews; study design; grant writing; institutional review board applications; data collection and analysis; dissemination of study findings; and the implementation of findings in teaching, research, and practice. For example, in an ethnonursing study of culturally congruent end-of-life care among rural Appalachians, an MSN student and a PhD student first participated in participant interviews with a research mentor and then conducted several such interviews independently. This three-member team then collaborated on data analysis and dissemination of the findings. The PhD student also helped write a grant proposal based on the needs assessment from the study.

Exemplar 4: Webinars/Seminars

Numerous webinars and seminars are available to teach nursing students, nursing faculty, practicing nurses, and advanced practice nurses about cultural competence and the culture care theory. Across the United States, more than 1,550 nurses and students have participated in such seminars. Based on the abundant evaluation feedback, webinars and face-to-face seminars effectively teach evidence-based and best practices that promote cultural competence and CCC in an efficient and cost-effective manner (Andrews & Collins, 2015).

Exemplar 5: Simulation

Nursing simulation is an important and growing part of clinical learning. The new International Nursing Association for Clinical Simulation and Learning (INACSL) Standards of Best Practice for Simulation incorporate a holistic view of clients that recognizes "...the interconnectedness of body, mind, spirit" (as cited in Lioce et al., 2013, p. S17) and the importance of environmental context. This interconnectedness encompasses how patients experience care from a cultural standpoint. Because simulation is used throughout nursing curricula in most undergraduate and graduate (MSN/DNP) clinical courses, combining cultural competence education with simulation work would facilitate the distribution of transcultural nursing education throughout the curriculum.

Exemplar 6: Domestic Immersion Experiences

International immersion experiences provide unique, effective opportunities for students to gain cultural competence (Larsen & Reif, 2011). However, given the economic and time constraints of modern nursing schools and students, domestic immersion and service-learning experiences present a feasible and effective alternative for increasing students' cultural competence (Kardong-Edgren, 2007). Regional immersion/service-learning projects allow students, nurses, and faculty to explore in-depth cultural knowledge of cultural groups with whom they may work, teach, or care for in practice. Seeing firsthand the health disparities experienced by vulnerable groups in their community frequently inspires learners to engage in local efforts to promote culturally congruent care and contribute to their neighbors' health and wellbeing.

Exemplar 7: Certification

Nursing certification is recognized as promoting "...excellence in nursing and health care globally" (American Nurses Credentialing Center [ANCC], n.d.). The Transcultural Nursing Society (TCNS) offers nurses worldwide the opportunity to earn basic (CTN-B) or advanced (CTN-A) transcultural nurse certifications. These designations recognize the nurse's commitment to contributing to the health and wellbeing of a global population in a culturally congruent and equitable manner (TCNS, n.d.).

Exemplar 8: Distance Scholarship

Culturally competent and congruent nursing care is needed in urban and rural settings locally, regionally, nationally, and internationally. To meet this need, faculty, students, and practicing nurses must be educated in and mentored/co-mentored in transcultural nursing at academic institutions at every degree level including associate, baccalaureate, master's, doctorate in nursing practice, and PhD, and in a variety of practice contexts such as acute care and community settings. Interactive distance technologies such as webinars, online courses, Skype, Go-to-Meeting, and Google Docs are essential for reaching nurses who live and work in remote locations. As technology continues to advance, new and creative methods will further facilitate distance teaching and mentoring in transcultural nursing education and scholarship worldwide.

ACADEMIC-PRACTICE PARTNERSHIPS

Teaching nurses cultural competence and CCC builds an initial knowledge base. However, academic-practice partnerships move nurses from learning about culture care to identifying actual cultural challenges in their practices, engaging in research, and then applying theory and research to address these challenges. Academic partners are nursing faculty who contribute their expertise in research processes, grant opportunities, and collaborative teaching and mentoring. Practice partners are nurses who contribute their expertise by identifying actual cultural challenges in their practices and continually grounding the research design, processes, and findings for application within the realities of the practice setting. As scholarship is generated nursing practice is transformed. Based on the research evidence, clinical nurses are able to improve their cultural competence and are empowered to change policies and practices to promote culturally congruent care for people, families, and communities. Faculty subsequently use these experiences and research findings to model and teach theory and research applications for real-world practice to undergraduate and graduate students. Through creative collaboration, all partners help build knowledge for the discipline of nursing.

For example, the nursing staff of a regional children's hospital and faculty at an area university collaborated to address a clinical challenge. Guided by the CCT and using the ethnonursing research method, they sought to discover culturally congruent care practices for Hispanic and underserved (educationally and financially) Caucasian children and their families (Mixer, McArthur, et al., 2013). As the partners formulated and conducted the research study, the institutional expertise and perspectives produced stronger research than would have been accomplished separately. The academic partners taught the nursing staff how to analyze articles and conduct a review of the literature; the practice partners immediately disseminated literature review findings to staff nurses. The combined expertise of the partners facilitated timely human subjects approval from both institutions resulting in a more robust data collection and analysis that led to the discovery of covert cultural data. As the findings were disseminated through professional presentations and publications, collegial feedback confirmed the value and strength of theory/research applications that integrate academic and practice perspectives.

This academic-practice partnership yielded mutual benefits. After forming an institutional cultural competence committee, practice partners began implementing policy changes to promote culturally congruent care. Numerous graduate students learned project management skills and strategies for applying theory and research to nursing practice. Several nurses have since started graduate work and are currently conducting their own research projects. Many staff members have continued developing their cultural knowledge and have used it to adjust their nursing care. This partnership model also fulfilled a portion of each institution's mission for community service and research engagement.

While combining academia and practice resources promotes cultural competence and culturally congruent care for all persons, partners do face challenges. Engaging in research through academic-practice partnerships is a lengthy process requiring a long-term commitment (Davidson & Bowden, 2011). Similar to reports in the literature, these participants discovered that it was challenging to find a time when academic-practice partners could meet. Partners worked to balance time demands of the academic calendar with the schedules of practicing nurses (Gorman et al., 2008). In this example, many staff were initially interested in participating. However, as the months passed, the number of participants decreased until only a core group committed to the success of the project and partnership remained.

Colearning and collaboration among educators, researchers, theorists, and practitioners are critical as each partner brings personal nursing knowledge that should be shared, acknowledged, and integrated among the other partners. This process requires strong co-mentoring relationships (Mixer et al., 2012). The organizational and practice implications generated by scholarship from academic-practice partnerships can directly contribute to agencies' efforts to promote quality patient care through research. Working together, practice and academic partners can examine the relationship between culturally congruent patient factors and organizational and patient outcomes. Combining the shared expertise of nurses in academia and practice can help make cultural competence and CCC a realistic part of everyday healthcare for people, families, and communities.

CONCLUSION

Nurse educators are called to teach the culture care theory to ignite students' analysis and synthesis of its contributions to nurses' ability to provide culturally congruent care. The ultimate goal of teaching CCT in nursing education is to contribute to the health and wellbeing of all people.

Using a theoretical framework such as the CCT—which has been used and tested for more than 50 years in nursing in settings around the globe—teaches students, faculty, and nurses to provide care based on current evidence and best practices discovered through research, rather than relying solely on rich clinical experiences. The CCT provides a holistic means to understand the range of factors that influence teaching culture care and a practical framework to teach culture competence and CCC in any setting.

DEDICATION

This book chapter is dedicated to Dr. Madeleine Leininger for her inspiration and mentorship in the culture care theory and ethnonursing method, and to the many mentors/comentors, research participants, and students who contributed to my journey in transcultural nursing and life itself.

ACKNOWLEDGEMENT

The author gratefully acknowledges the assistance of doctoral student Cecily Strang for her invaluable assistance in preparing this book chapter.

DISCUSSION QUESTIONS

1. Describe your plans for implementing culturally congruent care into your teaching/learning/practice environment.
2. Compare and contrast research findings in Table 12-1 with the characteristics of your teaching/learning/practice environment. In which areas are you doing well? What areas need improvement?
3. Using the culture care decision and action modes in Table 12-2, create recommendations to provide culturally congruent care in your teaching/learning/practice environment.

4. Examine the benefits and challenges of academic-practice partnerships. Consider how such partnerships could be used to promote cultural competence and culturally congruent care in your region.
5. Using the teaching culture care exemplars, design a plan to promote cultural competence and culturally congruent care in your teaching/learning/practice environment.
6. Reflect on the care constructs in Table 12-3. Consider which constructs are similar to your values, beliefs, and practices related to providing care in your caring context/setting.

REFERENCES

American Nurses Association (ANA). (2010). ANA receives grant to support nurses' cultural competency. Retrieved from http://nursingworld.org/HomepageCategory/NursingInsider/Archive_1/2010-NI/Jan10-NI/ANA-Receives-Cultural-Competency-Grant.html

American Nurses Credentialing Center (ANCC). (n.d.). Retrieved from http://www.nursecredentialing.org/

Andrews, M. M. (2012). Culturally competent nursing care. In. M.M. Andrews & J. S. Boyle (Eds.), *Transcultural concepts in nursing care* (6th ed., pp. 17–37). Philadelphia, PA: Lippincott, Williams & Wilkins.

Andrews, M. M., & Collins, J. (2015). Using the culture care theory as the organizing framework for a federal project on cultural competence. In M. R. McFarland & H. B. Wehbe-Alamah (Eds.), *Culture care diversity and universality: A worldwide nursing theory* (3rd ed.). Burlington, MA: Jones & Bartlett Learning.

Barrett, E. A. M. (2009). What is nursing science? In P. G. Reed & N. C. Shearer (Eds.), *Perspectives on nursing theory* (5th ed., pp. 644–660). Philadelphia, PA: Lippincott, Williams & Wilkins.

Bond, J. B., & Saucier, J. K. (2003). Teaching philosophy of science in nursing doctoral education. *Journal of Nursing Scholarship, 35*(1), 87–91.

California Endowment. (2003). *Principles and recommended standards for cultural competence education of health care professionals.* Woodland, CA: Author.

Campinha-Bacote, J. (2012). The process of cultural competence in the delivery of healthcare services. Retrieved from http://www.transculturalcare.net/Cultural_Competence_Model.htm

Chinn, P. L. (2005). From the editor: Praxis. *Advances in Nursing Science, 28*(1), 1.

Chinn, P. L., & Kramer, M. K. (2011). Nursing's fundamental patterns of knowing. In *Integrated theory and knowledge development in nursing* (8th ed., pp. 2–23). St. Louis, MO: Elsevier Mosby.

Davidson, M. M., & Bowen, N. (2011). Academia meets community agency: How to foster positive collaboration in domestic violence and sexual assault work. *Journal of Family Violence, 26*(4), 309–318.

DeGroot, H. A. (2009). Scientific inquiry in nursing: A model for a new age. In P. G. Reed & N. C. Shearer (Eds.), *Perspectives on nursing theory* (5th ed., pp. 417–433). Philadelphia, PA: Lippincott, Williams & Wilkins.

DeKeyser, F. G., & Medoff-Cooper, B. (2009). A non-theorist's perspective on nursing theory: Issues of the 1990s. In P. G. Reed & N. C. Shearer (Eds.), *Perspectives on nursing theory* (5th ed., pp. 59–68). Philadelphia, PA: Lippincott, Williams & Wilkins.

Embler, P., Mixer, S. J., & Gunther, M. (In press). *End-of-life culture care expressions, meanings, patterns, and practices among Yup'ik Eskimo.* Manuscript submitted for publication.

Fawcett, J. (2009). From a plethora of paradigms to parsimony in worldviews. In P. G. Reed & N. C. Shearer (Eds.), *Perspectives on nursing theory* (5th ed., pp. 216–220). Philadelphia, PA: Lippincott, Williams & Wilkins.

Gorman, G., Forest, J., Stapleton, S. J., Hoenig, N. A., Marschke, M., Durham, J., Suarez, M. L., & Wilkie, D. J. (2008). Massage for cancer pain: A study with university and hospice collaboration. *Journal of Hospice and Palliative Nursing, 10*(4), 191–197.

Institute of Medicine. (2010). The future of nursing: Leading change, advancing health. Robert Wood Johnson Foundation Initiative on the Future of Nursing at the Institute of Medicine. Retrieved from http://www.iom.edu /reports/2010/the-future-of-nursing-leading-change-advancing-health.aspx

International Council of Nurses. (2012). *The ICN code of ethics for nurses.* Geneva, Switzerland: Author.

Kardong-Edgren, S. (2007). Cultural competence of baccalaureate nursing faculty. *Journal of Nursing Education, 46*(8), 360–366.

Larsen, R., & Reif, L. (2011). Effectiveness of cultural immersion and culture classes for enhancing nursing students' transcultural self-efficacy. *Journal of Nursing Education, 50*(6), 350–354.

Leininger, M. M. (2006a). Culture care diversity and universality theory and evolution of the ethnonursing method. In M. M. Leininger & M. R. McFarland (Eds.), *Culture care diversity and universality: A worldwide nursing theory* (2nd ed., pp. 1–42). Sudbury, MA: Jones and Bartlett.

Leininger, M. M. (2006b). Ethnonursing research method and enablers [Revised reprint]. In M. M. Leininger & M. R. McFarland (Eds.), *Culture care diversity and universality: A worldwide theory of nursing* (2nd ed., pp. 43–82). Sudbury, MA: Jones and Bartlett.

Lioce, L., Reed, C. C., Lemon, D., King, M. A., Martinez, P. A., Franklin, A.E., ... & Borum, J. C. (2013). Standards of best practice: Simulation standard III: Participant objectives. *Clinical Simulation in Nursing, 9*(6S), S15–S18. Retrieved from http://download.journals.elsevierhealth.com/pdfs/journals/1876-1399 /PIIS1876139913000753.pdf

Mixer, S. J. (2008a). *Nursing faculty care expressions, patterns, and practices related to teaching culture care.* Doctoral dissertation. Retrieved from http://works.bepress .com/cgi/viewcontent.cgi?article=1000&context=sandra_mixer

Mixer, S. J. (2008b). Use of the culture care theory and ethnonursing method to discover how nursing faculty teach culture care. *Contemporary Nurse Journal: Advances in Contemporary Transcultural Nursing, 28*(1–2), 23–36.

Mixer, S. J. (2011). Use of the culture care theory to discover nursing faculty care expressions, patterns, and practices related to teaching culture care. *Online Journal of Cultural Competence in Nursing and Healthcare, 1*(1), 3–14.

Mixer, S. J., Burk, R. C., Davidson, R., McArthur, P., Abraham, C., Silva, K., & Sharp, D. (2012). Transforming bedside nursing care through practice-academic co-mentoring relationships. *Journal of Nursing & Care, 1*(3). doi: 10.4172/jnc.1000108

Mixer, S. J., Lasater, K. M., Jenkins, K. M., Burk, R. C., Oliver, M. K., Meyer, M., Cruze, C., & Mills, J. (2013). Preparing a culturally competent nursing workforce. *Online Journal of Cultural Competence in Nursing and Healthcare, 3*(4), pp. 1–14. doi:10.9730/ojccnh.org/v3n4a1

Mixer, S. J., McArthur, P., Sylvia, K., Carson, E., Sharp, D., Chadwick, J., Davidson, R., Abraham, C., Burk, R., & Newby, H. (2013). *Culture care of Hispanic and underserved Caucasian children and families.* Unpublished research study, College of Nursing, University of Tennessee and East Tennessee Children's Hospital, Knoxville, TN.

Mixer, S. J., McFarland, M. R., Andrews, M. M., & Strang, C. W. (2013). Exploring faculty health and wellbeing: Creating a caring scholarly community. *Nurse Education Today. 33*(12), 1471-1476. Advance online publication. doi: 10.1016/j.nedt.2013.05.019

Newman, M.A. (2009). Prevailing paradigms in nursing. In P. G. Reed & N. C. Shearer (Eds.), *Perspectives on nursing theory* (5th ed., pp. 221–226). Philadelphia, PA: Lippincott, Williams & Wilkins.

Reed, P. G. (2009). Nursing: The ontology of the discipline. In P. G. Reed & N. C. Shearer (Eds.), *Perspectives on nursing theory* (5th ed., pp. 614–620). Philadelphia, PA: Lippincott, Williams & Wilkins.

Schultz, P. R., & Meleis, A. I. (2009). Nursing epistemology: Traditions, insights, questions. In P. G. Reed & N. C. Shearer (Eds.), *Perspectives on nursing theory* (5th ed., pp. 385–394). Philadelphia, PA: Lippincott, Williams & Wilkins.

Silva, M. C., Sorrell, J. M., & Sorrell, C. D. (2004). From Carper's patterns of knowing to ways of being: An ontological philosophical shift in nursing. In P. G. Reed, N. B. Crawford Shearer, & L. H. Nicoll (Eds.), *Perspectives on nursing theory* (4th ed., pp. 259–270). Philadelphia, PA: Lippincott, Williams & Wilkins.

Tinkle, M. B., & Beaton, J. L. (2004). Toward a new view of science: Implications for nursing research. In P. G. Reed, N. B. Crawford Shearer, & L. H. Nicoll (Eds.), *Perspectives on nursing theory* (4th ed., pp. 191–200). Philadelphia, PA: Lippincott, Williams & Wilkins.

Transcultural Nursing Society (TCNS). (n.d.). Certification in transcultural nursing. Retrieved from http://tcns.org/Certification.html

Wehbe-Alamah, H., McFarland, M., Macklin, J., & Riggs, N. (2011). The lived experiences of African American women receiving care from nurse practitioners in an urban nurse-managed clinic. *Online Journal of Cultural Competence in Nursing and Healthcare, 1*(1), 15–26. doi:10.9730/ojccnh.org/v1n1a2

Culture Care Education and Experiences of African American Students in Predominantly Euro American Associate Degree Nursing Programs

Lana M. deRuyter

INTRODUCTION

A large majority of African Americans in the United States have African ancestors who were brought to the Americas during the period of the Atlantic slave trade. Historians are not certain of the number of Africans who were brought to the Americas as slaves because reliable records were often not kept. Firm data on the number of persons *illegally* transported do not exist. In spite of these limitations, historians have tried to estimate the number of Africans who arrived as slaves from the 1500s to the mid-19th century and believe that there were between 10 and 12 million people transported against their will (Palmer, 2000). Other sources have estimated between 3.5 million to 24 million slaves were brought to the Americas during the slave trade (Curtin, 1969).

Once in the New World, the African people developed and maintained cultural traditions that met their needs. For example, the family was the basis of their social organization. This was accomplished with a strong development of kinship ties that united members of their ethnic group. African people who were brought to the Americas as slaves were often deeply religious; many of them worshipped a supreme god and others had additional or lesser/secondary deities. Their African roots and religious beliefs determined when their activities such as when planting seasons, harvest time, or naming of children would take place. Not surprisingly, the African peoples who were transported to the Americas brought and kept very strong family and religious traditions with them (Palmer, 2000).

In the United States, the descendants of these proud peoples have continued to grow and flourish. Demographic populations in the United States have continued to shift precipitating ever-larger numbers of African American applicants to nursing programs. Although African Americans are enrolling in predominantly Caucasian associate degree nursing programs, a gap remains in the percentage of African American nurses in comparison to their demographic representation in the overall population of the United States (Glanville, 2003).

Nursing as a profession is committed to meeting the needs of all of the populations it serves (American Association of Colleges of Nursing, 2004). A commitment to culturally diversifying the nursing profession, therefore, requires at its core the completion of a generic prelicensure nursing program by larger numbers of African American students. As nursing programs become more ethnically diverse, it becomes important for educators to be able to understand and support the basic cultural needs of the students being taught. This shift toward increased diversity in enrollments for historically Euro American associate degree nursing programs precipitates the need for learning about and understanding the culture of African American students.

The worldview of African American nursing students in predominantly Euro American associate degree nursing programs was explored in the ethnonursing study discussed in this chapter. The theoretical framework used was Leininger's Theory of Culture Care Diversity and Universality guided by the Sunrise Enabler. Interviews were conducted with 9 key informants and 19 general informants from eight associate degree nursing programs located in southeastern Pennsylvania and southern New Jersey. The cultural and social structure dimensions of the Sunrise Enabler (educational factors, economic factors, political and legal factors, cultural values, kinship and social factors, religious factors, and technological factors) were explored in order to understand and explicate the cultural context of the worldview of African American associate degree nursing students.

PURPOSE OF STUDY AND DOMAIN OF INQUIRY

The purpose of this ethnonursing study was to discover, describe, and systematically analyze the culture care educational expressions, beliefs, and practices of African American nursing students in predominantly Euro

American academic environments located in eight schools in southeastern Pennsylvania and southern New Jersey. The domain of inquiry (DOI) was the culture care expressions, beliefs, and practices related to the educational experiences of African American nursing students within the context of these predominantly Euro American nursing programs. The research focus was to discover the educational experiences, practices, and patterns of culture care in this population of nursing students. The goal of the study was to discover new nursing knowledge using the culture care theory with implications for nursing practice, theory, and education for diverse cultures.

CULTURAL AND SOCIAL STRUCTURE CONTEXTS

According to Lassiter (1999), the African American family is an extended kinship network with strong bonds and flexible family roles: "Roles played by members are determined by ability rather than gender or marital association" (p. 43). The informants in the study confirmed these statements by their responses. In addition, when asked about their social life while in school, they universally answered that they ". . .don't have a social life" while in nursing school.

A 20-year-old informant when discussing kinship and family stated that her mother, stepfather, and 16-year-old brother all lived close by. During the interview, she indicated that she saw her family much more before starting the nursing program but that she made a point of visiting as often as she could. These visits are a priority for her, even though she was a single parent working to complete her education. When discussing her social life and responsibilities as a single parent, she stated:

> I have a network of friends that . . . like whenever I need help, they're always there for me. If I need her to watch my son, she'll watch him for me. . . . as for a social life, I don't have one.

A 51-year-old informant said that she did not have any family living in the immediate area; her parents still live in Africa but visit her every year for about 6 weeks. She came to the United States in 1977 and has five children of her own: One son living in a Northern state, another son in a Southern state, and three others still living at home. Family was a priority even to her while she was in school.

When discussing kinship and family, another 36-year-old key informant noted that she did not get to see her family often anymore but stated:

> We get together, we eat, we laugh, and we tease. I have five brothers, two sisters, and I'm the youngest. I have two sons, they are nine and seven, and I have a 43-year-old [husband] that acts like one.

Ethnohistory

Historically, African American students were denied the same educational opportunities as Euro American students. After the Civil War when slavery was legally abolished, the Reconstruction Act sanctioned former slaves the right to vote and to participate in government. The Thirteenth Amendment abolished slavery in 1865 and in 1866 the Fourteenth Amendment prevented states from depriving anyone of life, liberty, or their property without due process of the law. Southern states imposed serious restrictions on African Americans regarding ownership of property, legal and constitutional rights, and education (Bardolph, 1970). In 1875, the Civil Rights Act was passed to give African Americans greater rights as citizens. However, in the Southern states most African Americans were denied their civil rights and remained segregated and impoverished. Due to these conditions, many African Americans left the South and moved to Northern urban areas of the United States (Glanville, 2003). As late as during the 1940s, approximately 1.5 million African Americans (15% of the African American population) left the Southern states (Glanville, 2003; Jaynes & Williams, 1989). According to Glanville, this move to the Northern states was considered a *positive* by most of the relocating populations. Nevertheless, many African Americans still dealt with poverty and encountered the many problems of fragmented urban life as well as remaining in either overt or covert segregation.

During the early years of the 20th century, educational opportunities for African Americans were compromised due to segregated school systems: Black schools were given less funding and often provided students with a suboptimal education, resulting in poor job opportunities, low wages, and continuing poverty (Glanville, 2003). In 1954, the U.S. Supreme Court ruled against public school segregation. This ruling did have some impact on primary and secondary education for African American students during the 1960s. After the Civil Rights movement in the United States, the major focus for Blacks in postsecondary schools and higher education shifted toward vocational training. According to Glanville, the rationale at that time was that if African Americans could learn a trade they would be able to improve their socioeconomic status and become more self-sufficient. Although this emphasis persisted for a number of years, African Americans have since risen above this limited vision, receiving collegiate education in all university majors including nursing. Nevertheless, significant ethnic, racial, and gender gaps remain among graduates with higher degrees. In the United States, African Americans continue to be underrepresented in many professions, particularly notable in the profession of nursing (p. 41).

Minority registered nurses remain underrepresented in the current nursing workforce—a disparity in numbers that only adds to the escalating nursing shortage. In 2000, 4.9% of the nursing workforce (registered nurses and licensed practical/vocational nurses) listed their race/culture as Black/African American; by 2004 that percentage had dropped to 4.6% or 122,495 nurses (U.S. Department of Health and Human Services [USDHHS], Health Resources and Services Administration [HRSA], 2004). The RN and LPN workforce is slowly becoming more diverse over time. The proportion of non-White RNs increased from 20% to 25% during the past decade (USDHHS, 2013a) which included 9.9% African Americans (USDHHS, 2013b). The proportion of men in the RN workforce increased from 8% to 9% during this same time period (USDHHS, 2013b). A key characteristic of the nursing shortage is the inadequate numbers of minority registered nurses in the profession.

Environmental Context

In stating that they "...don't have a life, many nursing program informants stressed that they have put their life on hold while attending nursing school; this has been very hard on them and their families. The importance of family life and support was strongly emphasized by all informants throughout the study. All were commuting students attending nursing programs in suburban settings; the context of their care environment included their home lives, jobs, and the nursing program and college campus social and political activities. None of the informants were politically active in their college community. Most indicated that they went to class or lab and did not have time to participate in social or political activities on campus. One nursing student admitted that he attended one soccer game in the past year because he knew one of the other college students who was playing, but even then he arrived late and could not stay for the entire game.

Cultural diversity on campus at their respective colleges or in their nursing programs were described as nonexistent. One 36-year-old general informant stated, ". . .You know, if you look at percentages and numbers . . . no, it's not diverse." Another key informant stated:

> It [the college] is diverse. I notice quite a few Blacks. I have noticed Indians. But men of different cultures are rare in nursing. I think it's a general cultural thing, especially as you look at it from a . . . you know, a predominantly White school. In a big way I think coming from an African culture, you find that people are . . . they're less direct in communication. So sometimes somebody will tell you . . . oh, it's okay, [for a male nurse to care for the patient] but it's really not okay. So that really bothers me. In my culture, things are very clearly stated.

Throughout the study, informants discussed their environment at home and at the college; overall, most students stated they felt safe on their campuses. They also described generally feeling safe going to their clinical rotations. Some were not as comfortable about their home [neighborhood] environment, however. A 31-year-old general informant stated, ". . .Yeah, I don't [feel safe]. No. I try not to [go out at night]. When I come from a walk, I just run to the door." Another 31-year-old general informant stated she was very worried about her home [neighborhood] environment but was determined to keep her family safe and finish school; she relocated while still in school to help protect her children.

Another 30-year-old general informant stated:

> Yeah. I think the environment where I'm at right now . . . it's okay, but I feel like I can't let my children too much out of my sight in the area we're in. You know, they have their quiet months and then you have the months where I guess there's a lot of activity in the city and everybody wants to act up at the same time. On my block it seems like, you know, because the people see you, they know you, so they don't bother you.

The environmental context concerns were based mostly on the informants' places of residence and not their college campuses. Those who described living in an environment that was unsafe usually resided in an inner city neighborhood. Some informants acknowledged that they did not plan on living in their current location for much longer—only until they could finish school and become employed as a registered nurse.

REVIEW OF LITERATURE

The literature review revealed a dearth of research in the area of culture care educational expressions, beliefs, and practices of African American associate degree nursing students in predominantly Euro American programs. In order to discover the characteristics of the DOI, the literature review focused on associate degree nursing programs; ethnohistory of African American education; relevant literature; and research conducted with African American college and nursing students.

Associate Degree Nursing Programs

The associate degree nursing (ADN) movement in the early 1950s ". . .took form in the crucible of a persistent fear that the nation was not recruiting and educating enough young people to provide the nurses we would need" (Haase, 1990, p. 11). Nursing had a reform group intent on moving nursing education away from hospital-based programs, where most nurses were then educated, and into institutions of higher education. The United States was focused more than ever on education as a means of solving social issues and health problems. Nurse leaders soon realized that educational reform had an optimal opportunity to succeed. For many years, nurse leaders and educators had pushed for nursing education within collegiate settings and away from service agencies, but this type of reform had been consistently opposed by physicians and hospital administrators, who argued that nurses were exhibiting little more than self-interest (Haase, 1990). With most hospital-based diploma programs closed, nursing education is primarily in the collegiate environment. Community colleges have become the primary educators of associate degree nurses, while 4-year colleges and universities have developed associate, baccalaureate, master's, and doctoral programs for nurses.

Initiated as a research project in response to societal needs, ADN programs have had a significant impact on the profession of nursing and nursing education. By 1980, 47% of nurses qualified to take state licensing examinations were graduates of 2-year ADN programs. At the time of the study, there were 701 community college ADN programs, with 60% of all new nurses and 73% of the nursing graduates in rural settings being educated in these programs (American Association of Community Colleges, 2004). The ADN program has made a substantial contribution to nursing education in the United States. The National Organization for Associate Degree Nursing [N-OADN] (1998) stated:

> Associate Degree Nursing (ADN) education provides a dynamic pathway for entry into registered nursing (RN) practice. It offers accessible, affordable, quality instruction to a diverse population.

ADN education has continually evolved to reflect local community needs and healthcare trends. ADN graduates are prepared to function in multiple healthcare settings, including community practice sites. They possess a core of clinical nursing knowledge common to all entry-level nursing graduates and have continuously demonstrated their competency for safe practice by passing the National Council Licensure Examination for Registered Nurses (NCLEX-RN).

Associate degree programs have recruited students for nursing who might otherwise have chosen different careers. Men, single parents, minority students, and others select an ADN program when other programs have more restrictive admission criteria, are more expensive, or require a longer completion time (Haase, 1990). The majority of ADN graduates are adult learners who have been established as an integral part of their communities and exhibit a commitment to lifelong learning through continuing education offerings, certification credentialing, and ongoing formal education (N-OADN, 1998, p. 1) and who provide a stable workforce within the community.

The comprehensive review of the literature on the domain of inquiry specific to associate degree nursing programs identified only 82 published items in professional journals, news journal articles, and newspaper articles, along with 490 dissertation studies covering every theme relating to associate degree nursing. In regard to minority populations in associate degree programs, 23 dissertations addressed minority students and only 3 were identified as research with or about African American students in associate degree programs.

Hunt (1992) conducted a study on the perceptions of student retention in associate degree nursing programs by the directors of those programs. A random sampling of 250 directors of National League for Nursing (NLN)–accredited associate degree programs was conducted to identify information on student attrition rates, the involvement of the institution on retention, and the types of institutions administering the programs. The results of this study indicated that the mean attrition rate from the first to second year of the program was 20.5%. The study also found that the directors believed the most influential negative factor contributing to attrition was conflict with jobs and class schedules; financial aid was second; and inadequate counseling and support systems were third. The directors rated a caring and supportive faculty as one of the most important positive elements for the retention of nursing students. In this study, more than 92% of the campuses had implemented a program designed to improve the retention rates of their students (Hunt, 1992).

Sims' (1996) van Manen phenomenological study on Black women's experiences at predominantly Euro American schools of nursing indicated that nursing education and nursing research should focus efforts on evaluating nursing curricula that support diversity and multiculturalism in nursing education. Eighteen Black women graduates from associate degree nursing programs in the North and South Carolina area participated in taped audio interviews. Three major patterns and nine relational themes emerged. The three major patterns were *getting in*; *getting through*; and *getting out*. The nine relational themes were *coexisting*; *proving self*; *hiding self* (including *avoiding self-disclosure*); *avoiding the instructor* (some students had been LPNs and did not want their instructor to know their background); *making sacrifices*; *dealing with stress* (including threats to racial identity and cultural values, and threats to their pattern of living); *being treated differently*; *seeking and gaining support from religion, family members, each other, and advice from those they considered "trailblazers"*; and *determination* (identified by new graduates) (Sims, 1996).

Flinn (2000) conducted a study to identify, describe, and analyze multicultural teaching strategies being used by five nurse educators in associate degree nursing programs. This study identified 155 discrete multicultural education teaching strategies used by these educators. Five major categories were identified with all of the teaching strategies incorporated: *Sharing knowledge, working in groups, asking questions, developing relationships,* and *teaching psychomotor skills.* Flinn found that ". . .teaching that is culturally responsive occurs when there is equal respect for the backgrounds and contemporary circumstances of all learners, regardless of individual status and power" (p. 24). In addition, the goal of *good* teaching ". . .is to assist students to achieve their fullest potential. A goal of *multicultural* teaching is to create learning environments so that students from diverse cultural groups will have an equal opportunity to learn" (p. 43). This is a relevant study that supports the need for educators to understand and be aware of the cultural care values and lifeways of their students in order to offer culturally competent teaching strategies.

Stewart (2001) looked at retention strategies and attrition rates for African American associate degree nursing students. This study combined quantitative and qualitative methodologies. Quantitative data collected from the deans and directors of 11 ADN programs in South Carolina were analyzed and compared with the qualitative perspectives from minority students in one of the programs. Fourteen percent of the nursing students enrolled in these programs were African American; retention rates for these students ranged from 17% to 83%. To decrease attrition, the nursing programs implemented a variety of retention strategies. Regression analysis from the study indicated that there were no statistically significant relationships between the retention rates and the strategies for admissions/recruitment; orientation; and academic support initiated in the study by the programs. However, the study showed a statistically significant negative relationship between retention rates and student support.

Butters (2003) conducted a study of retention in ADN programs that also evaluated the retention of minority students. This quantitative and qualitative study used a survey and interviews with a small group of "successful" second-year associate degree nursing students at six institutions in Massachusetts with 268 completed surveys returned. There were only 79 minority students in the cohort that completed the survey. The survey results identified environmental factors as significant in attrition for both majority and minority students. Students identified difficulty in finding time for study along with the need to balance the responsibilities of family and work. Butters identified the importance and necessity to decrease the disproportion of minorities in the nursing profession. She also recognized the possibility of bias in her research with regard to interviewing students from other races and age groups, in that she was the researcher and a Caucasian female at least a generation older than most of the students. Butters was also disappointed that more minority students did not volunteer to be interviewed:

> I was disappointed that more minority participants did not volunteer to be interviewed, but I cannot be surprised. I arrived at the participant programs as a person unknown to the students who would fill out the survey and volunteer for the interview. How could the student know whether I came from an "external-insider" or "external-outsider" approach? For most of the participants, the day of the survey administration was the only time they would ever have contact with me as a person and a researcher. When I presented these findings to two student groups as a member check, I noticed that only one student of color, and no White, responded to any assertions concerning disproportion of minorities in the nursing field. Except for the one comment noted above, it was as though I had not discussed the topic.
>
> . . . Perhaps this is an example of support for Barbee's assertion (1993) that the culture of caring in nursing makes discussion about racism in nursing an unbearable topic. I would suggest a more long-term and comprehensive research approach for the future. The problem of minority disproportion in the nursing ranks will not be solved quickly or easily. Nursing education could become involved in research about students in their own states, and maintain, update, and analyze information on a regular schedule. (p. 200)

Butters' (2003) approach to her research from the external-insider and external-outsider perspective was congruent with Leininger's etic and emic perspectives and the Stranger-to-Trusted-Friend Enabler from the culture care theory.

Jackson (2003) also conducted a study on predictors of first-semester attrition with associate degree nursing students using Tinto's student integration model of persistence as the framework for a retrospective correlational study conducted to determine if such variables as English proficiency, weekly hours of employment, financial resources, and past academic achievement could differentiate between passing and failing in the first semester of an ADN program. This study, which was conducted at a multi-campus community college, demonstrated a significant correlation with preadmission English proficiency and nursing students' first semester success in a generic associate degree program in Florida. Based on this, the researchers recommended raising the admission grade point averages above the minimum "C" then required by the program. This study did not specifically address culturally diverse students or African American nursing students.

Rudel (2004) conducted a qualitative van Manen phenomenology study to gain a better understanding of how nontraditional associate degree nursing students perceived nursing education. The study was conducted in a Midwestern community college with six nontraditional ADN students and identified three major themes: *Retention*; *faculty characteristics*; and *challenges related to the lack of applications by faculty of adult learning theory*. Recommendations were that by embracing the learning principles for adult learners, faculty could facilitate a more positive learning experience for students (Rudel, 2004). The study did not address culturally diverse or African American students, but the results are relevant because they support the need for faculty to better understand the students and facilitate a more positive and congruent learning process.

Ethnohistory of African American Education

African Americans comprise one of the largest ethnic minority groups in the United States, accounting for 13.1% of the total population (U.S. Department of Commerce, Census Bureau, 2010). Although a few Africans arrived in the Americas prior to the 15th century, most Africans were brought as slaves to the mainland colonies of Central and South America by the Spaniards. Forms of servitude existed among many of the African ethnic groups, and the slave trade to the Americas was facilitated by the existence of such slavery practices and by a slave trade inside Africa. Debtors and persons convicted of certain crimes would be forced into slavery as punishment, but these individuals had the expectation that their freedom could be restored. While the slave trade to the Americas did not develop solely because slavery existed in Africa, the African collaboration with European slave traders made this type of business mutually beneficial. As noted earlier, an estimated 10 to 12 million Africans arrived as slaves from 1502 to the mid-19th century (Kelley & Lewis, 2000).

During the second half of the 17th century, the ". . .enslavement of people solely on the basis of race occurred in the lives of African Americans" (Kelley & Lewis, 2000, p. 63). For the first time, the dominant English came to view Africans not as *heathen people* but as *Black people*, and also began to describe themselves not as *Christians* but as *Whites*. It was a momentous step from saying that Black persons *could* be enslaved to saying that Negroes *should* be enslaved. In addition, those who wrote these colonial laws moved to make slavery not only *racial* but also *hereditary*. Under English common law, a child inherited the legal status of the father (p. 68). Hereditary enslavement based on skin color became a bitter reality in the New World by 1650. As a result, the Africans brought to the Americas faced significant personal and cultural challenges.

"Not surprisingly, the African peoples who came to the Americas brought very strong family and religious traditions with them" (Kelley & Lewis, 2000, p. 4). The worldview of African Americans in the United States stems from their cultural heritage and their life experiences. According to Tamela Heath (1998), author of a chapter in *African American Culture and Heritage in Higher Education Research and Practice*, ". . .ways of being, feeling, and knowing are shaped by many things, not the least of which is one's social and cultural experiences" (Freeman, 1998, p. 33).

Historically, African American students were denied the same educational opportunities as Euro American students. ". . .The evolution of education for African Americans is a narrative of their struggle for development in educational opportunity, [and] political, economic and social advancement" (Mungazi, 1999, p. 125). Attitudes and political views during the post–Civil War years had serious implications for the impeded development of education for African Americans. The South became more deeply fixed in its beliefs of the Black man as an inferior being who did not merit equal treatment as a citizen. At the same time, national leaders in the North were trying to convey the idea of racial equality. By 1878, the District of Columbia and 14 Southern states had passed legislation that authorized separate schools for White and Black children. The philosophy of separate but equal educational facilities expressed in legislation became firmly established. At the same time, states like Florida passed laws that made it a crime for any school to enroll both Black and White students in the same school. In a court decision of 1896, the U.S. Supreme Court put its stamp of approval on the principle of separate schools.

Established soon after the Civil War for Black students, Berea College in Kentucky was integrated by 1908, having disregarded the practice of segregation in defiance of the state law mandates. Berea filed a lawsuit against the state when it was ordered to segregate, arguing in court documents that the participation by the races at the school was purely voluntary and that there was no tension or hostility between the students. The college further recommended the integration of educational facilities on a voluntary basis serve as a model for other institutions. However, the ruling by the Kentucky Court of Appeals was upheld by the U.S. Supreme Court and Berea College was ordered to segregate its students (Mungazi, 1999). Nevertheless, the Berea College decision had a tremendous impact on the character of education for African Americans in the United States.

Clearly, segregated school systems created new problems, especially in regard to the education of African Americans. For the next 60 years, school districts were structured on the precept of segregation as "separate but equal." African Americans recognized inequalities in their schools and the negative psychological effects of being segregated were being identified. The *McLaurin vs. University of Oklahoma Board of Regents* case was the first in which the U.S. Supreme Court actually addressed the effects of segregation on African American students and marked a new way of thinking for the high court. Thereafter, court decisions and subsequent social and political actions brought the full Constitutional rights of citizenship for African Americans closer to reality. In 1954, in the case of *Brown vs. the Board of Education of Topeka*, Chief Justice Earl Warren wrote the unanimous decision:

> Segregation of White and Colored children in public schools has a detrimental effect upon the Colored children. The impact is greater when it has the sanction of the law, for the policy of separating the races is usually interpreted as denoting the inferiority of the Negro group. Segregation with the sanction of law, therefore, has a tendency to retard the educational and mental development of Negro children and deprive them of some of the benefits they would receive in a racially integrated school system. We conclude that in the field of public education the doctrine of "separate but equal" has no place. Separate educational facilities are inherently unequal. (Fellman, 1976, p. 138)

This decision was definitely a high point in the advancement of education for African Americans. Its intention was that no state legislature could pass laws permitting segregation in public schools (Mungazi, 1999).

Subsequently, two revolutionary initiatives gave a significant push to African Americans and other minorities to enroll in postsecondary education. These programs dramatically changed both the number of minority applicants and their geographical distribution throughout U.S. higher educational institutions. The first initiative occurred in 1945 with the passage of a GI bill that included educational benefits. The rationale for first GI bill was to keep the millions of returning veterans from overwhelming the job market after World War II—which would have seriously disrupted the national economy. In spite of its practical goal, the first GI bill

> enabled hundreds of thousands of veterans, including thousands of African American and Hispanic veterans, many the first in their families, to attend college independent of scholarship or previous educational achievement. The GI bill was a true educational revolution that structurally changed American higher education. (Wilson, 1994, p. 195)

The second initiative occurred in 1964 with the passing of the Civil Rights Act. Executive Order 11246 established the Affirmative Action, Upward Bound, Special Services, and Talent Search initiatives. In 1965, 600,000 African Americans were in college with 65% at historically Black colleges, but by 1980 African American enrollment had doubled to 1.2 million with only 20% of this number attending historically Black colleges (Wilson, 1994). In 1980, the majority of African American undergraduate student enrollment was in community colleges. Because of their policies of open admission, community colleges were more accessible to minorities whose primary and secondary educational preparation was often not sufficient to qualify them for entrance into 4-year colleges. In more recent decades, African American college enrollment has been trending away from the South and into the North and West where the majority of community colleges are located. "Community colleges, while increasing access to post secondary education, did not significantly contribute to improving baccalaureate degrees for minority populations" (deRuyter, 2008, p. 27). Most African American community college students aspire to complete a Bachelor of Arts or Bachelor of Science degree; however, fewer than 15% actually transfer to a 4-year school and fewer still ever graduate from the community college (Wilson, 1994).

Although the legal restrictions on access to schooling and postsecondary education have been lifted in the United States, remnants of racism still exist at the structural core of the education system (Freeman, 1998). The traditional educational setting is often incongruent with the African American culture in which their styles of being and knowing are embedded (deRuyter, 2008). This incongruity has been detrimental to the development of both cognitive and affective outcomes for African American students (Freeman, 1998) as reflected by their poor graduation rates and limited academic development (Stikes, 1984).

"Institutional emphasis on traditionalism in many areas such as the organization of the college; its delivery system for services; the administration, management and supervision of students; teaching methods; interpersonal relations; students' coping strategies; and students' learning styles create problems for different minority students, who often feel lost on predominantly Euro American campuses" (deRuyter, 2008, p. 28). Students become entangled in conflicts about cultural values with administrators, faculty, staff, and fellow students; they also experience conflicting pressures from college values and from families and their cultural expectations (Maynard, 1980). ". . .This destructive conflict need not exist. Educational programs for Blacks and Whites can co-exist in harmony with appropriate recognition of differing cultural values" (Stikes, 1984, p. 121). The cultural care educational expressions, beliefs, and practices of African American nursing students in predominantly Euro American associate degree programs still needs to be discovered and understood.

Relevant Literature

Minority registered nurses are underrepresented in the nursing workforce and this disparity adds to the escalating nursing shortage. In 2000, 4.9% of the nursing workforce listed their race/culture as Black/African American; by 2004 that percentage had dropped to 4.6% (USDHHS, 2004). In spite of their small numbers, practicing minority nurses have made significant contributions in the provision of healthcare services and are leaders in the development of models of care that address the unique needs of minority populations (Simmons, 2002). However, persistent underrepresentation of minorities in nursing education perpetuates the disparity of minorities entering the nursing workforce (U.S. Department of Health and Human Services, Bureau of Health Professions, National Advisory Council on Nurse Education and Practice, 2000). Efforts to identify cultural and educational barriers that influence African American students and methods to facilitate their recruitment and retention in basic and graduate nursing education programs are clearly needed.

Overall, minority nurses place a higher value on advanced education than their Euro American counterparts; 48.1% of African American nurses acquire baccalaureate or graduate degrees in nursing compared to 41.8% of Euro American nurses (Sullivan, Dole, & Rogers, 2004). Identifying minority students' culture care expressions, beliefs, and practices may help to improve completion rates in nursing programs. Improving completion rates of culturally diverse students will increase the representation of minorities in the nursing profession.

Research Studies

African American College Students

The postsecondary educational research literature review supports the influences of faculty on student retention. A focus-group study of minority students about what factors contributed to the retention of African American students in a 4-year postsecondary institution was conducted by Wynetta (1999) over one semester with a total of 120 students. This study found that African American students entering predominantly White public institutions bring with them a strong heritage that does not match the institution's culture and environment (Wynetta, 1999). Low retention rates and the complexities of their cultural heritage were deterrents to the students' degree attainment, pointing to the ". . .importance of effective strategies to foster retention to degree completion" (p. 30). The students in the study groups indicated that faculty mentoring was one of the important factors lending toward their retention. They also indicated that same-race faculty mentoring was not as important as having access to a faculty person from their field of study and supportive of their culture.

Recommendations from that study suggested mentoring relationships be developed that are beneficial to both faculty and students and that ". . .future research should also determine the extent to which majority faculty feel culturally competent to effectively mentor minority students" (Wynetta, 1999, p. 38). Such research would significantly transform institutional practices and improve the prospect of retaining African American students through to degree completion. This study identified how essential it is for faculty to strive for cultural competence to achieve African American student retention by understanding the cultural worldview and culture care values, beliefs, practices, and lifeways of African American students.

Understanding, valuing, listening, and responding to culturally diverse students' culture care needs are central to improving diversity in nursing. New and nontraditional paths in nursing education can be explored that encourage more diversity in the nursing workforce by understanding the culture care meanings attached to activities, events, behaviors, knowledge, and rituals. The Sullivan Commission's report on diversity in the health-care workforce identified the lack of minority health professionals as compounding the ". . .nation's persistent racial and ethnic health disparities" (Sullivan et al., 2004, p. i). Given that studies have consistently documented that racial minority health professionals are more likely to return to their communities and provide health care (Coffman, Rosenoff, & Grumbach, 2001; Moy & Bartman, 1995; Stinson & Thurston, 2002; Tucker-Allen, 1989), the Institute of Medicine (2003) recommended increased numbers of minority health professionals as a key strategy toward eliminating health disparities. The College Board (1999) report stated:

> Until many more underrepresented minority students from disadvantaged, middle class, and upper-middle class circumstances are very successful educationally, it will be virtually impossible to integrate our society's institutions completely, especially at leadership levels. Without such progress, the United States also will continue to be unable to draw on the full range of talents in our population during an era when the value of an educated citizenry has never been greater. (p. 11)

The United States has a very diverse society; educational differences have the potential to become progressively larger and more problematic if not effectively addressed. Educators, legislators, and educational policymakers know that eliminating disparities in education has become a moral and pragmatic imperative (College Board, 1999).

African American Nursing Students

A comprehensive search of the literature regarding the domain of inquiry did not identify any studies conducted on the culture care of African

American associate degree nursing students. However, studies focused on racial and ethnic minority students that investigated barriers to success and perceptions of experiences influencing success in nursing programs have been conducted. Many of these studies were carried out in 4-year baccalaureate nursing programs, but a few were conducted in associate degree programs that have relevance to this study. In addition, some research with African American postsecondary students has been conducted in predominantly Euro American institutions; these lent support to the need for the study discussed in this chapter.

Buckley (1980) identified the impact faculty had on African American nursing student retention. This early research acknowledged that a faculty commitment to Black nursing students was a positive factor affecting retention of African Americans in the program. This study was conducted in only one 4-year baccalaureate nursing program, limiting the transferability of the findings to all predominantly Euro American programs. Tucker-Allen (1989) acknowledged the lack of research on what African American nursing students believe would best serve their nursing educational needs and highlighted the problem of inadequate numbers of practicing African American nurses and the substantially negative impact this had upon disadvantaged African Americans' access to the healthcare system. Tucker-Allen also held that the lack of African American nurses affected the educational system due to the ". . .low number of African American nurses who are prepared to become teachers in schools of nursing" (p. 396).

In the 21st century, this disparity continues to affect the nursing educational system. Hyche-Johnson (1995) surveyed 202 generic baccalaureate nursing students and interviewed 12 junior and senior African American nursing students who perceived barriers to success in the nursing program. The barriers identified by the students in this study were primarily external and stemmed from the higher educational structure or the inflexibility of the nursing program; the courses and course sequencing; the rigidity of the rules and regulations in the program; and inadequate financial resources needed to complete the program. This study also found that the faculty recognized institutional constraints to a greater extent than Euro American students but less than Black students:

> Faculty members' perceptions of students' attitudes, feelings, and behaviors failed to take into consideration the fact that behavior, attitudes, perceptions, and feelings arise out of past experiences, observations of the experiences of other similar people, magazines, media, and shared life experiences by family and friends. (Hyche-Johnson, 1995, p. 166)

This discovery was significant when viewed in the context of providing a culturally competent education to students. Barriers alone did not impede some African American students but rather how the students viewed those barriers. Generally successful students had higher SAT scores or strong cognitive skills; noncognitive factors such as racism, self-concept, leadership skills, realistic self-appraisal, community service, long-term goal-directed behavior; and a strong support system played significant roles in student success. This small-sample study was significant in that the importance of noncognitive variables for success in nursing programs was acknowledged and identified. Elling and Furr (2002) supported this finding by noting the importance of studying the culture associated with student populations in order to meet their cultural needs, develop effective interventions, and improve retention.

Kersey-Matusiak (1999) conducted a study in a 4-year Catholic college to identify the factors that minority students perceived as influencing their success in college by using combinations of quantitative and qualitative methodologies. The Students' Perceptions Questionnaire (SPQ) distributed to 58 female and 2 male minority nursing student participants used a two-part method. The first part requested biographical data and the second part requested responses from the students on a 36-item perception scale about personal ambition, goal commitment, sociocultural integration, alienation, academic satisfaction, institutional support, and personal attributes. The quantitative findings of this study found no significant correlation between any of the demographic variables, grade-point averages (GPAs), or personal attributes; there were no significant differences between Black students and other minority groups or successful and unsuccessful students based on their GPAs. Qualitative data from face-to-face interviews revealed positive perceptions about the participants' academic satisfaction and their support from faculty.

This study demonstrated that faculty influenced the experiences of students and supported the findings from the early study by Buckley (1980). However, approximately 50% of these minority students felt that they were not integrating with the Euro American students on campus (Kersey-Matusiak, 1999). This study was conducted with baccalaureate students in a 4-year institution and has not been replicated with associate degree nursing students.

Coffman, Rosenoff, and Grumbach (2001) conducted a study to determine the reason for the lack of diversity in nursing by comparing the racial and ethnic composition of the registered nurse (RN) workforce with the general and work-age (20 to 64 years) populations in California. This retrospective study used the demographics from the National Sample Survey of Registered Nurses collected in 1996 to evaluate racial and ethnic groups in the highest educational levels attained by Californians aged 24 through

39 years over a 12-month period. Degrees grouped by category included nursing; other health fields; physical and biological sciences; and other.

Data was also obtained from the California Postsecondary Education Commission (CPEC), the state agency that collects educational data. The results of the study clearly indicated that African Americans and Latinos were under-represented among the California RN workforce, 93.5% of whom were women. Euro American female college graduates were ". . .56% more likely than Latina graduates were to receive degrees in nursing" (Coffman et al., 2001, p. 266). Gaps in educational attainment by minority students accounted for much of nursing's lack of diversity (Coffman et al., 2001).

The several limitations in this study included that it was conducted in one state; used graduation and degree data that covered only 1 year in that state; integrated all minorities in the analysis; and did not evaluate any one minority population in-depth. As this was a retrospective study, the interpretation of the data was confined to what was available to the researchers and the assessment and interpretation may not have accurately reflected the actual data. The study also did not take into consideration any qualitative factors, such as cultural perceptions of nursing, family support, role models, or counseling about entry into the profession of nursing.

The study findings revealed that to improve the representation of minorities in nursing, new and innovative programs to enhance educational attainment among minority populations of students were necessary, and identified the need to develop comprehensive and coordinated approaches to close the gaps in educational attainment as a method to improve diversity in nursing. These approaches needed to include qualitative factors such as understanding the culture care values, needs, worldviews, and lifeways of minority students.

Gardner (2005) conducted a qualitative phenomenology study at three 4-year public universities in California to identify the barriers influencing the success of minority students in predominantly Euro American nursing programs. Eight themes were identified: *Loneliness and isolation; differentness; absence of acknowledgment of individuality from teachers; peers' lack of understanding and knowledge about cultural differences; lack of support from teachers; coping with insensitivity and discrimination; determination to build a better future;* and *overcoming obstacles* (p. 151). The data from this research with 15 racial and ethnically diverse students illuminated the ". . .need for educators to become more knowledgeable about the challenges and needs of minority nursing students" (p. 161).

Jeffreys (2004) determined that the conceptual models and frameworks developed by several researchers to explicate student attrition had limited relevance to nursing students. Due to the lack of a relevant model to study nursing students, Jeffreys developed the NURS model to provide a framework with which to examine retention in undergraduate nursing students. Student characteristics such as age, ethnicity and race, gender, language, educational experiences, and family background were components of the model. Cultural values, beliefs, self-efficacy, and motivation are also considered important variables for retention and attrition. Jeffreys stated that while nurse educators are in a position to positively influence student retention, insight into interactive variables and the students' perspective is necessary in order to design supportive retention strategies.

THEORETICAL FRAMEWORK

The Theory of Culture Care Diversity and Universality was the framework used to guide this study and to discover the worldview, beliefs, values, and meanings of informant lifeways (2002b). The researcher believed that using the theory would provide optimal guidance to discover the cultural beliefs, values, and meanings related to the education of nursing students participating in the study. The researcher used the Sunrise Enabler and four assumptive premises adapted from Leininger (2002b) to study the major constructs of the theory and discover the cultural and social structure factors that influenced the culture care expressions, beliefs, and practices related to the educational experiences of participant African American nursing students within the context of their predominantly Euro American nursing programs.

RESEARCH QUESTIONS

For this study, the following research questions were developed:

1. What are the culture care educational expressions, beliefs, and practices of African American students in predominantly Euro American associate degree nursing programs?
2. What are the culture care supportive or facilitative acts or mutual decisions that help African American students in predominantly Euro American associate degree nursing programs reorder, change, or restructure their care patterns and practices for beneficial educational outcomes?
3. In what ways do cultural, social, religious, economic, technological, educational, and political factors influence the educational care expressions, beliefs, and practices of African American nursing students within the environmental context of a predominantly Euro American associate degree nursing program?

ORIENTATIONAL DEFINITIONS

For this qualitative ethnonursing study, the following orientational definitions were used as a guide to discover the culture care phenomena within the context of the study:

- **Environmental context**: Refers to the totality of the experience of a 2-year community college, 4-year college, or university that offers associate degree nursing programs, including the organizational factors, social factors, and the cultural background of the student body and faculty (adapted from McFarland, 1995, p. 17).
- **Educational health and wellbeing**: Refers to a state of wellbeing in which there is a continuous successful progression and ultimate completion of the associate degree nursing program (adapted from Leininger, 2002b, p. 84).
- **Culture care**: Refers to the subjectively and objectively learned values, beliefs, and lifeways that assist, facilitate, or enable caring acts toward self or African American students to participate, complete, and graduate from a predominantly Euro American associate degree nursing program (Leininger, 2002b, p. 83).
- **Culture care education**: Refers to the education that is based on culturally specific teaching and education that assists, supports, facilitates, or enables African American associate degree nursing students to maintain their educational health and wellbeing by progressing through the nursing program to completion to improve their human condition and lifeways (adapted from Leininger, 2002b, p. 84).
- **African American**: Nursing students who identify their culture as Black or African American.
- **Euro American**: Nursing students who identify their culture as Caucasian or White non-Hispanic.
- **Associate degree nursing program**: A 2-year college-based nursing curriculum that leads to licensure as a registered nurse. The curriculum can be completed in a community college or a 4-year college or university.
- **Predominantly Euro American nursing program**: For the purposes of this study, a predominantly Euro American nursing program is one that identifies greater than 60% of the student body as Euro American or White non-Hispanic.
- **Emic**: Refers to the African American associate degree nursing students' view and knowledge about culture care educational expressions, beliefs, and practices (adapted from Leininger, 2002b, p. 84).

- **Etic**: Refers to an outsider's (Euro American nursing faculty) professional knowledge, generalized view, or universal view of the educational expressions, beliefs, and practices of African American associate degree nursing students (adapted from Leininger, 2002b, p. 84).

ASSUMPTIVE PREMISES OF THE RESEARCH

Assumptions regarding the research design, its organization, and data processing are inherent in ethnonursing research. According to Leininger (2002a) ". . .culture is a very powerful and comprehensive construct that influences and shapes the way people know their world, live, and develop patterns to make decisions relative to their life world. Culture is known as the blueprint to guide human lifeways and actions and to predict patterns of behavior or functioning" (p. 9).

Leininger (1991, 2002b) formulated 13 assumptive premises for the theory of culture care to use as guides to systematically study and support the theory, position, tenets, and hunches. This study sought to discover and examine knowledge that would add substantively to four of the assumptive premises of the culture care theory which were used as guides to support the general purposes of this study:

- Culturally-based care is the broadest holistic way to know, explain, interpret, and predict beneficial and desirable nursing education care practices for African American associate degree nursing students in predominantly Euro American programs (derived from Leininger, 1991).
- Culture care concepts, meanings, expressions, patterns, processes, and structural forms of care for African American associate degree nursing students vary transculturally with diversities and some universalities (adapted from Leininger, 2002b, p. 79).
- Cultural care beliefs, values, and practices of African American associate degree nursing students in predominantly Euro American programs are influenced by the worldview, religious, political, educational, technical, and ethnohistorical dimensions of their culture (adapted from Leininger, 1991).
- The ethnonursing qualitative research method provides a means to accurately discover and interpret emic and etic embedded complex and diverse cultural data (adapted from Leininger, 2002b, p. 84).

METHODOLOGY

The ethnonursing method was used in this study of African American nursing students within the environmental context of predominantly Euro

American associate degree nursing programs located in the Eastern area of the United States. This method enabled the researcher to use:

> . . .data collection methods of participant observation in selected cultural activities and in-depth interviewing of the members of the subculture, as well as supplementary methods . . . to learn from informants the meaning that they attach to their activities, events, behaviors, knowledge, rituals, and other aspects of their lives. (Munhall, 2001, p. 278)

The ethnonursing research method was developed to study nursing phenomena from a nursing perspective (Leininger, 1991). It is a method that facilitates the discovery of data as it relates to the Theory of Culture Care Diversity and Universality. ". . .Knowledge of cultures with their care needs using the Culture Care Theory has become a major and unique emphasis in nursing as a means to know and help cultures" (Leininger, 2006, p. 3). Ethnonursing is a qualitative process that focuses on a naturalistic, open discovery, and largely inductive method to document, describe, explain, and interpret informants' worldview, meanings, symbols, and life experiences (Leininger, 1991, 2002b, 2006). This method focuses on ". . .learning from the people through their eyes, ears, and experiences and how they made sense out of situations and lifeways that were familiar to them" (Leininger, 1991, p. 79). Ethnonursing methodology facilitates knowing from an *emic* perspective about the knowledge and practices related to lifespan experiences. The ethnonursing research process was designed and has been used to build the body of transcultural nursing knowledge and to guide the culture care practices of nurses in clinical practice. It was an appropriate method for the study in that it allowed the researcher to get an in-depth emic understanding of the culture care educational expressions, beliefs, practices, and worldview of African American nursing students. Culturally congruent educational practices were discovered by exploring the culture care educational expressions, beliefs, practices, and experiences of African American nursing students. The ethnonursing method provided a richer, more focused nursing perspective for the study.

Sample

A letter describing the study was sent to the deans/directors and chairs of associate degree nursing programs in southern Pennsylvania, central and southern New Jersey, and northern Delaware. The deans/directors and chairs of the colleges with associate degree nursing programs in Pennsylvania and New Jersey verbally agreed to distribute this information (letter) to their student body. The demographics of the colleges in the study

Table 13-1 Student Demographics of Colleges

School	Caucasian (%)	African American (%)	Total Number of Students
1	79	13	2,723
2	60	24	2,787
3	69	9	8,860
4	81	3	9,596
5	74	9	6,022
6	78	5	7,019
7	65	8	2,681
8	85	8	35,000

are found in **Table 13-1**. After institutional review board (IRB) approval, a written agreement with the associate degree programs was obtained.

The letter distributed to students gave a brief description of the study, explaining that the researcher was a doctoral nursing student requesting to interview students from one to three times during the study for 45 to 90 minutes. In addition, the letter indicated that any student self-identifying as African American or Black who wished to participate in the research study could contact the researcher, the dean/director, or the dissertation chair. Snowball sampling was used to recruit additional informants for this study. Informants were recruited into the study until data saturation was reached.

Data Collection Procedure

Data obtained from field notes, observations, journals, and semi-structured interviews with informants over a period of 2 years. Data were also collected using the Observation–Participation–Reflection Enabler during student meetings, class meetings, or social events where students in associate degree programs gathered. One to three interviews each lasting from 45 to 90 minutes were conducted with each informant depending on their status as either a key or general informant. In-depth interviews were usually conducted on a one-to-one basis, but at times involved more than one informant due to informant schedules and time constraints, until saturation was reached. Audio-taped recordings of informant interviews, field journal notes, and the record of the researcher's feelings and reactions while with the informants were all transcribed on a regular basis and analyzed. This concurrent data collection and analysis occurred throughout the entire study.

All interviews with both key and general informants were used to identify, clarify, and explore areas in the domain of inquiry (DOI). At the beginning of each initial interview, the purpose of the study was explained and each informant was asked permission to tape the interview. Leininger's Stranger-to-Trusted-Friend Enabler was used to determine the progression with the informants. Care behaviors, attitudes, and expectations were discovered by the researcher with the use of this enabler. The researcher's stranger-to-trusted-friend relationship with the informants early and throughout the study assisted in gathering accurate and in-depth data. The transcribed data were dated and coded with a pseudonym for each informant after every interview to protect the informants' confidentiality. An open-ended interview guide was used to initiate each interview, but the information obtained during the interview further guided the interview process, follow-up interviews, and any subsequent contacts with informants.

Human Subjects Considerations

Informed consent was obtained from the informants both verbally and in writing at the beginning of the study. Verbal and written explanations of the plan and purpose of the study were provided to all informants. A signed consent was obtained from each informant with the assurance of confidentiality, privacy, and anonymity during data collection, assessment, evaluation, and presentation of the study. All informants were told that quotations would be used in reporting data for the final report and in any publications or presentations but without names or identifiers attached.

As most community colleges do not have an IRB, letters of permission were obtained from the dean, director, chair, or other appropriate individual at each participating community college associate degree nursing program with students in the study. If the college had an IRB, permission to conduct the study was sought and obtained from that board.

Data Analysis and Criteria

Leininger's Four Phases of Ethnonursing Qualitative Data Analysis ". . .provide a systematic data analysis when thoughtfully used" (Leininger, 2002b, p. 95). Leininger's Criteria for Qualitative Paradigmatic Studies (credibility, confirmability, meaning-in-context, recurrent patterning, saturation, and transferability) were used to evaluate the research data (Leininger, 2002b, p. 88).

Credibility of the data refers to how truthful, accurate, or believable the findings of the study are from the standpoint of the informants and the researcher. Direct experiences of the researcher with informants and the explanations and clarifications by the informants of situations or events substantiated the credibility. *Confirmability* was accomplished by reaffirming what the researcher saw, heard, and experienced regarding the culture care educational values, beliefs, practices, and experiences of the informants within the domain of inquiry using the researchers' observations and informants' explanations or restatements about specific aspects in the study. The researcher confirmed all data by asking for clarification and paraphrasing information provided by each informant during the interviews.

The *meaning-in-context* criterion focused on how African American students interpreted and understood their culture care educational values, beliefs, practices, or experiences. The interpretations and meanings that were related to experiences, communications, activities, and situations by the informants within the specific environmental context of a predominantly Euro American associate degree nursing program provided the meaning-in-context for this study.

Recurrent patterning was identified by the patterns and themes that repeated over time and reflected the consistency or lifeways and behaviors of the African American nursing students in the study. By confirming findings with key and general informants, patterns and themes that encompassed both the diversity and universality of the students were revealed from the interviews. *Saturation* occurred when the researcher ceased to obtain new data about the phenomena of the culture care education values, beliefs, practices, and experiences of the African American nursing students and by obtaining consistent information from additional informants. *Transferability* of the findings from this completed study may have a similar meaning in another context or situation such as associate degree nursing programs in another part of the country or with nursing students from other cultures or nursing programs.

RESULTS AND FINDINGS

The DOI for this study was the culture care expressions, beliefs, and practices of African American nursing students in predominantly Euro American associate degree nursing program. The presentation of the study findings is focused on three universal themes and eight care patterns discovered during the study. The researcher discovered the students' success in their nursing educational program was based on their *strength of purpose, determination, persistence, endurance,* and *optimism*. Individually, they expressed how having optimistic goals helped them to be successful. Overall, religion was an integral part of their worldview, giving them a path for optimism, focus, and guidance. Family and kinship relationships influenced everything they did as their lives revolved around not only their nuclear families but their extended families as well. Descriptors and direct quotes from the study are used to support the themes and patterns presented.

Three universal themes emerged from analysis, creative reflection, and synthesis of the culture care educational expressions, beliefs, practices, and experiences of African American nursing students in predominately Euro American associate degree nursing programs.

Universal Theme 1: Care, understanding, and spirituality by family, friends, and faculty are essential for meaningful educational experiences for African American students.

This universal theme was discovered from the expressions and responses of the informants. The care patterns that support this theme were: *A pattern of caring and understanding by family, friends, and faculty is essential; a pattern of education as valued and sought after;* and *religion and spiritual beliefs as an essential part of life.*

Care Pattern 1a: A Pattern of Caring and Understanding by Family, Friends, and Faculty is Essential

This care pattern emerged from the descriptions of how support, caring, and empathy were essential to achieving positive and meaningful outcomes in the informants' nursing education. As described by one key informant, her mother was her role model throughout childhood and continued to provide care and understanding for the informant as she pursued her nursing education. The informant felt this support was essential in order for her education to be meaningful to her. Another informant described how important encouragement, caring, and support from her family has been:

> I was blessed with a wonderful grandmother, a wonderful mother. My grandmother taught us a lot and she was always very caring. And she was just constantly giving me encouragement to pick myself up a little bit. And she was healthy for me.

Another stated:

> I feel like sometimes I feel like I have a heavy financial responsibility because my mom watches my son when I'm in school, so I work. Raising my son, invested in being a mother, a caregiver, a good provider for my son is my role. . . . But sometimes I feel like she wished she could have done what I've done. . . . I think she views me as beautiful. . . . I know she's proud of me. Sometimes she might not verbalize it, but I know she's proud of me. And . . . beautiful, smart, independent, she knows that I'm independent everything that she wanted me to be, a young lady.

Care by faculty was also viewed as necessary and important for a meaningful educational experience. One informant simply stated that she needed a caring faculty person to ". . .listen to me. Asking, trying to understand me, so that they can basically know the care that I need." She felt that if the faculty did not talk to her and listen to what she was saying, they would not be able to help her with her education. Another felt she has been very fortunate in her education: ". . .I don't really come across teachers or faculty members who just don't care. I really mean it." Support by faculty (as well as family and friends) was seen as essential to be successful, help alleviate stress, and survive each semester.

The informants found noncaring expressions were more difficult to articulate and define. However, they described concepts such as *only doing their job; impatient; rigid; harsh; is interested; you don't matter as an individual; not taking time to hear what someone is saying; arrogant;* and *ignorant to your feelings* as noncaring expressions. When discussing noncaring experiences they had endured during their lives and within the environmental context of their associate degree program, the informants were able to articulate noncaring expressions more readily. One informant expressed her frustration with faculty not picking up on her confusion in class and not understanding her as an individual:

> I like teachers that don't try to lump all the students together, like a majority. I like professors that will look at different people and see somebody and say maybe, you know, they may be confused or they might have had a problem, and you know they might seek them out. When they don't, it is noncaring. I just like when the teacher realizes that they're dealing with individuals in a group all of the time. And just take the group, you know, as individuals; just. . . they wouldn't think it's interracial. They are individuals.

A male informant recalled a time when he felt very discouraged and that his teacher did not care about his learning. He had been paying attention in the class, but had difficulty understanding some of the concepts; his questions went unanswered by the teacher during the class. He recalled:

> He didn't care what I did. I ask a question and not understand what was said. During the lecture I was thinking and had questions. Questions about the class . . . about five minutes were left and I've got two questions and he won't call on me. When I got my questions asked, he just looked at me and then the second time he told me, "No more questions; oh, I told you that already." He didn't care.

Two other informants were very clear in their description of a noncaring clinical faculty:

> Well, our first semester, you know, our first semester we were both in the same clinical group at the same clinical site with the instructor.

And she was very . . . she was cold. A lot of people would tell us, "Oh, you know what, my nursing instructor helped us do this." For us, it was all research and procedure, and you did it wrong or you did it right. She, like, really belittled us and there wasn't a lot of encouragement from her at all. I mean it really makes us appreciate our clinical instructors now who are a lot warmer and more encouraging, because from her. . . . I mean, she almost made me want to quit the program. We're just learning. Everything a mistake was made in, it was the end of the world.

Care Pattern 1b: A Pattern of Education as Valued and Sought After

Informants described many reasons why they chose the educational path of an associate degree nursing program which included factors such as time, cost, and recommendations by co-workers. Education was viewed, valued, and sought after as a means to improve themselves and their lives. Two informants expressed that determination and the importance of education and career were essential to being able to continue in the nursing program; one said:

> And you have to be strong. You actually have to want this because there's no way you can put yourself through all of what you're going through and not really want this career. Because there's no way you would stay in it if you didn't really want to be there. Like if it just didn't matter to you, I think it would be so much easier for you to just walk away.

The second informant shared:

> Even with me going to school, I look at it that I'm not doing it just for me; I'm doing it for all of us. And it's on a number of levels. I'm doing it because, yes, financially it will better us. But, I'm also doing it because one day they [her children] will be faced with the decision to go to school or not . . . and people look at it differently and it really shouldn't make a difference. You should just go. But, you know, depending on finances, depending on what your mindset is at that time, you're making a decision. And I want them to say, "You know what, it wasn't easy, but Mom did it." So on that level, I'm also moving towards the mark for that reason. I plant the seed within myself that this is what I'm doing, period, and end of story. No ifs, ands, or buts. I rarely say anymore . . . ". . .oh, *if* I become a nurse." I don't even say it. I think that that's negative. "*When* I become a nurse" is what I say.

Previous educational accomplishments of the informants also signified the value placed on education with two informants holding master's degrees in other fields; 10 holding bachelor's degrees; two with non-nursing associate degrees; and five with 1 to 2-plus years of collegiate coursework prior to attending their current nursing program. Eleven of the informants were working in health care including seven certified nursing assistants and one licensed practical nurse. All informants acknowledged a desire to progress forward with more nursing education after obtaining their associate degree. One informant stated:

> And I also look forward on the same note . . . educators are very special individuals because they are facilitating others to go and help. So I am not opposed to, God willing, when I get past my associate degree, BSN, looking into masters so that I could possibly at some point in time, in my life become an educator.

Informants described a variety of educational experiences, life events, and some noncaring behaviors they perceived as barriers prior to or during their nursing program. One informant described growing up in an inner-city neighborhood with gangs, drugs, graffiti, and intermittent attendance at school. He stated that he was never sure when he walked out his front door whether he would be shot or mugged. He had been in a gang and had also tried drugs while growing up. The informant believed that he learned to read in elementary school somewhat but his reading skills did not extend beyond that level. He stated that when he did go to class, textbooks for the class often were not available. His parents were divorced and he was the oldest of three children. He related that he did not attend his high school graduation because he did not think he had graduated but only found out when he was notified at the end of that summer to pick up his high school diploma.

This same informant was able to relate his frustration at what he called "being duped" about how other people live when he realized that not everyone lived like his family in his neighborhood. He met a girl in a bar one night and was invited back to her home outside of the city. He was amazed that these homes were not attached to each other and had grass around them. He realized at that point that this was what he wanted and enrolled in the community college. When he started classes at the community college, he then realized that he was unable to read and write and do math. He related that he was so determined to have one of those houses that he sat up at night and taught himself how to read, write, and do math. He was successful in his courses at the community college and graduated with an associate degree. He was then able to go to a 4-year college and get a bachelor's degree. Even with his bachelor's degree, he was still seeking a career that had meaning for him and found nursing was his calling. He was very clear that the quality of his secondary [high school] education was a significant barrier to his adult education.

Barriers to educational care for the informants in this study varied greatly, from difficult secondary educational experiences to the problems of being a nursing student while working and meeting family obligations. Informants continually discussed the importance of support and care from family and faculty along with the self-determination to successfully complete the program.

Care Pattern 1c: A Pattern of Religion and Spiritual Beliefs as an Essential Part of Life

Informants articulated the significance of their religious beliefs. For many, religion was viewed as an essential component for meaningfulness with their experiences and a way to achieve or maintain focus while in their educational program. While not all informants professed following an organized religion, their spiritual beliefs were deeply felt and important elements in their lives. For one key informant, religion was not a formal process; she stated:

> Not of the world, you know, but of my personal belief, my personal feelings of what I believe . . . I can feel it, with my heart. I just know that there is a spiritual being we call God in the United States in America. But all across the world, God is called something else. I only use that terminology, God, because everybody else uses that word. I don't know if it's God, Allah, or Buddha. I don't know. I just say that He knows because He lives. He or She or whatever. . . . I just know it's there. Whatever it is . . . that we don't have it by chance.

It was clear during the discussions that the informants believed *faith* and *beliefs* were important to them as individuals and as nurses. One informant indicated that while she identified with the Catholic religion and observed significant holidays such as Easter, Christmas, Lent, and Advent, and while she was strict at home, she did not go to church regularly every Sunday. She did feel that her religion helped her in nursing by giving her a moral compass to use when working with people, stating, ". . .I believe that most nurses do, and should have some kind of religious grounding."

Another informant stated that religion ". . .means everything. It's my life. Like if I was taking my last breath, I would say 'God, I don't know what to do. Is this the right thing?'. . . I need Him every day." She also believed that her religious beliefs helped her succeed in school: "Uh-hum. If I don't pray then I am afraid that I will be . . . a failure. God like would punish. Yeah, Lord, please, I can pray now."

Universal Theme 2: For African American students professional and generic health and illness beliefs are holistic concepts incorporated into all aspects of life including pursuing a professional nursing education.

This theme was discovered from the African American nursing students' cultural care expressions, patterns, lifeways, and practices while in their nursing program. The patterns of care that supported this theme were: *A pattern of health and illness beliefs as holistic concepts incorporating physical, spiritual, emotional, and mental aspects of life*; and *a pattern of technology as important to daily life, health, and health care.*

Care Pattern 2a: A Pattern of Health and Illness Beliefs as Holistic Concepts Incorporating Physical, Spiritual, Emotional, and Mental Aspects of Life

This pattern was developed from informants' responses related to the categories of *cultural beliefs and practices, health-related beliefs and illness-related beliefs,* and *environmental context and concerns.* Most informants described health and illness as including physical, spiritual, emotional, and mental components. Informants described *illness* as being physical ailments such as diabetes, cancer, heart disease and high blood pressure as well as emotional or psychological conditions such as lack of spirituality, mental distress, and lack of emotional tranquility. Many indicated that they put their faith and trust in God and prayed to stay healthy.

When discussing treatment of illness, some informants acknowledged having incorporated folk care remedies into their lives, whereas others chose to "ignore," to some extent, what they were taught by their parents, grandparents, friends, and relatives. Acknowledging that they generally did not practice the cultural folk care remedies taught them, most agreed that when sick they would treat themselves before they call a physician or nurse practitioner. One informant stated:

> It's hard because definitely what you learn in nursing school for African American[s] is [that they are] mainly [at] high risk for cardiovascular disease. All these diseases are exactly what's in my family. So me being in nursing school is just like . . . I know exactly why it's like that. Because you eat unhealthy food and you don't exercise. I see what's going on. But then when you go to nursing school, I'm like . . . okay, I know why this happened. So I mean I try, for the most part, since I've started nursing school, I've tried to have a lifestyle change as far as fruits and vegetables.

Health-related beliefs and practices were more easily articulated by informants born and raised outside of the United States. They described culture-specific or family-specific folk medicine practices using herbs, leaves, fruits, and spices and other substances administered as teas, soups, inhalations, or topical applications. Other folk remedies for health restoration, such as garlic, vinegar, and hot coffee, were described by informants born in the United States. Although folk remedies were passed on from their parents (usually mothers or grandmothers), most informants did not use these remedies all the time. Some informants had only vague recollections about what remedies they had been told would help to restore health. One informant shared his belief that the folk medicine and herbs that his father took in Kenya worked well to resolve sinus infections, stating, ". . .A lot of traditional medicine . . . it's a tradition that's carried down through the generations, so this medicine is handed down from father to the son, what works. Different kinds of medicines. And different herbs." Another informant described different folk remedies that she had been was taught would improve health, sharing that when her parents visited from Nigeria they brought her some of the herbs her mother used—one herb in particular, ". . .what we have like Hebba leaf. We have some, what you call grass roots. I don't know. There are special ones that they use. And in our culture that is what we do." Yet another informant grew up in Haiti and was taught by her mother to use oil of palm to treat a cold. She used this remedy before she went to a physician and had been doing so since she was very young. She did not really believe that special foods improved health other than simply eating healthy with fruits and vegetables. Still another informant from Granada stated:

> Well, I know that, for instance, if you have a cold, we like in the Islands we always have oranges . . . we peel the orange, we like dry the skin. You know, leave it out to dry in the sun and if you have a cold, you boil theorange peel, whatever, and drink that. That's the cold remedy right there.

She also described a folk remedy her mother used for asthma when she was growing up:

> I still remember how to make homemade concoctions. She [her mother] gave my niece, who is now 21, who still is a chronic asthmatic . . . when she was a baby, she would give her hot coffee, hot black coffee when she'd see her changing. . . . my youngest one is an asthmatic now. And from remembering how my mom used to say, . . . "She looks dusky," I've learned how to watch my son's skin changes and I know when this boy is getting ready to go into a full-blown asthma attack.

This same informant recalled her mother using other home remedies:

> She'd cook . . . had to get an onion and a lemon and a sugar and she had a glass full. She covered the onion and the lemon up. And overnight all

of that juice would mix . . . then she'd pour in the sugar and mix it up. And we had to drink it. And the mutton is . . . what is that stuff they rub on you? VapoRub. It did. That's what she would use to mix with the fat and whatever and it was VapoRub. It made our noses run, smelled like God knows what, but it worked. It worked. It worked.

Several other informants recalled similar remedies used by their mothers or grandmothers which involved the use of garlic or vinegar. One informant who was born in Nigeria talked about some of the folk medicine used by her family, ". . .Like, for example, my grandmother she has one for vomiting a lot, and she would use objects such as ashes and put them in the water. And you would just drink it and the vomiting stopped. Yes, it's not charcoal; it is white ashes."

The majority of the informants expressed a clear understanding of the meanings of professional care, generic care, health, illness, and wellbeing, and their related cultural beliefs. Most viewed health and wellbeing as physical, emotional, and spiritual harmony; others described health in specific terms. One informant viewed health as the ". . .absence of illness. Oh, health, just. . . I want to say feeling good about yourself like . . . like being able to like function every day physically, mentally, spiritually." Another informant described health and wellbeing as follows:

They're a little bit different. I guess health would be . . . I guess it would kind of be like your nutritional status. I don't know if you'd be healthy, but you may have a degree of health. I think health is like the nutritional . . . like if you were to do a lab test . . . that would measure the health. A person's wellbeing is more subjective, it's more like their whole, you know, like their whole self. You know, spiritual, and emotional . . . that would kind of be like their wellbeing, you know.

Most informants defined and described illness in terms of nonphysical holistic elements such as lack of spirituality, lack of peace, lack of emotional tranquility, and mental distress along with the physical symptoms. One informant stated, ". . .Loneliness, lacking peace is illness. And a big piece is to be at peace with yourself. To have people around you that know you and understand you and that you understand and can talk to you. Illness, of course, physical illness is breakdown of the immune system." Another informant believed that ". . .illness means there. . . whether it's physically or mentally, something's wrong—something out of the norm, out of whack. Some of the things can be remedied and others can't."

Other descriptors of illness by informants included illness as stress, death, and sadness; having some deficiency or a disease process such as diabetes or mental disease; suffering as with cancer; or being handicapped (wheelchair) or totally physically dependent on the care of others. Most informants held values and beliefs about health and illness that were holistic. Their descriptions of their health and illness beliefs and practices provided an in-depth understanding of how they viewed, valued, and responded to episodes of illness in their lives.

Informants overwhelmingly believed that general health is a harmony between the physical, emotional, and spiritual aspects of life. Most believed that physical health meant that one does not have a disease. A few others believed that a person can have a chronic disease and still be healthy as long as the disease was properly treated. *Proper treatment* was identified as Western medicine. To maintain health or stay healthy, informants expressed the importance of exercise and a healthy diet that included fruits, vegetables, and protein foods such as chicken, fish, and beef. Several informants believed cultural foods to be healthier. Cultural foods and beliefs about home remedies and health were very clear to one informant, who stated, ". . .Well, where I'm from [Granada], we cook every day. Everything is healthy. Nothing is frozen, not even our chicken. Everything is from the garden and we don't eat any canned food or stuff."

Care Pattern 2b: A Pattern of Use of Technology as Important to Daily Life, Health, and Health Care

This pattern was discovered from the responses to researcher questions about the social structure factors of *technology* and *technology factors* in daily life and health care. Informants generally believed that technology was a good and necessary tool overall. All informants stated they used technology every day, describing their use of computers, microwave ovens, cellular phones, personal digital assistants, digital video recorders and players, and many other forms of technology, but not all were comfortable with all forms of technology. One general informant described her reaction to her first online course experience: ". . .I haven't got comfortable with that yet. Yes, yes. I'm learning it. I will jump on there, but in my mind I'm quivering."

With regard to health, illness, and health care, the informants generally agreed that technology was also a beneficial and necessary tool in the treatment of illness. Their experiences using technology for clinical rotations included computers for electronic documentation and in medication administration. They noted the ability of healthcare providers and clinicians to quickly access medical, laboratory, and X-ray information as excellent for use in practice. They believed technology can decrease medical errors, help healthcare providers do a better job treating patients, and provide clarity and legibility when documentation is electronic. A few of the informants expressed caution that, if not used properly, technology could "depersonalize" patient care. One general informant discussed technology in health care by stating:

> Technology will play a huge part in health care in the near future. And a lot of these things have already started to show up in nursing homes and hospitals and things like that. And I think it's going to definitely provide better care. It will allow nurses to provide better care and doctors as well.

Another informant described illness treatment and beliefs in her village in Kenya:

> Basically, initially, like the days of my mom, they used to go to like...the elder people who are herbalists, they know all the types of plants in the forest and what they can do. Now because of the technology from the West, it is different back there.

Universal Theme 3: Care expressed through social interactions, financial support, resources, and scheduling is viewed as significant to beneficial educational outcomes for African American students.

The patterns of care that supported this theme were: *A pattern of expected social interactions by family, friends, religion, and school resulting in lack of self-care; a pattern of nonuse of college resources in place for students;* and *a pattern of financial resources as important for education.*

Care Pattern 3a: A Pattern of Expected Social Interactions by Family, Friends, Religion, and School Resulting in Lack of Self-Care

This pattern was derived from informants' responses about the cultural context of their worldviews, lifeways, and cultural beliefs. Informants described daily schedules that were so full that they were unable to fit in a "social life" which was perceived as a major conflict with their general lifeways. The majority of informants often expressed during the interviews that they "...don't have a life." One informant shared the following about her social life and her responsibility as a single parent:

> I have a network of friends that . . . I'm the kind of person where I'll meet some people that I know that will be my friend. Like, if I'm your friend, you'll also be my friend in return. So by befriending these kinds of people, like...whenever I need help, they're always there for me. And

> I have this one particular friend Tasha. Anytime she needs anything, I'm there for her. So I feel like . . . I feel like I just have to do things for them so . . . It's hard to explain. . . . And in return, if I need her to watch my son, she'll watch him for me. . . . as for a social life, I don't have one.

Another informant described the frequency of her family interactions:

> I think my grandmother would say 'not enough.' She has to call me. . . she called me two weeks ago and said. . . .'what are you doing? I haven't seen you in a long time.' And a long time for her would be three weeks. Just because I've been really busy and I just have problems doing other things. And then sometimes my godmother would say. . .you haven't been here in two weeks. And I say. . .my godfather will actually say it after three days. . .he hasn't seen me in three days. . .he's like. . . 'where have you been?' He told me to get out the other day, and then he wanted me to come back.

All informants described significant changes in their lives since starting the nursing program, in that their daily schedules and lifeways had been drastically altered by attending school. They almost unanimously indicated that social life was nonexistent. A few admitted that they were told that they would have a very intense 2 years in the program, but both general and key informants acknowledged they had not believed the program would be as intense as it was found to be. One shared how he felt:

> Nursing school is very, very difficult. And of course it's not like going to college. . .It's different. I went to college. . . .basically just a honeymoon. College was easy. Psychology was easy. I have a Master's degree in psychology....I mean every other degree in college to me, was easy; nursing school is completely different. I work well under pressure. But I came into nursing school and boy it was challenging.

Another informant agreed ". . .I have never spent as much time with my master's program as I have in the nursing program. I just did it and I graduated with a 3.8 in my master's program. It's just amazing . . .yes, nursing is difficult. People who aren't in it don't realize it."

Family was viewed as a life priority but balancing family obligations and school, made social time with family and friends severely limited. Informants were very clear that family responsibilities were a significant part of their lifeways and worldview. One informant talked about financing nursing school; he already had a 4-year degree in accounting and was working full-time as a certified nursing assistant while going to school for his third or fourth career. Another informant described how he financed school and how he handled his job and school, "You know, I have a home equity loan.... it's different when you live at home with your parents than when you have like a mortgage, car payments, credit card bills.... You have to pay your bills too, so you work full-time."

Informants repeatedly indicated that they believed one could not separate self from family and that family was important for support and positive outcomes. However, cultural beliefs and practices, including family responsibilities, required a time commitment that impacted their daily schedules and encroached on time for study. Prior to starting nursing school, informants had routine visits on an almost daily basis with certain family and friends; now, however, visits were shorter and much less frequent. Informants indicated that family also expressed that they had insufficient socialization with them. One general informant shared that her grandmother, godparents, and godsisters had expressed to her that she was not "around enough" now that she was in school.

Some informants did not have any immediate family living in the nearby vicinity, but extended family had always been included in their social interactions. Informants emphasized that support and care from family, including socialization, were essential to the meaningfulness of their educational experiences and how important family social interactions were to their daily lifeways and to maintain kinship. One informant shared, "We get together, we eat, we laugh, we tease. I have five brothers and two sisters." Another shared, "I am from the river country in Africa. River state is actually an Africa culture. You just believe that [about] family situations and you know family is very, very important. You cannot separate yourself from family. We believe in that strongly." Still another informant described that he grew up in Kenya where family and kinship were very important, ". . .So it's definitely a very caring community. You know, when one person is in need, you gather around them and they provide that. . . . They don't have to be [blood] relatives."

In regard to care of self, nearly all informants responded that they had not cared well for themselves since starting school. Some informants acknowledged trying to take an hour now and then, but generally admitted having not taken good care of themselves after starting their nursing program. Informants identified the importance of caring for self but acknowledged that their own self caring actions were very limited while attending school because of the demands and time constraints attached to work, school, and family responsibilities. One key informant described how she cared for herself:

> Awfully. One of my clinical instructors also a coworker she just reamed me forever and ever. I don't. . .take care of myself and I

always take care of other people, like I don't do what I say. I had not been for two years to my doctor. I was in the bed at 2 a.m. and up at 5a.m. My doctor, because I have high blood pressure said. . . 'He's like. . .are you crazy? You need to find another way because you are stressing yourself out.' So, no, I don't take care of myself. I was so busy taking care of everything else and everybody else, you know.

Care Pattern 3b: A Pattern of Nonuse of College Resources in Place for Students

This pattern was developed from responses by informants regarding *resources, economic factors,* and *environmental context and concerns.* Informants identified the importance of having resources for positive educational outcomes and were able to describe college resources available to students, even though they admitted not using them unless mandated by their own curriculum. Other resources, such as learning resource centers, test-taking tutorials or software packages, tutoring, college-sponsored minority student-support organizations, and academic support services were not used. Informants indicated that they would be comfortable using the resources but their schedules did not permit time to take advantage of them. Resources informants did utilize were personally developed such as peers, self-selected study groups or a study buddy, and occasionally, if necessary, a course instructor or faculty member. One general informant said, ". . .They have tutoring, but I can never get an appointment at the time I can go . . . I usually reach out to peers and co-workers. One of those people who pretty much understand the material, I'll ask them a question."

Most informants identified not using any of the resources provided by the college for them specifically as minority students or even as generic college students except for what was mandated within the curriculum of their program. One informant acknowledged, ". . . I know we do have a few resource programs such as at the learning center. I've never used any of them, but I know they're there" but also admitted that using resources was a necessity for positive outcomes in school. Another student informant stated:

> I would probably ask a peer first. I'm not. . .not too big on e-mailing instructors because I feel like. . . I don't like to be even asking for help. I usually never ask for help, but it would have to be a big serious issue for me to ask the instructor. No. I have never used any of the resource programs here at the college.

Informants clearly believed that resources to help them be successful in their education were very important, yet they still did not use any of the nonmandatory college-provided resources for their academic programs.

One other informant stated, "...boy those are so nice, I just wish I had the time. But that would be the only time I ever thought about the resources, I never got . . . just no time." Another shared that she knew the college had resources for students, but stated, ". . .I haven't used any. They do have the learning center over there which is very helpful. But I get things better on my own. . . .And if I don't understand, I'll read it again and ask somebody to explain it."

Care Pattern 3c: A Pattern of Financial Resources as Important for Education

This pattern was identified from the responses of the informants to researcher questions regarding the cultural and social structure dimensions of *economic care factors* and *environmental context*. Informants described their difficulty in meeting financial responsibilities while working long hours and not caring for themselves. All informants described in some way how the economics of going to school while keeping up a home and job negatively affected their self-caring actions.

One informant acknowledged that the school helped her to obtain a position as an extern in a hospital in addition to providing financial aid and student loans that enabled her to continue taking classes. Another informant also indicated that she had both grants and loans. She was very clear on how her school schedule affected her work schedule:

> I have grants and loans. It's kind of hard to maintain a schedule [at work] when they are constantly changing the curriculum and the schedule or whatever. So I had to like cut back hours and on the second part of the semester I had to cut back another day and hopefully I can add on [another day]— you know, somewhere else pick up time.

A 41-year-old male nursing student stated, ". . .I have loans and I had a nursing grant the first year because the school provided it to me. I worked full-time and at the end of the [first] year, my application for the grant was denied. I didn't qualify." He discussed that his financial obligation to his family required that he work full-time while in school but this made financing school more difficult because it made him ineligible to continue to receive the grant money for school and he had to take out a loan for his second year of school. Yet another informant said that she took out student loans because there was no funding that she was aware of from her nursing program.

Financing school was clearly a significant burden for the informants. While financial aid in the form of grants and scholarships might be available for many of them, the majority of the informants did not pursue or investigate how to obtain this type of funding. Those who did follow up on the information for scholarships and grants found the complexity of the application and the time required to complete the application prohibitive.

Financial responsibilities and locating or worrying about sources of funding for school were seen as significant factors affecting the students' daily lives. More than half of the informants in the study worked 40 hours per week while attending nursing school in order to meet their family financial obligations. Discussions regarding finances revealed that even when given information about grants and scholarships, many of the informants did not follow through or complete necessary forms to due personal time constraints. Both key and general informants repeatedly discussed how their schedules did not allow enough time for meeting all their obligations and responsibilities.

Barriers to educational care for the informants in this study varied greatly, from difficult secondary educational experiences to the problems of being a nursing student while working and meeting family obligations. Informants continually discussed the importance of support and care from family and faculty in addition to their own self-determination to successfully complete the program.

In summary, African American students in predominantly Euro American associate degree nursing programs identified and described in rich detail how important care by family, friends, and faculty was in their lives for meaningful, positive, and beneficial educational outcomes. They provided insights into the social and cultural expectations held by their families and by themselves as well as their cultural health and illness beliefs as African American students while attending a nursing program. They described their daily lifeways, worldviews, expectations, and experiences within academia from secondary education through postsecondary nursing education. Together, three themes were discovered that provided eye-opening insight into the daily lives, expectations, experiences, values, and beliefs of African American nursing students attending predominantly Euro American associate degree nursing programs.

DISCOVERIES FOR CULTURE-SPECIFIC CARE

Supported by Leininger's Theory of Culture Care Diversity and Universality, Leininger's three major nursing care modes of decision and action were used to discuss the study findings to help nurse educators provide culturally congruent education. These three nursing care modes of decision and action assisted the researcher in focusing on appropriate, congruent, satisfying, safe, and beneficial measures for the population being studied

(Leininger, 2002b, p. 78). These modes are cultural care preservation and/or maintenance; cultural care accommodation and/or negotiation; and cultural care repatterning or restructuring (Leininger, 2002b, p. 78).

Culture Care Preservation and/or Maintenance

According to Leininger (2002b), culture care preservation and/or maintenance is those "...assistive, supportive, facilitative, or enabling professional actions and decisions that help people of a particular culture to retain and/or maintain meaningful care values and lifeways for their wellbeing, to recover from illness, or to deal with handicaps or dying" (p. 84).

In order to preserve or maintain meaningful care values and lifeways for African American students during their nursing education, nurse educators need to first have a sincere desire to provide culturally congruent education to all nursing students. In order to accomplish this, nurse educators need to embrace a method or process early in the students' first academic semester to identify cultural values, meanings, beliefs, and practices. A significant finding with this study was the *importance and expectation of care* (viewed as *support and involvement by family, friends, and faculty*) in maintaining *meaningful educational experiences*. One of the expectations of study informants was *facilitation* of their learning by their nursing faculty. In many associate degree programs, the didactic component of the nursing curriculum is taught to small groups or sections of students. This practice lends itself to faculty being able to *meet with students on a one-to-one basis* and *learn who they are as individuals* so a personalized facilitation of student learning can be initiated. According to Cerbin (2000):

> I am suggesting that what is important is not just what students know, but how they think with what they know. A teacher who is attuned to students' thinking will make different decisions about what to tell students and how to support the development of their understanding, than a teacher who simply lectures according to pre-planned and inalterable syllabus. (p. 17)

It is also worthwhile and beneficial for the nurse educator to *identify the religious factors, beliefs, and practices that maintain healthy interactions* for African American students within the environmental context of the nursing program. The influence of religious beliefs on meaningful educational activities was a finding in this study that supported the existing literature regarding the importance of religion in the lives of many African Americans. Many informants indicated during their interviews that they incorporated prayer and spiritual thoughts into their educational actions and practices. Nurse educators should be *sensitive to and aware* of this practice in both the class-room and the clinical settings. In order to preserve and maintain meaningful culture care educational experiences for African American students, nurse educators need to know what those practices, experiences, and expectations are so as to *encourage* or facilitate these activities.

Many informants discussed difficulty in meeting expected family obligations as well as their curricular requirements. Offering open house or informational orientation sessions for family and friends prior to or early in the nursing program would provide them with a better understanding of the requirements and demands being placed upon the student. These events would thereby preserve the support and understanding from family and friends that students need and desire in order to have meaningful and beneficial educational experiences.

Culture Care Accommodation and/or Negotiation

The assistive, facilitative, enabling actions that help students to adapt or negotiate the educational environment of an associate degree program toward meaningful, beneficial, and culturally congruent educational outcomes requires the nurse educator to be open to recognizing that cultural diversity exists and to modifying educational practices to meet students' unique characteristics and cultural backgrounds. The first step to accommodation and/or negotiation in providing culturally congruent education to a diverse population of nursing students is a sincere willingness by the nurse educator to view the academic environment from a different perspective both in the classroom and in the clinical environment. Culturally meaningful educational experiences begin with the nurse educator's desire to provide culturally congruent education (deRuyter, 2008). In order to provide culturally congruent education to students, nurse educators need to understand their own cultural beliefs, values, and practices before they can identify and understand those of their students. The significance of care, understanding, and patience by faculty was an important finding in this study. Informants expressed their expectations of care by faculty as needed for positive, meaningful educational experiences.

In order to accommodate and/or negotiate educational care for African American students, faculty must be sensitive to the various factors relating to family, jobs, religious beliefs, and cultural expectations of students in the nursing program. Students' expectations about the nursing program are that faculty will support them, are interested in teaching them as individuals, and will facilitate their learning. Nurse educators should not make the assumption that all cohorts of students should be treated the same. This study identified diverse backgrounds and educational experiences among African American nursing students along with their universal and diverse views, beliefs, and values. An accommodation to learning styles and scheduling issues requires an understanding of the individual student's learning needs and expectations. Instructional methods that can be used to meet the needs of a diverse class of students also need to be identified.

Culture Care Repatterning and/or Restructuring

Culture care repatterning and restructuring for new, different, and beneficial educational outcomes for African American students will require nurse educators and students to better understand one another. The nurse educator must have a sincere desire to better understand students before any change or intervention can take place. Many nurse educators are very comfortable with their specific teaching strategies. They teach the content the same way each year by updating only their subject matter, not their teaching strategies. Nurse educators need to reflect on their own strategies as well as their own cultural views, beliefs, and values in order to better understand how their teaching strategies and other actions affect student actions, interactions, and outcomes.

Before repatterning and restructuring can occur, a rapport between students and faculty members must be established within a mutually trusting relationship. Informants indicated their reluctance to bring their discomfort to the attention of their nursing professor during class whenever teaching methods were not culturally congruent or comfortable. The vulnerability of students fearing reprisal from faculty members under such circumstances was clearly identified in the study data. One way to minimize or overcome student reluctance to seek assistance is for students and faculty to work toward knowing one another. As described earlier, one-on-one meetings between faculty and students are a new way to develop understanding between individuals and enable them to share their cultural values and beliefs. Once faculty and student become somewhat familiar with one another, the exchanging of ideas, values, and beliefs can begin to occur; faculty and student can then review responsibilities, expectations, and requirements and assess any repatterning or restructuring of lifeways, daily schedules, or practices that would support a more meaningful educational experience.

NURSING IMPLICATIONS

Nursing care has moved toward evidence-based practice and best practices in all areas of the profession; they are equally important in the culture care education of nursing students. This study sought to understand the culture care educational experiences of African American students in predominantly Euro American associate degree nursing programs in order to better understand ways to support or facilitate decisions that would enable culture care preservation and/or maintenance; accommodation and/or negotiation; or repatterning and/or restructuring of administrative or teaching methods for optimally beneficial educational outcomes. The study found that nurse educators not only need to teach students how to provide culturally congruent care and practice in a culturally aware and sensitive environment, but that faculty themselves must also teach the art and science of nursing using these approaches. Review of the literature revealed that health care provided by clinicians from the same cultural, ethnic, and racial background as patients creates a culturally congruent context which leads to a more satisfying healthcare experience that results in better healthcare outcomes. Yet, the nursing profession has less than half the percentage of minority nurses practicing within its ranks than are represented in the general population (USDHHS, 2004). This disparity needs to be resolved. Ways to retain minority students in nursing programs, decrease attrition rates, and recruit minority students into programs need to become a priority for the nursing education profession as a whole. Studies such as this one, which provide a better understanding of the cultural beliefs, values, and lifeways of minority students, are a strong start.

Implications for Nursing Theory

This study confirmed the four assumptions of the culture care theory used for the study on which this chapter is based:

- Culturally-based care is the broadest holistic way to know, explain, interpret, and predict beneficial and desirable nursing education care practices for African American associate degree nursing students in predominantly Euro American programs.
- Culture care concepts, meanings, expressions, patterns, processes, and structural forms of care for African American associate degree nursing students vary transculturally with diversities and some universalities.
- Cultural care beliefs, values, and practices of African American associate degree nursing students in predominantly Euro American programs are influenced by the worldview, religious, political, educational, technical, and ethno historical dimensions of their culture.

- The ethnonursing qualitative research method provides a means to accurately discover and interpret emic and etic embedded complex and diverse cultural data.

The environmental and cultural context of predominantly Euro American associate degree nursing programs for African American nursing students provided rich data regarding cultural experiences, beliefs, values, practices, and cultural perspectives. All informants in this study indicated they were very comfortable in their colleges and the environmental context of the associate degree program did not pose a conflict. In addition, this study supported the findings of the few studies about associate degree programs that had been conducted with African American students regarding the identification of job conflicts, family responsibilities, and difficulties with time and scheduling (Butters, 2003; Hunt, 1992; Sims, 1996).

The first assumption—that culturally-based care is a holistic way to know, explain, interpret and predict beneficial and desirable nursing education care practices—was supported by the study data. The assumption that culture care concepts, meanings, expressions, patterns, processes, and structural forms of care for African American associate degree nursing students varied transculturally with diversities and some universalities, was also supported as reflected in the universal themes and supporting care patterns described. The additional findings of this study regarding informants' lack of utilization of college resources and their disregard of information about obtaining grants and scholarships was unexpected. These are significant findings for legislators, administrators, deans, and directors of nursing programs that could impact future plans for funding of nursing education and resources. The assumption that the ethnonursing qualitative research method provides an accurate means to discover and interpret the emic and etic embedded complex and diverse cultural data of the study was supported and further contributed to the body of transcultural nursing knowledge.

Implications for Nursing Education and Practice

Nurse educators can begin to identify culturally congruent educational practices in the classroom and clinical settings that would enhance and support a more diverse student population. New and unusual teaching strategies can be identified, developed, and implemented that would accommodate the educational learning styles of a more diverse student nurse population. The ethnonursing qualitative research method provided an accurate means to discover and interpret the emic and etic embedded complex and diverse cultural data of the study, thus contributing to the body of transcultural knowledge. The emerging themes of overwhelming daily schedules for many students and the lack of utilization of college resources provides nurse educators with data that can assist in future decisions by college and schools of nursing regarding student scholarship and grant funding and the development of future college resources.

Implications for Nursing Research

This study's findings affirm the need for additional research in similar contexts with other minority populations of nursing students in predominantly Euro American associate degree nursing programs. The findings in this study involved one specific population of students; it is important that additional studies be conducted to discover and identify the culture care educational experiences of other minority populations of nursing students. The integration of evidence-based nursing and educational best practices into nursing programs requires that nurse educators have evidence for the development of culturally congruent nursing curricula and teaching contexts.

This research study provides the basis for future transcultural ethnonursing studies in nursing education to be conducted in other parts of the United States. Recommendations for future research studies include:

- Conduct studies with other minority populations, such as Hispanic Americans, Native Americans, Asian Americans, and Pacific Islanders.
- Perform comparison and contrast studies of culture care education and experiences with predominantly Euro Americans and minority populations.
- Investigate ways to repattern/restructure nursing program curricula so as to provide culturally congruent educational access to college resources.
- Explore processes that would assist minority nursing students to identify, complete, and successfully obtain financial aid for their education.

Increasing the number of nurse educators from all cultural backgrounds is essential to the future of the nursing profession. In order to increase the number of culturally diverse nursing faculty, more nurses from all minorities need to enroll in and graduate from nursing programs. Research studies with diverse populations of nursing students will provide information for nurse educators to use for review and updating of nursing curricula. Teaching from curricula that are culturally congruent and integrate cultural diversity is key to help lessen the disparate number of minority nurses in the profession.

CONCLUSION

Nurse educators need to learn about and understand the cultural views, beliefs, values, and expressions of their diverse minority students in order to better understand how their teaching strategies and actions affect student actions, interactions, and outcomes. Before repatterning and restructuring can occur, a rapport between individual students and faculty members must be established that leads to trusting and mutually beneficial relationships. Informants in this study indicated their reluctance to mention their discomfort in class when teaching methods were not culturally congruent and comfortable to the attention of their nursing professors. The vulnerability of students fearing reprisal from faculty members when educational teaching methods caused discomfort was a clear finding in the study data.

One way to diminish students' reluctance in broaching this topic is for students and faculty to begin to know one another better. One-on-one meetings between faculty and student is an approach that can facilitate the mutual understanding of both individuals as well as their unique cultural values and beliefs. Once they become trusted friends, the faculty and student can begin an open exchange of ideas, values, and beliefs about their respective responsibilities, expectations, and requirements, and can then work together toward any accommodation or repatterning of lifeways, daily schedules, or practices that would support a beneficial and meaningful educational experience for the student. Administrative discussions regarding repatterning and restructuring of decisions and actions, nursing program curricula, or teaching methods are also needed based on an internal faculty as well as general student body assessment and review of the combined data findings.

Schedules, responsibilities, and obligations of students make attending traditionally-delivered nursing programs difficult for a number of students. By identifying the personal and professional needs of nursing students, program administrators can begin to identify and develop creative methods of providing nursing education in associate degree nursing programs. Use of technology in the form of online courses, video conferencing, expanded simulation experiences, and alternate scheduling of didactic face-to-face classes—in addition to new and creative teaching methods not yet identified—all need to be considered.

APPENDIX 13-A: DERUYTER'S MODEL OF CULTURE CARE EDUCATION

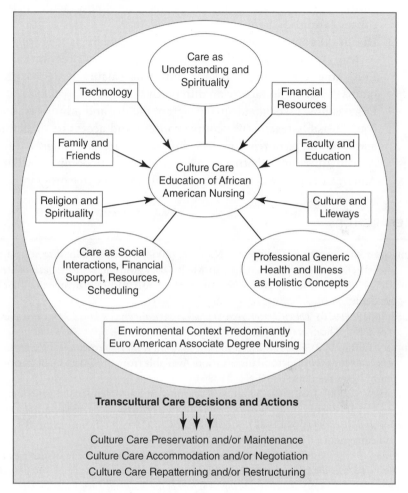

Appendix 13-A deRuyter's Model of Culture Care Education
Copyright © L. deRuyter (2003). Adapted from Leininger, M. M. (1991). *Culture care diversity and universality: A theory of nursing.* New York, NY: National League for Nursing.

DISCUSSION QUESTIONS

1. Discuss how the financial and emotional stressors/family demands identified by African American study informants affected their academic success in the associate degree nursing program. What changes could be made by students and faculty to reduce these stressors?

2. Discuss the value of faculty *caring* for African American and other minority students in predominately Euro American associate degree and/or baccalaureate degree programs. How could faculty better convey caring and support to these students?

3. Discuss the implications of perceptions of faculty as *noncaring* by African American and other minority students in predominately Euro American associate degree and/or baccalaureate degree programs. What could faculty do differently?

4. Discuss how associate degree program faculty and administrators could feasibly restructure course content and access to academic and financial resources toward being more culturally congruent for African American and other minority students in predominantly Euro American associate degree and/or baccalaureate degree programs.

REFERENCES

American Association of Colleges of Nursing. (2004, March 8). Nursing shortage fact sheet. http://www.aacn.nche.edu/Media/Backgrounders/shortagefacts.htm

Buckley, J. (1980). Faculty commitment to retention and recruitment of Black students. *Nursing Outlook, 28,* 46–50.

Bardolph, R. (1970). *The civil rights record: Black Americans and the law, 1949–1970.* New York, NY: Thomas Crowell.

Butters, C. R. (2003). *Associate degree nursing students: A study of retention in the nursing education program.* Doctoral dissertation. Available from ProQuest Dissertations and Theses database (UMI No. 3108614).

Cerbin, W. (2000). Investigating student learning in a problem-based psychology course. In P. Hutchings (Ed.), *Opening lines: Approaches to the scholarship of teaching and learning* (pp. 11–22). Menlo Park, CA: Carnegie Foundation for the Advancement of Teaching.

Coffman, J. M., Rosenoff, E., & Grumbach, K. (2001). Racial/ethnic disparities in nursing. *Health Affairs, 20*(3), 263–272.

College Board. (1999). *Reaching the top: A report of the National Task Force on Minority High Achievement.* New York, NY: Author.

Curtin, P. (1969). *The Atlantic slave trade.* Milwaukee, WI: University of Wisconsin Press.

deRuyter, L. (2008). *Culture care education and experiences of African American students in predominantly Euro American associate degree nursing programs.* Doctoral dissertation. Available from ProQuest Dissertations and Theses database (UMI No. 3303013).

Elling, T. W., & Furr, S. R. (2002). African American student in a predominantly White university: Factors associated with retention. *College Student Journal, 36*(2), 188–202.

Fellman, D. (1976). *The Supreme Court and education.* New York, NY: Teachers College Press.

Flinn, J. B. (2000). *Multicultural education teaching strategies used by select nurse educators.* Doctoral dissertation. Available from ProQuest Dissertations and Theses database (UMI No. 9938271).

Freeman, K. (Ed.). (1998). *African American culture and heritage in higher education research and practice.* Westport, CT: Praeger.

Gardner, J. (2005). Barriers influencing the success of racial and ethnic minority students in nursing programs. *Journal of Transcultural Nursing, 16*(2), 155–162.

Glanville, C. (2003). People of African American heritage. In L. Purnell & B. J. Paulanka (Eds.), *Transcultural health care: A culturally competent approach* (2nd ed., pp. 40–53). Philadelphia, PA: F. A. Davis.

Haase, P. T. (1990). *The origins and rise of associate degree nursing education.* New York, NY: Duke University Press.

Heath, R. (1998). African American students and self-concept development: Integrating cultural influences into research and practice. In K. Freeman (Ed.), *African American culture and heritage in higher education research and practice* (pp. 33–42). Westport, CT: Praeger.

Hunt, L. B. (1992). *A study of student retention in associate degree nursing programs as perceived by their directors.* Doctoral dissertation. Available from ProQuest Dissertations and Theses database (UMI No. 9530568).

Hyche-Johnson, M. (1995). *Student and faculty perceptions and responses to barriers to African American nursing students' persistence to graduation.* Doctoral dissertation. Available from ProQuest Dissertations and Theses database (UMI No. 9617874).

Institute of Medicine. (2003). *Unequal treatment: Confronting racial and ethnic disparities in health care.* Washington, DC: National Academy Press.

Jackson, D. K. (2003). *Predictors of first semester attrition and their relation to retention of generic associate degree nursing students.* Doctoral dissertation. Available from ProQuest Dissertations and Theses database (UMI No. 3076647).

Jaynes, D., & Williams, R. (1989). *A common destiny: Blacks and American society,* Washington, DC: National Academy Press.

Jeffreys, M. R. (2004). *Nursing student retention: Understanding the process and making a difference.* New York, NY: Springer.

Kelley, R. D., & Lewis, E. (2000). *To make our world anew: A history of African Americans.* New York, NY: Oxford University Press.

Kersey-Matusiak, G. M. (1999). *Black students' perceptions of factors related to their academic and social success in a predominately White undergraduate nursing program at a private Catholic college.* Doctoral dissertation. Available from ProQuest Dissertations and Theses database (UMI No. 9938679).

Lassiter, S. M. (1999). Black is a color, not a culture: Implications for health care. In S. Tucker-Allen & E. Long (Eds.), *Recruitment and retention of minority nursing students* (pp. 43). Lisle, IL: Tucker.

Leininger, M. (1991). *The theory of culture care diversity and universality.* New York, NY: NLN Publications.

Leininger, M. M. (2002a). Transcultural nursing and globalization of health care: Importance, focus, and historical aspects. In M. M. Leininger & M. R. McFarland (Eds.), *Transcultural nursing: Concepts, theories, research, & practice* (3rd ed., pp. 3–43). New York, NY: McGraw-Hill.

Leininger, M. M. (2002b). Part I: The theory of culture care and the ethnonursing research method. In M. M. Leininger & M. R. McFarland (Eds.), *Transcultural nursing: Concepts, theories, research, & practice* (3rd ed., pp. 71–116). New York, NY: McGraw-Hill.

Leininger, M. M. (2006). Culture care diversity and universality theory and evolution of the ethnonursing method. In M. M. Leininger & M. R. McFarland (Eds.), *Culture care diversity and universality: A worldwide nursing theory* (2nd ed., pp. 1–41). Sudbury, MA: Jones and Bartlett.

Maynard, M. (1980). Can universities adapt to ethnic minority student needs? *Journal of College Student Personnel, 21*(5), 398–401.

McFarland, M. R. (1995). *Cultural care of Anglo and African American elderly residents within the environmental context of a long-term care institution.* Doctoral dissertation. Available from ProQuest Dissertations and Theses database (UMI No. 9530568).

Moy, E., & Bartman, B. A. (1995). Physician race and care of minority and medically indigent patients. *Journal of the American Medical Association, 273*(19), 1515–1520.

Mungazi, D. (1999). *The evolution of educational theory in the United States.* Westport, CT: Praeger.

Munhall, P. L. (Ed.). (2001). *Nursing research: A qualitative perspective* (3rd ed.). Sudbury, MA: Jones and Bartlett.

National Organization for Associate Degree Nursing (N-OADN). (1998). Position statement in support of associate degree as preparation for the entry-level registered nurse. Retrieved from http://www.noadn.org/positionstatement.htm

Palmer, C. A. (2000). The first passage: 1502–1619. In R. D. Kelley & E. Lewis (Eds.), *To make our world anew: A history of African Americans* (pp. 3–52). New York, NY: Oxford University Press. Retrieved from http://www.questia.com

Rudel, R. J. (2004). *Nontraditional students in associate degree nursing: Perceived factors influencing retention and empowerment.* Doctoral dissertation. Available from ProQuest Dissertations and Theses database (UMI No. 3162921).

Simmons, F. (2002). Developing a diverse nursing workforce. *Gastroenterology Nursing, 25*(6), 263–266.

Sims, G. P. (1996). *The experience of becoming a white nurse: A phenomenological study of Black women's experiences at predominantly schools of nursing.* Doctoral dissertation. Available from ProQuest Dissertations and Theses database (UMI No. 9623606).

Stewart, C. G. (2001). *Retention of African American students in associate degree nursing programs in South Carolina technical colleges.* Doctoral dissertation. Available from ProQuest Dissertations and Theses database (UMI No. 3036240).

Stikes, C. S. (1984). *Black students in higher education.* Carbondale, IL: Southern Illinois University Press.

Stinson, M. H., & Thurston, N. K. (2002). Racial matching among African American and Hispanic patients and physicians. *The Journal of Human Resources, 37*(2), 410–428.

Sullivan, L.W., Dole, R., & Rogers, P. (2004). *Missing persons: Minorities in the health professions.* Washington, DC: The Sullivan Commission.

Tucker-Allen, S. (1989). Losses incurred through African American student nurse attrition. *Nursing & Health Care, 10,* 395–397.

U.S. Department of Commerce, Census Bureau. (2010). State and county quick facts. Retrieved from http://quickfacts.census.gov/qfd/states/00000.html

U.S. Department of Health and Human Services, Bureau of Health Professions, National Advisory Council on Nurse Education and Practice. (2000). *A national agenda for nursing workforce racial/ethnic diversity.* Washington, DC: Author.

U.S. Department of Health and Human Services, Health Resources and Services Administration. (2004, March). The registered nurse population: National sample survey of registered nurses. Retrieved from http://bhpr.hrsa.gov

U.S. Department of Health and Human Services, Health Resources and Services Administration. (2013a, April). The U.S. nursing workforce: Trends in supply and education: Results in brief. Retrieved from http://bhpr.hrsa.gov/health-workforce/reports/nursingworkforce/nursingworkforcebrief.pdf

U.S. Department of Health and Human Services, Health Resources and Services Administration. (2013b, April 26). The U.S. nursing workforce: Trends in supply and education [PowerPoint presentation: Slide 11]. Retrieved from http://bhpr.hrsa.gov/healthworkforce/reports/nursingworkforce/nursingworkforcebrief.pdf

Wilson, R. (Ed.). (1994). *Minorities in higher education.* Phoenix, AZ: Oryx Press.

Wynetta, L. Y. (1999). Striving toward effective retention: The effect of race on mentoring African American students. *Peabody Journal of Education, 74*(2), 27–44.

Chapter 14

Culture Care Diversity and Universality: A Pathway to Culturally Congruent Practices in Transcultural Nursing Education, Research, and Practice in Australia

Akram Omeri

> *Care is the essence of nursing and a distinct, dominant, central and unifying focus.*
>
> (Leininger, 2002a, p. 192)[*]

DEDICATION

Madeleine M. Leininger

July 13, 1925–August 10, 2012

Madeleine Leininger's original and pioneering work created a pathway for furthering the development of the discipline of nursing by establishing transcultural nursing as a *foundation for an authentic area of practice* through which nurses may directly contribute to the wellbeing of the world's populations by the application of her culture care theory to nursing education, research, and practice.

---

*Leininger, M. M., *Journal of Transcultural Nursing 13*(3) pp. 189–192, Copyright 2002a by Sage Publications. Reprinted by Permission of SAGE Publications.

This chapter is a tribute on behalf of those nurses from Australia who believe in her theory and I hope will continue to use it and to the all the faculty and clinicians who continue to eagerly seek mentors to study cultures in a nation such as Australia, which is truly *a nation of immigrants*.

It is also my personal tribute to the founder of the discipline of transcultural nursing, who not only advocated transcultural caring but also cared and shared her passion with me and allowed me to use her legacy to enrich the lives of other nurses just as she did for me.

INTRODUCTION

Transcultural nursing has been interpreted in Australia as a mixture of ideas, terminologies, and policies. The principles and policies of multiculturalism as established by the Australian government attempt to take into account cultural, linguistic, and lifeways practices. These policies have had a major impact upon the provision of *culture care* in nursing practice, education, research, and leadership. However, terms such as *multicultural, crosscultural nursing, transcultural nursing*, and *international nursing* have been used interchangeably in nursing and healthcare practice, education, research, and journal publications to describe educational and experiential study and learning related to the discipline of transcultural nursing.

This chapter describes the application and use of Leininger's Theory of Culture Care Diversity and Universality in transcultural nursing education, research, and practice in Australia. Research studies that have used Leininger's culture care theory with her ethnonursing research method and have generated new transcultural nursing knowledge relevant to diverse practice settings in Australia are presented as exemplars. The author asserts that transcultural nursing is a formal, legitimate, and essential field of nursing study, research, practice, and administration in multicultural Australia and will explicate how Leininger's culture care theory provides for the growth of transcultural nursing knowledge in order to provide culturally appropriate nursing care for the benefit of the cultural and linguistically diverse populations in Australia.

PURPOSE AND GOAL

The purpose of this chapter is twofold. The first is to report on the findings from the use of *culture care theory* in the development of transcultural nursing education, research, and practice in Australia. The many pathways and possibilities for promoting transcultural nursing in education and research with implications for the delivery of nursing care to diverse populations in diverse care settings in Australia and in culturally meaningful, congruent, and safe ways are examined. The second purpose is to map and record Madeleine Leininger's contribution to Australian nursing.

The importance of culture-specific and culture-universal care toward the goal of improving nursing practice in multicultural Australia using Leininger's Theory of Culture Care Diversity and Universality is presented by:

- Sharing evidence-based knowledge relating to the state of transcultural nursing education, research, practice, and administration/ leadership in Australia
- Examining and reviewing multicultural trends and implications for cultural diversity, fairness, and equal opportunity in multicultural Australia through transcultural nursing research informing nursing and healthcare practices
- Reporting on existing survey findings regarding the status of existing transcultural nursing education programmes in Australian nursing schools
- Reporting the findings of research related to experiences of immigrant nurses in the workforce in Australia
- Examining findings/outcomes of research that have used Leininger's culture care theory and the application of these findings to nursing practice and in the provision of culturally congruent care in Australia

Australia's population in 2012 was determined to be approximately 22,785,055 people. The 2011 Australian census revealed that 26% of Australia's population was born overseas and an additional 20% had at least one overseas-born parent (Australian Bureau of Statistics [ABS], 2012). Persons born in the United Kingdom continue to be the largest group of overseas-born residents, accounting for 5.3% of Australia's total population in June 2011, followed by persons born in New Zealand (2.5%); China (1.8%); India (1.5%); Vietnam and Italy (0.9% each); and Aboriginal and Torres Strait Islander people (2.5%) (ABS, 2012). These figures highlight the cultural diversity that exists throughout Australia.

This evidence supports the author's view that Australia is a cosmopolitan heterogeneous nation with a distinct multicultural identity. The cultural pluralism of the nation is founded on the ethnic and cultural diversity of the people and the interplay between two exceedingly diverse groups: The *indigenous* people and the *immigrant* people. Nevertheless, it is an anomaly that Australia's institutions have remained monocultural in nature, reflecting the Anglo-Celtic origins of the population majority culture; the argument is made here that Australia's core institutions need to change to reflect the multicultural nature of the population (Omeri, 1996). With such a wide diversity of cultures, *culture care* is an essential construct for the delivery of nursing care using the application of Leininger's culture care theory (CCT) as the means to discover the knowledge essential for providing culturally congruent and meaningful care.

The nation's culturally diverse society has been increasingly recognized by the government through the implementation of advanced multicultural policies (Commonwealth of Australia, National Multicultural Advisory Council, 1999; Garrett & Lin, 1990). From a historical perspective, Australia's policies on immigration have evolved in response to social changes, the global human rights movement, and a commitment to the development of society as a whole (**Table 14-1**). After 1947, Australia's policies on immigration shifted between phases of assimilation, integration, multiculturalism, and mainstreaming, and have now moved forward to a status of inclusiveness and being united in diversity (Castle, 1999; Commonwealth of Australia, 1989; Davidson, 2000).

In health care, two distinct key policy principles have emerged from the numerous multicultural policies developed since 1980 to deal with Australia's diversity. The first is *access and equity* which in practice means equality of access to health services for all. The second is *inclusiveness* which when applied in practice means the provision of culturally appropriate services to meet the needs of people from culturally and linguistically diverse backgrounds.

However, in nursing and health care, diversity management has been limited to ethno-specific services and cultural assessments to identify recipient country of origin, religion, language spoken, and the possible need for interpreters (Maltby, 1999; Omeri, 1997). Omeri and Hamilton (1996) concluded that the links between policy and practice, and more specifically between nursing education and practice, are abysmal and merely rhetorical. The obvious diversity of Australia's population is not reflected in the provision of healthcare services, including nursing services. Improved transcultural education for students and a closer connection between education, practice, and policy for nursing services through the application of knowledge derived from the culture care theory has not come to fruition despite significant efforts since 1990 by members of the transcultural nursing (TCN) movement (Omeri, 2003b).

Table 14-1 Periods of immigration and policy development

Years	Policy	Features	Health policy implication
1945–70	Assimilation	Predominantly White Australian Anglo-Saxon policies	Absence of government assistance
1970–80	Integration	White Australia Policy relaxed and gradually abandoned	Relevant services provided
		Some cultural characteristics tolerated	Welfare needs of migrants being addressed
1980–89	Multiculturalism	Pluralistic approach to immigration	Provision of various health services
		Policies to limit discrimination on racial and ethnic grounds	Equality of access to culturally appropriate services
		Cultural and ethnic diversity becoming more accepted in Australian society	
		Cultural identity, social justice and economic efficiency were adopted	
1983	Mainstreaming	Redirecting service delivery from marginal to a central base	Promotion of culturally sensitive health services
		Concern of government institutions based on social equity and access; economic efficiency and cultural identity	Equality of access to health services by immigrants

(continues)

Table 14-1 Periods of immigration and policy development (*continued*)

Years	Policy	Features	Health policy implication
1999	Inclusiveness	Diversity	Promotion of culturally sensitive health services
		Multicultural policies built upon civic duty, cultural respect, social equity and productive diversity	Equality of access to health services by immigrants
		The term multiculturalism to remain Inclusiveness	
2000–06	United in Diversity	National agenda for a multicultural Australia	Main components of *Multicultural Australia: United in diversity policy 2003–2006* with responsibility, respect, fairness, and benefits for all
		Policy framework including:	
		All Australians are expected to have a "…loyalty to Australia and its people, and respect the basic structures and principles underpinning our democratic Society. These are: Constitution, parliamentary democracy, freedom of speech and religion, English as the National language, the rule of law, acceptance and equality" (Commonwealth of Australia, 2003:6)	
		The Rudd Labor Government and Gillard Labor Government reaffirmed their support for the relevance and constitution of Australia's Multiculturalism Policy	

Source: Commonwealth of Australia (1999, 2003, 2007b, 2008b). Garrett, P. & Lin, V. (1990). Ethnic health policy and service development. In J. Reid, & P. Trompf (Eds.), *The health of immigrant Australia: A social perspective* (pp. 339–382). Sydney: Harcourt Brace, Jovanovich.

LEININGER'S THEORY IN AUSTRALIAN NURSING EDUCATION, RESEARCH, AND PRACTICE

Given the widely diverse and multicultural population, the nursing profession in Australia needs the philosophy and tenets of the culture care theory to develop new knowledge to ensure effective, safe, and culturally meaningful nursing care practices that would embrace the multicultural key principles of access, equity, and inclusiveness set forth in national policies. Research as part of nursing curricula in undergraduate and postgraduate courses using Leininger's theory and the ethnonursing research method would facilitate development of cultural competence among all levels of Australian nursing practice. Transcultural curricular content would promote nursing scholarship, help generate transcultural research, engender the publication of studies reflecting Australia's multiculturally diverse population, and build the image of Australian nursing as having global influence.

Culture Care in Australian Nursing Education

Leininger's work became visible in Australia in the mid-1980s and marked the beginning of scholarship in transcultural nursing. Several published authors began using the term *transcultural nursing* in their writings without apparent use of the culture care theory or the ethnonursing research method as a theoretical basis (Idrus, 1988; Kanitsaki, 1988). Thereafter, a number of misconceptions and misunderstandings about the nature of transcultural nursing soon became apparent: First, the idea that it was possible to work with people from different cultural backgrounds without any transcultural nursing preparation to provide culture-specific care to diverse clients; and second, that experience working with any single cultural group was sufficient preparation to be a transcultural nurse. These misconceptions were based upon misinterpretations of the significance of the transcultural discipline to nursing education, research, and practice (Omeri, 1996).

Questions arose as to what nursing students were actually being taught. The National Review of Nursing Education in Australia in 2002 reported on surveys of universities and colleges of nursing in Australia to determine the extent of multicultural nursing education (Commonwealth of Australia, 2002). Three specific surveys were conducted between 1991 and 2003 in an attempt to build upon the original 2002 survey, and to inform the nursing community of the survey results.

Guided by Leininger's transcultural nursing and human care view, Omeri (1991) undertook her own survey of transcultural course content in undergraduate and graduate nursing education to establish the extent to which Australian nursing students were being prepared in transcultural care. The survey revealed that formal preparation in transcultural nursing was not available; nurses were graduating from universities and schools of nursing with inadequate and minimal preparation in transcultural nursing and were thus unprepared for nursing practice within intensely multicultural communities. Nurses confronted by and involved in the provision of nursing care to clients from diverse cultural backgrounds were unable to provide culturally appropriate and meaningful nursing care and nursing practices remained essentially monocultural (Omeri, 1991). The results of this first survey also showed a lack of faculty prepared in transcultural nursing as well as minimal commitment by nursing faculties to initiate such educational training.

D'Cruz and Tham (1994) reported their findings from a comparative study of cultural characteristics of general practice nurses (including students). In conjunction, these findings presented a profile of hospital patients in comparison to the general population from the State of Victoria, Australia, between 1985 and 1989. The cross-cultural nursing content in university nursing preregistration programs in Victoria was also analyzed. [Preregistration corresponds to prelicensure or generic BSN programs for students with no previous formal nursing qualifications, for enrolled nurses (LPN/LVN), and/or for psychiatric/mental health/mental deficiency nurses who would like to become eligible to register with the Nursing and Midwifery Board of Australia as a Registered Nurse (Flinders University, 2013).] This survey also demonstrated the cultural heterogeneity of the local population underscoring the importance of recognizing diversity in populations from Western countries. However, analysis of nursing curricular content in Victoria revealed only ad hoc minimal content relating to cross-cultural issues across all levels of nurse education. The findings of the D'Cruz and Tham (1994) study supported a prior study by Tham (1993) who reported that very little attention was given to cross-cultural issues in nursing education and asserted the importance of discovering whether and how cross-cultural issues were being addressed in nursing curricula. "These results demonstrate the necessity for healthcare professionals to be prepared transculturally to provide knowledgeable culturally-specific care" (Ray, 1994, p. 45). The researchers recommended that nurses and other healthcare workers undertake appropriate courses covering cultural perceptions of illness and health.

Pinikahana, Manias, and Happell (2003) were prompted by the observation that terms like *cultural pluralism*, *cultural diversity*, and *multiculturalism* were widely used in *policy and political structures.* However, consistency of meaning in the use of these terms among *academics* was lacking even though these concepts are critically important for understanding the cross-cultural relationships essential for nursing practice in a culturally diverse society. The authors concluded that "...although the introduction of transcultural dimensions together with the principles of sociology into the nursing curriculum provides an opportunity for nurses to perceive and respond to different patient behaviours in increasingly multicultural societies, it has not been sufficient to understand the complexities of the modern health care system" (p. 153).

The findings of these surveys suggested that many universities did not include transcultural nursing modules in their undergraduate nursing curricula. It would also appear that the concept of *transcultural nursing* was being variably defined and interpreted. It was evident that the approach to developing transculturally prepared nurses was inconsistent across and within institutions.

Culture Care in Australian Nursing Practice

Madeleine Leininger asserted that care is the essence of nursing and its dominant, distinctive, and unifying feature (Leininger, 1991b, 2006a; McFarland, 2010). She noted that care is complex, elusive, and often embedded in social structure and other aspects of culture and that patterns of care are diverse and take different forms and expressions and some are universal (Leininger, 1991b, 2002b, 2002f, 2006a; McFarland, 2010).

Leininger's culture care theory allows for the comparative study and analysis of diverse cultures and subcultures in the world with respect to their caring values, expressions, and health–illness beliefs and patterns of behaviour in order to discover human care diversities and universalities. Based on this knowledge, ways to provide "...culturally congruent care to people of different or similar cultures, in order to maintain or regain their wellbeing or health, or to face death in a culturally appropriate way" may be developed (Leininger, 1991b, p. 45). The goal of the theory is the provision of culturally congruent care to people that is beneficial, fits with, and is useful to the client, family, or cultural groups' healthy lifeways (Leininger, 1991b, 2002f; McFarland, 2010).

Leininger (1992) stated that *cross-cultural nursing* is not the same as *transcultural nursing*. Cross-cultural nursing focuses on using anthropological concepts, theories, and research in nursing and is based on applied medical or anthropological concepts that cannot lead to the development of research-based transcultural nursing knowledge (Leininger, 1995c, 2002d, 2002f, 2006a). To address these problems, nursing academics needed to refine their attitudes about the importance of cultural care in nursing education and practice by introducing more transcultural nursing content into nursing curricula. Transcultural nursing uses concepts to explore cultural phenomena (Leininger, 2002f) and "...focuses on generating culture care knowledge and using this knowledge in nursing within practices" (p. 39).

The growing worldwide trend toward multiculturalism challenges nurses to provide safe, appropriate, and culturally meaningful care to the world population regardless of their geographical location. To achieve this goal and provide this new and culturally appropriate care, transcultural nursing knowledge and an understanding of the cultural care values, beliefs, and practices of the people are urgently needed (Leininger, 2006a; McFarland, 2010).

Culture Care in Australian Nursing Research

The first transcultural nursing study in Australia, *The Use of Leininger's Culture Care Theory and the Ethnonursing Research Method with Yugoslav Immigrants in an Inner City Community, NSW Australia,* was undertaken by Omeri (1992) and was the first to use Leininger's Theory of Culture Care Diversity and Universality and the ethnonursing research method with the enablers. It was a mini-study conducted in partial requirement for completion of a Summer Special Course in Transcultural Nursing and Human Care taught by Professor Madeleine Leininger in 1992 at Wayne State University, College of Nursing, Detroit, Michigan.

The purpose of the mini-study was to discover care meanings and expressions relating to health and illness as expressed by key and general informants who were immigrants from Yugoslavia and regular clients of the local community centre. Four key and six general informants were interviewed using open-ended questions as well as the Observation–Participation–Reflection Enabler (OPR); Leininger's Stranger-to-Friend Enabler; Leininger's Phases of Ethnonursing Data Analysis Guide as an Enabler; Leininger–Templin–Thompson Ethnocript Qualitative Software (LTT); the Life History Health Care Enabler; Cultural Care Values and Meanings; the Culturological Care Assessment Guide; and the Generic and Professional Care Enabler Guide (Leininger, 1985, 1988b, 2002e, 2006b).

Dominant culture care values and beliefs discovered for the migrants from Yugoslavia included *involvement with family and community*; *respect for elders*; *duty and obligation to kin*; *feelings of national/cultural identity*; and *belief in a magic woman* (a *Rajacka*, in Macedonian) for folk healing. Folk healing was an extremely important discovery; combining folk and generic care for this community was an essential caring mode. Improved adherence to professional care in more meaningful and effective ways could improve care among the Yugoslav community through culturally congruent ways of combining professional and generic folk healing. Religiosity was also discovered to be an important element to care for this community as well as a source of cultural identity.

The Theory of Culture Care Diversity and Universality (Leininger, 1991b) was used as the conceptual and theoretical guide to discover the worldview, cultural values, and lifeways of Iranian immigrants in New South Wales (NSW), Australia, in the Omeri (1996) dissertation study *Transcultural Nursing Care Values, Beliefs, and Practices of Iranian Immigrants in NSW Australia*. This doctoral thesis was the first transcultural nursing study completed in Australia to use the culture care theory and ethnonursing research method.

The purpose of the study was to discover, explicate, analyze, and describe the culture care meanings and experiences of Iranian immigrants. It was predicted that these care meanings and expressions of the Iranians *as immigrants* had been influenced by and derived from their then currently shared cultural values, beliefs, and practices; their worldview, social structure features, language, and cultural values rooted in their ethno-historical past, and their current lifeways in NSW, Australia. These care meanings and expressions were discovered as:

- *Care* meant family and kinship ties (*hambastegie*) as expressed in daily lifeways and interactions with family, friends, and community;
- *Care* as expressed in carrying out traditional urban gender roles (*role-zan-o-mard*) (*Azadie zan*) as well as in fulfilling emerging new role responsibilities related to equality for Iranian immigrant women; and
- *Care* as preservation of Iranian identity (*inhamoni, hamonandi*) as expressed in traditional cultural events and health care practices (Omeri, 1996).

Brooke (1996) conducted a mini-ethnonursing TCN study in Australia endeavouring to discover, describe, and analyze care values, beliefs, and practices relating to immunization by Lebanese Muslim immigrants in New South Wales, Australia entitled *An Inquiry into the Way in Which Childhood Immunisation Is Viewed by People of Lebanese Muslim Background Living in Australia*. The researcher used the ethnonursing research method to explore the importance of care related to immunization knowledge of informants relating to vaccines, diseases, side effects, and contraindications. The study findings revealed the significance of the status and role of general practitioners in the delivery of immunization care for Lebanese Muslims. However, nurses were not generally identified as a significant group for having a primary role in the provision of immunization services but were regarded highly for their support to parents and for giving information regarding the sequence and schedule of vaccinations. Therefore, understanding culture and applying this understanding to nursing practice is integral in the provision of nursing and health care (Brooke & Omeri, 1999).

Culture Care in Australian Nursing Literature

Omeri and Ahern (1999) explored discoveries relating to the importance of culturally meaningful strategies to enhance recruitment and retention of Australian indigenous nursing students. Their study proposed a number of change strategies to facilitate this process including faculty prepared in transcultural nursing; faculty learning Aboriginal languages; changes in curricular philosophy and content to incorporate historical and cultural evidence relating to Aboriginal and Torres Strait Islander people; transcultural nursing research promoting respect and understanding for Aboriginal cultures; and development of culturally congruent educational strategies. This study has been cited by National Health and Medical Research Council (Australia), other government documents, and health-related and academic publications that address the importance of culture care.

Omeri, Malcolm, Ahern, and Wellington (2003) documented findings from their systematic review of literature that explored the implications of cultural diversity in academia across a number of countries and disciplines. This review examined both research and descriptive papers in order to capture a broad range of ideas; many of these research findings focused on university experiences of indigenous students, local students from non-English-speaking backgrounds, and international students. The review findings had implications for improved teaching-learning strategies to enhance the educational experiences of students and proposed methods that could assist educators from academic settings with a culturally diverse mix of students. Omeri (2003b) addressed the challenges of cultural diversity in nursing practice and examined the significance of research-based transcultural nursing in the evolutionary change context occurring in Australia with regard to multicultural policy. Transcultural nursing research builds upon existing nursing knowledge to provide evidence for advanced transcultural nursing practice; research-based transcultural nursing practices were examined and discussed.

Omeri, Lennings, and Raymond (2006) reported findings from their study about understanding Afghan refugees' perspectives on their experiences when resettling to New South Wales and accessing health services in that context. The study utilized qualitative research methods, including focus groups and semi-structured interviews with members of the Afghan community and those organizations and individuals serving the healthcare needs of Afghan people. The researchers sought to identify the beliefs and practices of the Afghan people and how these influence the way they access health services. The ultimate goal was to develop culture-specific strategies to improve healthcare services for the Afghan refugee community in culturally accessible and meaningful ways. Major themes discovered in the analysis of the participant interview data were *emotional responses to trauma, immigration and resettlement,* and *culture-specific health maintenance strategies.* Impediments to care included cultural views about mental illness, cultural and general barriers affecting the accessibility and appropriateness of Australian health and welfare services, and cultural factors influencing health outcomes (Omeri, Lennings, & Raymond, 2004).

Transculturalism in the Australian Nursing Workforce

A review of the literature could not identify any nursing publications specifically using the culture care theory and the ethnonursing research method to study Australian workforce issues. Most published articles used *multicultural nursing* and *diversity* with occasional references to *transcultural nursing* without expanding or using the culture care theory or the ethnonursing method for research. The articles discussed in the following paragraphs are based on research that used other theories or methods to study specific issues related to the workforce, implications for immigrant nurses, and abuses in the workplace.

Pittman and Rogers (1990) conducted two surveys in 1989 to collect information about cultural characteristics and perceptions of nurses on the General, Psychiatric, Mental Retardation and State Enrolled Nurses' Registers in Victoria. This study identified growth in the multicultural nature of the nursing population: Almost 60% of Survey 1 respondents were born in English-speaking countries (United Kingdom, New Zealand, United States, Canada, and South Africa), 25% in the Asian region; 1% in Australia; and the rest in 48 other non-English-speaking countries. In Survey 2, 21% of respondents were born overseas in 48 different countries. More than 60 languages were fluently spoken and more than 40 languages were spoken at home by nurses who participated in both surveys.

In Survey 1, racial prejudice and discriminatory practices were identified from responses to an open-ended question about nursing difficulties encountered in practice associated with the respondent's cultural background. Content analysis of these responses revealed six main categories of difficulty: Discrimination; registration [licensing] difficulties; language problems; different professional practices; nursing in a multicultural society; and being seen as a threat.

Jackson (1996) examined three elements within the multicultural workplace: Comfort, safety, and migrant nurses. Migrant women from non-English-speaking backgrounds participated in this phenomenological study of their experiences working as nurses in the NSW healthcare system. The women described feelings of displacement in many aspects of life, and these feelings were compounded by feeling uncomfortable in a culturally hazardous work environment. For participant women, *the need to belong* and *to have a place* emerged as compelling and important. The author concluded that in order to belong or take one's place, there needs to be acceptance by those who already have a place. In nursing, this means acceptance into the local nursing culture by local nurses.

Omeri and Atkins (2002) sought to understand immigrant nurses' experiences and their underrepresentation in the nursing workforce. Using a Heideggerian phenomenological approach, the purpose of the study was to explore, describe, and analyze the lived experiences of the immigrant nurses. Issues in recruitment and retention of immigrant nurses, cultural factors influencing interaction and communication, response of the host-country nurses, and cultural factors in the practice of nursing were investigated though naturalistic interviews. The findings were:

- *Professional negation*: Experiences in lack of support;
- *Otherness:* Experiences in cultural separateness and ultimate loneliness; and
- *Silencing*: Experiences in language and communication issues.

These nurses experienced marginalization and their contributions were undervalued. They were denied participation above the lower employment ranks and were undermined in their professional roles in multicultural work settings. This study highlights the social and cultural distance that persists between nurses from the dominant culture and immigrant nurse graduates from culturally and linguistically diverse backgrounds (Jupp, 1990; Martin, 1978). The findings have implications for current issues related to nursing workforce shortages.

The Omeri and Atkins (2002) study and the study by Jackson (1996) are major contributions to the body of transcultural nursing knowledge regarding the lack of *culture care* for immigrant nurses in a much neglected nursing care culture. These studies lend support for further work to explore how we engage with others when *the other* is perceived to be different. In this regard, Canales (2000) had proposed a theoretical framework for analyzing how we engage with others, and described *othering* as *exclusive* and *inclusive* processes that expand the boundaries of understanding and interaction with those perceived as different. Canales put forward the view that our perceptions of differences are not unchanging but are altered by time, distance, and perspectives. Her proposed framework provides initial direction for self-exploration of attitudes, beliefs, and assumptions about *the other* and the effects these personal views have on interactions with colleagues and patients, caregiving, and healthcare delivery.

These study findings contribute to the existing body of transcultural nursing knowledge and research, lending support for the development of transcultural nursing knowledge that is truly global and could serve as a means to overcome cultural differences.

CULTURALLY COMPETENT CARE

There has been steady growth in Australia in the movement among professional nurses and midwives toward developing competency standards for nursing and midwifery practice. The most significant early work was undertaken by the Australian Nursing Council Inc. (ANCI; 2002) which initially developed the Australian National Competency Standards for the Registered Nurse in 1990 through a group known as the Australian Nurse Registering Authorities Advisory Council (ANRAC, 2002). Later on, these standards became the ANCI Competencies but they are now known as the Australian Nursing and Midwifery Council (ANMC; 2006) Competency Standards for the Registered Nurse. The ANMC has also developed competency standards for enrolled nurses (ENs) [similar to licensed practical or vocational nurses or LPNs/ LVNs in USA]; registered midwives (RMs) [similar to certified nurse-midwives or CNMs in USA]; and nurse practitioners (NPs). These standards are those that the RN, RM, and EN are expected to demonstrate on entry to practice and are said to "...provide the framework for assessing competence but also serve to communicate to consumers the standards they can expect" (ANMC, 2002, as cited in Chiarella, 2006, p. 1).

Universities use standards in developing nursing curricula and to assess student and program performance (ANMC, 2006). The ANMC defines competency as "...an attribute of a person which results in effective performance" (ANMC, 2002, as cited in Chiarella, 2006, p. 2). The ANMC (2006) National Competency Standards for Registered Nurses remain as the core competency standards that all registered nurses must be able to demonstrate. The competencies are consistent across the competency standards documents for enrolled nurses, registered nurses, and midwives. The competency standards for each professional group (EN, RN, and RM) are organized into a number of domains, each with a series of corresponding statements or descriptors that include professional practice; critical thinking and analysis; provision and coordination of care; and collaborative and therapeutic practice. The competencies are used as the basis for all undergraduate programs, and all nursing undergraduate curricula are required to demonstrate that graduates from the program will be able to meet the competency standards. However, the sensitivity of the competencies in reflecting the complexity of nursing care for differing cultural groups has been raised as a concern (Chenoweth, Jeon, Goff, & Burk, 2006).

Regulatory authorities in Australia also set standards of competency that regulate the behaviour of nurses and under which they are held accountable to the community for the delivery of high quality, safe, and effective work practice (ANCI, 2002; Chiarella, 2006). From a regulatory perspective, although the ANMC competency standards were already endorsed by all state and territory regulatory authorities, the National Review of Nursing Education (Commonwealth of Australia, 2002) initiated by the Department of Education, Science, and Training took a more formalized and national approach and recommended that nationally agreed-upon principles should be developed to underpin state and territory nursing legislation that should include requirements for "...assessment against the ANCI competencies for initial regulation of registered and enrolled nurses" (p. 120).

Transcultural nurses are ready to take the lead through consultation and research to assist and inform ANCI Competency Standards with an Australian perspective that not only demonstrates commitment to our national policies but also to practices that would be culturally congruent with professional care practices in a discipline of nursing envied by all (McFarland & Eipperle, 2008; Omeri, 2003b).

CULTURALLY SENSITIVE CARE

The International Council of Nurses (ICN) uses these words to encompass the diversity of nursing and the people they serve in the world:

> *[Nurses are] everywhere.*
> *From African villages to other remote outposts you will find them.*
> *Yet, they struggle equally at the heart of the most deprived and forgotten blighted urban ghettos.*
> *In the most populous metropolitan centres of the world they are on the cutting edge of research, at the core of the most advanced technology.*
> *They speak every language. Their history started the moment humans first felt the need to care for each other.*
> *They attend the unempowered, and they speak for them, demanding that prevention, care, and cure be the right of every human being.*
> *United they are a single voice.*
> *Their message reaches the most influential leaders in international capitals as well as the chieftains of tribal clans.*
> *The strength of their numbers and their unified determination to make change is a powerful weapon, a weapon that will be used in the coming century to bring healthcare to humanity worldwide.*
> *They are nurses, the health professionals who can make the greatest difference in the world of certain change.*
> (International Council of Nurses as cited in Pratt, 1995)

To make the *greatest difference* nurses need to be prepared in transcultural nursing in a multicultural world to provide culturally congruent care.

Preparation in transcultural nursing will equip them to make cultural assessments and to know culture care values, beliefs, and practices of clients in order to provide culturally congruent care. Leininger (2002c) held that nurses needed creative and different approaches to make *care* and *culture* needs meaningful and helpful to clients. Three theoretically predicted decision and action modes of the culture care theory were defined as follows (Leininger, 1991a, 1991b, 2002f):

- Culture care preservation and/or maintenance: Referred to those assistive, supportive, facilitative, or enabling professional acts or decisions that help cultures to retain, preserve, or maintain beneficial care beliefs and values or to face handicaps and death.
- Culture care accommodation and/or negotiation: Referred to those assistive, accommodating and/or facilitative, or enabling creative provider care actions or decisions that help cultures adapt to or negotiate with others for culturally congruent, safe, and effective care for their health and wellbeing, or to deal with illness or dying.
- Culture care repatterning and/or restructuring: Referred to those assistive, supportive, facilitative, or enabling professional actions and mutual decisions that would help people to reorder, change, modify, or restructure their lifeways and institutions for better (or beneficial) healthcare patterns, practices, or outcomes (Leininger, 1991a, 1991b, 1995a, 2002f).

Leininger's (1991a, 1991b) Theory of Culture Care Diversity and Universality provides the means to discover knowledge about culture care from a nursing perspective for all cultures and forms the basis for cultural competency in nursing practice. The theory challenges nurses to discover specific and holistic care as known and used by cultures over time in different contexts; both *culture* and *care* are held to be central and critical nursing constructs.

FOUNDING THEORIST DR. MADELEINE LEININGER

After her initial visit in 1960, Leininger made 15 additional trips to Australia; during these visits, she mentored many Australian nurses. Her contribution to transcultural nursing was recognised at the 26th Annual International Transcultural Nursing Society Conference in 2000 when she was awarded a Life Fellow of the Royal College of Nursing, Australia and was identified as a Distinguished Visiting Scholar—the first time this award was bestowed on anyone from outside Australia. The October 2003 issue of the Australian journal *Contemporary Nurse* was dedicated to Leininger in recognition of her pioneering work and consultations with Australian nurses in supporting and promoting transcultural nursing education, research, and practice (Omeri, 2003a, 2003b).

Reflections, Experiential Learning, Reflective Practice

I would like share my personal journey with TCN and acknowledge my indebtedness to Madeleine Leininger, for her personal support and guidance so generously given. I have had the opportunity to test and apply her theories and concepts in my work and the privilege of adding to the body of transcultural knowledge that may be applied in nursing practice.

Undertaking transcultural nursing studies and research with leading nurse theorist Professor Madeleine Leininger in 1992 and 1994 was an extraordinary experience for which I was humbled and grateful. The experience was invaluable in helping me to plan and introduce courses in transcultural nursing at Cumberland College of Health Sciences and the University of Sydney. It gave me the knowledge and the confidence not only to design and teach transcultural nursing courses, but to supervise students in transcultural nursing research.

Since then I have designed and taught other transcultural nursing courses with a focus on Leininger's culture care theory (Leininger, 1978, 1991b, 2002f; McFarland, 2010) in other universities integrated with the educational and teaching philosophies of the chosen schools of nursing. Other TCN models have been added to my teachings such as Andrews and Boyle (2012); Campinha-Bacote (1998); Giger and Davidhizar (1999); Papadopoulos (2006); and Purnell and Paulanka (2008). I have taught the course and conducted workshops in transcultural nursing for faculty and clinicians in Dar Al Hekma, School of Nursing, Jeddah, Saudi Arabia and have presented scholarly lectures at the Universities of Central England in Birmingham, the University of Middlesex, Centre for Transcultural Research, and De Montfort University in Leicester, United Kingdom. Undertaking studies in transcultural nursing research was key to my ongoing professional achievements in transcultural nursing in Australia and internationally. In addition, I have continued to teach, conduct research, and perform consultations in transcultural nursing, and have been able to reach clinicians worldwide via the Internet since 2009.

Leininger's Legacy

In their tribute to Madeleine Leininger, Daly and Jackson (2003, pp. xiii–xiv) summarized her phenomenal contribution to transcultural nursing by the following words:

> *Madeleine Leininger's pioneering work, which resulted in her theory of transcultural nursing, became the seminal body of knowledge about culture care from a nursing perspective. Leininger developed the Theory of Culture Care Diversity and Universality in nursing in the early 1950s, along with over 30 distinct*

concepts and many principles to guide nurses in transcultural nursing. The theory was to discover what is universal (or commonalities) and what was diverse about human care values, beliefs and practices, and was critical for a future body of transcultural nursing knowledge. Madeleine Leininger's theory of transcultural nursing has stood the test of time. From its framework, worldwide research has demonstrated a value, approachability, and appeal of the theory that crosses cultural borders. Today Leininger's Sunrise Enabler cognitive map is used worldwide by many graduate and undergraduate students.

The purpose of Leininger's theory is to discover human care diversities and universalities in relation to worldview, social structures, and other dimensions, and then to discover ways to provide culturally congruent care to people of different or similar cultures in order to maintain or regain their wellbeing or health, or to face death in culturally appropriate ways (McFarland, 2010, p. 458).

The goal of the theory is to improve and to provide culturally congruent care to people that is beneficial and will fit with and be useful to the client, family, or culture group's healthy lifeways (Leininger, 1991b). A central thesis of Leininger's culture care theory is that if the meaning of care can be fully grasped, the wellbeing or health care of individuals, families, and groups can be predicted and culturally congruent care can be provided (1991b). Leininger viewed *care* as one of the most powerful constructs and the central phenomenon of nursing, and held that detailed and culturally-based caring knowledge and practices should distinguish nursing's contributions from those of other disciplines (1988a, 1994).

Leininger (1991b, 2002f; McFarland, 2010) found that care is largely an elusive phenomenon often embedded in cultural lifeways and values. However, culture care holding knowledge provides a sound basis for nurses to guide their practice in the provision of culturally congruent care and culture-specific therapeutic ways to maintain health, prevent illness, heal, or help people face death (Leininger, 1994). Leininger believed that because culture and care knowledge are the broadest and most holistic means to conceptualize and understand people, they are central to and imperative to nursing education and practice (Leininger, 1991b, 1995a, 1995b, 2002f, 2006a; McFarland, 2010). From these premises, Leininger developed the culture care theory.

Leininger (1985, 1991b) favoured qualitative ethnomethods—especially ethnonursing—to study care and to discover people-truths or the views, beliefs, and patterned lifeways of people. During the 1960s, the theorist developed the ethnonursing research method to study culture care phenomena specifically and systematically. This method focuses on the classification of care beliefs, values, and practices as cognitively or subjectively known by cultures (or cultural representatives) through local emic people-centered language, experiences, beliefs, and value systems about actual or potential nursing phenomena such as care, health, and environmental factors (Leininger, 1991b, 1995a, 1995b, 2002f, 2006c).

Leininger defined transcultural nursing as *a major area of nursing that focuses on the comparative study and analysis of diverse cultures and subcultures in the world with respect to their caring values, expressions, and health–illness beliefs and patterns of behaviour* (Leininger, 1978, 1991b, 2002f; McFarland, 2010). Transcultural nursing goes beyond a state to awareness to that of using *culture care* nursing knowledge to practice culturally congruent and responsible care (Leininger, 1991b, 1995a, 1995b).

Leininger predicted a new kind of nursing practice that reflects different nursing practices that are culturally defined, grounded, and specific to guide nursing care provided to individuals, families, groups, and institutions. She stated that because culture and care knowledge are the broadest and most holistic means to conceptualize and understand people, they are central to and imperative to nursing education and practice (Leininger, 1991b, 1995a, 1995b, 2002f, 2006a). Leininger predicted that for nursing to be meaningful and relevant to clients and other nurses in the world, transcultural nursing knowledge and competencies will be imperative to guide all nursing decisions and actions for effective and successful outcomes (Leininger, 1996a, 1996b, 2002f).

Leininger described the transcultural nurse generalist as ". . .a nurse prepared at the baccalaureate level who is able to apply transcultural nursing concepts, principles, and practices that are generated by transcultural nurse specialists" (Curren, 2006; Leininger, 1995b, 2002c). The transcultural nurse specialist is prepared in graduate programs and receives in-depth preparation and mentorship in transcultural nursing knowledge and practice. The specialist has acquired competency skills through post-baccalaureate education. This specialist has studied selected cultures and is highly knowledgeable and theoretically-based about care, health, and environmental factors related to transcultural nursing perspectives (Leininger, 1989). This individual also values and uses nursing theory to develop and advance knowledge within the discipline of transcultural nursing which Leininger (1995b, 1995c) predicted must be the focus of all nursing education and practice (McFarland, 2010).

Leininger (1991a, 1995a, 1995b, 2002f) stated that the goal of the culture care theory is to provide culturally congruent care (Curren, 2006). She maintained that nurses cannot separate worldviews, social structures, and cultural beliefs (folk or professional) from health, wellness, illness, or care when working with cultures because these factors are closely linked.

Culturally congruent care is what makes clients satisfied that they have received good care; it is a powerful healing force for quality health care. Quality care is what clients seek most when they come for services from nurses, and it can be realized only when culturally derived care is known and used.

Leininger's Voice

The first International Transcultural Nursing Society conference held in Australia was at Cumberland College of Health Sciences of Health Sciences, The University of Sydney, Australia on July 13-14, 1992. This conference constituted a significant historical breakthrough in Australian nursing and made many participants more aware the significance of transcultural nursing to an increasingly multicultural country, but also the academic and professional implications for education, research, and practice. The following is a summary of Madeleine Leininger's message to the conference delegates; it constitutes her message to Australian nurses and to nurses of the world.

Madeleine Leininger's Message

Predicting that future studies will be guided by the Theory of Culture Care Diversity and Universality, Dr. Leininger foresaw that all Australian nurses would be involved in transcultural nursing and finding creative ways to apply research findings in practice and education. In her Oration to Cumberland College (Sydney), Leininger (1992) expressed the hope that Australian nurses would seek to establish global networks with other nurses to share transcultural nursing research, education, and practice knowledge. She urged Australian nurses to develop a global perspective and—a truly caring—transcultural nursing focus that she claimed is imperative for teaching nursing.

Based upon common links and bonds transculturally-prepared nurses, in Dr. Leininger's vision of the future, would avoid destructive tendencies by respecting and valuing the contributions of one another and embracing not only nurses of differing cultures but also non-nurses; they would lead by example—sharing in a common nursing humanity. Dr. Leininger saw compassionate caring with a transcultural nursing focus as the means to ameliorate suffering in the world's populations. She identified that much had yet to be learned about diverse human cultures and the ways that professional nurses may help as caregivers. She also claimed that from a transcultural nursing perspective issues of social justice, abuse, and violence are within its scope and can be applied in finding ways to best help people suffering violence, deprivation, and social and legal injustices. Dr. Leininger stated that a major goal of transcultural nursing was to provide culturally congruent care and that the key to achieving this was through transcultural nurses serving as role models, "...[helping] others value, appreciate, and understand people of diverse and similar cultures in the world" (Leininger, 1992).

In closing, Dr. Leininger asserted that ". . .while nursing today remains one of the greatest and most influential professions in the world," it needs to be well grounded in ". . .transcultural nursing education, research, practice, and in multicultural public relations activities" to reach its potential as a force for good in the world (Leininger, 1992). She expressed her best wishes for the further development of transcultural nursing in Australia and predicted that its contribution will continue to grow worldwide.

THE FUTURE OF THE CULTURE CARE THEORY AND ETHNONURSING RESEARCH METHOD IN AUSTRALIA

As nurses discover the client's particular cultural orientation, they learn from the client ways to provide sensitive, compassionate, and competent care that is beneficial and satisfying to the client. Gaining a deep appreciation for cultures with their commonalities and differences is one of several goals of transcultural nursing. At the same time, the nurse discovers many nursing insights about her or his own cultural background and how to use such knowledge appropriately with clients in a particular community, hospital, or other kinds of healthcare settings.

However, progress in the application of transcultural nursing remains slow. Leininger attributed this to the need for transcultural nursing education and listed the following primary reasons for the delayed progress:

- The lack of sufficient numbers of qualified transcultural nursing faculty in schools of nursing;
- The failure of academic nurse leaders to value, recognize, and promote transcultural nursing in schools of nursing;
- The dominance of monocultural and traditional nursing curricula;
- The lack of significant funding to support transcultural nursing education, research, and curricular changes;
- The dominance of biomedical and psychological content in nursing education;
- The fear of moving to use transcultural content; and
- Cultural ignorance, prejudices, and biases among faculty and administrators (Leininger, 1995b, pp. 33–34, 53).

In Australia, although culture care services are used by nurses or other healthcare practitioners, much more research is needed to address a number of culture care and culture-specific issues that go beyond such services. *Mainstreaming* as an ideology adopted [by Australia] in 1986, sought to strengthen the base of multiculturalism by changing government service provision for immigrants from a *marginal* to a *central* concern of government institutions. Based on the assumptions that the immigrants' needs for social services were no different from other persons in the community and that compensatory measures could be adopted to reduce these disadvantages, the government hoped to improve accessibility to hospital facilities (Garret & Lin, 1990). However, the use of terms such as *ethnic minority* is innately discriminatory and separatist as *minority* denotes being below some other, or being *other*. Taking a more positive view, the author makes recommendations to involve cultures holistically, including all Australians, without dividing people into dominant and minority cultures.

With the culture care theory, nurses can think about differences and similarities and the beliefs, practices, and lifeways of clients. Nurses learn to value understanding people regarding their special needs and concerns and to develop different ways to assist their diverse clients. These concerns underpin the following recommendations for the future of the Theory of Culture Care Diversity and Universality in Australian nursing.

Recommendations

Recognizing Australia as one of the world's most multicultural nations and having advanced multicultural policies, the author draws upon her personal experiences as an immigrant to Australia; as a person who has firsthand experiences working with multicultural communities in Iran, Lebanon, United Kingdom, United States, and Saudi Arabia as well as in Australia; and also as a scholar who has used and applied the culture care theory clinically, academically, and professionally.

The author has demonstrated through research that culture care theory is the most comprehensive worldwide nursing theory that emphasizes the concepts of culture and care as its two major constructs. These two major constructs when studied through research can lead to essential culture care knowledge that, when applied, can facilitate healing in culturally congruent ways, in harmony with the cultural care values and beliefs of clients and their families.

The first recommendation is that Australian nurses pursue the culture care theory as a framework to develop their capacity to advance culture care knowledge and to apply it in their practice in order to appropriately meet the care needs of individual clients, families, communities, and organizations in culturally meaningful ways to the satisfaction of clients. Support for my recommendations as expressed by Leininger (2006a) are:

- The culture care theory has been thoughtfully constructed and refined over the past 3 decades to discover transcultural nursing care phenomena that are rooted in diverse cultures. *It has stood the test of time.* The theory offers a broad and comprehensive means to study human beings and culture care and can be used in any culture or subculture in the world to discover culture care differences and similarities in a systematic and rigorous way;
- The culture care theory is comprehensive, holistic, and broad in scope and yet can explicate specifics of an individual, family, group, community, or institution;
- The culture care theory is used to focus on social structure dimensions but also to study total cultures, incorporating the broadest conceptual and theoretical perspectives to discover the totality of how a culture knows and experiences caring from their emic perspectives;
- The culture care theory was designed to be used primarily from an inductive emic focus to generate knowledge using the ethnonursing method within the qualitative paradigm; and
- The culture care theory is important to generate knowledge of human care patterns and themes that are congruent with the cultural lifeways, values, beliefs, practices, and meanings of individuals and groups (Leininger, 1991c, pp. 391–414).

In addition, the author adds:

- The culture care theory has the capacity to make a fundamental change in Australian nursing from a largely monocultural profession to a multicultural one—to make *culture care the essence of nursing.*
- A *duty of care* must be accomplished and met by all nurses as specified in the report on Nursing Education Review (Commonwealth of Australia, Department of Employment, Training and Youth Affairs (Australia) [DETYA], 2002). The culture care theory with constructs of culture and care assists nurses to realize the importance of care in caring for culturally diverse communities in Australia.
- The culture care theory is suited to the context of multicultural Australia because it
  - Is comprehensive, practical, and culturally appropriate;
  - Has stood the test of time, with revisions;

- Has been used globally and has been used to study diverse cultures; and
- Addresses many cultural constructs that are essential to be known by nurses in practice, education, research, and administration.

Nursing in Australia has other mandates to follow:

- Australia is a signatory to the 1951 refugee convention for support of refugees who need to be cared for in culturally sensitive and respectful ways and be given a home (The United Nations, Office of the United Nations High Commissioner for Refugees, Refugee Convention, 1951).
- Australia is a member country and is committed to the Alma Ata Health for All by 2000 and Beyond consensus, also known as the Declaration of Alma-Ata (Butler, 2000, 2007; World Health Organization, 1978).
- The International Transcultural Nursing Society statement of commitment to human rights regarding the provision of culturally appropriate care (www.tcns.org).

Leininger (2006b) foresaw that many ethical and moral problems would arise in the 21st century because of culture value conflicts and clashes between clients and healthcare providers. There will be some who will lay claim to or try to rename transcultural nursing without acknowledging the nearly 6 decades of work by transcultural nurse leaders. Interprofessional jealousy, envy, and struggles for status recognition along with a lack of professional honesty and integrity, may be encountered. True scholars and honest users of transcultural nursing knowledge will always value the contributions of our pioneering Leader and her followers.

CONCLUSION

In this chapter, trends in the application and use of the culture care theory have been examined in regard to the pursuit of effective transcultural nursing education, research, practice, and administration in the context of multicultural Australia. Some multicultural policies presented have influenced the growth and evolution of transcultural nursing and evidence-based research in Australia. A few nursing faculties in Australia established transcultural nursing through courses of study which opened opportunities for nurses to undertake research relating to diverse cultures in various healthcare settings and to share their findings with the global community of nurses through publications and presentations to inform nursing practice.

Through the lens of culture care theory, the future looks exceedingly promising for nursing practice, research, education, and leadership. Should the nursing profession in Australia chose to follow this pathway and realize its potential to offer culturally specific nursing care to the Australian community, it would make a major contribution toward assisting the nation to realize ". . .the principles of social justice, equality of access to services, including health and economic efficiency, and to demonstrating Australia's commitment to equality in health care and *a fair go* for all Australians" (Bullivant, 1986; Commonwealth of Australia, Office of Multicultural Affairs, 1989) as expressed in its multicultural policies.

ACKNOWLEDGMENTS

I would like to acknowledge those who have shaped my thinking while contemplating and writing this chapter. This gratitude extends to students, colleagues, friends, and mentors and to those whose path-finding research provided the intellectual foundation and motivation for establishing transcultural nursing in Australia.

- Special acknowledgement and thanks to the management and staff of the former Cumberland College of Health Sciences, School of Nursing, The University of Sydney—in particular Faith M. Jones (HOS), Verna Rice, Kay Plymat, and Patricia Malcolm, for their support throughout the years.
- Special thanks to Elizabeth Percival and Elizabeth Foley and the Executive of the Royal College of Nursing, Australia (RNCA [now known as the Australian College of Nursing]) for supporting the move to place transcultural nursing in nursing education, research, and publishing on the national nursing agenda and for establishing a national network for TCN to inform nursing practices.
- Special thanks to Professor Beverly Horn and the Executive Committee of the Transcultural Nursing Society for their past support.

I wish to also acknowledge my students who have inspired me to continue to promote TCN through research; special thanks to Lynnette Raymond, Debra Prior, and Deborah Brooke. My heartfelt appreciation to the many friends and colleagues who have inspired me to continue my work in TCN and especially:

- Helen Hamilton, friend, keen editor, and mentor;
- Dr. Marilyn R. McFarland for her support and friendship as a collaborative researcher and co-publisher;

- Dr. Rosalie Pratt for her endless support and wise counsel in my endeavours to find pathways for establishing transcultural nursing and in my struggles to maintain and advance it in Australia;
- Dr. Anne McMurray for her research mentorship; and
- The late Dr. Anna Frances Wenger, who gave me endless support in research and by her presence in 1998 in sharing my achievements when I received the Leininger Award.

An additional note of appreciation to editors Dr. Marilyn R. McFarland and Dr. Hiba B. Wehbe-Alamah, together with Marilyn Eipperle, MSN, RN, FNP-BC, CTN-A, for inspiring me to write my chapter in this special text which will hopefully be an important and useful addition to transcultural nursing knowledge in Australia and globally.

My deepest appreciation to my dear family who have shared my journey in transcultural nursing over the past many decades.

DISCUSSION QUESTIONS

1. Discuss what cultural diversities exist in Australia.
2. Explain and discuss factors in Australia leading to the development of multicultural policies as an over-arching framework.
3. Discuss how multiculturalism and related policies differ from related policies in other countries such as the United States, Canada, and nations of the Middle East, Europe, Africa, and Asia. Discuss underlying reasons based on the social structure dimensions of Leininger's Sunrise Enabler.
4. Discuss the transcultural challenges faced by Australian nurses.
5. Identify the role of Leininger and McFarland in promoting transcultural nursing in Australia.
6. What factors have hindered the progress of transcultural nursing in Australia? Discuss whether and how they remain relevant for Australia.

REFERENCES

Andrews, M. M., & Boyle, J. S. (2012). *Transcultural concepts in nursing care* (6th ed.). New York, NY: Lippincott Williams & Wilkins.

Australian Bureau of Statistics (ABS). (2012). Census: Basic community profile. Census of population (Catalogue/s 3101.0 & 3218.0). http://www.abs.gov.au/ausstats/abs@nsf/web

Australian Nursing Council Incorporated (ANCI). (2002). *Principles for the assessment of national competency standards for registered and enrolled nurses.* Canberra, Australia: Author.

Australian Nursing and Midwifery Council (ANMC). (2006). *National competency standards for the registered nurse.* Dickson, ACT, Australia: Author.

Australian Nurse Registering Authorities Conference (ANRAC). (2002). *Vol. 1: Nursing Competencies Assessment Project. Vol. 2: The Project Report. Vol.3: Assessment and Evaluation.* St. Lucia: Queensland, Australia: Research Unit, Education Department, University of Queensland.

Brooke, D. A. (1996). *An inquiry into the way in which childhood immunisation is viewed by people of Lebanese Muslim background living in Australia: Using Leininger's culture care theory and mini-ethnonursing research method.* Doctoral thesis, The University of Sydney, NSW, Australia.

Brooke, D. A., & Omeri, A. (1999). Beliefs about childhood immunisation among Lebanese Muslim immigrants in Australia. *Journal of Transcultural Nursing, 10*(3), 229–236.

Bullivant, B. M. (1986). Getting a fair go: Case studies of occupational socialization and perceptions of discrimination in a sample of seven: Melbourne High School. *Human Rights Commission, Occasional Paper No. 13* (pp. 252–253). Canberra, Australia: Australian Government Publishing Service.

Butler, C. D. (2000). Inequality, global change and the sustainability of civilisation. *Global Change and Human Health, 1*(2), 156–172.

Butler, C. D. (2007). Globalization, population, ecology, and conflict [Editorial]. *Health Promotion Journal of Australia, 18*(2), 87–89.

Campinha-Bacote, J. (1998). *A culturally competent model of care* (third edition). Cincinnati, OH: Transcultural C.A.R.E Associates.

Canales, M. (2000). Othering: Towards an understanding of difference. *Advances in Nursing Science, 22*(4), 16–31.

Castle, S. (1999). Globalisation, multicultural citizenship and transnational democracy, part 1: Debating the migrant presence (pp. 31–41). In, G. Hage & R. Couch (Eds.), *The Future of Multiculturalism: Reflections on the Twentieth Anniversary of Jean Martin's The Migrant Presence.* Research Institute for Humanities and Social Sciences, University of Sydney.

Chenoweth, L., Jeon, Y-H, Goff, M., & Burk, C. (2006). Cultural competency and nursing care: An Australian perspective. *International Nursing Review, 53*(1), 34–40.

Chiarella, M. (2006). *An overview of the competency movement in Australian nursing and midwifery.* Sydney, Australia: Nursing and Midwifery Office, NSW Health and Faculty of Nursing, Midwifery & Health, University of Technology. Retrieved from http://www.health.gov.au/resources.nursing/pdf

Commonwealth of Australia. (2002). *National review of nursing education: Multicultural nursing education.* Canberra, Australia: Commonwealth (Australia) Department of Education, Science and Training. Retrieved from wysiwyg://9/http://www.dest.gov.au/highered/nursing/pubs/multi_cultural/4.htm

Commonwealth of Australia, Department of Employment, Training and Youth Affairs (Australia) [DETYA], 2002). *Commonwealth of Australia Gazette.* Canberra, Australia: Author.

Commonwealth of Australia. (2003). *Multicultural Australia: United in Diversity: Updating the 1999 New Agenda for Multicultural Australia: Strategic directions for 2003–2006.* Canberra, Au: Author.

Commonwealth of Australia, Department of the Prime Minister and Cabinet, Office of Multicultural Affairs. (1989). *National agenda for a multicultural Australia: Sharing our future.* Canberra, Australia: Australian Government Publishing Service.

Commonwealth of Australia, National Multicultural Advisory Council. (1999). Australian multiculturalism for a new century: Towards inclusiveness. http://www.immi.gov.au/fact-sheet/ 06evolution

Curren, D. (2006). Clinical nursing aspects discovered with the culture care theory. In M. M. Leininger & M. R. McFarland (Eds.), *Culture care diversity and universality: A worldwide nursing theory* (2nd ed., pp. 159–180). Sudbury, MA: Jones and Bartlett.

Daly, J., & Jackson, D. (Eds.). (2003). Preface: Transcultural health care: Issues and challenges for nursing [Special issue]. *Contemporary Nurse: Advances in Contemporary Transcultural Nursing, 15*(3), 161–350.

Davidson, A. (1999). Migrants, citizenship and the new civics, part 4: Multicultural routes (pp. 245–252). In G. Hage & R. Couch (Eds.), *The Future of Multiculturalism: Reflections on the Twentieth Anniversary of Jean Martin's The Migrant Presence.* Research Institute for Humanities and Social Sciences, University of Sydney.

D'Cruz, J. V., & Tham, G. (1994). *Nursing and nursing education in multicultural Australia: A Victorian study of some cultural, curriculum and demographic issues.* Melbourne, ACT, Australia: David Lovell.

Flinders University, Undergraduate Programs, Bachelor of Nursing. (2013). Retrieved from http://www.flinders.edu.au/courses/undergrad/bngu/

Garrett, P., & Lin, V. (1990). Ethnic health policy and service development. In J. Reid & P. Trompf (Eds.), *Health of immigrant Australia: A social perspective.* Sydney, NSW, Australia: Harcourt Brace Jovanovich.

Garrett, P. & Lin, V. (1990). Ethnic health policy and service development. In J. Reid, & P. Trompf (Eds.), *The health of immigrant Australia: A social perspective* (pp. 339–382). Sydney: Harcourt Brace, Jovanovich.

Giger, J. N., & Davidhizar, R. E. (1999). *Transcultural nursing assessment and intervention* (3rd ed.). New York, NY: Mosby.

Idrus, L. (1988). Transcultural nursing in Australia: Response to a changing population base. In M. J. Morse (Ed.), *Recent advances in nursing: Issues in cross-cultural nursing* (pp. 81–91). Edinburgh, UK: Churchill Livingston.

Jackson, D. (1996). The multicultural workplace: Comfort, safety and migrant nurses. *Contemporary Nurse, 5*(3), 120–126.

Jupp, J. (1990). Two hundred years of immigration. In J. Reid & P. Trompf (Eds.), *Health of immigrant Australia: A social perspective.* Sydney, Australia: Harcourt Brace Jovanovich.

Kanitsaki, O. (1988). Transcultural nursing: A challenge to change. *Australian Journal of Advanced Nursing, 5*(3), 4–11.

Leininger, M. M. (1978). *Transcultural nursing concepts, theories, & practices.* New York, NY: Wiley & Sons.

Leininger, M. M. (1985). Transcultural care diversity and universality: A theory of nursing. *Nursing and Health Care, 6*(4), 202–212.

Leininger, M. M. (Ed.). (1988a). *Care: Discovery and uses in clinical and community nursing.* Detroit, MI: Wayne State University Press.

Leininger, M. M. (Ed.). (1988b). Leininger's theory of nursing: Cultural diversity and universality. *Nursing Science Quarterly, 1*(4), 152–160.

Leininger, M. M. (1989). Transcultural nurse specialists and generalists: New practitioners in nursing. *Journal of Transcultural Nursing, 1*(1), 4–16.

Leininger, M. M. (1991a). Becoming aware of types of health practitioners and cultural imposition. *Journal of Transcultural Nursing, 2*(2), 32–49.

Leininger, M. M. (1991b). *Culture care diversity and universality: A theory of nursing.* New York, NY: National League for Nursing Press.

Leininger, M. M. (1991c). Looking to the future of nursing and relevancy of culture care theory. In M. M. Leininger (Ed.), *Culture care diversity and universality: A theory of nursing* (pp. 391–414). New York, NY: National League for Nursing Press.

Leininger, M. M. (1992, July 13–14). Some reflections and message to the 1992 transcultural nursing conference participants at Cumberland College of Health Sciences, The University of Sydney. *Transcultural Nursing Conference Proceedings,* pp. 1–4.

Leininger, M. M. (1994). Transcultural nursing: A worldwide imperative. *Nursing and Health Care, 15*(5), 254–257.

Leininger, M. M. (Ed.). (1995a). Overview of Leininger's culture care theory. In: *Transcultural nursing: Concepts, theories, research, & practices* (2nd ed., pp. 93–114). New York, NY: McGraw Hill.

Leininger, M. M. (Ed.). (1995b). Transcultural nursing: Importance, history, concepts, theory, and research. In: *Transcultural nursing: Concepts, theories, research, & practices* (2nd ed., pp. 3–54). New York, NY: McGraw Hill.

Leininger, M. M. (Ed.). (1995c). Transcultural nursing perspectives: Basic concepts, principles, and culture care incidents. In: *Transcultural nursing: Concepts, theories, research, & practices* (2nd ed., pp. 57–92). New York, NY: McGraw Hill.

Leininger, M. M. (1996a). Future directions for transcultural nursing in the 21st century. *International Nursing Review, 44*(1), 19–23.

Leininger, M. M. (1996b). Major directions for transcultural nursing: A journey into the 21st Century. *Journal of Transcultural Nursing, 7*(2), 37–40.

Leininger, M. M. (2002a). Culture care theory: A major contribution to advance transcultural nursing knowledge and practice. *Journal of Transcultural Nursing, 13*(3), 189–192.

Leininger, M. M. (2002b). Essential transcultural nursing concepts, principles, examples, and policy statements. In M. M. Leininger & M. R. McFarland (Eds.), *Transcultural nursing: Concepts, theories, research, & practice* (3rd ed., pp. 45–69). New York, NY: McGraw-Hill.

Leininger, M. M. (2002c). The future of transcultural nursing: A global perspective. In M. M. Leininger & M. R. McFarland (Eds.), *Transcultural nursing: Concepts, theories, research, & practice* (3rd ed., pp. 577–595). New York, NY: McGraw-Hill.

Leininger, M. M. (2002d). Part 1. The theory of culture care and the ethnonursing research method. In M. M. Leininger & M. R. McFarland (Eds.), *Transcultural nursing: Concepts, theories, research, & practice* (3rd ed., pp. 71–98). New York, NY: McGraw-Hill.

Leininger, M. M. (2002e). Transcultural nursing: Curricular concepts, principles, and teaching and learning activities for the 21st century. In M. M. Leininger & M. R. McFarland (Eds.), *Transcultural nursing: Concepts, theories, research, & practice* (3rd ed., pp. 527–561). New York, NY: McGraw-Hill.

Leininger, M. M. (2002f). Transcultural nursing and globalization of health care: Importance, focus, and historical aspects. In M. M. Leininger & M. R. McFarland (Eds.), *Transcultural nursing: Concepts, theories, research, & practice* (3rd ed., pp. 3–43). New York, NY: McGraw-Hill.

Leininger, M. M. (2006a). Culture care diversity and universality theory and evolution of the ethnonursing method. In M. M. Leininger & M. R. McFarland (Eds.), *Culture care diversity and universality: A worldwide nursing theory* (2nd ed., pp. 1–41). Sudbury, MA: Jones and Bartlett.

Leininger, M. M. (2006b). Envisioning the future of culture care theory. In M. M. Leininger & M. R. McFarland (Eds.), *Culture care diversity and universality: A worldwide nursing theory* (2nd ed., pp. 389–394). Sudbury, MA: Jones and Bartlett.

Leininger, M. M. (2006c). Ethnonursing research method and enablers. In M. M. Leininger & M. R. McFarland (Eds.), *Culture care diversity and universality: A worldwide nursing theory* (2nd ed., pp. 43–81). Sudbury, MA: Jones and Bartlett.

Maltby, H. J. (1999). Interpreters: A double-edged sword in nursing practice. *Journal of Transcultural Nursing, 10*(3), 248–254.

Martin, J. (1978). *The migrant presence: Australian responses, 1947–1977: Research report for the national population inquiry.* Sydney, Australia: Allen & Unwin.

McFarland, M. R. (2010). Madeleine Leininger: Culture care theory of diversity and universality. In A. M. Tomey & M. R. Alligood (Eds.), *Nursing theorists and their work* (7th ed.). St. Louis, MO: Elsevier.

McFarland, M. R., & Eipperle, M. K. (2008). Culture care theory: A proposed practice theory guide for nurse practitioners in primary care settings [Special issue]. *Contemporary Nurse: Advances in Transcultural Nursing, 28* (1–2), 49–63.

Omeri, A. (1991). *Educating nurses in multicultural Australia: Survey of nursing curricula to determine status of transcultural nursing education.* [Unpublished]. Centre for Nursing Research. W.H.O. Collaborating Centre for Nursing Development in Primary Health Care, Cumberland College of Health Sciences, The University of Sydney.

Omeri, A. (1992). *The use of Leininger's culture care theory and the ethnonursing research method with Yugoslav immigrants in an inner city community, NSW Australia* [Unpublished mini-study]. Detroit, MI: Wayne State University.

Omeri, A. (1996). *Transcultural nursing care values, beliefs and practices of Iranian immigrants in NSW Australia.* Doctoral thesis, University of Sydney, Sydney, NSW, Australia.

Omeri, A. (1997). Culture care of Iranian immigrants in NSW Australia: Sharing transcultural nursing knowledge. *Journal of Transcultural Nursing, 8*(2), 5–16.

Omeri, A. (2003a). Dedication: Advances in contemporary transcultural nursing [Special issue]. *Contemporary Nurse, 15*(3), ii.

Omeri, A. (2003b). Meeting diversity challenges: Pathways of advanced transcultural nursing practice in Australia [Special issue]. *Contemporary Nurse: Advances in Contemporary Transcultural Nursing, 15*(3), 175–187.

Omeri, A., & Ahern, M. (1999). Utilising culturally congruent strategies to enhance recruitment and retention of Australian Indigenous nursing students. *Journal of Transcultural Nursing, 10*(2), 150–155.

Omeri, A., & Atkins, K. (2002). Lived experiences of immigrant nurses in New South Wales, Australia: Searching for meaning. *International Journal of Nursing Studies, 39*(5), 495–505.

Omeri, A., & Hamilton, H. (1996). Transcultural nursing: Fact or fiction in multicultural Australia. In A. Omeri & E. Cameron-Traub (Eds.), *Transcultural nursing in multicultural Australia* (pp. 37–52). Canberra, Australia: Royal College of Nursing.

Omeri, A., Lennings, C., & Raymond, L. (2004). Hardiness and transformational coping in asylum seekers: The Afghan experience. *Diversity in Health and Social Care, 1*(1), 21–30.

Omeri, A., Lennings, C., & Raymond. L. (2006). Beyond asylum: Implication for nursing and healthcare delivery for Afghan refugees in Australia. *Journal of Transcultural Nursing, 17*(1), 30–39.

Omeri, A., Malcolm, P., Ahern, M., & Wellington, B. (2003). Meeting the challenges of cultural diversity in the academic settings. *Nurse Education in Practice, 3*(1), 5–22.

Papadopoulos, I. (2006). *Transcultural health and social care: Development of culturally competent practitioners.* London: Churchill Livingstone.

Pinikahana, J., Manias, E., & Happell, B. (2003). Transcultural nursing in Australian curricula. *Nursing and Health Sciences, 5*(2), 149–154.

Pittman, L., & Rogers, T. (1990). Nursing: A culturally diverse profession in a monocultural health system. *The Australian Journal of Advanced Nursing, 8*(1), 30–38.

Pratt, R. (1995). *Australian nursing: Illuminating—illuminating. Forty-third annual oration.* Sydney, Australia: New South Wales College of Nursing, Australia.

Purnell, L. D., & Paulanka, B. J. (2008). *Transcultural health care: A culturally competent approach.* Philadelphia, PA: F. A. Davis.

Ray, M. R. (1994). Book review [Review of *Nursing and nursing education in multicultural Australia,* by J. D'Cruz & G. Tham]. *Journal of Transcultural Nursing, 5*(2), 44–45.

Tham, G., & Royal Melbourne Institute of Technology, Faculty of Nursing. (1993). *Culturally sensitive nursing management: Developing a patient profile.* Faculty of Nursing, RMIT Bundoora Campus, Bundoora, Vic.

The United Nations, Office of the United Nations High Commissioner for Refugees. (1951). The 1951 Convention relating to the Status of Refugees. Retrieved from http://www.unhcr.org/pages/49da0e466.html

World Health Organization. (1978, September 6–13). Report of the International Conference on Primary Health Care, Alma-Ata, USSR, sponsored jointly with the United Nations Children's Fund. Geneva, Switzerland: Author. Retrieved from http://www.who.int.hpr/NPH/docs/declaration_almaata.pdf

Application of Culture Care Theory to International Service-Learning Experiences in Kenya

Linda D'Appolonia Knecht
Colleen Knecht Sabatine

> *It is impossible to provide culturally congruent care without first understanding the culture of the people you are caring for.*
> —(U.S. nursing student in Kenya)

INTRODUCTION

In a global society, it is imperative that nurses develop the values, beliefs, and practices necessary to provide nursing care that is culturally congruent within their professional nursing practice. International service-learning experiences provide opportunities for nursing students to develop cultural understanding and competency, grow personally and professionally, and become engaged citizens within a multicultural society. As one student reflected upon returning from an international service-learning course to Kenya:

> I have never been outside the U.S. and believe that the learning that happened on this trip has developed a call within me to continue to

have a service-driven heart and a new sense of citizenship not only back here in the U.S. but as a global citizen. (student comment 1)

In response to rapid globalization and an increased focus on global health, universities are expanding opportunities for students to engage in international study. Semester or year-long study-abroad programs have been the traditional design of international experiences for students. Nevertheless, there is growing interest in short-term experiences, particularly in disciplines such as nursing, where longer engagement in international study poses time and financial challenges (Donnelly-Smith, 2009). Faculty-led, short-term immersion service-learning experiences in international settings are a valuable curricular design that provides opportunities to expand students' worldviews and advance their knowledge, skills, and values related to globalization and cultural care.

This chapter provides a reflection of a journey by a faculty member and a former nursing student in the development and implementation of international service-learning experiences in Kenya for nursing students from a mid-sized Midwestern university in the United States. This process has been enhanced and enriched by integrating the constructs of Leininger's (1997, 2002b, 2002c, 2006a, 2006b, 2006c) Theory of Culture Care Diversity and Universality (also known as the culture care theory (CCT)) to guide planning; implementing (pre-travel, intra-travel, and post-travel); and evaluating international service-learning elective courses. Integral to the culture care theory is the focus on diversity and commonalities in culture and care (Leininger, 1997). Leininger's Sunrise Enabler depicts multiple social structure dimensions of the theory that influence and explain health and wellbeing.

REVIEW OF THE LITERATURE

With increased globalization and a growing need for nurses to care for people of diverse cultures at home and abroad, there has been an expanded focus on the development of cultural competencies in undergraduate and graduate nursing education programs. The expectation of cultural competency as an essential component in nursing education is supported by multiple U.S. organizations, including the American Association of Colleges of Nursing (2008a, 2008b, 2009), the American Association of Community Health Nursing Educators Education Committee (2009), the National League for Nursing (2009), and the National League for Nursing Accrediting Commission (2008). Nursing standards of practice and codes of ethics address expectations regarding cultural competency in nursing practice and are used to guide nursing education (American Nurses Association, 2004; Douglas et al., 2011; International Council of Nurses, 2006).

Nursing programs continue to seek effective strategies to support nursing students to develop the attitudes, knowledge, and skills needed to provide culturally congruent care. The wide variety of strategies utilized in nursing education include case studies; simulations; readings; multimedia and other presentations; role play; self-reflection exercises and projects; guided local, national, and international clinical/experiential experiences; and others (American Association of Colleges of Nursing, 2008c; Grant & Letzring, 2003). International study provides opportunities for unique multicultural and cross-cultural learning experiences. Understanding the value and contribution of various educational strategies in the development of cultural competencies of nursing students is a needed—and therefore recommended—focus for future research (Grant & Letzring, 2003; Kardong-Edgren & Campinha-Bacote, 2008).

International educational experiences are recognized as a valuable strategy to enhance cultural understanding and clinical practices; however, traditional semester-long study-abroad courses can be challenging to fit into nursing curricula. Increasingly, nursing programs are choosing to offer short-term experiences to provide students with international study experiences. Designing international experiences with a service-learning perspective provides an additional dimension to learning. Service-learning is defined as ". . .a teaching and learning strategy that integrates meaningful community service with instruction and reflection to enrich the learning experience, teach civic responsibility, and strengthen communities" (National Service-Learning Clearinghouse, n.d.). Service-learning experiences are developed through collaborative efforts between the academic and community institutions, ". . .relying upon partnerships meant to be of mutual benefit" (Gelmon, Holland, Driscoll, Spring, & Kerrigan, 2006, p. v). The inclusion of service-learning enriches the international experience by directly engaging students with individuals in the community. The service-learning experience described in this chapter is supported by the constructs of the cultural care theory which provides a guiding framework for faculty and nursing students seeking to understand cultural, healthcare, and nursing needs from the insiders' perspective of the healthcare system and local communities in Kenya. Culturally congruent care experiences have therefore been planned and implemented collaboratively with members from the local Kenyan communities visited.

Research evidence supports that engagement in short-term immersion international service-learning experiences enhances the cultural competence of students and the discovery of similar and diverse student outcomes that have been reported using anecdotal evidence and quantitative and qualitative methodologies (Amerson, 2010, 2012; Casey & Murphy, 2008; Green,

Comer, Elliot, & Neubrander, 2011; Jones, Ivanoc, Wallace, & VonCannon, 2010). Cultural competency prior to and following international service-learning experience has been measured by a number of different surveys. Amerson (2010) noted that undergraduate nursing students completing a community health clinical experience that integrated service-learning projects (domestic and abroad) demonstrated increased cultural competency based on results from surveys using Jeffreys' (2006) Transcultural Self-Efficacy Tool (TSET). Bentley and Ellison (2007) reported students who completed an elective international service-learning course showed improved scores on the Inventory for Assessing the Process for Cultural Competence Among Health Care Professionals developed by Campinha-Bacote (as cited in Bentley & Ellison, 2007). Green et al. (2011) noted increased student competency scores on the Cultural Competence Behavior Scale of the Cultural Competence Survey (Schim, Doorenbos, Miller, & Benkert, 2003) following an international service-learning experience.

Through international educational experiences, nursing students have had opportunities to study constructs of the culture care theory and the values, beliefs, and practices used to provide culturally congruent care (Allen, Berry, Knecht, & Whitehill, 2012). Leininger (1997) emphasized the importance of having students reflect on knowing and examining their own cultural values, beliefs, and practices as well as their cultural biases and ethnocentric views. In a study by Fennel (2009), students responding to a survey following an international study abroad program indicated that the experience broadened their worldview. Other students completing international experiences have reported personal growth (Kollar & Ailinger, 2002; Zorn, 1996) including reexamination of their own values and personal biases (Haloburdo & Thompson, 1998; Ryan, Twibell, Brigham, & Bennett, 2000).

The literature reports increased student awareness of both cultural similarities and differences following international study (Casey & Murphy, 2008; Haloburdo & Thompson, 1998; Ryan et al., 2000). Through these international experiences, students recognize similarities and discover diverse ways of caring, particularly in environments with limited resources (Bosworth et al., 2006; Casey & Murphy, 2008; Green et al., 2011; Haloburdo & Thompson, 1998; Jones et al., 2010). Being immersed in a different culture provides students with opportunities to learn the effect of these dimensions toward influencing health and care. Students completing academic international experiences have reported expanded knowledge regarding social and environmental factors influencing health and wellbeing (Haloburdo & Thompson, 1998; Jones et al., 2010) and increased confidence in integrating culturally competent nursing practices in the care of diverse cultures (Bosworth et al., 2006; Haloburdo & Thompson, 1998; Kollar & Ailinger, 2002).

PURPOSE AND RATIONALE

The purpose of this chapter is to provide examples of how the culture care theory can be used for planning, implementing, and evaluating international service-learning courses. Using the culture care theory as the guiding framework in an international service-learning course provides students with opportunities to gain cultural competence congruent with the purpose of the cultural care theory which Leininger (2006a) has stated is "... to discover, document, know and explain the interdependence of care and culture phenomena with differences and similarities between and among cultures" (p. 4). Immersion experiences such as the Kenyan service-learning course allow students to use a naturalistic process of open discovery in a largely unknown environmental context to discover, document, know, and explain diverse cultural lifeways and care values, beliefs, and practices.

Students are provided opportunities to develop cultural holding knowledge and explore diverse worldviews. Foremost, students explore the ethnohistory of the many cultures that coexist in Kenya. As the course progresses, students explore their own worldviews and lifeways which leads to the discovery of common and diverse care views, values, and beliefs. Students are then prepared and encouraged to discover, compare, and document the culture care expressions, beliefs, and practices from their own cultures and the diverse Kenyan cultures.

HISTORICAL BACKGROUND

The Department of Nursing at a Midwestern university in the United States and St. Mary's Mission Hospital system in Kenya, along with an associated Kenyan high school, have built a partnership over a 5-year period based on commitment, respect, and caring as the foundation for the alliance. The ability to build trusting and working relationships, value various perspectives, and appreciate cultural similarities as well as differences supports partnership development. Successful international partnerships are sustained not only by the goals of individual partners but also by the establishment of shared goals.

To explore and initiate the development of a partnership with the St. Mary's Mission Hospital organization, two nursing faculty members from the Midwestern university first traveled to Kenya. In the following year, the principal nurse tutor from the Kenyan mission hospital came to the university in the United States. During these two initial exchanges, caring relationships were developed. There was expanded appreciation, knowledge, and respect with regard to the social structures and environmental contexts influencing health and wellbeing, care, nursing education, and the nursing profession in each culture.

In subsequent years, five faculty-led, short-term elective international courses have been implemented, with additional courses planned. Undergraduate and graduate students engage in clinical, educational, and cultural experiences at St. Mary's rural and urban hospitals, the affiliated high school, outreach clinics, and local orphanages. A variety of cultural excursions provide further opportunities for cultural exchanges and learning. Nursing faculty and students continue to work to discover, document, know, and explicate the universal and diverse culture care expressions of the Kenyan people served by the mission organization in order to gain insight into culturally congruent care. Partnership and course development are evolving processes aimed toward strengthening the partners' mutual understanding of their cultural care expressions, beliefs, values, and practices. It is also a mutual goal to enhance learning outcomes for nurses from Kenya and the United States and to minimize cultural pain, imposition, and unintended negative outcomes.

COURSE DEVELOPMENT FOCI

The course development foci were developed around the following reflective points:

- Use of the Theory of Culture Care Diversity and Universality as a framework to guide the development of Kenyan international service-learning courses
- Integration of the Theory of Culture Care Diversity and Universality and ethnonursing research method into the student experiences during the Kenyan international service-learning course
- Observations of diverse cultural expressions, values, beliefs, worldviews, lifeways, and culture-specific care practices by Kenyan and U.S. staff, patients, students, and nurses throughout the experience of the service-learning course

THEORETICAL FRAMEWORK

Use of the Theory of Culture Care Diversity and Universality (culture care theory) as a guiding framework for international service-learning experiences allows for open discovery of care and culture. Students are challenged to discover worldviews through exploration of culture care universalities and diversities (Leininger, 2006a). Guided by faculty, students use the culture care theory and elements of the ethnonursing research method to discover, document, and explain care differences and commonalities observed throughout the experience.

Orientational definitions are incorporated in the pre-travel teaching and preparation, intra-travel experiences and discussion, and the post-travel reflection and documentation. The following orientational definitions from Leininger's culture care theory have been adapted for use within the service-learning course to facilitate students to discover, document, know, and explain Kenyan cultures, lifeways, worldviews, and care practices:

- *Care*: The concept of care is abstract, yet concrete, with elements of assistive, supportive, and enabling efforts that benefit the health and lifeways of those encountered during service-learning courses in Kenya (adapted from Leininger, 2006a, p. 12).
- *Culture*: Observed and shared ideas, decisions, and actions fundamental to the lifeways, values, beliefs, and norms of the Kenyan and U.S. cultures which are shared, learned, and transmitted during service-learning courses (adapted from Leininger, 2006a, p. 13).
- *Generic/folk or emic care*: The traditional, indigenous, or tribal care values, beliefs, and practices that are cultural influencers on health beliefs, illness, and wellness evidenced throughout the Kenyan service-learning course experiences (adapted from Leininger, 2006a, p. 14).
- *Professional or etic care*: The care knowledge and practices of students, educators, and healthcare providers from the United States, as well as the Kenyan healthcare providers, educators, and leaders, that have been learned through institutional or formal educational processes (adapted from Leininger, 2006a, p. 14).
- *Ethnohistory*: The past and present facts, events, and instances including, but not limited to, past colonialism; political and tribal conflicts; environmental and resource issues; endemic disease prevalence; and ongoing efforts to deal with significant poverty that have influenced the lifeways and cultural care expressions, values, beliefs, and practices of the Kenyan people and which continue to affect their health and wellbeing (adapted from Leininger, 2006a, p. 15).
- *Culturally congruent care*: Care knowledge, decisions, and actions that not only improve health and wellbeing or prevent illness and disability, but also are sensitive to and harmonious with the cultural care values, beliefs, and practices of those encountered through St. Mary's Mission Hospital organization (adapted from Leininger, 2006a, p. 15).
- *Culture shock*: [The experience of a] student, faculty member, or Kenyan who is unsettled or unable to respond appropriately to a situation because the views, practices, or lifeways expressed, encountered, or observed are conflictingly strange and unfamiliar. Cultural shock is experienced in a variety of ways when a person is unable to

know what to say or how to act in a situation that is shocking to them (adapted from Leininger, 2002b, p. 50).

- *Ethnocentrism*: "Refers to the belief that one's own ways are the best, most superior, or preferred ways to act, believe, or behave" (Leininger, 2002b, p. 50).
- *Western cultures and values*: "Refers to those cultures that value and use modern technologies and that are industrialized. Western cultures are known for their emphasis on being efficient and using scientific equipment that makes them *progressive* or *modern*" (Leininger, 2002b, pp. 50–51).
- *Non-Western cultures and values*: "Refers to those cultures that have traditional values and lifeways and rely less on modern technologies. Non-Western cultures have a rich, traditional philosophy of life that is supported by symbols, beliefs, and different patterns of living and dying" (Leininger, 2002b, p. 50).
- *Cultural imposition*: "Refers to the tendency of an individual or group to impose their beliefs, values, and patterns of behavior on another culture for varied reasons" (Leininger, 2002b, p. 51).
- *Cultural pain*: "Refers to the suffering, discomfort, or being greatly offended by an individual or group who shows a great lack of sensitivity toward another's cultural experience" (Leininger, 2002b, p. 52).

The Sunrise Enabler (illustrated in the *Leininger's Enablers for Use with the Ethnonursing Research Method* chapter) is a pictorial representation of the culture care theory ". . .used as a major guide . . . to explore comprehensive and multiple influencers on care and culture" (Leininger, 2006a, p. 24). Students are challenged to discover ways to provide culturally congruent care and are encouraged to use Leininger's Sunrise Enabler with the three care modes of action and decision which are:

- *Culture care preservation and/or maintenance*: "Refers to those assistive, supportive, facilitative, or enabling professional actions and decisions that help people of a particular culture to retain, preserve, or maintain beneficial care values and lifeways for their wellbeing, to recover from illness, or to deal with handicaps or dying" (Leininger, 2002c, p. 84).
- *Culture care accommodation and/or negotiation*: "Refers to the assistive, accommodating, facilitative, or enabling professional actions and decisions that help people of a designated culture (or subculture) to adapt to or to negotiate with others for meaningful, beneficial, culturally congruent, and safe care for health and wellbeing or to deal with illness or dying" (Leininger, 2002c, p. 84).

- *Culture care repatterning and/or restructuring*: "Refers to the assistive, supportive, facilitative, or enabling professional actions and decisions that help clients reorder, change, or modify their lifeways for new, different, and beneficial healthcare patterns, practices, or outcomes" (Leininger, 2002c, p. 84).

Theoretical assumptions of the culture care theory are also useful when adapted to guide faculty and students in the process of developing cultural competencies through international learning experiences. In addition, culturally competent care needs to be evidence based. According to Melnyk and Fineout-Overholt (2011), the use of "...*evidence-based theories* [emphasis added] (i.e., theories that are empirically supported through well-designed studies) also should be included as evidence" (p. 5), which also includes the Theory of Culture Care Diversity and Universality. Select theoretical assumptions from the culture care theory have, therefore, been integrated into the international service-learning experience in Kenya; these are:

- "Care is the essence and the central dominant, distinct, and unifying purpose in nursing" (Leininger, 2006a, p. 18).
- Commonalities and diveralities exist between the U.S. and Kenyan care expressions, meanings, patterns, and practices (adapted from Leininger, 2006a, p. 18).
- Care values, beliefs, and practices are influenced by and rooted in the worldview, social structure factors, ethnohistorical, and environmental contexts of the people cared for within the context of the Kenyan service-learning course (adapted from Leininger, 2006a, p. 19).
- Generic (emic) and professional (etic) care practices can be discovered and integrated into the provision of culturally congruent care within the St. Mary's Mission Hospital system in Kenya (adapted from Leininger, 2006a, p. 19).
- "Culturally congruent and therapeutic care occurs when culture care values, beliefs, expressions, and patterns are explicitly known and used appropriately, sensitively, and meaningfully with people of diverse or similar cultures" (Leininger, 2006a, p. 19).

Components of the culture care theory including orientational definitions, the Sunrise Enabler, the three modes of care action and decision, and specified or adapted theoretical assumptions are beneficial to faculty and students engaging in the Kenyan service-learning experience. The process of discovery, documentation, and explanation of Kenyan cultures, lifeways, worldviews, and care practices is not accomplished solely during the immersion period of the service-learning experience, but also along the continuum of experiences before and after travel.

THE COURSE SEQUENCE

The planning, implementation, and evaluation processes for the international service-learning nursing course in Kenya may be applicable and adaptable to other programs and other international experiences. Planned educational activities from pre-travel through post-travel are supported by Koskinen and Tossavainen (2004) who noted that the findings of their study ". . .underline the importance of considering an international exchange programme as a continuum consisting of orientation, study abroad, and reentry debriefing" (p. 119) to support development of cultural competencies. Examples of assignments and course activities during pre-travel, intra-travel, and post-travel from the Kenyan service-learning course sequence are described.

Course Planning

Grant and Letzring (2003) reported on the shortage of faculty expertise in transcultural nursing necessary to support nursing students' development of cultural competencies. As with other faculty who may be planning or implementing an international educational experience, the faculty member who developed the elective nursing course in Kenya had not participated in an international course as part of her nursing education nor had she been formally educated in transcultural care. Multiple faculty development resources were utilized to develop and implement the international service-learning course. During the initial planning phases, faculty efforts focused on extensive preparatory readings related to international service-learning, transcultural care, culture care theory, and global health. The course faculty member attended multiple conferences related to international health and international education networking, learning from the expertise of other nursing faculty experienced in international study and transcultural care nursing.

In preparing to lead an international nursing course, it was important to gain holding knowledge specific to the culture and setting of the intended educational experience. The Sunrise Enabler provided a framework to guide understanding of the cultural, social structural, environmental, and historical contexts influencing the health and wellbeing of Kenyans in addition to the professional status of nursing and the healthcare system in Kenya. Kenyan books, journal articles, online newspapers, and other relevant literature by Kenyan authors as well as by non-Kenyan authors were read or reviewed. Kenyan faculty and students provided additional information and understanding regarding their country of origin. Internet websites for the Kenyan embassy, the Centers for Disease Control and Prevention, the World Health Organization, the U.S. Department of State, YouTube, and others were accessed as resources by faculty and students to increase holding knowledge about the nation, people, and culture of Kenya.

In addition to gaining cultural knowledge, it is important to evaluate one's own values, beliefs, attitudes, and biases when developing cultural competencies (Andrews & Boyle, 2008; Leininger, 2006c). A faculty-only immersion experience (without students) provided opportunities for examination of their own worldviews, cultural biases, ethnocentrisms, and cultural competencies. Throughout the initial visit, the focus was on gaining an understanding of the similarities and differences among the cultures of the United States and Kenya and their unique cultural expressions of caring, nursing practices, nursing education, and health care. Collaborative planning for future student experiences by U.S. and Kenyan nurse educators, administrators, and others directly involved in the course development and implementation partnership emerged based on their mutual understanding of the mission and goals; respect for similarities and differences; and sharing of resources and decision making.

Key constructs of the culture care theory were integrated into the course syllabus, objectives, and assignments. The following course description includes a focus on culture, care, and culturally congruent practices:

> This course provides the student an international academic service-learning experience working with the various cultural backgrounds of the people of Kenya. The student will travel for two to three weeks to underserved areas of Kenya. The student will apply the culture care theory and/or other transcultural nursing models while participating in academic and service-learning activities. Students will participate in direct care and teaching activities in hospitals, clinics, health centers, schools and other settings with culturally diverse populations. Emphasis is on exploration of care, culture, cultural interchanges with Kenyans, provision of nursing care, and a focus on culturally congruent nursing practice. (University of Michigan–Flint, 2013, p. 2)

Course objectives further support the application of the culture care theory and include the following:

- Apply culture care theory and/or other transcultural nursing models to the provision of nursing care in diverse healthcare settings
- Incorporate an understanding of influences of culture and diversity, various healing modalities, diverse beliefs regarding health/illness, and diverse ways of caring in providing culturally appropriate care
- Utilize the process of creative and critical thinking to develop strategies and adapt clinical skills to address issues of scarce resources, social injustice, health disparities, and/or ethical dilemmas while

    providing care to individuals served by St. Mary's Mission Hospital and associated schools and orphanages

- Demonstrate strategies for effective verbal and nonverbal communication techniques, including the use of translators
- Develop an awareness of the environmental, educational, economic, political, legal, kinship, spiritual, ethical, social structure, and kinship factors affecting the health and wellbeing of the people of Kenya
- Reflect on the relationships between learning, service, and global citizenship
- Accept responsibility for examining one's own value system within the role of the professional nurse and global health needs
- Identify ways to integrate lessons learned regarding transcultural care in Kenya to nursing practice in the United States (University of Michigan–Flint, 2013, p. 4)

Course Implementation

Recruitment of students for an international travel course includes developing a written course overview for distribution through email, in flyers, and at informational meetings. The course overview provides an opportunity for faculty to state the foci of the course design related to service-learning and to explicate content about the culture care theory. Dimensions of the Sunrise Enabler are used to provide students with an overview of the course context. A brief ethnohistory of the mission hospital system in Kenya is provided. Use of theoretical constructs such as care, culture, cultural diversities and commonalities, and culturally congruent care are integrated into the overview. Through this overview, students begin to understand that the foci of the course are learning about cultural diversities and similarities and the provision of culturally congruent care using a service-learning approach.

    Students are invited to informational meetings which allow faculty to provide more in-depth descriptions and engage in discussions about the course context than is possible in a two- to three-page written overview. During these informational meetings, the history of the ongoing partnership with the mission hospital in Kenya and the importance of building a sustainable collaboration are emphasized. Cultural artifacts such as pictures, craftwork, and clothing are displayed. A student PowerPoint presentation from a previous excursion is shown to the prospective students. This presentation reflects the environmental context of the course, examples of care experiences, and visual representations of cultural diversities and commonalities. Previous course alumni are invited to the informational meetings to share their own past student perspectives.

As part of the application process, interested students are asked to a write short essay about their motivation or rationale for wanting to participate in the Kenya course and why they would be a suitable candidate. Faculty members subsequently interview each applicant in person or by telephone. Prospective students examine their worldviews and personal goals, first through written and verbal application processes, and later with preparatory assignments and activities. Each student reflects about his or her personal strengths and any apprehensions that may bear upon the experience. About being open and ready to engage in the international experience, one student stated:

> Traveling to another country and being immersed in their culture is the best way to learn about cultural competence and it is a very humbling thing. Your perceptions of your own daily life are changed when you live a day in the life of someone else so different. I look forward to going from an outsider, there to learn and grow about different places and different people, to an insider participating in the growth and learning of the people in the community by focusing on our similarities. This experience will touch me and change me in a way that no [other] class can. It will shape me into the healthcare professional that I will be in just 8 more months! And because of the experience, the people that I meet, and the way my perceptions will change, I will be that much more of a resource to my community. . . (student comment 2)

Pre-travel

Pre-travel preparation is an important component of international educational experiences and supports enhanced student experiences and outcomes, including growth in cultural competencies. Structured assignments and preparatory activities during the pre-travel time period are designed to support students' reflections about their own cultures, values, beliefs, and biases. These assignments and activities enable students to develop skills in recognizing and appreciating cultural similarities and diversities; identifying factors influencing health and wellbeing; and exploring care expressions, values, beliefs, and practices across cultures. Pre-travel preparation begins upon selection of students and continues until their arrival in the international setting, typically occurring over a period of one or two academic semesters prior to travel. One academic course credit is assigned to the pre-travel phase in recognition of the time commitment required for preparation.

Students selected to participate in the international elective course engage in both structured and independent pre-travel preparation during which time they design and lead classroom presentations about Kenya. Leininger's Sunrise Enabler provides a framework for the topics covered which include geographical/environmental context; ethnodemographics, cultural values, and languages; history and political system; educational, religious, and spiritual factors and influences; legal and economic factors; technological factors; and healthcare system/care practices, major health challenges, and diseases. Previous students have been creative in their presentations, using audio and video clips, web resources, and other ways to explore and share aspects of the Kenyan culture prior to travel. The influences of these lessons are reflected in the post-presentation discussions about diverse expressions of health and wellbeing and some of the anticipated care experiences. All PowerPoint presentations and course overviews are posted on the university's electronic interface [BlackBoard] which serves as a repository for the course documents and as a means to build holding knowledge of the Kenyan culture. Classroom presentations are enriched when alumni from previous trips and/or individuals from Kenya attend and participate in the discussions. Faculty members also have provided traditional Kenyan foods for students to sample at these gatherings.

In addition to the group sessions, other student pre-travel expectations include independent preparatory work (refer to the list on the electronic database) geared toward gaining an understanding and appreciation of cultural and social structure factors that influence the health and wellbeing of the diverse peoples of Kenya. Learning strategies include recommended readings and review of multimedia content. Readings from the culture care theory and transcultural nursing, professional nursing literature, and a wide range of academic disciplines are used to support students' preparation. The cultural and social structure dimensions within the Sunrise Enabler provide the framework for the development of the preparatory reading list and other activities.

Language preparation is not a requirement for the course but is encouraged. Both English and the national language Kiswahili are official languages in Kenya. English is the primary language in the Kenyan educational system; thus students and faculty can usually communicate well with the nurses, doctors, students, and staff at St. Mary's. However, many of the hospital patients and younger orphans do not communicate well in English; most often they speak in Kiswahili which for them may be a second language with their tribal language as primary. Students and faculty participating in the Kenyan service-learning experience are provided with fundamental resources and reference cards containing some essential Kiswahili. As it is culturally regarded as a sign of respect for outsiders to use basic Kiswahili greetings and phrases when in Kenya, gaining some familiarity with the indigenous language and other customs is integrated into the students' pre-travel preparation.

Initiating the pre-travel phase one or two semesters prior to traveling allows students time to seek funding support for the cost of the course. In the past, students have applied for scholarships to partially cover these costs; some have also performed independent and group fundraising. Activities such as fundraising, applying for scholarships, obtaining supplies, and securing donations also provide students with opportunities for reflection and discussion about their motivations for participating in the course and their anticipations about experiential service-learning. The pre-travel phase is brought to a close with a final "packing party." This event is a gathering of faculty, students, and supportive family members and friends who assist with organizing and packing supplies, donations, and other items which will be used or distributed during the course travel period. Additionally, this event provides an opportunity for students and supporters to have any final questions answered, express feelings and personal bonds, and further develop the team spirit being shared.

Pre-travel preparation must be adjusted to fit the schedules of the students and faculty. Barriers such as physical location, timing of activities, and other commitments can complicate the pre-travel phase of an international service-learning course. Pre-travel planning, preparatory activities, and meetings are essential to provide students and faculty with opportunities to enhance self-reflection and build holding knowledge as the basis for a meaningful learning experience in Kenya. The pre-travel period is an important course component contributing to the development of cultural competencies throughout the international service-learning course.

Intra-travel

Nursing students spend 2 to 3 weeks with nursing faculty during the intra-travel portion of the international service-learning elective course. Students are afforded a variety of clinical opportunities while in Kenya which reflect adaptations to the capacities of the individual site locations and also allows for the areas with the greatest need to be served. There are similarities and differences within each course that permit such flexibility along with continuity for projects that have been mutually planned by nursing faculty from the United States and their Kenyan colleagues. Clinical experiences include providing inpatient and outpatient care at St. Mary's Mission Hospital, health exams, screening, and health education and promotion activities at a high school for destitute and/or orphaned children, orphanages, and outreach clinics.

During the international experience, students provide care, share meals, and participate in cultural excursions together with colleagues from the partner mission hospital. These shared experiences have afforded students opportunities for interaction with local care providers and to explore ways in which social structural dimensions (e.g., environment, language, and spiritual factors; economic and political factors; and the ethnohistory of the hospital) influence patient health and wellbeing as well as the functional systems of nursing and health care in Kenya. Nursing students from the United States work directly with Kenyan nurses, physicians, and other healthcare providers at hospital, clinic, and community settings to promote self-learning related to the following theoretical assumption: There are both generic and professional care practices to be discovered and integrated through the provision of culturally congruent care within the St. Mary's Mission Hospital system in Kenya (adapted from Leininger, 2006a, p. 19). Students have frequently commented about the adaptability and the skill of nurses and healthcare providers in administering care in circumstances with limited resources and technology, as expressed by the following observation:

> I watched clinician after clinician, and person after person, provide care using the resources they had. . . . Making the resources available stretch just a little more to help just one more person, they all just did what needed to be done and found ways that I couldn't even begin to imagine to do it. (student comment 3)

In resource-limited healthcare settings, students are provided with opportunities to focus on the dimensions of nursing assessment and care that are less dependent on technology. For example, students have provided care focused on physical comfort measures, appropriate touch, presence, and therapeutic verbal and nonverbal communication. One student wrote:

> I learned how to rely on assessment skills and focus less on technology. This is something that is taught in nursing school again and again but when we go to clinical (in the U.S.), the technology is always there. With this experience, I was truly able to understand . . . [what it means to provide care without reliance on technology]. (student comment 4)

Performing health screening and health promotion care for orphaned and/or destitute children has provided nursing students with opportunities to discover the meaning of health and wellbeing from the perspective of Kenyan students' worldview. It also offers an opportunity to provide culturally congruent nursing care to an ostensibly healthy, albeit vulnerable population. The high school healthcare experience is planned in collaboration with the high school administration and various Kenyan partners. The care provided assists in meeting the health needs of the Kenyan students and provides meaningful learning experiences for the nursing students.

Nursing students encounter such clinical challenges as determining an appropriate course of action and decision when a health screening result indicates the need for treatment or follow-up care that is not readily available or affordable. Students and faculty have worked together with their Kenyan partners to discover culturally congruent care actions within the accessible or available resources.

Graduate students have been assigned to conduct in-depth interviews with clients and Kenyan care providers guided by the Sunrise Enabler and Leininger's Inquiry Guide (Leininger, 2002a, pp. 137–141). This assignment has enabled students to expand their understanding of the worldview and culture care needs of the people interviewed. Subsequently, graduate students have worked together to create a PowerPoint presentation synthesizing their cultural assessment interviews. These syntheses reflect discoveries of cultural similarities and differences regarding care values, beliefs, and practices; assets as well as challenges; and implications for future nursing care.

Nursing students and Kenyan healthcare providers work together to provide health care at urban and rural hospitals, orphanages, and outreach clinics. Students as well as faculty have encountered situations leading to culture shock, such as extremely impoverished living conditions. One student wrote:

> The most difficult part of the journey was the slum orphanage clinic.
> . . . the sheer number of children sleeping in one room was hard to take
> in. These things you hear about or see on television, but in that mo-
> ment standing there seeing it with my own eyes sent pain and helpless-
> ness through my heart. (student comment 5)

Faculty must be prepared to recognize and support students who may be examining and dealing with their emotions, interpretations, and reactions to such experiences as culture shock. Support measures incorporated by faculty in the past have included one or more of the following: Acknowledgement of emotions and feelings; maintaining presence; active listening; assistance with interpreting the situation/events; encouraging journaling, peer support, and group discussion; and encouraging discussion with Kenyan colleagues.

International service-learning experiences provide opportunities for students to examine the concepts of cultural imposition and/or cultural pain. One student wrote:

> It was important when going into the hospital or doing outreach clin-
> ics to remember that things are not done the same way as back home.
> One of the most important things to do was to take cues from Kenyan

> healthcare providers and most importantly your patient. I was very
> conscious of not making the patient or those that I was working with
> [feel] uncomfortable. (student comment 6)

By anticipating the potential for culture shock, cultural imposition, and cultural pain faculty, students, and Kenyan partners work to address immediate situations and minimize negative effects. Informal as well as formal discussions, interactions, and activities between and among faculty, nursing students, and Kenyan care providers provide opportunities to enhance intercultural dialogue, debriefing, and learning. These reflections from diverse perspectives offer insights and understanding related to care experiences, similarities, and differences among and between the respective cultures, and increase awareness of the complex dimensions influencing health, health care, and the nursing profession. The developed partnership has enhanced this reflective process, which is consistent with the theoretical assumption that "...care values, beliefs, and practices are influenced by and rooted in the worldview, social structure factors, ethnohistorical and environmental contexts" (adapted from Leininger, 2006a, p.19). Over the years, a core group of Kenyan doctors, nurses, and staff have become particularly involved and familiar with the nursing students and faculty from the Midwestern university. Because the transition from stranger to friend took place (Leininger, 2006b, p. 51), sensitive issues can be more confidently addressed with one another knowing that a cultural *faux pas* is not intentional and, therefore, does not become a missed opportunity for continued sharing and learning.

As friendships within the partnership have developed, students and faculty are now routinely invited to cultural activities within and outside of the hospital system by Kenyan healthcare providers. Contact information is often exchanged between students, faculty, and Kenyans. This has permitted the development of relationships and interactions—some that have often persisted for years—which in turn have enhanced cultural understandings and strengthened the partnership.

In addition to group reflection activities, students are required to maintain a written reflective journal throughout their time in Kenya. Journaling provides opportunities for self-reflection; exploring emotions and feelings; examining values, beliefs, and practices; and creating connections among service, clinical and cultural experiences, and learning. Instructions for the individual journal include:

> Students are required to create their own individual reflective journal
> regarding their experiences in Kenya. Journals provide a reflection of lessons
> learned, challenges, insights, concerns, and analysis of experiences.

The journal should reflect connections to the course objectives but is not limited to a focus on the course objectives. (University of Michigan–Flint, 2013, p. 6)

Portions of the individual journals are subsequently used post-travel to complete an individual self-analysis paper and to develop a group project about their collective international service-learning experiences which are both then submitted to the faculty.

By experiencing immersion in a culture different than their own, students develop and expand their worldviews, cultural knowledge, and awareness. Students gain and share new understandings and demonstrate skills and competencies related to culture care. Throughout the intra-travel experience, learning is enhanced by the use of the culture care theory to guide exploration and discovery of culture and culture care. The theory provides a guiding framework for the provision of culturally congruent nursing care, intercultural interactions, and individual and group reflections regarding the international service-learning and cultural experiences.

Post-travel

Upon their return from Kenya, students continue to reflect upon their care experiences, the culture that they have left, and the culture to which they are returning. Individual and group coursework is completed during the post-travel period. Individually, students examine and describe their learning through a self-reflection paper based on course objectives and individual goals and objectives. Collectively, students work to produce a PowerPoint presentation, poster, written group journal, YouTube video, photo journal, or other product demonstrating analysis and synthesis of their individual reflections about their cultural and care experiences and learning. In addition to fulfilling a course requirement, these educational products are used for multiple purposes, including conference, student group, and pre-travel informational session presentations, and are shared with the collaborating partners in Kenya.

Faculty and student share contact information and many maintain communication with one another through email, personal meetings, or social media. A post-travel group meeting provides another opportunity for further reflection about their international learning experiences. Students and faculty discuss worldviews, cultural similarities and differences, and how new learning is being or may be applied to current nursing practice and future nursing careers.

Students are asked to share any conflicts and challenges that may have emerged from their international experiences or reentry to their own culture. Students often note their own decreased usage or wastage of resources (water, food, energy) after returning home. Some have provided examples of multiple ways they found to reduce waste and reuse supplies in their clinical settings and have encouraged their clinical colleagues to do the same. Students returning from Kenya have frequently commented on missing the openness and welcoming nature of the Kenyan people. As an example, one student wrote:

> The people of Kenya are some of the most open, and welcoming that I ever met. Coming home and walking by people on the sidewalk or in the store and them not even acknowledging my presence was a little odd for me. (Student comment 7)

Student growth in cultural competency and their enhanced ability to provide culturally congruent care has been evident in verbalizations, observed actions, and written individual and group work. Students gain an appreciation for the development of cultural competencies as an ongoing process rather than a short-term outcome. For example, one student commented, "...I always considered myself a pretty open-minded, culturally competent individual; after the trip to Kenya, I understand how much I still have to learn about the world" (student comment 8). Students have demonstrated evidence of an expanded worldview, attainment of new perspectives on global issues, cultural appreciation, cultural understanding and competence, expanded communication skills, and development as citizens within a multicultural world. They frequently reflect on their commitment to nursing as a profession:

> The process of learning through service in Kenya was a challenging experience, but my cultural awareness was exponentially increased by the end of my trip. . . . My enthusiasm to be a nurse has never been greater since my experiences in Kenya. (student comment 9)

Additional opportunities to reflect and grow from the experience come from sharing examples of the intra-travel experience with others. Family and friends are often anxious to learn of student and faculty experiences. Discussions of the experiences initially aid the student or faculty to establish lasting memories and reflections of the course. Over time, it is anticipated that the nursing students will reflect upon their experiences to enhance the cultural competence they initially developed during the course.

CARE ACTION AND DECISION MODES

Throughout the Kenyan service-learning course, the culture care theory has been used as a guide to discover, evaluate, and implement culture-specific care. University faculty and students and the Kenyans partners benefit from the collaborative partnerships which promote a mutual exchange of culture care beliefs, values, patterns, and practices that lead to the provision of culturally congruent care through the use of the three culture care action and decision modes (preservation and/or maintenance, accommodation and/or negotiation, and repatterning and/or restructuring).

During the travel experience, nurses, doctors, and staff from the Kenyan mission hospital and the university faculty and students share knowledge and mutually discover care values, beliefs, and practices. The mutuality of these exchanges has been shown in student reflections. One student noted, "...I found that staff members at St. Mary's were just as eager to learn what I had to say, as I was of them. It was a constant flow of conversation" (student comment 10). Another student wrote:

> I signed up for this trip thinking to myself, "I can't wait to go help make a small difference in their lives," but never expected for them to get the short end of the stick, because I got so much more from them than I gave. (student comment 11)

The three care modes are used throughout the interactions among the Kenyan healthcare providers, Kenyan people, and the nursing students. Culture care preservation and/or maintenance are used when the students identify and support beneficial professional actions and decisions within the Kenyan health system. An example of a preservation care practice in the St. Mary's Mission Hospital system is the expectation that mothers will stay at the bedside and provide basic care for their young children. Students reflected on the value of this practice for the child, the parent, and the healthcare system. This practice was preserved and/or maintained when Kenyan staff and nursing students supported mothers in the care of their children while in the unfamiliar environment of a hospital.

Culture care accommodation and/or negotiation are those facilitative, safe, and caring professional practices that occur when Kenyan nurses and doctors work side-by-side with nursing faculty and students. Examples of this include hand hygiene practices and the use of universal precautions by nursing faculty and students during direct patient care and the role modeling of these practices. Resources for basic hand hygiene practices and personal protective equipment are not as readily available as in the United States. Thus the university students and faculty learn resourcefulness from the Kenyans' attention and diligence to maximizing resources. University students and faculty soon realize that supplies such as exam gloves and sterile gauze are scarce and, therefore, valuable. Disposable alcohol swabs are expensive and create packaging waste compared to large containers of alcohol and rolls of cotton. During one particular course session, the Kenyan healthcare staff began to demonstrate greater attention to hand hygiene practices and use of universal precautions. The Kenyan nurses and doctors accommodated their hand hygiene practices and universal precautions measures to those role-modeled by U.S. nursing students and faculty, and nursing faculty and students accommodated their care practices after becoming more aware of and resourceful in their use of the limited healthcare supplies available in Kenya.

Working together with Kenyan healthcare clinicians provides opportunities for nursing faculty and students from the United States to learn from practice situations in which outcomes may be improved through culture care repatterning and/or restructuring. For example, the parents of an infant with jaundice were reluctant to allow treatment due to their belief that their child would "die from pneumonia" unless swaddled. Students recognized the need for culture care repatterning and/or restructuring in order to effectively care for the child and family. Students encountered multiple clinical situations in which professional care was sought very late in the disease process, after generic care did not suffice as the sole treatment. Students inquired about how to effectively promote positive care outcomes by integrating culturally appropriate professional care practices with generic care practices at an earlier time.

Further opportunities for nursing students to gain understanding and use culture care repatterning and/or restructuring in their nursing practice occurred while conducting health fairs at St. Mary's high school for orphaned and destitute children. Many of the high school students reported having no previous health screening or preventive health care. The nursing students found it challenging to provide culturally congruent care or to assist the high school students to repattern some of their harmful self-care practices to improve health outcomes discovered during screenings because of the limited resources available. The health fairs also provide the high school students with opportunities to ask questions about such topics as personal care, HIV/AIDS, infectious disease, and sexual health. Many myths and false beliefs on these and other topics have been addressed through the nursing students' efforts to repattern the high school students' knowledge and subsequent generic care practices.

The St. Mary's system in Kenya and the nursing program in Midwestern United States continue to build their partnership based on mutual respect and acceptance of culture care beliefs, values, and practices. Through this alliance, Kenyan care providers, U.S. university faculty, and students continue to have opportunities for expanded learning about one another's traditional and professional healthcare systems. Leininger's (2006c) care action and decision modes provide theoretical guidance to provide care to meet the healthcare needs of diverse individuals, groups, or institutions.

IMPLICATIONS FOR FUTURE COURSES/EXPERIENCES

Personal and professional growth, including development of cultural competency, is a lifelong process. Nursing alumni, practicing nurses, and other healthcare providers have frequently expressed an interest in participating in international nursing or interdisciplinary healthcare experiences. The Theory of Culture Care Diversity and Universality (culture care theory) is a useful guide to plan, implement, and evaluate international service-learning experiences outside of the academic setting.

One of the challenges to implementing an international experience for nursing alumni, practicing nurses, and other healthcare providers is making adaptations during the pre-travel phase. The selection and preparation of students and other participants that take place prior to travel are essential to the overall learning experience, the anticipated culturally congruent care experiences, and the ongoing partnership development. In the academic setting, this preparation is structured and assigned with course credit. Outside of the academic setting, careful consideration is needed to select participants with the commitment to engage in the essential preparation necessary to participate in the international experience in a way that is culturally congruent and supportive of the international partnership.

CONCLUSION

International service-learning experiences are valuable approaches in nursing education to promote and enhance the development of cultural competence. Use of the culture care theory provides a guiding framework to plan, implement, and evaluate international educational experiences. At the conclusion of an international course, one student wrote, "...the difference between learning this [influence of culture and diversity on health and wellbeing] in class and learning it hands-on was that it [international course] made the culture real" (student comment 12).

Through international service-learning experiences, nursing students engage with others in their professional journey toward providing culturally congruent care which is essential for a global society. Students examine culture care theoretical assumptions related to the essence of nursing; commonalities and diversities of care values, beliefs, and practices; and the influence of worldviews, social structure factors, ethnohistorical, and environmental contexts of health. Students explore and implement ways of caring, with a focus on nontechnological aspects of care and are provided opportunities to examine their own worldviews and lifeways as well as those of diverse cultures. They consistently share that their appreciation for and knowledge of human similarities and differences are enhanced. Through immersion in a culture significantly different from their own, students seek to understand multiple cultural dimensions affecting the health and wellbeing of individuals and populations. Students are prepared and challenged to discover, compare, document, and know culture care expressions in other cultures, such as the Kenyan culture, as well as their own. Students express having taken the lessons learned and integrating them into their personal lives, clinical practices, and home cultures after a short-term international service-learning immersion experience. As one student reflected, "This trip has made more changes to me as a person than I am able to write, but I believe actions speak louder than words, so hopefully my changes are evident to those around me" (Student comment 13).

An ongoing challenge is to engage in international learning in a way that is culturally congruent, promotes and sustains partnerships, and advances the nursing profession toward meeting the care needs of people from diverse cultures. The use of the Theory of Culture Care Diversity and Universality (culture care theory) provides a guide to plan, implement, and evaluate such international learning experiences.

DEDICATION

We dedicate this chapter to:

- Family and friends who have encouraged and supported our travel, viewing our world from various perspectives, and the value of life and caring;
- Nursing colleagues Maureen Tippen, for sharing her expertise in developing and implementing international service-learning study for nursing students; Marilyn McFarland for her guidance and gentle teaching of the culture care theory; Margaret Andrews for her administrative support and commitment to transcultural nursing; and, to all the students who have also become our teachers;
- Dr. Rev. Bill Fryda who promoted the initiation of our partnership by saying:
  "Come with a receptive mind to what the experience might offer you, what our staff can teach you, and what you might be able to offer from your own background. Just your presence is what we look forward to. Welcome!"
- Francis Muthiri who has been the cornerstone of our St. Mary's Kenyan partnership.

DISCUSSION QUESTIONS

1. Discuss the potential value of short-term international experiences in promoting the development of cultural competencies in nursing students.
2. Discuss the potential benefits of designing an international experience from a service-learning perspective.
3. Discuss strategies to enhance student readiness to engage in international study during the pre-travel phase of the course.
4. Discuss strategies to integrate the reflective process during the intratravel phase of the course.
5. Discuss strategies to minimize the negative effects of culture shock experienced by immersed students.

REFERENCES

Allen, M., Berry, L., Knecht, C., & Whitehill, D. (2012). *Exploration of developing cultural competencies in nursing students through short-term international immersion course.* Unpublished master's thesis, University of Michigan–Flint.

American Association of Colleges of Nursing. (2008a). Cultural competency in baccalaureate nursing education. Retrieved from http://www.aacn.nche.edu/Education/pdf/competency.pdf

American Association of Colleges of Nursing. (2008b). The essentials of baccalaureate education for professional nursing practice. Retrieved from http://www.aacn.nche.edu/education-resources/baccessentials08.pdf

American Association of Colleges of Nursing. (2008c). Tool kit of resources for cultural competent education for baccalaureate nurses. Retrieved from http://www.aacn.nche.edu/education-resources/cultural-competency

American Association of Colleges of Nursing. (2009). Establishing a culturally competent master's and doctorally prepared nursing workforce. Retrieved from http://www.aacn.nche.edu/education-resources/cultural-competency

American Association of Community Health Nursing Educators Education Committee. (2009, Fall). Essentials of baccalaureate nursing education for entry level community/public health nursing. Retrieved from http://www.achne.org/files/EssentialsOfBaccalaureate_Fall_2009.pdf

American Nurses Association. (2004). Code of ethics for nurses with interpretative statements. Retrieved from http://www.nursingworld.org/codeofethics

Amerson, R. (2010). The impact of service-learning on cultural competence. *Nursing Education Perspectives, 31*(1), 18–22.

Amerson, R. (2012). The influence of international service-learning on transcultural self-efficacy in baccalaureate nursing graduates and their subsequent practice. *International Journal of Teaching and Learning in Higher Education, 24*(1), 6–15.

Andrews, M. M., & Boyle, J. S. (2008). *Transcultural concepts in nursing care* (5th ed.). Philadelphia, PA: Wolters Kluwer/Lippincott, Williams & Wilkins.

Bentley, R., & Ellison, K. J. (2007). Increasing cultural competence in nursing through international service-learning experiences. *Nurse Educator, 32*(5), 207–211.

Bosworth, T., Haloburdo, E., Hetrick, C., Patchett, K., Thompson, M. A., & Welch, M. (2006). International partnerships to promote quality care: Faculty groundwork, student projects, and outcomes. *Journal of Continuing Education in Nursing, 37*(1), 32–38.

Casey, D., & Murphy, K. (2008). Irish nursing students' experiences of service-learning. *Nursing and Health Sciences,10*(4), 306–311. doi: 10.1111/j.1442-2018.2008.00409.x

Donnelly-Smith, L. (2009). Global learning through short-term study abroad. *Peer Review, 11*(4), 12–15.

Douglas, M. K., Pierce, J. U., Rosenkoetter, M., Callister, L. C., Hattar-Pollara, M., Lauderdale, J., . . . Pacquiao, D. (2011). Standards of practice for culturally competent nursing care: A request for comments. *Journal of Transcultural Nursing, 20*(9), 257–269. doi: 10.1177/1043659609334678

Fennel, R. (2009). The impact of an international health study abroad program on university students from the United States. *Global Health Promotion, 16*(3), 17–23. doi: 10.1177/1757975909339766

Gelmon, S. B., Holland, B. A., Driscoll, A., Spring, A., & Kerrigan, S. (2006). *Assessing service-learning and civic engagement.* Providence, RI: Campus Compact.

Grant, L. F., & Letzring, T. D. (2003). Status of cultural competence in nursing education: A literature review. *Journal of Multicultural Nursing & Health, 9*(2), 6–13.

Green, S., Comer, L., Elliott, L., & Neubrander, J. (2011). Exploring the value of an international service-learning experience in Honduras. *Nursing Education Perspectives, 32*(5), 302–307.

Haloburdo, E., & Thompson, M. A. (1998). A comparison of international learning experiences for baccalaureate nursing students: Developed and developing countries. *Journal of Nursing Education, 37*(1), 13–21.

International Council of Nurses. (2006). The ICN code of ethics for nurses. Retrieved from https://www.icn.ch/about-icn/code-of-ethics-for-nurses/

Jeffreys, M. R. (2006). *Teaching cultural competence in nursing and health care.* New York, NY: Springer.

Jones, E. D., Ivanov, L. L., Wallace, D., & VonCannon, L. (2010). Global service-learning project influences culturally sensitive care. *Home Health Care & Management Practice, 22*(7), 464–469. doi: 10.1177/1084822310368657

Kardong-Edgren, S., & Campinha-Bacote, J. (2008). Cultural competency of graduating U.S. bachelor of science nursing students. *Contemporary Nurse, 28*(1-2), 37–44.

Kollar, S. J., & Ailinger, R. L. (2002). International clinical experiences: Long-term impact on students. *Nurse Educator, 27*(1), 28–31.

Koskinen, L., & Tossavainen, K. (2004). Study abroad as a process of learning intercultural competence in nursing. *International Journal of Nursing Practice, 10*, 111–120.

Leininger, M. M. (1997). Classic article: Overview of the theory of culture care with the ethnonursing research method. *Journal of Transcultural Nursing, 8*(2), 32–52.

Leininger, M. M. (2002a). Culture care assessments for congruent competency practices. In M. M. Leininger & M. R. McFarland (Eds.), *Transcultural nursing: Concepts, theories, research, & practice* (3rd ed., pp. 117–143). New York, NY: McGraw-Hill.

Leininger, M. M. (2002b). Essential transcultural nursing care concepts, principles, examples, and policy statements. In M. M. Leininger & M. R. McFarland (Eds.), *Transcultural nursing: Concepts, theories, research, & practice* (3rd ed., pp. 45–69). New York, NY: McGraw-Hill.

Leininger, M. M. (2002c). Part 1. The theory of culture care and the ethnonursing research method. In M. M. Leininger & M. R. McFarland (Eds.), *Transcultural nursing: Concepts, theories, research, & practice* (3rd ed., pp. 71–116). New York, NY: McGraw-Hill.

Leininger, M. M. (2006a). Culture care diversity and universality theory and evolution of the ethnonursing method. In M. M. Leininger & M. R. McFarland (Eds.), *Culture care diversity and universality: A worldwide nursing theory* (2nd ed., pp. 1–41). Sudbury, MA: Jones and Bartlett.

Leininger, M. M. (2006b). Ethnonursing: A research method with enablers to study the theory of culture care. In M. M. Leininger & M. R. McFarland (Eds.), *Culture care diversity and universality: A worldwide nursing theory* (2nd ed., p. 43–81). Sudbury, MA: Jones and Bartlett.

Leininger, M. M. (2006c). Selected culture care findings of diverse cultures using culture care theory and ethnomethods. In M. M. Leininger & M. R. McFarland (Eds.), *Culture care diversity and universality: A worldwide nursing theory* (2nd ed., pp. 281–305). Sudbury, MA: Jones and Bartlett.

Melnyk, B. M., & Fineout-Overholt, E. (2011). *Evidence-based practice in nursing and healthcare: A guide to best practices* (2nd ed.). Philadelphia, PA: Wolters-Kluwer /Lippincott, Williams & Wilkins.

National League for Nursing. (2009). A commitment to diversity in nursing and nursing education. Retrieved from http://www.nln.org/aboutnln/reflection_ dialogue/refl_dial_3.htm

National League for Nursing Accrediting Commission. (2008). NLNAC 2008 standards and criteria: Baccalaureate. Retrieved from http://www.nlnac.org/manuals /SC2008.htm

National Service-Learning Clearinghouse. (n.d). What is service-learning? http://www .servicelearning.org/what-service-learning

Ryan, M., Twibell, R., Brigham, C., & Bennett, P. (2000). Learning to care for clients in their world, not mine. *Journal of Nursing Education, 39*(9), 401–408.

Schim, S. M., Doorenbos, A. Z., Miller, J., & Benkert, R. (2003). Development of a cultural competence assessment instrument. *Journal of Nursing Measurement, 11*(1), 29–40.

University of Michigan–Flint. (2013, Spring). *NUR381: International nursing: Kenya* [Syllabus]. Flint, MI: Department of Nursing, University of Michigan–Flint.

Zorn, C. (1996). The long-term impact on nursing students of participating in international education. *Journal of Professional Nursing, 12*(2), 106–110.

Chapter 16

The Greek Connection: Discovering the Cultural and Social Structure Dimensions of the Greek Culture Using Leininger's Theory of Culture Care: A Model for a Baccalaureate Study-Abroad Experience

Muriel Larson

INTRODUCTION

In her classic article "Overview of the Theory of Culture Care with the Ethnonursing Research Method," Dr. Madeleine Leininger wrote "…care and culture were two phenomena in nursing that had not been formally and systematically studied" (1997, p. 32). She maintained that heretofore culture had not been seen as important and that caring was mostly "a rhetorical cliché," adding, "Care and culture were the invisible and unknown phenomena that had been patently ignored as essential knowledge and skills to advance nursing as a discipline and profession" (p. 32). Leininger also believed that the world was rapidly becoming a "global community" and that by the year 2010, nurses would need to possess knowledge of diverse cultures in order in order to provide culturally congruent care to clients. Her Theory of Culture Care Diversity and Universality and the enablers therein are recognized worldwide as invaluable to the practice of nursing in diverse settings and with diverse populations in the world. The world has, indeed, become a global community, and Leininger's vision for a theory that related culture and care has led the way to establishing the discipline of transcultural nursing (Leininger, 1997).

The focus of this chapter is to share a project that has used Leininger's Theory of Culture Care Diversity and Universality for the past decade with baccalaureate students from the Midwestern United States as a framework for a university/college international travel study-abroad course in Greece for an interim session during the month of January. The purpose of "The Greek Connection: Embracing Transcultural Caring in Ancient and Modern Greece" course is for undergraduate students to gain an understanding of cultural competence. Greece was chosen because of its special interest to the author, who conducts the course. It is also a good starting point for baccalaureate students to understand the roots and history of Western civilization and their significance to U. S. history, not only in the arena of health care but also in regard to the cultural and social structure dimensions of Leininger's Theory of Culture Care Diversity and Universality as depicted in the Sunrise Enabler. In Greece, students can gain an understanding of the roots and history of Western civilization, the similarities and differences in comparison to the history of the United States, and the cultural and social structure dimensions of Leininger's culture care theory (CCT). These dimensions include technological; religious and philosophical; kinship and social; cultural values, beliefs, and lifeways; political and legal; economic; and educational factors along with the expressions, patterns, and practices of culture care.

The level of cultural understanding that students are able to obtain from this course is largely due to the guiding framework of the Theory of Culture Care Diversity and Universality and the Sunrise Enabler used during their first-hand experiences in Greece. As students travel through Greece throughout the month-long course, they work together to explore these cultural and social structure dimensions while gathering data through their observations of and interactions with the Greek people. The students record the data for each dimension in their individual bluebooks and share their results in a formal presentation to Greek students and other invited guests and partners while still in Greece and again at the end of the course to fellow students in the United States. Together, the bluebook and presentations represent a significant portion of the academic course grade. The eyes and minds of the students are opened to the Greek culture throughout this exploration, first with Leininger's culture care theory and the Sunrise Enabler, and later when using the three nursing care modes of decision and action to guide their application of the collected data into practice.

The Greek Connection course content does not require that students actually conduct ethnonursing research or use the ethnonursing research method. However, they are guided toward understanding key constructs of the culture care theory, the three nursing care modes of decision and action, and the meaning of culturally congruent care. Culturally congruent care, according to Leininger (2006a), "…refers to culturally-based care knowledge, acts, or decisions used in sensitive and knowledgeable ways to appropriately and meaningfully fit the cultural values, beliefs, and lifeways of clients for their health and wellbeing, or to prevent illness, disabilities, or death" (p. 15).

Leininger's definition of culturally congruent care incorporated culture care in a way that facilitates a naturalistic and open discovery process, permitting the *emic* (insiders') viewpoints and the *etic* (outsiders') perspectives to come forth. The students understand that they are "outsiders" in the Greek culture as they learn what cultural or generic care practices are valuable to the Greek people and which need to be maintained, negotiated, or changed. They also examine the professional practices that affect care and health outcomes in Greece.

The Greek Connection has its own roots in Sioux Falls, South Dakota, which grew following the author's initial exploration of Greece as a graduate student in 1995, 1998, and 1999. On the premise that Greece would be an exceptional country and culture for baccalaureate students to study using Leininger's Theory of Culture Care Diversity and Universality, the course was developed and submitted to the Curriculum Council at Augustana College, Sioux Falls, and the Board for the Upper Midwest Association for International Education (UMAIE), a consortium for the development of undergraduate courses for international studies. The Greek Connection was offered for the first time in January 2004, and in 2013 the tenth consecutive academic year culminated with more than 200 baccalaureate students having studied in Greece using Leininger's culture care theory.

Over the duration of The Greek Connection course, outstanding partnerships have been developed with nurses and professionals from many places and institutions in Greece. In Athens, these partnerships have included the University of Athens, the Red Cross Hospital, Henry Dunant Hospital, the Technical Educational Institute, and the Athens Medical Group; the hospitals in Amfissa and Argos; and the Hellenic Nurses Association, the University of Crete, and the Community Health Center in Harakas in Crete. Outside the formal partnerships, countless people in Greece have welcomed students from the United States, bringing focus to another enabler from Leininger's culture care theory: Stranger-to-Trusted Friend. By the end of the course and their time in Greece, the students have many new friends and often report that they "know Greece"—a compliment to the people of Greece and to the professionals, institutions, and organizational entities that assisted in their learning process.

THE COURSE IMPLEMENTATION

The purpose of "The Greek Connection: Embracing Transcultural Caring in Ancient and Modern Greece" course is to enhance cultural competence through the acquisition of knowledge and understanding about the Greek culture—a culture that is different from, yet similar to, the student's own— and to share that knowledge and understanding with healthcare students, providers, and other interested people. The first objective in the course is to become culturally competent both personally and professionally through the use of Leininger's Theory of Culture Care Diversity and Universality and the Sunrise Enabler. When approaching cultural competence, Leininger (1991) suggested that nurses "…begin with their own domain of interest or inquiry" (p. 50). Students prepare themselves for the course by reading assigned texts on Greek history and culture, writing a reflection paper about these readings, and developing a site report that they will present in Greece at the subject location.

For the site report assignment, each student is assigned to an archeological site that will be visited while in Greece. The assignments are randomly made well in advance of travel to Greece; each student is required to prepare a researched site report prior to departure. The student must provide each class member and our guide in Greece with a copy of the paper. Students find the time and effort required to complete the assignments pre- and post-travel very rewarding and worthwhile. Once each student arrives at her or his "own site" in Greece, preparatory research and "the story" about that site are shared from an archeological, historical, or mythological/folklore perspective.

The second part of the course provides students with early steps toward developing cultural competence during a 1-month cultural immersion experience in Greece. Through this immersion experience, students acquire cultural knowledge and understanding that are useful in building a network of trusting friendships that exemplify Leininger's belief that the world is a global community. As people are approached and engagement with them takes place, trusting relationships begin to develop. Dialogues and conversations occur that focus on exploring what health and human caring mean to individuals as citizens of a global community. Students learn how values and beliefs are enacted in daily lifeways and quickly discover that cultures are more alike than different, supporting the first tenet of Leininger's theory that people are more similar than different (Leininger, 2006a, p. 18) and her belief that we are all citizens of a global community (Leininger, 2006b, p. 391). Trust is a natural part of caring—genuine caring—which happens when one reaches out and seeks to learn about another's life and what is important to that person in that life.

Students are assigned to groups that meet together in Greece to discuss assigned research articles, primarily from the *Journal of Transcultural Nursing*, such as "Cultural Care of Older Greek Canadian Widows within Leininger's Theory of Culture Care" by Rosenbaum (1990). The students prepare for these conversations while traveling in Greece, first in small groups that facilitate eventual larger group discussion sessions in a "roundtable" format. Students are expected to read all of the assigned articles and to work in their small groups to prepare for and facilitate the large-group discussions, and to develop questions for their fellow classmates to address during the roundtable sessions.

Students enroll in The Greek Connection as an interim session elective. The course is excellent for nursing majors, but is open to interdisciplinary student members who have followed the appropriate admission process as determined by the UMAIE Board and Consortium. Leininger's Theory of Culture Care Diversity and Universality with the Sunrise Enabler have proved to be excellent guides for professionals in all healthcare disciplines to understand social structure dimensions and culture care. Students are provided with an orientation to the course via a webinar that prepares them for the activities they must complete before leaving for Greece in early January.

The description for "The Greek Connection: Embracing Transcultural Caring in Ancient and Modern Greece" is intended to be inviting to the student searching for an exciting way to spend the January interim term. The course description reads as follows:

> Health care as we know it today has its roots deeply embedded in a rich history. Recorded history and myth provide us with much knowledge about health practices that date back to ancient Greece and the Healing Temples of Askelpios. Exploring the contributions of ancient and modern Greece enhances our understanding and appreciation of the

history of health, healing, and wellness. Leininger's Theory of Culture Care provides the theoretical framework for this course. This theory is grounded in cultural anthropology and features broad cultural and social dimensions that offer diverse ways of exploring a culture. These dimensions are technology, religious, and philosophical factors; kinship and social factors; cultural values and lifeways; political and legal, economical and educational factors. Leininger believed that providers of health care must understand the cultural and social factors in order to provide culturally congruent care in a work that has become a "global community" (1997). Using her model, this immersion experience in Greece will provide a student with a deeper understanding of the cultural diversities and similarities that have existed over time, as well as in our present era, not only in matters of health and healing, but in all aspects of daily life. (Augustana College, 2004, pp. 1–2)

The course goals and objectives are stated as:

Goal 1. To experience a cultural immersion experience in Greece.
Objectives: The student will be able to:

- Apply Leininger's Theory of Culture Care Diversity and Universality in a diverse cultural setting, using dialogue with key and general informants, on-site exploration and observation, and participate in structured class activities that highlight the theory.
- Describe the Greek culture through the lens of the Sunrise Enabler.
- Reflect on one's own personal journey as a member of the "global community."

Goal 2. To examine the historical connection between ancient and modern healthcare practices using Leininger's Theory of Culture Care Diversity and Universality with the Sunrise Enabler.
Objectives: The student will be able to:

- Identify specific Greek contributions to health and healing through background research, readings, and visits to ancient sites.
- Compare and contrast modern and ancient healthcare practices in Greece and the United States.
- Gain an appreciation for the heritage that the ancient Greeks left to the Western world. (Augustana College, 2004)

Information from cultural observations, reflections, and notes from conversations or other interactions with the Greek people during their month-long course is recorded by students in their bluebooks along with other subjective and objective data gathered. With Leininger's culture care theory and the Sunrise Enabler, data related to the cultural and social structure dimensions are used to consider specific avenues of transcultural and nursing care modes of decision and action. The Sunrise Enabler is also used as a guide for the student's final presentation at the end of the January term. Discovering the cultural and social structure dimensions in the context of both ancient and modern health care for Greece and the United States gives students, faculty, and Greek partner members' insight into the similarities and differences of each culture as part of the global community. As Leininger (1994) stated:

> . . .knowledge of any culture has become essential today to function with people in diverse cultures and society in general to become and remain an effective nurse. For without such knowledge and sensitivity, nurses will encounter a host of intercultural problems and stressors without understanding the why of the stressors and will be unable to take appropriate actions. (p. 19)

This chapter does not describe a specific ethnonursing research project, but rather provides a narrative of the development of a course guided by the use of Leininger's Theory of Culture Care Diversity and Universality that enhances baccalaureate students' understanding of a culture different from, yet similar to, their own through immersion study in Greece. The course design could be implemented with any culture or in any diverse setting to accomplish many of the same goals and objectives presented.

LET THE SUN RISE: THE SUNRISE ENABLER

Newspaper sports columnist Mitch Albom spent time at Brandeis University with his 78-year-old sociology professor Morrie Schwartz, who was dying from amyotrophic lateral sclerosis, generally known as ALS or Lou Gehrig's disease (www.webmd.com). Morrie reflected:

> The problem, Mitch, is that we don't believe we are as much alike as we are. Whites and Blacks, Catholics and Protestants, men and women. If we saw each other as more alike, we might be very eager to join in one big human family in this world, and to care about the family the way we care about our own. (Albom, 1997, p. 156)

Leininger's research enablers have been very useful for "…teasing out hidden and complex data … through facilitating informants to share their ideas in natural and casual ways" (Leininger, 2006a, p. 24). One of Leininger's enablers is the Sunrise Enabler, "…developed as a conceptual holistic research guide ... to help researchers discover multiple dimensions related to the theoretical tenets of the theory of culture care" (Leininger, 1997, p. 40).

The Sunrise Enabler (**Figure 16-1**) depicts the multifaceted dimensions of culture that are essential for cultural and knowledge and understanding. These factors include technological factors; religious and philosophical factors; kinship and social factors; cultural values and lifeways; political and legal factors; and economic and educational factors. Collectively, they are "...powerful explanatory forces that explain health and wellbeing" (Leininger, l997, p. 36). The students in the Greek Connection course focus on all of these factors during their explorations of the cultural practices in ancient and modern Greece as well as when comparing the United States and Greece. Using the Sunrise Enabler was very helpful to the author in guiding the students through the process of understanding the Greek culture.

The Sunrise Enabler is an excellent guide for baccalaureate students who are beginning their exploration of culture care. The image of the sunrise provides both aesthetic value and holistic application for students; they remember the model. During a month of immersion within the Greek culture, students quickly learn to use the enabler as a guide when meeting

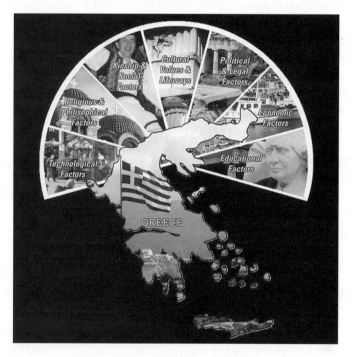

Figure 16-1 Greek social structure model
Adapted from Leininger (2006a). Copyright © M. Larson (2013).

with informants and asking them to share their stories related to their cultural and social values, beliefs, and practices. In Leininger's (1997) well-known statement, "…Let the sun rise figuratively means to have nurses open their minds in order to discover many different factors influencing care and ultimately the health and wellbeing of clients" (p. 40). The theorist reaches to students at intellectual and emotional levels as they reach out to embrace transcultural caring in ancient and modern Greece (Augustana College, 2004).

Data that have been discovered by student cohorts from their experiences while in Greece are presented in the following pages and highlight the social structure dimensions and culture-specific values, beliefs, practices, lifeways, and worldviews of the Greek people and their culture.

Technological Factors

Greece has modern healthcare facilities that use and value technology.

> Large city hospitals (*nosokomeios*) have specialized units that use modern technology for monitoring of patients and diagnosing disease in their laboratories. They have high-tech systems for reaching out into the rural areas of the country to those who have limited access to quality health care. Researchers are connected to each other, not only in Greece but across country boundaries through the use of Internet, Skype, and other high-tech modalities. (personal communication, student A)

> The use of technology in the ancient world was observed at archeological sites where "modern" plumbing is evident, water systems, drainage, storage, and heated baths can be found. Amazing structures for theater, government, and athletics are found through [out] ancient Greece further evidence of the use of technology that has a long and amazing history, preserved for all of history by the Greek people who value and maintain these artifacts for the world through the use of modern technology. (personal communication, student B)

Religious and Philosophical Factors

> Ninety-eight percent of the population in Greece today is Greek Orthodox. Faithful worshippers and fellow believers gather together to share in the sacraments of the church with the Orthodox priest central to the community of believers. Students are introduced to monastic life through visits to monasteries and direct visits with monks and nuns.

Many of the churches and monasteries were built during the Byzantine period and in these peaceful places, students can reflect on the history of the early church as depicted with beautiful and meaningful mosaics of the life and death of Jesus Christ, His disciples, and the Virgin Mary. (personal communication, student C)

Icons can be found in many locations—in hospitals, schools, public places, and, of course, churches. The Greek Orthodox do not believe that Christ should be depicted in anything three-dimensional, and thus, the history and art of iconography is an area of interest to the student studying in Greece. Replicas can be purchased almost anywhere; originals can be enjoyed and admired in the beautiful museums of Athens and of Greece. (personal communication, student D)

In ancient Greece, worship to many gods took place in splendid and huge temples. The importance of religion in the ancient world is evident all around us as we visit the archeological sites. We learn that the ancient people before the time of Christ understood their world through a multi-god system that did not include a personal relationship with one God. Through visiting some of the sites where St. Paul preached, students review the difficult spread of Christianity in Greece, adding understanding in their own spiritual journey. (personal communication, student E)

Kinship and Social Factors

Family life in Greece is very obvious and very important. Historically Greece [sic] families have been strongly patriarchical, however, women have a very important role in family, also, and children are valued as a part of the family. It is not uncommon to see children with their grandparents, and they are open, demonstrative, and caring. Growing old in Greece generally means that you will be cared for by your family, although there is some evidence of the church getting involved in providing for long-term care needs. First and foremost, the family is in charge. Families frequently have owned businesses for decades, and in some cases (such as olive groves) the family may have owned the business for over a century. (personal communication, student F)

Greek people love food and love to be together in the *tavernas* to eat, sing, and dance. Good Greek wine is enjoyed with their meals, and it is not uncommon for a dinner meal to begin late and end even later. Food and fellowship with each other provides a very festive environment, contrary to what we in America might settle for—fast food—eaten quickly! (personal communication, student G)

Cultural Values and Lifeways

The cultural values in Greece are intimately connected to the history of the country and hence, we can learn a great deal about the lifeways of Greece by studying the archeological sites and its remnants of ancient civilization. Family and community life is obvious as we tour each site, following the footsteps of the Mycenaean and Minoan cultures. We also see the struggle that took place to establish and maintain a democracy, a very high value in the history of Greece. Food, family, community, drama, scholarship, health, art are all values in this culture, in ancient times and now. History writes a script for us to learn from and to add to in a setting where all that is a part of freedom is a highly valued and sought after value. (personal communication, student H)

Political and Legal Factors

Greece has a fascinating political history, claiming to have been a democracy for over 2500 years. Gaining or maintaining this freedom is the focal point for many Western civilization classes, embracing such historical events as the Persian War, the Classical Age of Greece, the great thinkers of Greece, the political influence of theater and drama, and the conversations that took place in the *agoras* of major cities. Students can stand where Socrates spoke, see the prison where he drank hemlock, and [where] Paul addressed the Athenians on Mars Hill, with the approval but watchful eye of the government. (personal communication, student I)

Today Greece is a socialistic democracy, influenced by its geography, history, and the strong belief in freedom. Most public institutions are managed through the central government including the Minister of Education and the Minister of Health. Demonstrations are not uncommon in Greece with citizens rising up with their opinions. Occasionally these demonstrations result in destruction or injury, but are never directed toward the tourists who come to Greece. (personal communication, student J)

On several occasions students in the Greek Connection have been invited to meet with government officials and leaders. This affords the students with a rich opportunity to ask questions and receive responses that enable them to make more knowledgeable comparisons between the Greek and

U.S. governments. It has not been uncommon for local and national television stations to film these dialogues for later broadcast. The local newspaper in Crete as well as journalistic entities on the mainland have written about the student visits to Greece and their course activities.

Economic Factors

Greece is currently in a very unstable economic time. This instability does not impact the students who study there directly, [who are] ever treated with hospitality and respect. The last decade has found Greece in debt and struggling to maintain those things that are valuable to its citizens. The outcomes of this debt, the membership in the European Union, and the fate of austerity are yet to be seen. It has been evident that businesses and persons have suffered in all of this, especially in the years since the Olympics of 2004. (personal communication, student K)

The economical activities in Greece include the production of olives and products made from the olive, the production of wine, tourism to this beautiful country, and the continuing hope for a prosperous and peaceful future. Students quickly observed—and taste—the good things that are grown in Greece, and see that obesity is an uncommon entity in a culture that values being out of doors and eating the delicious fruits, vegetables, olives, fish, and so forth. While the Mediterranean diet is perhaps less central today than in the past, these good foods continue to frame the epicurean experience for the student. (personal communication, student L)

Educational Factors

The contributions to education from Greece date back to the scholars of the Classical Age and continue to this present day. Education is highly valued in Greece and most people are guaranteed a good education as a part of a democracy. Admission to a specific program at a university is dependent on one's achievement in the secondary school, so students work very hard to do their best. (personal communication, student M)

It is not uncommon to see parents or grandparents walking their children to school, nor is it uncommon to hear the sounds of children laughing and playing in and around elementary school playgrounds, sounds of children that are recognized around the world and that bring delight to the interested observer. The students in The Greek

Connection are invited to visit the public and private schools upon request, [and to] interact with the students from Greece, who delight in having "important visitors" from the United States of America. Similar to the U.S. today security issues are very important in Greece, [including] protecting children in school from uninvited disturbances. (personal communication, student N)

Scholarly research is a big part of the professional life of physicians, teachers, nurses, etc. Students become familiar with the educational opportunities at the university and post-graduate level. They learn about the studies that have been done or are in process at the University level, and see the connectedness of Greece with the scholarly 'global community' around them. Online exploration can easily connect the Greek Scholars with other scholars around the world. (personal communication, student O)

Nursing Care Modes of Decision and Action

As the students traveling in Greece become more knowledgeable about the social structure dimensions depicted in Leininger's Sunrise Enabler and the culture-specific care values, beliefs, and practices of Greece, they are guided to adjust their data collection efforts toward greater focus on individuals, groups, families, communities, or institutions. In this process, people must be valued, and differences (diversities) and similarities (universalities) must be recognized (Larson, 2000). A mental picture of the Greek culture is developed and students are able to "...tease out embedded or concealed care factors in the social structure factors" (Leininger, 1997, p. 41) that provide a wealth of information that will influence culturally congruent care. Leininger stated that care phenomena have been limited in nursing in the past because identifying and understanding care factors requires "...in-depth discovery in order to grasp the multiple and complex factors influencing care" (p. 41). As Leininger's culture care theory and the Sunrise Enabler become more familiar to students during their month of immersion in Greece, they are able to use both to identify culture care needs in Greece and to consider nursing care decisions and actions. The three modes of nursing care decision and action that the researcher can focus on are culture care preservation and/or maintenance; culture care accommodation and/or negotiation; and culture care repatterning and/or restructuring (p. 41). The following are brief examples of the three nursing care modes of decision and action as they relate to care and caring in the Greek culture.

Culture Care Preservation and/or Maintenance

Students studying in Greece recognize the importance of the culture care preservation and/or maintenance of the antiquities of ancient Greece for the world to appreciate and perhaps visit. Preserving these priceless artifacts comes at a high price to the Greek people, taking up valuable space that might otherwise be used for housing and agriculture in a country that has very limited available land and is locked in by the mountains and the sea. From a social structure perspective, the ethnohistorical, economic, and environmental benefits of maintaining these precious historical pieces of early civilization carry a price the Greek people are willing to pay. The preserved antiquities from the Athens Acropolis are now housed in a new state-of-the-art facility—The Acropolis Museum. Other outstanding museums can be found throughout the mainland, the Peloponnese Islands, and on Crete.

Culture Care Accommodation and/or Negotiation

Professional care decisions and actions involve working toward mutually agreeable culture care solutions for the many healthcare needs for diverse individuals and groups that exist in any country or culture. Negotiation and/or accommodation are important for the health and wellbeing of people in Greece. There is evidence that respiratory and gastrointestinal diseases among Greeks are increasing (World Health Organization [WHO], 2010), a finding that could be attributed to the overall prevalence of air pollution and the high rate of tobacco abuse (smoking) among Greek adults. In 2008, 60% of males and 30% of females were chronic tobacco users (WHO, 2010). Many *tavernas* have adopted no-smoking policies; cooperation with this policy is gaining acceptance, but a great deal of long-term habit change remains to be accomplished. Although research has shown the traditional Mediterranean diet to be nutritionally far superior (Paletas et al., 2010), fast food has permeated much of the world and Greece is no exception (De Vogliab, Kouvonenc, & Gimenod, 2011). According to the 2010 WHO report, negative health effects included elevated blood pressure in 40% of adults; a 20% rate of obesity in both genders; a 60% rate of overweight in males; and 51% rate of elevated cholesterol in males and females. Sedentary lifestyle was reported for 20% of adults, and there was a 58% morbidity rate from cardiovascular disease (WHO, 2010).

Culture Care Repatterning and/or Restructuring

Despite being the richest country in the Balkan region, life in Greece has often been difficult. The economics of the early 21st century have added to the concerns that the Greek people have had about their economic future.

Restructuring a society in such a way that poverty, powerlessness, and discrimination are no longer acceptable should be a goal in every nation. All citizens need to have a sustainable income to provide for their families and run their businesses, and countries need to solve the economic issues that prevent them from providing what is needed to manage the affairs of the state. A major factor in the Greek economic crisis is the large national debt and the shrinking middle class—problems not unfamiliar in the world at large. In the early 21st century, Greece faced major economic restructuring when the historical drachma currency was replaced with the euro, resulting in a 20% drop in the nation's gross domestic product (GDP) after 2007, necessitating an emotional culture care repatterning as well as a social and political one (Anonymous, 2013).

The nursing profession has always concerned itself with taking a leadership role in the changing of human experience. Nurses must continue in this endeavor as they make nursing care decisions and actions to promote culturally congruent care in what most certainly is a "global community" (Leininger, 1997).

CONCLUSION

Leininger predicted in the 1950s that the world would become a global community by 2010, and that all nurses would need to be able to provide culturally congruent care in the 21st century. Her pioneering work in the development of the Theory of Culture Care Diversity and Universality has given nursing a framework and a model that continue to guide transcultural nursing education, research, and practice, equipping nursing students and professional nurses with the knowledge and skills to provide care and caring to diverse people, groups, communities, and institutions.

> Care (caring) is the essence of nursing and a distinct, dominant, central, and unifying focus. Care (caring) is essential for wellbeing, health, growth, survival, and to face handicaps or death. Care (caring) is essential to curing and healing, for there can be no curing without caring. (Leininger, 1997, p. 39)

Dr. Athena Kalokerinou-Anagnostopoulou (2006) stated:

> Nurses must be able to care in culturally competent ways, and in a clinical practice discipline such as nursing there are limitless opportunities for exploring viable options to enrich the practice. Although theoretical knowledge learned from a textbook or in the classroom is important, nurses can learn a lot from each other and from their clients and families, but nurses must recognize their own ethnocentricity and know

which questions to ask. Nurses must value the skills, experiences, and practices that colleagues from other cultures bring and reflect on how this could be incorporated to improve the care of clients from other cultures. (p. 246)

The Theory of Culture Care Diversity and Universality is an excellent framework for an international immersion experience for baccalaureate students of nursing and other healthcare disciplines to address the need for culture care knowledge. "The Greek Connection: Embracing Transcultural Caring in Ancient and Modern Greece" is an exemplar for the application of culture care theory in nursing and healthcare education through an immersion study-abroad course. Over the span of one decade, students have seen with their eyes and "touched" the Greek culture guided by Leininger's Sunrise Enabler. Their "....minds have been opened in order to discover the many different factors influencing care and ultimately the health and wellbeing of clients" (Leininger, 1997, p. 40).

DEDICATION

It is with deep appreciation that I thank Dr. Madeleine Leininger for her encouragement in the development of "The Greek Connection: Embracing Transcultural Caring in Ancient and Modern Greece." The students who have gone to Greece and have used her theory have had an opportunity to have "…their minds opened as the rising sun" to the history, culture, and the people of Greece. The world is a far richer place due to the contributions of Dr. Leininger and her love of transcultural nursing.

ACKNOWLEDGMENTS

My appreciation is also extended to the people of Greece who have partnered with me for the past 10 years for their expert attention to the needs of my students as we traveled in Greece:

- Maria Gika, PhD, RN, The Red Cross Hospital
- Ioanna Christopoulou, PhD, RN, and Eleni Evagelou, PhD, RN, The Technical Educational Institute (TEI) in Athens
- Athena Kalokerinou-Anagnostopoulou, PhD, RN, Department of Nursing, University of Athens
- Yiannis Kalofissoudis, PhD, RN, Athens Medical Group
- Ada Markaki, PhD, RN, Christos Lionis, PhD, MD, and Foteini Anastasiou, PhD, MD, University of Crete, Department of Social and Family Medicine

- The citizens of Harakas and the Community Health Center of Harakas, Crete
- Irini Lemonari, Masters in Archeology, Athens, Greece
- Yoannis Patros, Athens
- Nikos Fragioudakis, Crete

A special thank you to Dimitri, Myrto, and Thalia Cocconi, and the staff at Educational Tours, Athens, for their management of our travel details for the past 10 years.

My thanks also to Dr. Marilyn McFarland, PhD, RN, FNP-BC, CTN-A, School of Health Professions and Studies, Department of Nursing, University of Michigan–Flint, for her thoughtful and thorough review of this chapter.

Finally, a very special thank you to the exceptional students from the Midwestern United States who have taken The Greek Connection course and have begun their journey into understanding the "global community" and Leininger's culture care theory. They share my love of Greece! A special note of appreciation to them for giving me permission to use excerpts from their bluebooks for writing this chapter and for future research.

DISCUSSION QUESTIONS

1. Discuss the ethnohistorical factors presented in this chapter about Greece and how they are affecting modern Greek culture, worldview, and lifeways.
2. Reflect on the Greek ethnohistory and compare these influences upon other cultures or cultural groups encountered in daily life; in the news media; and in entertainment and pop culture. Discuss the influence this knowledge and reflection has on your own worldview.
3. Discuss how these reflections contribute to your heightened cultural awareness and your own cultural competence.
4. Discuss how your cultural awareness and cultural competence can be applied to interactions or encounters at the individual, family, group, practice setting, and institutional levels in which you participate professionally and/or personally.

REFERENCES

Albom, M. (1997). *Tuesdays with Morrie*. New York, NY: Lippincott.

Anonymous. (2007). The Greek economy: Daring to hope, fearing to fail: Back to the source of the euro-zone crisis. *The Economist*. Retrieved from http://www.economist.com/blogs/freeexchange/2013/05/europes-spring-economic-forecasts

Augustana College, Sioux Falls, SD. (2004). *The Greek connection: Embracing transcultural caring in ancient and modern Greece* [Syllabus].

De Vogliab, R., Kouvonenc, A., & Gimenod, D. (2011). Globalization: Ecological evidence on the relationship between fast food outlets and obesity among 26 advanced economies. *Critical Public Health, Special Issue: Food and Public Health,* 4(21). doi: 10.1080/09581596.2011.619964

Kalokerinou-Anagnostopoulou, A. (2006). Cultural healthcare issues in Greece. In I. Papadopoulos (Ed.), *Transcultural and social care: Development of culturally competent practitioners* (p. 246). London, UK: Churchill Livingstone Elsevier.

Larson, M. M. (2000). *The Greek connection: The development of a model to study ancient and modern patterns of care in Greece using Leininger's theory of culture care diversity and universality.* Master's thesis, Augustana College, Sioux Falls, SD.

Leininger, M. M. (1991). *Culture care diversity and universality: A theory of nursing.* New York, NY: National League of Nursing Press.

Leininger, M. M. (1994). The tribes of nursing in the United States culture of nursing. *Journal of Transcultural Nursing,* 6(1), 18–22.

Leininger, M. M. (1997). Overview of the theory of culture care with the ethnonursing research method. *Journal of Transcultural Nursing,* 8(2), 32–51.

Leininger, M. M. (2006a). Culture care diversity and universality theory and evolution of the ethnonursing method. In M. M. Leininger & M. R. McFarland (Eds.), *Culture care diversity and universality: A worldwide nursing theory* (2nd ed., pp. 1–41). Sudbury, MA: Jones and Bartlett.

Leininger, M. M. (2006b). Envisioning the future of the culture care theory and the ethnonursing method. In M. M. Leininger & M. R. McFarland (Eds.), *Culture care diversity and universality: A worldwide nursing theory* (2nd ed., pp. 389–396). Sudbury, MA: Jones and Bartlett.

Paletas, K., Athanasiadou, E., Sarigianni, M., Paschos, P., Kalogirou, A., Hassapidou, M., & Tsapas, A. (2010, July 31). The protective role of the Mediterranean diet on the prevalence of metabolic syndrome in a population of Greek obese subjects. *Journal of American College of Nutrition,* 29(1), 41–5.

http://go.galegroup.com/ps/i.do?id=GALE%7CA232571688&v=2.1&u=lom_um ichflint&it=r&p=AONE&sw=w&asid=26e067195df5f14e9c3a2620375e6420

Rosenbaum, J. N. (1990). Cultural care of older Greek Canadian widows within Leininger's theory of culture care. *Journal of Transcultural Nursing,* 1(2), 37–47.

WebMD. (June 28, 2013). Amyotrophic lateralizing sclerosis. Retrieved from http://www.webmd.com/brain/tc/amyotrophic-lateral-sclerosis-als-topic-overview

World Health Organization (WHO). (2010). Programmes and projects: Global Health Observatory (GHO) country profile [Greece]: Non-communicable diseases country profile. Retrieved from http://www.who.int/nmh/countries /grc_en.pdf

Using the Culture Care Theory as a Guide to Develop and Implement a Transcultural Global Health Course for Doctor of Nursing Practice Students for Study in Italy

Rick Zoucha
Melanie Turk

> *Many users of the theory find it most meaningful and timely as*
> *our world becomes increasingly global and complex, requiring*
> *realistic and sensitive understanding of people.*
>
> (Leininger, 2002a, p. 192)*

INTRODUCTION

The United States has seen dramatic changes in the cultural make-up and demographics of its population. According to the 2010 Census, Hispanics are the fastest-growing population in the United States. It is predicted that major growth in non-White populations and a shift in the minority/majority demographic ratio will occur by the year 2042, making the current minority populations the new majority (U.S. Department of Commerce,

---

2010). Many of these shifting changes in the population will result from increased numbers of immigrants and refugees entering the United States. The U.S. Congress continues to debate the issue of immigration reform, which may ultimately affect whether still larger numbers of immigrants and refugees may be granted citizenship and/or residency as the future unfolds.

The reality of increased cultural diversity in the United States raises questions about the readiness of nurses to care for people who may have different cultural values regarding care, health, and wellbeing. For many years, schools of nursing in the United States have been seeking creative solutions to promote culturally congruent nursing care for *undergraduate* students. Transcultural nursing courses have been implemented in Bachelor of Science in Nursing (BSN) programs across the country. Programs that do not offer stand-alone transcultural nursing courses have set priorities that include creating conceptual threads related to culture in the BSN curriculum. This identified priority in nursing education has been supported by nursing accrediting bodies such as the National League for Nursing Accreditation Commission (NLNAC, 2008) and the American Association of Colleges of Nursing Commission on Collegiate Nursing Education (AACN, 2008).

The purpose, rationale, and focus of this chapter are to describe how Leininger's Theory of Culture Care Diversity and Universality has been used as the framework to develop and implement a transcultural and global health perspectives course primarily for Doctor of Nursing Practice (DNP) students. This course included focused objectives and content related to transcultural nursing, social justice, vulnerability, and concepts of global health. A unique addition to the course was the requirement for cultural immersion and fieldwork in a context other than the traditional U.S. health system within or outside the United States. Students who opted to study locally were required to conduct observational fieldwork with healthcare providers who do not fall within the traditional view of the U.S. or other Western health systems. Examples of nontraditional Western systems included visiting and observing a *currendera* (Mexican folk healer), a granny midwife, or a *shaman* (Native American healer). Students who chose to conduct fieldwork outside of the United States could travel to study abroad in Italy with the course faculty.

Promoting opportunities for DNP students to learn and study in healthcare environments outside their usual knowledge or comfort zone fosters the development of insight from such emic experiences. *Emic* refers to the *other* or *insider* worldview and, more specifically, to a unique view of health and wellbeing. Doctoral students often do not have many opportunities to consider health and wellbeing from a different context other than the U.S. healthcare system. As DNP students graduate and join the workforce, they will interact with, treat, and care for culturally diverse individuals, families, and communities. People who are culturally diverse, such as refugees and immigrants, may have a different view of health based on the health and belief systems that they know best. The "Transcultural and Global Health" course discussed in this chapter offered DNP students a theory-based perspective as well as a cultural immersion experience designed to help students develop into culturally competent transcultural advanced practice nurses.

REVIEW OF LITERATURE

At the time this course was developed, little information existed in the literature specifically about the use of Leininger's theory to guide the development and implementation of a culture care course for nursing students, and no literature was found that described using Leininger's theory solely for a graduate-level nursing course. Approaches for incorporating transcultural nursing concepts into nursing curricula based on Leininger's theory were located in an associate degree curriculum, a baccalaureate program, and an online course (Jeffreys & O'Donnell, 1997; Kleiman, Frederickson, & Lundy, 2004; Wendler & Struthers, 2002).

Jeffreys and O'Donnell (1997) discussed the importance of using a broad, generalist method to structure the teaching of culture care content to prelicensure students and utilized an approach that incorporated concepts on culture, health, and aging—coining the approach "Cultural Discovery." Designed to facilitate cultural assessment skills among first-semester associate degree nursing students, the learner-centered activities of Cultural Discovery were based upon Leininger's Acculturation Health Care Assessment Enabler for Cultural Patterns in Traditional and Nontraditional Lifeways (Leininger, 1991). Experiential learning was incorporated, and students first practiced interviewing each other using verbal and nonverbal communication techniques considered to be culturally appropriate. An interview with an elderly person of a different culture was then conducted. The students also reviewed the literature about the cultural background of their client and examined how the client's culture might affect beliefs about health care, behaviors, and needs. Final student papers revealed newly discovered awareness of the need for effective communication to learn about another's culture; personal unrecognized biases toward a culture different than their own; and a greater appreciation of culturally diverse values that may impact health-related behaviors (Jeffreys & O'Donnell, 1997).

In a baccalaureate nursing program, Leininger's Comparative Cultural Caring Model (Leininger, 2001) was used as the basis for infusing the concepts of cultural awareness, cultural sensitivity, and cultural competence throughout the curriculum (Kleiman et al., 2004). Experiential learning exercises were planned to acquaint students with the application of these three concepts. In the first exercise, students were divided into groups according to their cultural self-identification and asked to give a presentation about the cultural characteristics of their group, such as traditions, beliefs, cuisine, or clothing. Reported student outcomes included recognition that belonging to a certain cultural group may not necessarily reveal individual responses; open-mindedness is needed about cultural similarities or differences between nurses and patients; and each patient must be treated as a unique individual who may or may not follow the norms of their dominant cultural group. This approach to teaching cultural diversity in nursing care guided by the use of Leininger's Comparative Cultural Caring Model resulted in students' recognition that nurses must have an understanding of cultural influences on patients but that each patient is an individual who must be cared for according to the unique person that he or she is (Kleiman et al., 2004).

Matching the format of the DNP course to be described in this chapter, an online, asynchronous course for both undergraduate and graduate nursing students was developed to address cultural concerns in illness and health and was loosely guided by Leininger's culture care theory (Wendler & Struthers, 2002). Course objectives for the graduate students included analyzing theoretical approaches underpinning cultural congruence and synthesizing academic literature to enable culturally congruent health care. Student teams were created based on four cultural groups common to the region (African America/Black, Asian—particularly Hmong, Hispanic/Latino, and Native American). Teams worked to learn about their culture's history, life situations, and cultural approaches to health and illness through online discussions, assignments, cultural enhancement activities, and a final term paper. Students reported acquiring advanced skills in providing culturally competent health care; knowing more about needs of the four cultural groups studied; and being able to accomplish the course objectives at their own pace because of the online, asynchronous nature of the course.

Keeping with the notion that experiential learning is important when teaching transcultural nursing concepts, nursing curricula have incorporated study-abroad opportunities, which is a component of the DNP course discussed in this chapter. Two qualitative studies of study-abroad experiences found common themes among the students: experiencing personal growth from seeing how others live; recognizing their ethnocentrism; and developing an identity as a professional nurse (Edmonds, 2010; Walsh &

DeJoseph, 2003). Numerous benefits to nursing students studying abroad have been identified, including enhanced transcultural self-efficacy, a better grasp of the elements of cultural competence, and development of a global perspective of nursing (Edmonds, 2012).

Only one research study of a study-abroad experience was found that included some graduate nursing students (Carpenter & Garcia, 2012). A total of six master's or PhD students participated in one of two 4-week immersion experiences in Guadalajara, Mexico, during either 2007 or 2008 as part of a "Spanish for Healthcare Professionals" course. This study examined how the experience impacted students' cultural awareness, knowledge, attitudes, and skills. Students felt their beliefs were affected by their culture, experienced a strong respect for choices patients made that were impacted by their cultural beliefs, and reported an enhanced ability to work with people who are culturally different. Students also reported an increased cultural awareness; an enhanced knowledge of how the Mexican healthcare system differs from the U.S. healthcare system; and improved Spanish-speaking skills. The opportunity to offer health teaching in the communities of Mexico was reported as "life-changing" (Carpenter & Garcia, 2012, p. 88).

This review of the literature highlights that experiential learning is a critical component of courses designed to promote understanding of transcultural nursing care. Experiential learning took the form of classroom and clinical activities as well as study-abroad opportunities, resulting in significant positive outcomes for the participating students. The DNP course discussed in this chapter also incorporated a cultural immersion and experiential learning experience.

HISTORICAL BACKGROUND

The School of Nursing at Duquesne University has a long history of including transcultural and global health content in courses across its programs and has valued the inclusion of transcultural nursing concepts in courses beginning with a required transcultural nursing course for BSN students as early as 1998. In 2000, the school started a program awarding a post-master's certificate in transcultural nursing. During that same year, the school created an option to obtain a PhD in nursing with a transcultural nursing focus. This program integrated required courses from the transcultural nursing post-master's certificate program as cognates for this PhD course of study.

With the advent of the Doctor of Nursing program in 2008, it seemed reasonable to include a required core course in transcultural nursing and global health to fit with the research agenda and philosophy of the school.

These foci include a clinical and research focus on social justice, cultural competence, vulnerable populations, health disparities, and wellness within chronic illness.

The 2009–2014 strategic plan of the School of Nursing placed special emphasis on extending interactions with the local community while promoting a global approach to health, care, and nursing. The school has a more than 20-year history and sister school relationship with Universidad Politécnica de Nicaragua (UPOLI) in Managua, Nicaragua. For more than 10 years, the School of Nursing at Duquesne University sponsored a Center for International Nursing. The goal of the center was to promote international experiences and connections regarding health and nursing around the globe. For the majority of the center's years of operation, a major focus was on maintaining the relationship between the School of Nursing and UPOLI in Nicaragua. Undergraduate, graduate, and doctoral students engaged in study-abroad clinical and research experiences that included working in the nurse-run academic center in an urban Nicaraguan *barrio*. Historically, the majority of student experiences were focused toward the BSN program. There had been minimal School of Nursing–sponsored opportunities for graduate students to study abroad. It was limitedly possible for students in the transcultural nursing post-master's certificate and PhD programs to study abroad with a faculty member teaching one of the required courses from Duquesne University, but with the stipulation that the objectives of their planned research activities were being met. Only small numbers of graduate students have opted for this individualized version of study-abroad. Unfortunately, until 2009 there were no opportunities for graduate students to study abroad while taking a specific course from the School of Nursing.

In addition to student engagement and commitment to international nursing and healthcare opportunities, Duquesne nursing faculty participated in a variety of international short-term experiences. Several faculty from the School of Nursing have been invited as visiting scholars to share and exchange views of nursing knowledge in Puerto Rico, Ireland, Australia, Spain, Taiwan, Nicaragua, Korea, and Jordan. Faculty have also engaged in collaborative research with other schools of nursing on a variety of research studies such as breast cancer screening, cervical cancer, and issues related to mental health and illness in both Nicaragua and Jordan.

The Center for International Nursing was put on hiatus around 2004; however, international interest and experiences for students and faculty have continued. In response to subsequent changes in the School of Nursing's administrative structure, the Center for International Nursing was converted to a faculty committee called the International Nursing Committee. The focus and philosophy of this committee were similar to that of the Center, with the caveat that efforts were to be managed by a committee appointed to 3-year terms. The current work of the International Nursing Committee is to promote global and transcultural experiences for students and faculty.

Since 2004, there has been continued and renewed involvement with UPOLI in Nicaragua, as well as exploratory trips to Ireland, Nigeria, Liberia, and Australia. In addition, Duquesne University opened a campus in Rome in 2002, primarily to enable undergraduate students to study in Italy for one semester. Several undergraduate nursing students have taken advantage of this opportunity over the intervening years.

In 2012, a representative from the School of Nursing was invited to join a board for the Center for African Studies for the purpose of promoting a minor in African Studies to be offered across all the schools at the university. The idea was to create an interdisciplinary undergraduate minor of 12 to 15 credits that would include course selections from a variety of Duquesne schools. Accordingly, the School of Nursing planned to offer two courses in transcultural health care open to all majors, with other schools to concurrently offer a selection of courses open to a variety of majors with a specific focus on Sub-Saharan Africa. It was anticipated that one of the courses in this minor would include a clinical study-abroad experience in Africa. Future intentions include expanding this idea to include a minor or focus in African Studies for graduate students across the university.

With the rich history of involvement in international initiatives in the School of Nursing, it seemed logical to initiate a study-abroad program for graduate students. The "Transcultural and Global Health Perspectives" core course offered in the Doctor of Nursing program afforded graduate students opportunities to study abroad as part of a required course. Although the course itself was required, the study-abroad portion of the course was encouraged but not required. The course has been offered every summer since 2009, with more than 80 participating graduate students having taken advantage of the study-abroad opportunity. In 2009 and 2010, two nursing faculty members accompanied students to Montreal and Toronto in Canada. Students were purposefully placed into non-English-speaking environments to learn about the Canadian healthcare system and the role of nursing in that country. They were placed in the field, took notes, and interpreted those notes from the perspective of not knowing the language or the healthcare system.

In 2011, 2012, and 2013, two faculty from the School of Nursing (**Figure 17-1**) accompanied 12, 22, and 30 DNP and PhD students, respectively, to Rome in order to spend time in the field. The student experiences included cultural immersion, observation of care in both public and private healthcare institutions, and activities designed to enhance understanding of the influences of culture on health systems. Analysis and synthesis of student and faculty reflections in relation to the immersion experience within the Italian culture prompted nurse educators in one of the DNP student cohorts to recognize the importance of actively facilitating prelicensure students' transcultural learning opportunities with culturally diverse patients (Easterby et al., 2012). Another group of DNP students focused on cultural competence in nursing faculty—a journey, not a destination (Montenery, Jones, Perry, Ross, & Zoucha, 2013). Among a group of PhD students who took the course as a cognate, the need to learn about the cultural influences of individuals, communities, or families prior to including them in research was identified (Wolf et al., 2013). Two faculty members with 26 DNP and 4 PhD students returned to Rome and Palermo, Italy, for 10 days in the summer of 2013. The visit to Palermo, Sicily, provided an additional opportunity for students to learn about the unique inclusion of a hospital owned and operated by a U.S. organization functioning within the Italian healthcare system.

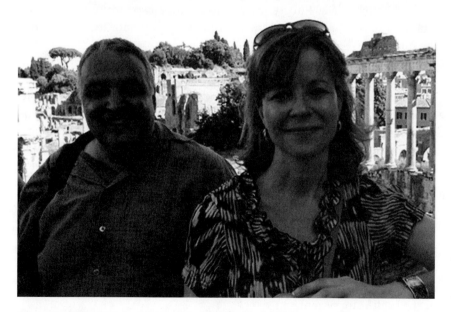

Figure 17-1 Dr. Rick Zoucha and Dr. Melanie Turk in Rome.
© R. Zoucha.

APPLICATION OF LEININGER'S THEORY

Leininger's Theory of Culture Care Diversity and Universality served as the framework for the development and implementation of the "Transcultural and Global Perspectives" course in the DNP program. The culture care theory is the outcome of decades of research and development during which Leininger and other transcultural nursing researchers studied more than 80 cultures and identified 172 care constructs (at last count) for use by nursing and other healthcare professionals (Leininger, 2006). Leininger predicted that *culture* and *care* were embedded in each other and could be understood in a cultural context. Therefore, the purpose of the theory is to discover, document, understand, and explain the interdependence of care and cultural phenomena with differences and similarities between and among cultures.

Leininger (2006) described two distinct systems of caring that existed in every culture she studied. The first system of caring is *generic* and is the oldest form of caring. Generic care, also referred to as *folk* or *emic* care, consists of culturally derived interpersonal practices which are considered essential for health, growth, and survival of humans (Leininger, 2002a). The second type of caring, also referred to as *professional* or *etic* care, is learned, practiced, and transmitted through formal and informal means of professional education such as schools of nursing, medicine, and dentistry (Leininger, 2006).

According to the culture care theory, three predictive cultural care modes of nursing decisions and actions may be derived from generic (emic) care and professional (etic) care knowledge (Clarke, McFarland, Andrews, & Leininger, 2009). The three cultural care modes are cultural care preservation and/or maintenance; cultural care accommodation and/or negotiation; and cultural care repatterning and/or restructuring (Leininger, 2006). Leininger (2002a) asserted in her theory that these three predicted modes of decisions and actions serve to guide judgments, decisions, and actions, and culminate in the delivery of culturally congruent care. Leininger (2002a) described culturally congruent care as beneficial, satisfying, and meaningful to the individuals, families, and communities served by nurses. She used the concept of cultural congruence to focus on acceptable (caring) behavior by nurses in practice, education, research, and administration.

The Sunrise Enabler depicts Leininger's theory as having seven cultural and social structure dimensions: technological; religious and philosophical; kinship and social; political and legal; economic; educational factors; and cultural values, beliefs, and lifeways (Leininger, 2006, p. 25). These social structure dimensions are usually embedded in cultures and are interrelated influencers or potential influencers on human care (Leininger, 2002b, p. 81). The three modes of nursing care decisions and actions are culture care preservation and/or maintenance; culture care accommodation and/or preservation; and culture care repatterning and/or restructuring. The modes "...come from data obtained from the upper and lower parts of the Sunrise Model [Enabler] providing a wealth of rich and meaningful data to guide certain care actions and decisions" (Leininger, 2002b, p. 82). The theory describes diverse healthcare systems as ranging from folk beliefs and practices to nursing and other healthcare professional systems often utilized by people around the world.

THE COURSE

The "Transcultural and Global Health Perspectives" course described in this chapter is a required core course in the Doctor of Nursing program at Duquesne University School of Nursing. The course explores the impact of globalization on health care and healthcare planning, and the need to design healthcare systems that are responsive to diverse cultural needs. The course foci include selected global health problems that are to be assessed in a multidisciplinary manner to ensure attention to the underserved and their complex cultural needs and requirements. Attention is directed at increasing the capacity of healthcare professionals to develop culturally sensitive healthcare systems (Duquesne University School of Nursing, 2013, p. 1).

The course goals and objectives, which were designed and framed using the cultural care theory as the framework, include the following:

- Identify global health problems and diverse cultural needs across various culture groups.
- Understand the utility of theories, models, and approaches in promoting health from a global perspective.
- Compare health systems across cultures for methods of success to facilitate positive health outcomes within the cultural context.
- Analyze caring practices in the context of comparative health systems through immersion in the cultural context in which they are occurring.
- Analyze evidence for practice to promote culturally congruent care from a global perspective and to influence health policy.

The course has been consistently scheduled for the 12-week summer session every year since 2009 and is taught completely online. Among the several assignments included in the course, there is one unique project that encourages students to participate in fieldwork. Students are taught how to do research-oriented fieldwork (observation and interpretation) through a series of readings and practical exercises. At the mid-point of the class (around week 6), two faculty members accompany the DNP (PhD cognate) students to Rome for a short-term (10–12 days) study-abroad experience. Students keep field notes of their observations using the Sunrise Enabler and culture care theory as guides. Students reflect on and keep notes about the experiences of being immersed in a non-English-speaking context and observe aspects of the Roman environment as they seek to understand the unique Roman/Italian worldview within the contexts of daily living and health. Their observations are based on the social structure factors of the Sunrise Enabler and include technological, religious and philosophical, kinship and social, political and legal, economic, educational factors, and cultural values, beliefs, and lifeways.

In addition to observations of daily life, students observe care provided by nurses and other healthcare professionals in both private and public hospitals. The Director of Nursing and/or a physician at the private and public hospitals provide formal talks and discussions about the Italian healthcare system and the role of nurses and other healthcare profession-als in that system. To help them understand the ethnohistory and religious aspects of the Roman and Italian cultures (as supported by the culture care theory and Sunrise Enabler), students are taken on an extensive and experiential view (literally) of ancient Rome, including the Coliseum and Roman Forum (**Figure 17-2**) by a professor of ancient Roman history. To

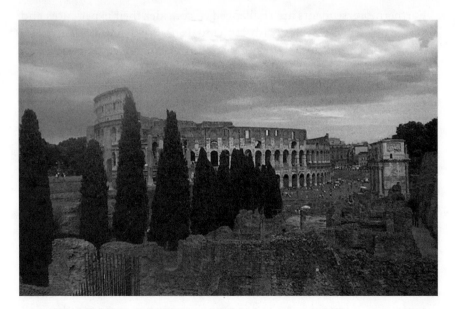

Figure 17-2 The Roman Forum and ruins.
© R. Zoucha.

help them understand the religious and faith expressions of the culture, students experience the Vatican museum and St. Peter's Basilica through the unique perspective of a Vatican art historian.

After the completion of the study-abroad portion of the course, students work on completion, analysis, and interpretation of their field notes either individually or in small groups. Students are asked to analyze and categorize their notes while looking for commonalities and diversities among and between their observations. From the identified categories, students endeavor to identify themes related to aspects of the Sunrise Enabler as a guide for analysis, then develop their interpretations into a written paper or publishable manuscript that loosely adheres to the following criteria:

- The paper/manuscript must begin with a summary and interpretation of fieldwork, followed by a written comparison of the observed Italian system of health and the influences of culture in relation to the U.S. healthcare system.
- Students are to critically frame discovered differences and similarities using Leininger's cultural care theory.
- Based on the constructs of the cultural care theory and Sunrise Enabler, as well as the three nursing care modes of decisions and actions, students are to apply their findings to the practice role of the DNP.

Furthermore, students are challenged to consider their experiences and observations when working with individuals, families, and communities who may come from a different system of health care but are accessing care within the U.S. healthcare system.

Since 2009, students have freely offered their views and evaluations of the course and study-abroad experience. Students over the past 5 years have expressed their evaluations of the course and study-abroad experience with reflective comments. One student from 2011 stated, "This course was a wonderful experience for me as I continue to understand culture and the healthcare practices of different places. This course afforded me the ability to understand the Italian healthcare system in more ways that I can think of; I hope to continue this journey in my future." Another student from 2013 said, "The cultural icon was a good start for exploring our own values, beliefs, and traditions. The readings were very valuable in stressing vulnerable populations, resilience, cultural awareness, and cultural competence, but I don't really think I totally got it until after the immersion experience in Italy." A second student from 2013 shared: "…we cannot ignore the increases of immigration and is time for nurses to come together and advocate for health care globally, regardless of background, socio-economic status, race, and so on." A third student from 2013 said:

> The study-abroad in Italy was simply phenomenal; an experience that will have a lasting impact both personally and professionally. Stretching beyond our daily levels of comfort/experience seems to always provide exceptional learning on multiple levels, often far beyond the scope of the primary intent of the planned activity. The trip certainly offered some opportunities for "stretching," for which I am grateful.

Evidence of further learning, evaluation, and implied meaning regarding the course has been exemplified by three groups of students since 2011 (approximately 15 in number) who have been published in nursing and healthcare journals. Another three groups of students (approximately 12 in number) are currently revising manuscripts based on their experiences from the 2013 study-abroad course for submission to publishers. In addition, the authors themselves are currently involved in a study entitled "Assessing Transcultural Self-Efficacy in Graduate Nursing Students," in which data are currently being analyzed.

CONCLUSION

The culture care theory and Sunrise Enabler were used as the framework and guide in the development and implementation of the "Transcultural and Global Health" course with a 12-week study-abroad immersion experience in Italy for Doctor of Nursing Practice students. The theory was instrumental in the overall development of the course goals and objectives as well as the unique assignments and study-abroad portion of the course. The study-abroad portion of the course offered an experiential view of culture through the lens of the culture care theory by promoting an understanding of technological, religious and philosophical, kinship and social, political and legal, economic, educational factors, and cultural values, beliefs, and lifeways of the Italian culture. As a framework, the theory challenged students to use their observations and insight as tools of learning, interpretation, and analysis. Students used every aspect of the theory to identify culture care knowledge in a meaningful way regarding the role of the DNP and the three nursing care modes of decisions and actions.

Using the modes of decisions and actions based on culture care knowledge may positively affect the health and wellbeing of individuals, families, and communities. The course and study-abroad experience in Italy may provide opportunities for students to transfer these unique experiences to people of diverse cultures when providing care within the U.S. health-care system. Students who engaged in experiential learning through the study-abroad portion of the course in Italy reported that they were deeply affected by their first-hand experiences, which have helped them recognize the importance of one's own culture to health and wellbeing.

ACKNOWLEDGMENTS

The authors would like to thank Duquesne University, School of Nursing, Office of International Programs, and the Duquesne University Rome Campus for their support in making the study-abroad experience a reality for graduate students in nursing.

DISCUSSION QUESTIONS

1. What impact do the changing demographics of the United States have on how nurse educators prepare DNP students for advanced practice in a variety of roles?
2. The profession of nursing endeavors to provide care that is culturally congruent. What challenges and solutions can be identified for educating Doctor of Nursing Practice students about transcultural nursing/constructs given the courses currently available to address their need to develop cultural competence and learn about global health concerns?
3. What is the value and potential impact of experiential learning in a study-abroad format on the overall development of DNP graduates?
4. How does the Theory of Cultural Care Diversity and Universality frame and inform the experiences of DNP students following their participation in the "Transcultural and Global Health" course and beyond?

REFERENCES

American Association of Colleges of Nursing. (2008). Cultural competence in baccalaureate nursing education. Retrieved from http://www.aacn.nche.edu/Education/cultural.htm

Carpenter, L. J., & Garcia, A. A. (2012). Assessing outcomes of a study abroad course for nursing students. *Nursing Education Perspectives, 33*(2), 85–89.

Clarke, P. N., McFarland, M. R., Andrews, M. M., & Leininger, M. M. (2009). Caring: Some reflections on the impact of the culture care theory by McFarland & Andrews and a conversation with Leininger. *Nursing Science Quarterly, 22*(3), 233–239.

Duquesne University School of Nursing. (2013). *Transcultural and global health perspectives* [Syllabus].

Easterby, L. M., Seibert, B., Woodfield, C. J., Holloway, K., Gilbert, P., Zoucha, R., & Turk, M. W. (2012). A transcultural immersion experience: Implications for nursing education. *Association of Black Nursing Faculty Journal, 23*(4), 81–84.

Edmonds, M. L. (2010). The lived experience of nursing students who study abroad: A phenomenological inquiry. *Journal of Studies in International Education, 14*(5), 545–568.

Edmonds, M. L. (2012). An integrative literature review of study abroad programs for nursing students. *Nursing Education Perspectives, 33*(1), 30–34.

Jeffreys, M. R., & O'Donnell, M. (1997). Cultural discovery: An innovative philosophy for creative learning activities. *Journal of Transcultural Nursing, 8*(2), 17–22.

Kleiman, S., Frederickson, K., & Lundy, T. (2004). Using an eclectic model to educate students about cultural influences on the nurse-patient relationship. *Nursing Education Perspectives, 25*(5), 249–253.

Leininger, M. M. (1991). Leininger's acculturation health care assessment tool for cultural patterns in traditional and non-traditional lifeways. *Journal of Transcultural Nursing, 2*(2), 40–42.

Leininger, M. M. (2001). A mini journey into transcultural nursing with its founder. *Nebraska Nurse, 34*(2), 16–32.

Leininger, M. M. (2002a). Culture care theory: A major contribution to advance transcultural nursing knowledge and practices. *Journal of Transcultural Nursing, 13*(3), 189–192.

Leininger, M. M. (2002b). Part I: The theory of culture care and the ethnonursing research method. In M. M. Leininger & M. R. McFarland (Eds.), *Transcultural nursing: Concepts, theories, research, & practice* (3rd ed., pp. 71–116). New York, NY: McGraw-Hill.

Leininger, M. M. (2006) Culture care diversity and universality theory and evolution of the ethnonursing method. In M. M. Leininger & M. R. McFarland (Eds.), *Culture care diversity and universality: A worldwide nursing theory* (2nd ed., pp. 2–41). Sudbury, MA: Jones and Bartlett.

Montenery, S., Jones, A., Perry, N., Ross, D., & Zoucha, R. (2013). Cultural competence in nursing faculty: A journey, not a destination. *Journal of Professional Nursing, 29*(6), 51–57.

National League for Nursing Accreditation Commission (NLNAC). (2008). *NLNAC accreditation manual: Assuring quality for the future of nursing education* (8th ed.). Atlanta, GA: Author. Retrieved from http://www.nlnac.org/manuals/NLNACManual2008.pdf

U.S. Department of Commerce, Census Bureau. (2010). Population. Retrieved from http://www.census.gov/newsroom/releases/archives/population/cb08-123.html

Walsh, L., & DeJoseph, J. (2003). "I saw it in a different light." International learning experiences of baccalaureate nursing education. *Journal of Nursing Education, 42*(6), 266–272.

Wendler, M. C., & Struthers, R. (2002). Bridging culture on-line: Strategies for teaching cultural sensitivity. *Journal of Professional Nursing, 1*(6), 320–327.

Wolf, K. M., Irwin, R. E., Houck, N. M., Kramer, N. P., Zoucha, R., Martin, M. B., Stayer, D., Turk, M. T., & Wills, J.S . (2013). Fieldwork as a way of knowing: An Italian immersion experience. *Online Journal of Cultural Competence in Nursing and Healthcare, 3*(3), 1–15.

Chapter 18

Using the Culture Care Theory as the Organizing Framework for a Federal Project on Cultural Competence

Margaret Andrews
John Collins

> *Theories are creative ways to discover new truths, refute inadequate explanations, and gain in-depth insights about a phenomenon in order to advance discipline knowledge and improve human conditions.*
>
> (Leininger, 1995, p. 93)[*]

INTRODUCTION

The purpose of this chapter is to describe the ways Leininger's Theory of Culture Care Diversity and Universality was used as the organizing framework for a federally funded cultural competence project (CCP) and to serve as an example for those wanting to write grant proposals using the culture care theory and/or the ethnonursing research method. Dr. Madeleine Leininger had challenged leaders and members of the Transcultural Nursing Society (TCNS) to seek external funding to support, in part, the strategic initiatives of the Society (http://www.tcns.org). To assure that a maximum number of nurses gained preparation in transcultural nursing, Dr. Leininger had suggested focusing on educational initiatives that would provide knowledge

---

[*]Leininger, M. M. (1995). *Transcultural nursing: Concepts, theories, research, & practices* (2nd ed.). New York, NY: McGraw-Hill Companies, Inc.

and skills in transcultural nursing for nurses who completed their formal nursing education without preparation in transcultural nursing and for students currently enrolled in undergraduate or graduate programs in nursing. A team of TCNS members that included Dr. Marilyn McFarland, Dr. Hiba Wehbe-Alamah, Dr. Margaret Andrews, along with Dr. Teresa Thompson, Dean of the Madonna University College of Nursing and Health, and several Madonna faculty and staff developed a grant proposal to fund a project aimed at developing the cultural competencies of nurses, nurse practitioners, nursing faculty, and nursing students (Andrews et al., 2011). Leininger's culture care theory and the body of transcultural nursing knowledge were used as foundations for the proposal, particularly for the key educational or training components. The theory integration into the project proposal and implementations are described throughout this chapter.

The goal of the Theory of Cultural Diversity and Universality is to use culture care research findings to provide "…specific and/or general care that would be culturally congruent, safe, and beneficial to people of diverse or similar cultures for their health, wellbeing, and healing, and to help people face disabilities and death" (Leininger, 2006a, p. 5). The grant writing team endeavored to submit a proposal that would provide nurses and nursing students with educational programs that would prepare them with a theoretically sound, evidence-based, and best practices background to support their individual nursing practices when caring for people with diverse cultural backgrounds across the lifespan, particularly those at risk for health disparities. Although Leininger used the term "…culturally congruent nursing care" in her theory and other writings (Leininger, 1995, 2002c, 2006a), the proposal writing team cited both *cultural congruence* and *cultural competence* in the grant proposal because the U.S. Department of Health and Human Services, Health Resources and Services Administration (USDHHS, HRSA) used the latter term in its funding opportunity guideline. The team believed that the federal definition of cultural competence was compatible with Leininger's theory and that using the language of the funder would increase the likelihood of receiving an award. In the funding opportunity guideline, cultural competence is defined as the "…ability to respect the beliefs, language, interpersonal styles, and behaviors of individuals, families and communities receiving care services as well as other health care professionals who are providing services. Cultural competence requires a willingness to draw on community-based values, traditions, customs, and to work with knowledgeable persons from the community in developing targeted interventions, communication, and other supports" (USDHHS, 2009, p. 86).

The proposal submitted to HRSA was entitled "Developing Nurses' Cultural Competencies: Evidence-Based and Best Practices" and was funded from July 1, 2008, to March 31, 2013, for the amount of $1,004,461. The University of Michigan–Flint (UM–Flint), in partnership with Madonna University, with the support of the TCNS and other organizations with missions that focus on developing nurses' cultural competencies, provided online and face-to-face educational offerings for nurses to enhance their cognitive, affective, and psychomotor cultural competencies and to develop their skills in addressing the health and nursing care needs of individuals, groups, and communities that are diverse, with special emphasis on those at risk for health disparities. The original grant proposal writing team, and those who joined them after the proposal was funded, together embraced Leininger's culture care theory as the theoretical framework to be used as the foundation for project implementation.

The CCP had four major objectives. First, the project provided nurses, nurse practitioners, nursing faculty, and nursing students with online and face-to-face educational opportunities to develop their cultural competencies using a train-the-trainer model. Second, the project provided electronic and print resources about culturally congruent and culturally competent nursing care based on theoretical, evidence-based, and/or best practices for nurses and nurse practitioners to access clinically when caring for patients/clients from diverse backgrounds. Third, the project focused on the preparation of nurse educators, advanced practice nurses, and administrators with the knowledge and skills necessary to use cultural competencies in clinical practice, teaching, administration, and research and to help them prepare for the Transcultural Nursing Society's certification examinations, at both the basic (CTN-B) and advanced (CTN-A) levels. Fourth, the project provided education aimed at development of the cultural competencies of students in undergraduate and graduate nursing programs. The specific project objectives are presented in Appendix 18-A at the end of this chapter.

METHODOLOGY

The methodology used for the CCP is threefold:

- The use of webinars and face-to-face educational offerings to educate nurses, advance practice nurses, and nursing faculty about cultural competence using a train-the-trainer model
- Dissemination of information electronically and in print formats
- Curricular infusion of content on cultural competence through the professional development of nursing faculty

After project faculty conducted faculty development programs and engaged in curriculum consultation, the participating faculty first offered faculty development sessions for other nursing faculty using a special toolkit for educators that used Leininger's Theory of Culture Care Diversity and Universality as an organizing framework; included Leininger's Health Care Assessment Guide for Cultural Patterns Traditional and Non-Traditional Lifeways (Leininger 2002a, pp. 139–141); and provided information about the Ethnonursing Research Method (Leininger, 2002b, 2006b). Second, participating faculty integrated cultural competence into the nursing curricula and programs of study at their respective colleges and universities. Third, they integrated cultural competence into the didactic and clinical courses and course syllabi for which they were responsible as teaching faculty, thereby developing the cultural competencies of undergraduate and graduate students in nursing.

OBJECTIVE 1: TRAIN-THE-TRAINER

A series of educational offerings focused on developing nurses' cultural competencies using a train-the-trainer model were provided by the project faculty; among them were some of the foremost transcultural nursing leaders in the United States including nursing experts on cultural competence who had authored textbooks and articles on transcultural nursing. A culturally competent nursing and healthcare workforce is needed to promote healthy lifestyle behaviors and choices that will reduce, and ultimately eliminate, health disparities. The focus of the educational offerings was on the relationship between nurses' cultural competencies and the reduction or elimination of health disparities across the lifespan, from infancy to old age. The project provided nurses with extensive online, print, and audiovisual resources on Leininger's theory; the ethnonursing research method; conducting a cultural or culturological assessment; providing culturally congruent and culturally competent nursing care; applying the theory using participants' real world clinical experiences; and case examples.

Leininger's theory guided the project toward increasing nurses' and other healthcare providers' holding knowledge about cultures they commonly encounter. The culture care theory also provided a systematic approach for the delivery of culturally congruent care using the social structure dimensions of the Sunrise Enabler and the three modes of nursing care decisions and actions of theory (Leininger, 2006a, p. 25). The purpose of the theory is to describe, explain, interpret, and predict human care phenomena related to diverse cultures in order to identify and document culture-specific care knowledge that fits with and is acceptable to people whom nurses serve (Leininger, 1995) and is reflected in the objectives of the CCP. The overarching aim of the CCP is to teach, share, articulate, communicate, and encourage nurses and nursing students as they progress on their individual

journeys toward becoming culturally competent nurses who provide culturally congruent nursing care.

Train-the-Trainer Educational Programs

From October 2008 to February 2013, a total of 37 educational programs
were offered both electronically and face-to-face by transcultural nursing
experts under the auspices of the University of Michigan–Flint, Madonna
University, the Transcultural Nursing Society, and several other organizations committed to the delivery of culturally competent and culturally congruent nursing and health care by nurses whose clinical practice, teaching,
research, and administration consisted of theoretically and/or evidence-
based best practices. Some course offerings were either solely funded by
the CCP and/or co-sponsored or co-funded by partnering organizations.

Participant institutions were from all regions of the United States:
Dartmouth-Hitchcock Medical, Center Clinical Educators, Dartmouth,
Massachusetts; Towson University School of Nursing, Baltimore, Maryland
from the North; SUNY Downstate Medical Center Faculty Students, New
York, New York; Home Care of Rochester Clinical Staff, Rochester, New
York from the East; Cleveland Clinic Nursing Staff, Cleveland Ohio; Detroit
Medical Center Clinical Staff, Detroit, Michigan; Crittenden Hospital
Clinical Staff, Rochester, Michigan; University of Michigan–Flint Nursing,
Flint, Michigan from the Midwest; University of Tennessee–Knoxville
School of Nursing, Knoxville, Tennessee; Vanderbilt University School
of Nursing, Nashville, Tennessee; East Tennessee Children's Hospital
Nurse Managers and Clinical Staff Knoxville, Tennessee; Florida Atlantic
University School of Nursing, Boca Raton, Florida; Baptist Health South
Florida Clinical Staff, Miami, Florida; University of Alabama School of
Nursing, Birmingham, Alabama; St. Luke's Episcopal Hospital Clinical
Staff, Houston, Texas from the South; and Lucille Packard Children's
Hospital Clinical Staff, Stanford University, Palo Alto, California; Brigham
Young University School of Nursing, Provo, Utah from the West. In addi-
tion, educational presentations were given at the Annual Conferences of the
International Annual Transcultural Nursing Society in Seattle, Washington;
Atlanta, Georgia; and Las Vegas, Nevada.

Project Faculty and Staff

Dr. Margaret Andrews, co-author of *Transcultural Concepts in Nursing Care*
(Andrews & Boyle, 2012) and Project Director for the CCP, earned her PhD
in nursing with a specialization in transcultural nursing. John Collins,

currently a PhD student at Duquesne University in its Transcultural Nursing Program and co-author of this chapter, was the Program Manager for the CCP. He has formal academic preparation in both nursing and health education with special emphasis on cultural competency. The chapter authors and staff prepared the educational materials and taught the education programs.

Many of the project faculty were leaders and visionaries in transcultural nursing and expert teachers who hold faculty appointments at schools of nursing in U.S. colleges and universities and each was well-qualified to teach Leininger's Theory of Culture Care Diversity and Universality; ethnonursing research method; cultural or culturological assessment; and related topics. The project faculty included Drs. Josepha Campinha-Bacote, Peggy Chinn, Cheryl Hilgenberg, Susan Hasenau, Anne Hubbert, Marianne Jeffries, Stephen Marrone, Marilyn McFarland, Sandra Mixer (Project Education Consultant), Larry Purnell, Priscilla Sagar, John Vanderlaan (Project Webmaster), Hiba Wehbe-Alamah, the late Anna Frances Wenger, and Richard Zoucha. Some project faculty have developed their own theory or conceptual model(s) of cultural competence; however, each acknowledges having been significantly influenced by Dr. Madeleine Leininger, the culture care theory, and research findings pertinent to culture care. Administrative Assistant Kai Wright (graduate degree in health education with specialization in cultural competence) also delivered some of the educational programs and prepared electronic and print materials for trainees who participated in the educational programs. Other staff included an evaluation consultant, reference librarian, statisticians, and webmaster/informational technology consultant.

Recruitment

Informational announcements about planned presentations were dispersed in snowball fashion through professional networking, email messages, and telephone calls among friends of scholars; word of mouth by participants; and communication between and among sponsoring partner organizations and their websites and the CCP website (http://www.cultural-competence-project.org). As word spread, interested future attendees contacted staff offices with inquiries for additional details about the training sessions, and healthcare and educational institutions from across the United States made requests to plan on-site sessions for presentations by project faculty.

Education

The educational component of the project was designed in a train-the-trainer (TtT) delivery model. After completing a training program, each participant was asked to become a trainer by teaching a minimum of five nursing professionals in his or her professional network, i.e., the trainees became trainers. Many trainees offered educational sessions to more than five nurses and some adapted the content to include physicians; social workers; physical, occupational, and respiratory therapists; and other health professionals. This delivery method was employed so that the overall influence of the project would have continuing effects toward improving the cultural competence of nurses and other health professionals even after the funded project ended. Participants were asked to continue the training at their hospital, home health, public health, long-term care, or other healthcare agency, university, college, or related organization using the resources provided in the training sessions.

Participants were encouraged to continue the training, and this request to train was reinforced by providing the trainers with access to the complete presentation materials in a cultural competence toolkit. By offering a comprehensive toolkit, it was expected that participants would be prepared to continue the training without needing to conduct research and create the presentation slides, web links, handouts, pre/post-evaluation instruments, and associated training materials. The toolkits were created in collaboration with the project director, program manager, education consultant, project faculty, and staff and were used by the project faculty at the initial training workshops, and subsequently made available to those participants who agreed to continue the training for their peers and other groups or organizations within their professional network(s).

Toolkits were made available to trainees (future trainers) to facilitate their ability to teach colleagues when they returned to their respective institutions. The toolkits included resources such as references on Leininger's Theory of Culture Care Diversity and Universality; the Sunrise Enabler; the ethnonursing research method; cultural or culturological assessment; and foundational definitions of terms such as *culture* (ethnic and non-ethnic cultures and subcultures). Also addressed in these toolkits were such topics as cultural competence; culturally congruent nursing care; transcultural nursing; evidence-based and best practices in cultural competence; approaches to the development of cultural competencies; information on health disparities; pre- and post-evaluation forms; audiovisual and computer software on cultural competency development; health disparities, internet resources, PowerPoint slide presentation development; cultural assessment guides; and case scenarios for participant breakout and discussion sessions.

For each educational offering taught by project faculty, train-the-trainer toolkits with reference sources, evaluation instruments, and other useful information pertaining to the topic for use with their trainees were made available. Project faculty, the education consultant, and the project

IT/reference librarian shared references and instructional materials developed while preparing to teach the various educational offerings. By doing so, the project faculty and staff facilitated the ease of preparation for the trainees and thereby promoted the continued training of other nurses and healthcare professionals in a cascade fashion. The train-the-trainer cascade approach has been highly successful in perpetuating and sustaining the educational sessions throughout the project. After funding ended, trainees have reported that the training sessions and dissemination of educational resources has continued.

Global Outreach

Interest in the culture care theory, ethnonursing research method, cultural or culturological assessment, provision of culturally congruent and culturally competent nursing care, and related topics attracted participation by nursing professionals both in the United States and globally. Given that the CCP was funded by U.S. federal tax dollars, the training focused on U.S. nurses, nursing faculty, and nursing students; however, many of the educational programs included non-U.S. residents. Toolkits and other reference materials were made available at no cost to all who visited the CCP website (www.cultural-competence-project.org) and the *Online Journal of Cultural Competence in Nursing and Healthcare* (http://www.ojccnh.org). The project faculty and staff have responded to nurses from Australia, Canada, China, Denmark, Finland, France, Germany, Greece, Hungary, India, Indonesia, Israel, Italy, Japan, Malaysia, Mexico, the Netherlands, Poland, Portugal, Saudi Arabia, Spain, Sweden, Thailand, Taiwan, and the United Kingdom.

Measurement and Evaluation of Training Programs

To evaluate the train-the-trainer (TtT) model of delivery, participant institutions were asked to track the numbers and demographic backgrounds of trainees as well as the training sessions their trainees conducted after receiving their toolkits. The project's success in achieving the outcomes for the first educational objective was measured by counting the number of registered nurses and nurse practitioners, nursing faculty, nursing students, and other health professionals who participated in and successfully completed the educational offerings. To assess the effectiveness of the training in developing participants' transcultural self-efficacy, the Transcultural Self-Efficacy Tool (TSET; Jeffreys, 2006) was administered before each educational offering and 6 weeks after their training. The TSET is a reliable and valid instrument for measuring and evaluating participants' confidence or self-efficacy about carrying out or accomplishing nursing practices related to cultures and culture care. The 83 items of the TSET instrument are categorized into three general content areas or subscales—cognitive (25 items); affective (30 items); and practical/psychomotor (28 items)—and uses a 10-point Likert rating scale ranging from 1 (not confident) to 10 (totally confident).

The number of trainees who participated in the 37 webinars and face-to-face training programs over a 5-year period from July 2008 through March 2013 totaled 1,022 nurses, 114 nurse practitioners, 872 nursing faculty, and 293 nursing students. Additionally, 1,252 students at the University of Michigan–Flint and the University of Tennessee–Knoxville received training materials from the CCP bringing the total number of students trained to 1,545. The participants represented 45 of the 50 states and the District of Columbia. Given that nurse practitioners and nursing faculty are also registered nurses, to avoid double-counting, those individuals self-identifying as nursing faculty or nurse practitioners were placed in the appropriate category and were not included in the count for nurses. Although the funding announcement and objectives for the CCP included training solely for nurses, some host organizations that partnered with the CCP elected to include physicians; physical, occupational, and respiratory therapists; social workers; dieticians; and public health professionals in their training programs.

Using train-the-trainer methods, the project faculty trained 872 nursing faculty nationally, many of whom taught other faculty about cultural competencies and health disparities either in their home location or at another venue mutually agreed upon with the project staff. The faculty trainers and trainees reported that they formed cohesive bonds that frequently enabled them to collaborate on projects, co-teach courses, and/or assist one another in the search for new resources to support curriculum development (e.g., web-based resources, audiovisual and computer software related to cultural competencies).

OBJECTIVE 2: DISSEMINATION OF INFORMATION

Electronic and Print Dissemination

Electronic information and printed copies of presentation materials were disseminated as part of the train-the-trainer toolkits to webinars and face-to-face presentation participants as described. In addition, electronic resources were made available to persons or institutions that made inquiries by email, telephone, or the CCP website. The project website presents a graphic design reflecting racial, ethnic, gender, and other forms of diversity on the opening page, and has individual pages that include an overview of the project list-ing goals, project staff names, titles, and contact information; schedule for educational offerings; and an online registration option for webinars and face-to-face programs. In addition, there are links to other websites with information about Leininger's Theory of Culture Care Diversity and Universality; the ethnonursing research method; transcultural nursing; the Transcultural Nursing Society; and cultural competence. There also are links to sites about health disparities including the *Healthy People 2010*; Office of Minority Health; and other HRSA project websites. For more interactive formats, there are additional links to moderated discussion or chat rooms for nurses in practice settings, education, administration, and research. Also available on the project website are audiovisual resources; evaluation instruments and tools related to cultural competence measurements for use in practice, education, and research; annotated and categorized references on cultural competencies and teaching cultural competencies; and leading health indicators, risk factors, and health disparities. The project website also contains a section on evidence-based and best practices for nurses in prac-tice, education, research, and administration. Print and electronic resources pertinent to transcultural nursing and nursing cultural competence, as well as other related books and journal articles including resources for nursing education and practice, and books and articles related to health disparities, are listed by both title and author on the website for ease of identification.

Finally, information about the project and the project website have been disseminated to nurses and nurse practitioners through professional orga-nizations such as the American Association of Colleges of Nursing; National League for Nursing; Sigma Theta Tau International; National Organization of Nurse Executives; National Black Nurses' Association; National Hispanic Nurses Association; Transcultural Nursing Society; Arab American Nurses Association; National Organization of Nurse Practitioner Faculty; and related groups via their newsletters, websites, and other communication methods. Project staff have responded to requests for additional materials and in some instances have conducted research to assist nurses who have made inquiries about specific topics.

Creation of an Online Journal

The CCP staff did not initially plan to create a new journal; however, it soon became apparent that existing journals related to cultural competence and transcultural nursing were backlogged with manuscripts. To help alleviate this problem, the project team decided to establish the *Online Journal of Cultural Competence in Nursing and Healthcare* (*OJCCNH*) to facilitate the rate at which dissemination of new research and cultural competence information could transpire; encourage interaction between authors and readers; and provide experienced scholars and developing scholars (including students) with a venue for intellectual exchange. The *OJCCNH* may be accessed free of charge through the website (www.ojccnh.org).

The *OJCCNH* was established based on the principles of Leininger's Theory of Culture Care Diversity and Universality and her construct of collaborative care (Leininger, 2015). As a quarterly peer-reviewed publication, the *OJCCNH* provides a forum for the discussion of issues, trends, theory, research, evidence-based and best practices currently applicable to or about the provision of culturally congruent and competent nursing and health care for individuals, groups, communities, and organizations.

Philosophically, the CCP staff and *OJCCNH* editorial board members believe that a culturally competent nursing healthcare workforce is needed to promote healthy lifestyle behaviors and choices that will reduce, and ultimately eliminate, health disparities. They also posit that nursing as a theory-based humanistic discipline serves individuals, organizations, communities, and institutions. The *OJCCNH* seeks to disseminate scholarly work among nurses and other healthcare professionals through publication of articles on culturally competent and congruent care-based research, theory, education, practice, administration, and policy. Culturally competent care occurs when culture care values are known and serve as the foundation for meaningful care. Care is the core construct for the discipline of nursing, and human care is defined within the context of culture. This journal encourages dialogue representing diverse perspectives, fosters debate, and clarifies moral/ethical decision-making on related topics of interest and concern to promote health and wellbeing for all people.

The *OJCCNH* editorial board members endeavor to present different perspectives about the provision of culturally congruent and competent nursing and health care relative to contemporary trends and issues that influence clinical practice, administration, education, theory development, and research in nursing and health care. The interactive format of the journal encourages an in-depth, dynamic dialogue resulting in a comprehensive discussion of relevant topics and thereby contributes to the body of nursing and healthcare knowledge; provides a discussion forum about the implications of healthcare policy; promotes the overall wellbeing and health of people from diverse and similar cultures through the dissemination of nursing and healthcare knowledge; and promotes the reduction of health disparities in traditionally underrepresented and/or minority populations.

Since January 2011, the *OJCCNH* has been a means for the dissemination of information about cultural competence. The editorial board and peer reviewers comprise an internationally recognized group of individuals representing a variety of racial, ethnic, gender, religious, national origin, and academic backgrounds, and includes those with bachelor's, master's, practice doctorate (DNP), and research doctorate (PhD) degrees. The journal serves as a method for students and scholars to submit their work related to cultural competence issues, including articles and poster presentations.

Measurement and Evaluation of Dissemination

During the grant-funded period of the CCP, there were 39,896 hits on the project website, which exceeded the original projected number of 6,000 hits by more than six-fold. Website visitors are largely from the United States; visitors from other countries (presented in descending order by greatest frequency) include Canada, the Philippines, Australia, the United Kingdom, Finland, Brazil, Italy, Spain, Portugal, Colombia, Germany, Malaysia, India, Indonesia, Sweden, Thailand, Hungary, Israel, Mexico, Denmark, France, Poland, and Japan.

Twenty articles, 16 poster presentations, and 2 videos were published in the *OJCCNH* from the time of the inaugural issue in January 2011 to the end of the funded project in March 2013, including Dr. Madeleine Leininger's final recorded professional presentation and her last journal publication (Leininger, 2011). There were 15,243 articles, posters, and videos downloaded and 107,579 pages viewed. The journal is free, distributed globally to 132 countries and territories, and indexed in the CINAHL and EBSCOhost databases.

OBJECTIVE 3: PREPARATION FOR CERTIFICATION IN TRANSCULTURAL NURSING

The third objective of the CCP focuses on preparing nursing faculty with the knowledge and skills necessary to use cultural competencies in their practices, teaching, consultations, and research. To this end, faculty completed a series of three train-the-trainer graduate-level educational offerings that would prepare them for transcultural nursing certification examination and for training nursing faculty colleagues. The implementation of this objective needed to be addressed in a somewhat different method than was originally planned. The overarching emphasis of this objective was to provide current nursing faculty with the knowledge and skills necessary to use cultural competencies in their practices, teaching, consultations, and research that would prepare them for transcultural nursing certification. Certification is a highly honored distinction for nurses who pass the internationally recognized, comprehensive transcultural nursing certification examination offered under the aegis of the Certification Commission of the Transcultural Nursing Society. Although a series of graduate-level educational course offerings initially had been planned, implementation was not feasible due to two major factors: The cost of preparing and implementing this type of training was determined to be prohibitive; and faculty whom the project staff contacted indicated that they were unable to make the required time commitment due to the heavy teaching workloads at their respective colleges and universities.

To achieve this objective of preparing nurses for both the basic and advanced transcultural nursing certification examinations but by using a different methodology, Douglas and Pacquiao (2010) edited the *TCNS Core Curriculum Study Guide*. The grant faculty and staff made this guide available for direct distribution to nurses interested in the certification examination through the Transcultural Nursing Society as well as through supplemental publication in the *Journal of Transcultural Nursing*. Project funds were used to support the expenses associated with developing the guide. The newly revised and updated format of the transcultural nursing certification examinations have been used by the TCNS since 2010.

OBJECTIVE 4: STUDENT IMPROVEMENT IN TRANSCULTURAL SELF-EFFICACY

The project staff contacted nursing faculty in undergraduate and graduate nursing programs nationally to identify those who currently teach courses on cultural competence; transcultural, cross-cultural, or intercultural nursing; cultural diversity; and/or health disparities. Using quantitative and qualitative methods, faculty were surveyed to determine their needs regarding their own professional development opportunities for planning, implementing, and evaluating their course(s), and to identify necessary resources to support their teaching/learning needs. The project faculty, education consultant, and staff developed web-based resources designed to address these needs identified from the survey. Faculty members were also provided with the opportunity to make customized requests for searches on topics related to cultural competence and health disparities.

CONCLUSION

The purpose of this chapter was to demonstrate the use of Leininger's Theory of Culture Care Diversity and Universality as the organizing framework for a federally funded project to develop the cognitive, affective, and psychomotor cultural competencies of registered nurses, including staff RNs, nurse practitioners and other advanced practice nurses, nursing faculty, and undergraduate and graduate nursing students. Using a train-the-trainer model, leaders in transcultural nursing and cultural competence gave a series of webinars and face-to-face presentations that contained evidence-based and best practices for the provision of culturally competent and culturally congruent nursing and health care for individuals across the lifespan, families, groups, and communities. The authors hope that others will find the culture care theory and the ethnonursing research method useful in planning, implementing, and evaluating similar projects.

ACKNOWLEDGMENT

This chapter is based on grant number D11 HP09759 by the U.S. Department of Health and Human Services, Health Resources and Services Administration, July 1, 2008 to March 31, 2013.

DISCUSSION QUESTIONS

1. Discuss the benefits to nursing programs and their students derived from the train-the-trainer educational process for learning cultural competency knowledge and cultural assessment skills. How might this apply to your own program and students?
2. Discuss how your nursing program could use the Theory of Culture Care Diversity and Universality with the Sunrise Enabler as the overarching framework for the program.
3. Discuss how your nursing program could integrate cultural competency into the undergraduate and/or graduate nursing program courses (objectives and content).
4. Discuss how students and faculty could utilize the *Online Journal of Cultural Competence in Nursing and Healthcare* and the resources available via the cultural competence project website for their course development, assignments, and nursing practices.
5. Discuss how student and registered nurses at all levels of educational preparation can integrate the Theory of Culture Care Diversity and Universality with the Sunrise Enabler into their practices.
6. Discuss the value of Transcultural Nursing Certification (basic and advanced) for nursing faculty, students, and practicing registered nurses.

APPENDIX 18-A: OBJECTIVES OF THE CULTURAL COMPETENCE PROJECT

Objective 1: Prepare nurses to address the culture care needs of individuals, families, groups and communities at risk for health disparities by increasing the cognitive, affective, and psychomotor cultural competencies of 600 registered nurses and 100 nurse practitioners by offering a series of intensive continuing professional development programs using a train-the-trainer model, as measured by results on pre-test/post-test instruments for measuring cultural competencies.

Objective 2: Disseminate electronic and print resources on cultural competencies that are theoretically and evidence-based, best practices to at least 6,000 nurses and nurse practitioners to use when caring for diverse patients/clients.

Objective 3: Prepare 60 nurse educators, advanced practice nurses, and/or administrators with the knowledge and skills necessary to use cultural competencies in clinical practice, teaching, administration and research by completing a series of three graduate-level educational offerings which will contribute to their cultural competency and prepare them for the Transcultural Nursing Certification Examination.

Objective 4: Improve the cultural competencies of 600 students in undergraduate and graduate nursing programs by at least 15% over a baseline, as measured by the scores of graduates on selected instruments for measuring cultural competencies.

Copyright © M. Andrews and J. Collins, 2013.

REFERENCES

Andrews, M. M., & Boyle, J. S. (2012). *Transcultural concepts in nursing care* (7th ed.). Philadelphia, PA: Wolters Kluwer/Lippincott, Williams, and Wilkins.

Andrews, M. M., Cervantez Thompson, T. L., Wehbe-Alamah, H., McFarland, M. R., Hanson, P. A., Hasenau, S. M.,... Vint, P. A. (2011). Developing a culturally competent workforce through collaborative partnerships. *Journal of Transcultural Nursing, 22*(3), 300–306.

Douglas, M. K., & Pacquiao, D. F. (Eds.). (2010). Core curriculum for transcultural nursing and health care. Thousand Oaks, CA: Dual printing as supplement to *Journal of Transcultural Nursing, 21*(1), 317S–322S.

Jeffreys, M. (2006). *Transcultural self-efficacy tool Multidisciplinary healthcare provider.* New York, NY: Springer.

Leininger, M. M. (1995). *Transcultural nursing: Concepts, theories, research, & practices* (2nd ed.). New York, NY: McGraw-Hill.

Leininger, M. M. (2002a). Culture care assessments for congruent competency practices. In M. M. Leininger & M. R. McFarland (Eds.), *Transcultural nursing: Concepts, theories, research, & practice* (3rd ed., pp. 139-141). New York, NY: McGraw-Hill.

Leininger, M. M. (2002b). Part I: The theory of culture care and the ethnonursing research method. In M. M. Leininger & M. R. McFarland (Eds.), *Transcultural nursing: Concepts, theories, research, & practice* (3rd ed., pp. 145-156). New York, NY: McGraw-Hill.

Leininger, M. M. (2002c). Transcultural nursing and globalization of health care: Importance, focus, and historical aspects. In M. M. Leininger & M. R. McFarland (Eds.), *Transcultural nursing: Concepts, theories, research, & practice* (3rd ed., pp. 3-43). New York, NY: McGraw-Hill.

Leininger, M. M. (2006a). Culture care diversity and universality theory and evolution of the ethnonursing method. In M. M. Leininger & M. R. McFarland (Eds.), *Culture care diversity and universality: A worldwide nursing theory* (2nd ed., pp. 1-41). Sudbury, MA: Jones and Bartlett.

Leininger, M. M. (2006b). Ethnonursing research method and with enablers to study the theory of culture care. In M. M. Leininger & M. R. McFarland (Eds.), *Culture care diversity and universality: A worldwide nursing theory* (2nd ed., pp. 43-81). Sudbury, MA: Jones and Bartlett.

Leininger, M. M. (2011). Leininger's reflection on her ongoing father protective care research. *Online Journal of Cultural Competence in Nursing and Healthcare, 1*(2), 1-13.

McFarland, M. R., & Wehbe-Alamah, H. B. (2015). The Theory of Culture Care Diversity and Universality. In M. R. McFarland and H. B. Wehbe-Alamah (Eds.), *Culture care theory and universality: A worldwide nursing theory* (3rd ed.; Chapter 1).

U.S. Department of Health and Human Services (USDHHS), Health Resources and Services Administration (HRSA). (2009). Nurse education, practice, quality, and retention program. Retrieved from http://bhpr.hrsa.gov/nursing/grants/nepqr.html

Transcultural Nursing Course Outline, Educational Activities, and Syllabi Using the Culture Care Theory

Hiba B. Wehbe-Alamah
Marilyn R. McFarland

> *Transcultural nursing knowledge and practice have become*
> *global and essential imperatives, which are transforming the*
> *profession and related health practices into transculturalism. It*
> *is therefore imperative that transcultural nursing education be*
> *explicitly taught in undergraduate and graduate programs.*
> (McFarland & Leininger, 2002, p. 527)[*]

PROLOGUE

On a glorious snowy Michigan day, the following conversation occurred:

Hiba: Good morning, Marilyn!

Marilyn: Good morning, Hiba! One second, Rodney is handing me a cup of coffee in bed.

Hiba: Enjoy it! I am drinking a cup of Hot Cinnamon Spice tea. I just received a delivery of 16 tins.

Marilyn: Why so many?

---

[*]McFarland, M. R., & Leininger, M. M. (2002). Transcultural nursing: Curricular concepts, principles, and teaching and learning activities for the 21st century. In M. M. Leininger & M. R. McFarland (Eds.), *Transcultural nursing: concepts, theories, research, and practice* (3rd ed., pp. 527–561). New York, NY: McGraw-Hill, Companies, Inc.

Hiba: I had to stock up on brain fuel in preparation for my sabbatical writing. It seems to be working: I had a great idea today about the syllabi chapter.

Marilyn: What is it?

Hiba: Well, you know how we discussed including our undergraduate, graduate, and Taiwanese syllabi? Right? Well, I am thinking we can also elaborate on some of the educational teaching exercises we have used in our classes. What do you think?

Marilyn: Hiba, you are a genius! That's a great idea!

Hiba: Well, it takes one to know one, plus, I had a great teacher …

INTRODUCTION

One of the first and most important reasons for transcultural nursing education and concomitant culturally congruent practices is that our world has become intensely multicultural and will be ever more so in the future. This transformation necessitates that nurses become transculturally knowledgeable, sensitive, and competent (McFarland & Leininger, 2002, pp. 528–529). With increasing diversity in the United States and worldwide, there is a corresponding and growing interest for healthcare providers to deliver culturally congruent care to individual patients, families, organizations, and communities (Andrews & Friesen, 2011). More than 1 million nurses are expected to be needed to meet the nation's healthcare needs in 2014 according to the U.S. Department of Labor (Duphily, 2011; U.S. Department of Labor, 2005).

For nurses to deliver culturally congruent care, they need to receive formal transcultural education in the form of courses, workshops, conferences, mentoring, training, in-service programs, and other forms of continuing education. Academic faculty can play an important role in facilitating this process by preparing current and future generations of nurses to be culturally competent. This will necessitate the inclusion of transcultural educational content in both undergraduate and graduate curricula. Accordingly, transcultural concepts, theories, and models as well as cultural assessment and communication techniques could be offered in a transcultural course and/or threaded and reinforced throughout a formal nursing program.

PURPOSE AND GOAL

The purpose of this chapter is to share core content, transcultural exercises, outlines, and syllabi of undergraduate, graduate, and international transcultural nursing courses previously taught by the authors. The content of these courses was adapted using three different texts, one of which was the

2006 culture care theory book by Leininger and McFarland. Examples of transcultural educational activities that can be incorporated into instructional units are summarized. The ultimate goal is to assist nursing faculty and other nurses responsible for teaching transcultural nursing or cultural competence by providing resources that can be adapted to their own needs, purposes, and curricula.

BACKGROUND

Numerous resources exist to assist nursing and other educators in developing and implementing cultural competence and transcultural curricula. The American Association of Colleges of Nursing (AACN) has issued several documents that are designed to guide and facilitate the incorporation of cultural competency in nursing education at the undergraduate and graduate levels (**Table 19-1**). Douglas and Pacquiao (2010) published the *Core Curriculum for Transcultural Nursing and Health Care* which aimed to define the distinct body of knowledge and practice that encompasses transcultural nursing and health care. Many transcultural nursing scholars

Table 19-1 American Academy of Colleges of Nursing (AACN) Resources for Incorporation of Cultural Competencies in Undergraduate and Graduate Nursing Curricula

Resource	Direct Link
The Essentials of Baccalaureate Education for Professional Nursing Practice (AACN, 2008)	http://www.aacn.nche.edu /education-resources /baccessentials08.pdf
Cultural Competency in Baccalaureate Nursing Education (AACN, 2008)	http://www.aacn.nche.edu /leading-initiatives/education-resources /competency.pdf
Tool Kit of Resources for Cultural Competent Education for Baccalaureate Nurses (AACN, 2008)	http://www.aacn.nche.edu /education-resources/toolkit.pdf
Establishing a Culturally Competent Master's and Doctorally Prepared Nursing Workforce (AACN, 2009)	http://www.aacn.nche.edu /education-resources/CulturalComp.pdf
Tool Kit for Cultural Competence in Master's and Doctoral Nursing Education (AACN, 2011)	http://www.aacn.nche.edu /education-resources/Cultural_ Competency_Toolkit_Grad.pdf
The Essentials of Master's Education in Nursing (AACN, 2011)	http://www.aacn.nche.edu/education-resources/MastersEssentials11.pdf
The Essentials of Doctoral Education for Advanced Nursing Practice (AACN, 2006)	http://www.aacn.nche.edu /publications/position/DNPEssentials.pdf

Table 19-2 Selected Transcultural Online Resources

Resource	Direct Link
Transcultural Nursing Basic Concepts and Case Studies (2011)	http://www.culturediversity.org/index.html
The Office of Minority Health (2013)	http://minorityhealth.hhs.gov/templates/browse.aspx?lvl=2&lvlID=11
Transcultural Nursing Society (2013)	http://tcns.org/
Diversity RX (2013)	http://www.diversityrx.org/
National Center for Cultural Competence (n.d.)	http://www11.georgetown.edu/research/gucchd/nccc/
National CLAS Standards (OMH, 2013)	http://minorityhealth.hhs.gov/templates/browse.aspx?lvl=2&lvlID=15

contributed to various sections of this publication. This collective body of work, among others, is also intended to serve as the basis for basic and advanced Transcultural Nursing Certification granted by the Transcultural Nursing Society.

Numerous websites offer relevant educational materials that can be integrated into transcultural nursing or other interdisciplinary healthcare courses (**Table 19-2**). Cultural competency material can also increasingly be located on social media outlets such as YouTube, Facebook, and culturally focused and other blogs (**Table 19-3**) and therefore can be utilized as

Table 19-3 Selected Cultural Competency YouTube Videos

Video	Direct Link
The Power of Transcultural Nursing (2012, 11 minutes)	http://www.youtube.com/watch?v=6U3n4UF_XGg
Cultural Competence for Healthcare Providers (2009, 9 minutes)	http://www.youtube.com/watch?v=dNLtAj0wy6I
Weight Bias in Health Care (2009, 16 minutes)	http://www.youtube.com/watch?v=IZLzHFgE0AQ
Overcoming Cultural Stereotypes (2011, 12 minutes)	http://www.youtube.com/watch?v=MDw68BQxKEk
Cross-Cultural Patient Care Panel: Latino/Hispanic Patients (2012, 1.25 hours)	http://www.youtube.com/watch?v=V1hSBMboJfE
Cross Cultural Patient Care Panel: Islam and Muslim Patients (2011, 1.09 hours)	http://www.youtube.com/watch?v=n2AZPhP6dQc2009
Incompetent versus Competent Cultural Care (2010, 7.5 minutes)	http://www.youtube.com/watch?v=Dx4Ia-jatNQ

creative teaching methodologies or exercises. Nurses and other educators are encouraged to examine these resources as they embark on the journey toward developing their own curricula, courses, or syllabi.

CORE CONTENT

Regardless of the text selected by faculty when planning to teach either an undergraduate or a graduate transcultural nursing or healthcare course, the authors recommend inclusion of the following core content (modules): Introduction to transcultural nursing (TCN); TCN concepts; TCN theories and models; ethnonursing research method; cultural assessment; principles of transcultural communication; and application in clinical practice to specific cultural groups. This content can be further supplemented through journal articles and other readings to expand course content beyond the text selected for the course.

Introduction to TCN

This module may include a definition of transcultural nursing, some background about the historical development of the transcultural movement, and an acknowledgment of Dr. Madeleine Leininger as the founder of TCN. Leininger conducted seminal research and published extensively about her work as theorist, researcher, educator, international presenter, author, and founder of the Transcultural Nursing Society (TCNS) and the *Journal of Transcultural Nursing*.

TCN Concepts

Understanding basic TCN terminology and constructs is an important precursor to learning about cultural competence and delivery of culturally congruent care. The authors recommend that the following TCN concepts be introduced to students taking a TCN course: Culture, subculture, ethnicity, race, cultural shock, cultural pain, cultural conflict, ethnocentrism, cultural imposition, cultural blindness, cultural diversity, cultural universality, stereotyping, prejudice, discrimination, generic (folk) care, professional care, acculturation, enculturation, assimilation, and culturally congruent/sensitive care. Faculty may add additional constructs as indicated by the needs of their students or course objectives.

TCN Theories and Models

This module may discuss transcultural nursing theories and models beginning with Leininger's Theory of Culture Care Diversity and Universality, the first transcultural nursing theory, which was initially developed specifically for nursing but is now also used by other healthcare disciplines. Faculty are especially encouraged to address professional and generic care as well as the three culture care modes of decisions and actions and to advocate for their inclusion in clinical care planning. Other theories or models may also be presented in this module, such as the Process of Cultural Competence in the Delivery of Healthcare Services [Model] (Campinha-Bacote, 2002); Purnell Model for Cultural Competence (Purnell, 2002); Giger and Davidhizar Transcultural Assessment Model (Giger & Davidhizar, 2002); Spector's Health Traditions Model (2009); and Jeffreys' Cultural Competence and Confidence Model (2010).

Ethnonursing Research Method

Faculty may choose to present a brief or a detailed explanation of the ethnonursing research method depending on the purpose and goal of the course and the academic level at which it is being taught. However, special emphasis must be placed on the fact that the ethnonursing research method is the first research method developed specifically for nursing and for use in conjunction with a nursing theory (Leininger, 2006a, 2006b).

Cultural Assessment

Faculty members are encouraged to teach the principles of cultural assessment with foci on cultural self-assessment; cultural assessment of individuals, families, and communities; and organizational cultural assessment. Faculty may choose to introduce students to any combination of the following cultural assessment enablers and tools: Leininger's Sunrise Enabler; Acculturation Healthcare Assessment Enabler; Semi-Structured Inquiry Guide Enabler; and Life History Healthcare Enabler (Leininger, 2006b); Cultural Competence Assessment Instrument (CCA; Schim, Doorenbos, Miller, & Benkert, 2003); Inventory for Assessing the Process of Cultural Competence Among Healthcare Professionals-Revised (IAPCC-R; Campinha-Bacote, 2003); Transcultural Self-Efficacy Tool (TSET), Cultural Competence Clinical Evaluation Tool (CCCET), and Clinical Setting Assessment Tool—Diversity and Disparity (CSAT-DD; Jeffreys, 2010); Andrews and Boyle's Transcultural Nursing Assessment Guide for Individuals and Families, Transcultural Nursing Assessment Guide for Groups and Communities, and Transcultural Nursing Assessment Guide for Health Care Organizations and Facilities (Andrews & Boyle, 2012); and Giger and Davidhizar's Transcultural Assessment Model (Giger & Davidhizar, 2002).

Principles of Cross-Cultural Communication

Healthcare providers caring for people from diverse cultural backgrounds need to be prepared in cross-cultural communication principles and techniques to avoid cultural clashes and miscommunication and develop healthy and meaningful relationships with clients. It is recommended that faculty address cultural principles of verbal communication (how to address a client); appropriate use of interpreters or translators; and recognition and appropriate use of nonverbal communication including personal space, eye contact, touch, and silence (Andrews, 2012).

Application in Clinical Practice to Specific Cultural Groups

Faculty need to encourage and empower students to explore the cultural and generic (folk) care beliefs, expressions, and practices of common cultures within the geographical area of their professional practice. Once these cultures are identified and assessed, students can develop culturally congruent care decisions and actions for the provision of culturally sensitive care to members of these diverse groups. Faculty can be creative in how to approach this objective.

EDUCATIONAL ACTIVITIES

Some educational activities used by the authors in their undergraduate, graduate, and/or international transcultural courses are summarized in the following paragraphs. These exercises may be replicated or adapted as needed. All of these exercises have been and can be used in both face-to-face and online formats. Their level of complexity can be tailored to fit the academic level of the course and the needs of the students.

Stereotype, Prejudice, and Discrimination Activity

This educational activity is an adaptation of an exercise initially administered to one of the authors as a student in the PhD program at Duquesne University by Professor Joan Lockhart. The purpose of this assignment is to engage students in the discovery and discussion of personal and generalized stereotypes, prejudices, and discriminations. In its most currently adapted form, this exercise consists of faculty searching the Internet for four to eight pictures of interesting individuals, gathering brief information about them as depicted, inserting each as a numbered picture into a PowerPoint slide, and providing students with a handout (**Table 19-4**) containing a list of questions to be answered by each student. Some of these questions

Table 19-4 Table for Use with Stereotype, Prejudice, and Discrimination Activity

Picture Number	Person's Name	Where Does This Person Live?	Educational Background	Employment Status and Job Description	Marital Status (Single, Married, Divorced, Widow)	Does This Person Have Children and How Many?	What Does This Person Do for Fun?	Would You Be Friends with This Person? Why?

may include: *What does this person do for a living? What is this person's educational background? What does this person do for fun? Where does this person live? What is his or her marital status (including children, if any)? Would you be friends with this person, and why or why not?*

Students are asked to respond anonymously (for online courses, students are provided with the option to post their responses without personal identifiers) within seconds after seeing each picture and are encouraged to write down their honest first impressions. It is important for faculty to choose pictures that are open for interpretation and portray different activities, religions, and ethnicities. The authors have used photographs of well-groomed serial killers, international singers, Nobel Prize winners, family members, and individuals with tattoos (including a physician), body piercings, and/or dark sunglasses.

Once anonymous individual answers are collected, they are shared with the rest of the class members; similarities and diversities among the group's answers are identified and discussed. The instructor then reveals the correct identity of the individuals in the photographs. Students are consequently divided in groups and asked to reflect on the exercise and address specific questions in relation to stereotypes, prejudice, social justice, discrimination, and prevention of all of the above in the healthcare setting.

Cultural Self-Assessment and Cultural Assessment of Others

Discover Thy Cultural Self: Discovery of One's Own and Others' Cultural Values, Beliefs, and Practices

This exercise combines a cultural self-assessment and a cultural assessment of others. Seven open-ended questions were developed based on Leininger's culture care theory and Sunrise Enabler to help participants investigate their own cultural beliefs, values, and practices. When the exercise is conducted in a traditional face-to-face classroom format, each of these questions is written on a gigantic post-it sheet. Each sheet is taped to a space on one of the walls in the classroom. Students are asked to move among sheets and answer questions without reading classmates' responses. This part of the activity allows students to engage in a self-assessment of their own cultural values, beliefs, and practices. For the second part of the exercise, students and instructor review the collective responses to each question, identify similarities and differences, and discuss relevance to and implications for clinical practice. Eliciting student reflections about the importance of cultural self-assessment and the relationship to as well as the impact from conducting cultural assessments on others can be facilitated through such faculty-led discussions. Some of the questions used by the authors for this activity have included: *What cultural beliefs and values are important to you? What does family mean to you? What roles do family members play in your health care?*

Cultural Interview

Students are asked to conduct a cultural interview with a person from a diverse cultural background using their own culture-specific adaptation of Leininger's Suggested Interview Guide and Sunrise Enabler (Leininger, 2006b). Faculty may practice formulation of interview questions with students and provide guidance as to proper interviewing techniques. Students are encouraged to develop cultural care decisions and actions to preserve and/or maintain, accommodate and/or negotiate, and restructure and/or repattern some of their discovered interview findings. In addition, they are asked to synthesize similarities and differences between their own culture and that of the person interviewed. Students may present their findings in the format of a paper or a PowerPoint presentation to their student/class peers. International students, staff, or faculty members at the university may serve as potential informant/interviewee sources.

International Video-Conference

Faculty may plan for video-conferencing with international faculty and students across the globe. Free software such as Skype or Tango may be used to facilitate this activity; in addition, more sophisticated video-conferencing equipment may be available on the university campus or through businesses, hospitals, educational/conference centers, community colleges, or elsewhere. Face-to-face networking can occur with international faculty on campus or at conferences to facilitate and plan these types of shared activities.

One of the authors arranged for international video-conferencing via Skype on several occasions with groups of nursing students and faculty from Israel, students from Taiwan, and a family from Lebanon. Students were asked to prepare open-ended questions based on Leininger's Sunrise Enabler and the Semi-Structured Interview Guide in advance of the planned session. Following the video-conference, students were asked to reflect on their findings and experiences in writing.

On-Campus Cultural/International Activities

Faculty can take advantage of diverse cultural events held across campus and in the surrounding community as well as activities organized by the International Office or equivalent. The authors included in their syllabi opportunities for earning extra credit by participating in and reflecting on events organized by the school's Diversity Committee, Campus Common Read events, presentations by Fulbright Scholars, visiting professors, community members, and faculty or staff colleagues from other disciplines.

Students enrolled in transcultural courses taught by one or both authors engaged in the *Bafa Bafa* game, as well as discussions, video presentations, and live Skype interviews with authors or film-makers (*The Immortal Life of Henrietta Lacks* [Skloot, 2010] and *The Submission* [Waldman, 2011]) as well as numerous events offered during Campus Diversity Week.

Religious Panel Presentations and Discussions

For this activity, a religious panel comprised of community members representing the Jewish, Christian, Muslim, Hindu, Baha'i, and/or Jehovah's Witness faiths is convened. Representatives of other faiths have also been solicited without success thus far. Guests are each given 15 minutes to present major tenets of their faiths and discuss implications to the healthcare system. **Figure 19-1** is a sample letter sent to potential religious presenters containing specific guidelines regarding the content of their presentation. Students are typically asked in advance to prepare questions to ask the presenters. Following all of the speakers' individual presentations, a discussion session ensues during which students may pose questions to any of the religious panel members. A faculty member acts as a moderator and teases out similarities and differences among the diversely presented beliefs and practices. The event is usually videotaped. Students subsequently develop a written reflection about the overall experience and its implications to health care and their own role or practice.

Disability/Accessibility Exercise

This exercise instills awareness of challenges faced by individuals with varying forms of disability and addresses appropriate and inappropriate terminology, communication techniques, and culturally sensitive actions when interacting with a person or caring for a patient with a disability. A disability advocate was consulted in the development of this activity. The exercise consists of borrowing various forms of adaptive or assistive equipment from physical/occupational/speech/rehabilitative therapy academic units such as wheelchairs, walkers, canes, crutches, and transfer boards; wrist, knee, ankle, and foot braces, slings, wraps, or splints; adaptive eating equipment; and goggles with limited or no visibility. Assistance from a physical (or other) therapy department faculty member is solicited to help instruct students on safe and culturally appropriate use of the equipment.

Students are sent across campus with specific tasks to accomplish, including but not limited to using the restroom, purchasing meals, accessing different floors, using computer labs, and going in and out of buildings. Each student has the opportunity to experience a temporary disability, its related challenges, and other people's reactions. Before returning to class, students submit an electronic reflection about their experience.

Invitation to Join Religious Panel Presentation for NUR 369 Transcultural Health Care
Room: WSW 3203

November 8, 2012, from 10:00 am–12:00 pm

Greetings,

On behalf of the nursing department at the University of Michigan–Flint, I would like to thank you for making the time to educate our students about your cultural and religious beliefs and practices. Your audience will be composed of undergraduate students pursuing studies in diverse healthcare professions.

When you join us for the panel presentation, would you please briefly explain major tenets of your faith?

In addition, can you please touch on the healthcare-related implications or restrictions to the following? You may share a short 15 slides PowerPoint presentation if you desire (this is not a requirement).

- Touch, personal space, and eye contact
- Modesty/privacy/gender preference of healthcare provider (or is this not applicable?)
- Meals/Medications
- Care of dying patient
- Care of newborn
- Care of women during and after childbirth
- Organ donation/blood transfusion/cremation
- Religious practices associated with hospitalizations or surgery
- Any other issue health care providers should be knowledgeable about to provide culturally sensitive care to patients from your faith?

Our goal is to have our students empowered with knowledge necessary to provide culturally congruent care to all patients. Thank you for helping us achieve this goal. If you have any questions, please feel free to contact me at xxx-xxx-xxxx or hiba@umflint.edu

Thank you!

Dr. Hiba Wehbe-Alamah
Associate Professor
Department of Nursing, SHPS
University of Michigan–Flint

Figure 19-1 Sample letter sent to religious panel presenters

Upon returning to the classroom, the instructor engages the students in a discussion about their experiences and any lessons learned. A guest speaker either from the community or the campus office of accessibility services is invited to discuss implications for culturally competent communication and appropriate care practices by healthcare professionals.

Teaching Principles of Cultural Competence

This assignment is included in graduate-level courses and consists of having students synthesize and present educational material learned throughout the semester to a group of multidisciplinary healthcare professionals. However, the intended audience must include registered nurses, nursing faculty, nursing students, and/or nurse administrators. Students design their own PowerPoint presentations using established guidelines that address required content while encouraging creativity and interactive exercises. They secure their own audience, deliver and video-tape the presentation, then mail or electronically submit the video along with other required documents such as a self-reflection to the instructor for evaluation and grading.

STANDARDIZED CONTENT IN COURSE SYLLABI

Some of the standard content included in the authors' syllabi has been removed from the presented samples to avoid redundancy. Examples include policies related to academic integrity, honor code, school closings, accessibility services, Healthcare Insurance Portability and Accountability Act (HIPAA) statement, and technology requirements. Different schools may have their own corresponding language or mandates. Some additional standardized content developed by the faculty and integrated into in all course syllabi includes areas described in the following paragraphs.

Classroom and Online Etiquette (Netiquette)

As current and future healthcare professionals, we value, advocate, and exercise caring for patients. Throughout this course, we will demonstrate care and caring for each other. Thus, caring is exemplified by professional conduct that is courteous, respectful, absent of any tone or inference that may be perceived as rude, demeaning, dismissive, hurtful, or sarcastic.

It is very easy for comments to be misinterpreted in the electronic environment given that facial expressions cannot be seen for interpretation of visual cues. It has been estimated that 80% of interpersonal communication is nonverbal and conveyed through facial expressions and body language. When sending email or engaging in a discussion that presents an opposing or differing point of view to that of another course participant (including those of faculty), it is *essential* to maintain a tone that is both *respectful* and *courteous*. Expression of differences can be effectively communicated in a professional manner.

Caring is additionally expressed by:

- Being on time for class
- Silencing cellular phones
- Refraining from texting during class teaching time
- Staying for the duration of class

Paper Release Form

As part of maintaining our national credentialing, the Department of Nursing at the University of Michigan–Flint retains examples of exceptional work from all courses. If you are willing to allow your work to be used as an exemplar for both credentialing and future classes, you will need to submit a paper release form (included in the syllabus or course shell).

Email Communication

Students are expected to use UM–Flint Outlook email when communicating with one another or with the instructors; email is also accessible through BlackBoard via the communication/send email link. Email communication sent from personal accounts may end up in spam or junk folders of UM–Flint accounts.

Students are asked to address any questions or concerns to Dr. or Professor xxxxx at: xxxx@umflint.edu or xxx-xxx-xxxx. Faculty will make every attempt to check email daily and to respond within 24–48 hours. Email sent after 5:00 p.m. Friday evening and throughout the weekend will be responded to after 9:00 a.m. on Monday morning. However, faculty will take urgent calls or texts anytime on cell phones.

Students are required to enter their section number (Sect 1 or Sect 2) in their email subject heading when emailing/texting the instructor as more than one section of this class is offered at this time.

SAMPLE SYLLABI FOR UNDERGRADUATE, GRADUATE, AND INTERNATIONAL TCN COURSES

Appendix 19-A found at the end of this chapter is a syllabus prepared for a transcultural healthcare course taught by the authors in Taipei, Taiwan, to a group of international and Taiwanese students. The course was open to graduate and undergraduate students enrolled in National Yang Ming University. Prior to teaching this course, the authors visited different areas in Taipei and conducted a windshield survey (**Figure 19-2** and **Figure 19-3**) in an effort to learn about the Taiwanese culture.

Taiwanese students enrolled in the course acted as tour guides and gatekeepers. A trip to the Chinese medicine clinic provided a plethora of educational opportunities, pictures, and videos to incorporate both in the course taught in Taiwan and those taught in the United States. Examples from Taiwanese culture and pictures taken during outings were integrated into course educational materials. On course Day One, students had grouped

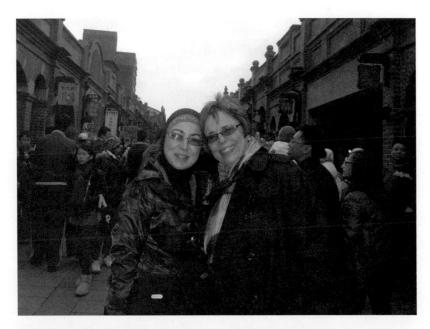

Figure 19-2 Dr. Hiba Wehbe-Alamah and Dr. Marilyn McFarland at a popular traditional shopping market in Taipei.

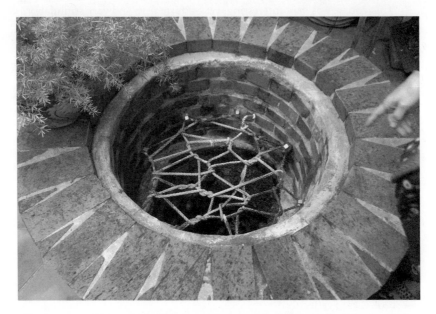

Figure 19-3 A well at an older Taiwanese home. Fish placed inside well were used by the owners as a warning system for poisoning attempt (e.g., if found dead and floating in water).

themselves in the classroom into two groups: Taiwanese and international. The authors proceeded to rearrange seating so that each Taiwanese student was paired with an international student for group activities and discussions.

The following are samples of journal reflections submitted by students enrolled in this course:

> The session was started with a self-introduction both by the two lecturers and the students. From the lecturers (Dr. Hiba and Dr. McFarland) introduction I have noticed the two unique cultures of each one. Dr. Alamah [sic] came from a long history of cross-cultural [descent] from Kuwait through Lebanon to Michigan in the USA. She has a wide range of exposer [sic] to different culture … It took her many years of learning and cultural exposer to become what she is today. On the other hand Dr. McFarland had very little exposer [sic] to other cultures. Because she lived in the same home that was handed down from her ancestors and her education was done not far from her home … But her enthusiasm and respect for other cultures had developed her to what she had become today … Putting these two unique backgrounds together already demonstrated what transcultural health care means on the outset. (Day 1 reflection)

> This course was very interesting, very informative and very stimulating. It will go a long way in the development of our health care services in our respective countries. I am very privileged indeed to have chosen to undertake this course. It has been one of my areas of great interest so build my knowledge and answers some of the many questions I have over the years. This course I believe will help a lot in my future strategies in addressing nursing development issues in my country. From this session I learnt that as professionals we need to consider seriously that, "No one choose to be born, let alone to the *race* they are, the *disability* they may have, or the *country* they live, or to the *socioeconomic* status they are brought up, and with the *skin color* they have. The decision was made by someone else. So each individual person deserves to be respected for who he or she is or has become. We need to respect how they respond to the different environment and environmental influences." Thank you very much Dr. Hiba and Dr. McFarland for the wonderful course and superb teaching skills and for teaching us a new skill in assessing our patients needs through the cultural assessment tool. (Day 3 reflection)

The authors teach a transcultural healthcare course in the undergraduate nursing program at their university. The syllabus prepared for this course is available via coded access to the electronic database for instructors. This course is one of the undergraduate nursing core courses required for graduation but is open to students enrolled in any major at the university as it fulfills the requirements for global study, civic engagement, and general education. Students taking this course include traditional and nontraditional learners, and most are declared prenursing majors. This course is taught in both face-to-face and online formats with *Transcultural Concepts in Nursing Care* (6th edition) by Andrews and Boyle (2012) as the required text. Students' course evaluations typically reflect appreciation for the educational content, interactive and engaging learning activities, interview and teaching opportunities, and their realizations of or accounts about how the course has transformed their own worldviews and nursing practices and is applicable to many circumstances throughout everyday life.

A transcultural healthcare course is also taught by the authors in the Doctor of Nursing Practice (DNP) graduate program, which is offered completely online and required for the BSN-DNP and MSN-DNP students at the University of Michigan–Flint. *Culture Care Diversity and Universality: A Worldwide Nursing Theory* by Leininger and McFarland (2006) is the required text for this course. Additional required readings include research, evidence-based, and other scholarly articles. This graduate course syllabus is also available via the coded access to the electronic database for instructors. Group projects provide an opportunity for some students to mentor others. All students conduct a peer review and grading of classmates' assignments. One of the challenges encountered in this course has been the different video formats used by students and other technological issues related to the cultural competence teaching assignment. Ongoing collaboration with the university's Office of Extended Learning continues to address ways to eliminate or reduce technical difficulties. Students' feedback during and at the completion of the course as well as ongoing instructor self-evaluation and reflection on teaching methods and approaches are taken into consideration when planning changes or revisions for future administration of this course.

TIPS FOR SUCCESS

The field of transcultural nursing is fluid and dynamic. However, there are basic principles, concepts/constructs, and competencies that should be acquired by all healthcare practitioners. Faculty members are encouraged to assess their existing curricula and develop a plan for teaching these and additional cultural competencies to their students. The authors recommend inclusion of transcultural healthcare core content at the beginning and throughout the entire curriculum. Flexibility, creativity, mastery in the use of existing resources, and networking with peers from similar or other disciplines through conference attendance and other venues are approaches faculty can utilize in order to design transcultural curricula that graduate culturally sensitive and competent healthcare providers.

The authors invite readers to share with them via email creative or innovative educational activities used in their teaching, suggestions for future improvements, or reflections related to the application of any of the exercises or assignments presented in this chapter. Nursing and other faculty may also access additional syllabi provided in the electronic test bank.

DISCUSSION QUESTIONS

1. Discuss your personal experiences with developing a transcultural course or curriculum.
2. Which of the presented educational activities can you adapt for use in your educational environment and how?
3. What are other creative strategies to teach transcultural nursing concepts/principles/competencies?
4. What facilitators/barriers do you envision faculty might face when planning interactive transcultural educational activities?

APPENDIX 19-A
NATIONAL YANG MING UNIVERSITY,
SCHOOL OF NURSING

Course Name: Course #:
Transcultural Health Care

Course Type: Elective   Course Level: Graduate

Credit: 1 credit   Class time: December 14–16, 2011

Classroom: Nursing Building Room #

Instructors:

Hiba Wehbe-Alamah, PhD, RN, FNP-BC, CTN-A
  Associate Professor, School of Health Professions and Studies
  Department of Nursing, University of Michigan–Flint
  Email: hiba@umflint.edu
  Skype: Hiba Wehbe-Alamah

Marilyn McFarland, PhD, RN, FNP-BC, CTN-A
  Professor, School of Health Professions and Studies
  Department of Nursing, University of Michigan–Flint
  Email: mmcf@umflint.edu
  Skype: marilynruth.mcfarland

A. COURSE DESCRIPTION

This course explores the unique interaction of culture and cultural values with health beliefs and the impact these have on the utilization of the health-care system. Leininger's Theory of Culture Care Diversity and Universality and the Sunrise Enabler are used as a basis for studying the relationship between culture and health. The various approaches necessary to provide culturally congruent care are explored. A focus is placed on the assessment and analysis of select cultural diversities as related to clinical practice.

B. COURSE OBJECTIVES

Upon completion of the course, students should be able to:

- Discuss the historical and theoretical development of transcultural nursing and health care
- Examine the concepts and principles in transcultural health care
- Describe the relevance of cultural diversities to healthcare delivery

- Explore methods to promote cultural competence in transcultural nursing and health care
- Describe effective use of transcultural communication principles
- Conduct a cultural assessment

C. SYLLABUS

Date	Topic	Hours	Instructor
12/14	Introduction to Transcultural Healthcare	6	Hiba Wehbe-Alamah, Marilyn McFarland
12/15	Transcultural Healthcare in Theory and Research Transcultural Communication	6	Hiba Wehbe-Alamah, Marilyn McFarland
	Transcultural Assessment		
12/16	Student Presentations and Evaluation	6	Hiba Wehbe-Alamah, Marilyn McFarland

D. EVALUATION

1. Class attendance/discussion (15%)
2. Class activities (15%)
3. PowerPoint presentation (40%)
4. Journaling (30%)

E. COURSE REQUIREMENTS AND EXPECTATIONS

The course requires advance preparation for each class meeting. For the most part, students will learn by engaging in classroom discussions and activities, at the individual or group level as part of student teams.

Students are expected to prepare readings and other required materials for class discussion. The willingness of all students to participate in class discussions, ask questions, and bring relevant issues to class will be critical for successful completion of this course. Class participation will be evaluated in the following ways:

- Students are expected to attend *every* session of this course and complete the assigned reading before the session.
- Students are expected to arrive for class on time and be ready to actively participate in class discussions and activities. *Students are asked to silence all cell phones.*

- Students *may use laptop computers during class for educational purposes only.*
- Students will be evaluated on both the quantity and quality of their participation in class discussions and classroom activities.

a. Class Materials and Instructional Strategies

Electronic copies of the class materials—including required readings, PowerPoint presentations, and articles—will be made available to students in both the English and Chinese languages prior to the beginning of the course. Students are expected to do the readings prior to coming to class. Instructional strategies include lecture discussions, interactive group activities, Socratic teaching, PowerPoint presentations, videos, and journaling.

b. PowerPoint Presentation

Students are expected to give a PowerPoint presentation based on a cultural interview conducted in class. The purpose of the presentation is to present the findings from a cultural assessment interview conducted with an individual from a particular cultural background, using a cultural assessment tool derived from Leininger's Suggested Inquiry Guide for Use with the Sunrise Model to Assess Culture Care and Health. The PowerPoint presentation should address the following topics:

- Ethnodemographics (2 points)
- Ethnohistory (2 points)
- Cultural values and customs (4 points)
- Religious/spiritual values, holidays, and customs (4 points)
- Generic care practices (4 points)
- Professional care practices (4 points)
- Culture care preservations and/or maintenance (3 points)
- Cultural care accommodation and/or negotiation (3 points)
- Cultural care repatterning and/or restructuring (3 points)
- Comparison of findings to own culture (2 points)
- Conclusion/most important lessons learned from course (2 points)
- Expected future application to practice (2 points)

On the day of the presentation, students are advised to arrive early to class and to upload and minimize their presentation on the classroom's computer in preparation for their presentation (and to ensure a smooth flow for all presenters) (2 points).

Creativity expressed in use of pictures, clipart, music, and other audiovisuals is encouraged (1 point).

A paper copy of the presentation and any references used for the presentation are to be handed in a folder to the instructors the day of the presentation for grading (2 points).

c. Journaling

Students are to engage in daily journaling activities following each class session, including the last session, covering student presentations. Journaling activity should include a brief summary of topics covered in class, lessons learned from lectures, group discussions and activities, and reflections on the overall experience. For the last day covering student presentations, journaling should also include a discussion of similarities discovered in student presentations (common themes) and overall impression of the course. Students should email both instructors their journals by Saturday, 10 a.m.

d. Academic Integrity

Students are expected to act in accordance with the National Yang Ming University policy on academic integrity. Cheating, lying, misrepresentation, or plagiarism in any form is unacceptable behavior. Specifically, the submitted written work must be the student's own. Direct quotations and specific concepts from sources should be footnoted.

F. COURSE SCHEDULE, READINGS, AND INSTRUCTIONAL ACTIVITIES

Session 1: December 14 (Wednesday)

Topic: Introduction to Transcultural Healthcare

Content may cover the concepts of culture, subcultures, transcultural nursing, transcultural healthcare, history of transcultural nursing development and contributions to transcultural healthcare, globalization, and the importance of transcultural healthcare in contemporary healthcare system. Transcultural Healthcare Concepts and Terminology: Content may cover ethnicity, cultural shock, cultural pain, cultural conflict, ethnocentrism, cultural imposition, cultural blindness, culture-bound, cultural diversity, cultural universality, stereotyping, discrimination, acculturation, enculturation, assimilation, and culturally congruent/sensitive care.

Readings

Leininger, M. M., & McFarland, M. R., (2002 [English], 2007 [Mandarin Chinese]). *Transcultural nursing concepts, theories, research & practice.* New York, NY: McGraw-Hill: Chapters 1 and 2. (Handout or electronic PDF English and Chinese versions provided.)

Instructional Activities

Self-introductions and ethnohistory (personal stories)
 Name tents
 Cultural self-assessment exercises: Know Thyself activity
 Stereotype activity
 Group discussion: Taiwanese versus American healthcare system, challenges, cultures served
 Homework: Journaling

Session 2: December 15 (Thursday)

Topic: Transcultural Healthcare in Theory and Research and Transcultural Health Care in Practice—Assessing the Cultural Healthcare Beliefs and Practices of People from Diverse Cultural Backgrounds and Implications for Clinical Practice

Content may cover Leininger's culture care theory; ethnonursing research method; Leininger's cultural assessment and research enablers; samples of ethnonursing transcultural studies conducted by lecturers; cultural competence development; diverse cultural beliefs and practices; cultural assessment tools and models to deliver culturally competent care; principles for culturological [cultural] assessment; principles for cross-cultural communication; and guidelines and application to clinical practice.

Readings

Leininger, M. M., & McFarland, M. R. (2002 [English], 2007 [Mandarin Chinese]). *Transcultural nursing concepts, theories, research, and practice.* New York, NY: McGraw-Hill: Chapter 3, Parts I and II; Chapter 4. (Handout or electronic PDF English and Chinese versions provided.)

Instructional Activities

Inquiry-guide practice
 Role play: Cultural interview practice in class [students interview each other in groups of two]
 Group discussion
 Homework: Journaling

Session 3: December 16 (Friday)

Topic: Student Presentations and Evaluation

Cross-cultural learning and exchange: Students to present results of cultural interview, a synthesis of most important lessons learned from course, and expected future application to clinical practice. Final words from lecturers.

Reading

Leininger, M. M., & McFarland, M. R., (2002 [English], 2007 [Mandarin Chinese]). *Transcultural nursing concepts, theories, research, and practice.* New York, NY: McGraw-Hill: Chapter 25. (Handout or electronic PDF English and Chinese versions provided.)

Instructional Activities

Student presentations
  Group discussions
  Course evaluation
  Homework: Email electronic copy of journal to both instructors after class is completed and no later than Saturday, 10 a.m.

REFERENCES

Andrews, M. M. (2012). Culturally competent nursing care. In M. M. Andrews & J. S. Boyle *Transcultural concepts in nursing care* (6th ed., pp. 17–37). Philadelphia, PA: Lippincott Williams & Wilkins.

Andrews, M. M., & Boyle, J. S. (2012). *Transcultural concepts in nursing care* (6th ed.). Philadelphia, PA: Lippincott Williams & Wilkins.

Andrews, M. M., & Friesen, L. (2011). Finding electronically available information on cultural competence in health care. *Online Journal of Cultural Competence in Nursing and Healthcare, 1*(4), 27–43.

Campinha-Bacote, J. (2002). The process of cultural competence in the delivery of healthcare services: A model of care. *Journal of Transcultural Nursing, 13*(3), 181–184.

Campinha-Bacote, J. (2003). *The process of cultural competence in the delivery of healthcare services a culturally competent model of care.* Cincinnati, OH: Transcultural C.A.R.E. Associates.

Douglas, M. K., & Pacquiao, D. F. (Eds.). (2010). Core curriculum for transcultural nursing and health care. Thousand Oaks, CA: Dual printing as supplement to *Journal of Transcultural Nursing, 21*(1).

Duphily, N. (2011). From clinician to academic: The impact of culture on faculty retention in nursing education. *Online Journal of Cultural Competence in Nursing and Healthcare, 1*(3), 13–21.

Giger, J. N., & Davidhizar, R. (2002). The Giger and Davidhizar transcultural assessment model. *Journal of Transcultural Nursing, 13*(3), 185–188.

Jeffreys, M. R. (2010). *Teaching cultural competence in nursing and health care* (2nd ed.). New York, NY: Springer.

Leininger, M. M. (2006a). Culture care diversity and universality theory and evolution of the ethnonursing research method. In M. M. Leininger & M. R. McFarland (Eds.), *Culture care diversity and universality: A worldwide nursing theory* (2nd ed., pp. 1–42). Sudbury, MA: Jones and Bartlett.

Leininger, M. M. (2006b). Ethnonursing research method and enablers. In M. M. Leininger & M. R. McFarland (Eds.), *Culture care diversity and universality: A worldwide nursing theory* (2nd ed., pp. 43–82). Sudbury, MA: Jones and Bartlett.

Leininger, M. M., & McFarland, M. R. (2006). *Culture care diversity and universality: A worldwide nursing theory* (3rd ed.). Sudbury, MA: Jones and Bartlett.

McFarland, M. R., & Leininger, M. M. (2002). Transcultural nursing: Curricular concepts, principles, and teaching and learning activities for the 21st century. In M. M. Leininger & M. R. McFarland (Eds.), *Transcultural nursing: Concepts, theories, research, and practice* (3rd ed., pp. 527–561). New York, NY: McGraw-Hill.

Purnell, L. (2002). The Purnell model for cultural competence. *Journal of Transcultural Nursing, 13*(3), 193–196.

Schim, S., Doorenbos, A. Z., Miller, J., & Benkert, R. (2003). Development of a cultural competence assessment instrument. *Journal of Nursing Measurement, 11*(1), 29–40.

Skloot, R. (2010). *The immortal life of Henrietta Lacks.* New York, NY: Crown Publishing/Random House.

Spector, R. (2009). *Cultural diversity in health and illness.* Upper Saddle River, NJ: Pearson Prentice Hall.

United States Department of Labor. (2005). *Monthly Labor Review, 28*(11), 1–18.

Waldman, A. (2011). *The submission.* New York, NY: Farrar, Straus and Giroux.

Chapter 20

Transcultural Nursing Certification: Its Role in Nursing Education, Practice, Administration, and Research

Priscilla Limbo Sagar

> *Transcultural healthcare will ultimately be heralded as one of the greatest breakthroughs in nursing and many health disciplines in the 21st century. As transcultural care knowledge is used in people care, the consumers will rejoice, for it will be the first time they can rely on culturally-based, culturally congruent, safe, and meaningful healthcare practices—a most welcome outcome.*
>
> (Leininger, 2006, p. 394)

INTRODUCTION

The mission and goals of most schools of nursing encompass lifelong learning. Early on, nursing students become aware of the need to further their education and training after program completion. Many nurses desire learning beyond entry level to hone their skills and adapt to the ever-changing healthcare delivery system. In its report entitled *The Future of Nursing*, the Institute of Medicine (2010) highlighted nurses' commitment to lifelong learning. *Certification* (in line with lifelong learning) is a process of granting recognition upon meeting criteria or standards of specialty practice (Fights, 2012; Kelly-Thomas, 1998). *Recertification* entails yet further commitment to lifelong learning and the enhancement of skills (Eisemon & Cline, 2006), maintenance of knowledge and competency (Accreditation Board for Specialty Nursing Certification, 2012), and keeping abreast of new developments in the field (McFarland & Leininger, 2002).

The American Nurses' Association (ANA, 1991, 1995, 2003), the American Association of Colleges of Nursing (AACN, 1998, 2008), and the National League for Nursing (NLN, 2009a, 2009b) have consistently advocated for cultural diversity and the integration of culturally congruent care in nurse–client interactions. Furthermore, accrediting bodies such as The Joint Commission (TJC), the Commission on Collegiate Nursing Education (CCNE), and the National League for Nursing Accrediting Commission (NLNAC) have included standards addressing cultural diversity and the inclusion of cultural competence in academic nursing curricula. These initiatives have gathered momentum since the promulgation of culturally and linguistically appropriate services (CLAS) mandates and guidelines (see Appendix 20-A at the end of this chapter) by the U.S. Department of Health and Human Services (USDHHS), Office of Minority Health ([OMH], USDHHS, OMH, 2000). This being the case, certification in transcultural nursing (TCN) deserves to be at the forefront of the thrust for culturally congruent care. Certification and recertification of transcultural nurses are global imperatives to provide culturally congruent, safe, and quality care (McFarland & Leininger, 2002).

PURPOSE/RATIONALE

This chapter explores specialty certification in nursing, a credentialing process that is aligned with lifelong learning. Lifelong learning is a concept that is woven throughout nursing curricula, encouraged and rewarded in practice and administration, and beginning to be investigated in research specifically in terms of patient outcomes and nurse satisfaction. This chapter also examines the history of certification in general and TCN in particular. It concludes with a vision of TCN where certification is recognized, sought, rewarded, and acknowledged for improvement of client outcomes and satisfaction. This author predicts a marked increase in the number of nurses seeking basic and advanced transcultural certification over the next 2 decades.

HISTORICAL BACKGROUND: SPECIALTY CERTIFICATION IN NURSING

The history of specialty certification dates back to 1946, when the American Association of Nurse Anesthetists (AANA) required certification for entry into nurse anesthesia practice (Wolgin, 1998). In 1966, the American Nurses' Credentialing Center (ANCC) reported that 111,164 nurses held certification in 16 specialties, including 2,078 nurses who obtained certification in staff development (Kelly-Thomas, 1998). Between 1990 and 2009, the ANCC certified more than 250,000 registered nurses and more than 75,000 advanced practice nurses (ANCC, 2009). The American College of Nurse–Midwives required certification in 1971; 3 years later, the ANA also began offering specialty certification examinations (Wolgin, 1998).

The American Nurses' Credentialing Center, a subsidiary of the ANA, is the most prestigious credentialing organization in nursing. In addition to offering specialty nursing certifications, the ANCC also developed the Magnet Recognition Program (MRP) which "...recognizes healthcare organizations for quality patient care, nursing excellence and innovations in professional nursing practice" (ANCC, 2012b, para 1). Consumers have come to depend on Magnet designation as the definitive credential for best quality nursing care practices.

The ANCC, in turn, is accredited by the Accreditation Board for Specialty Nursing Certification (ABSNC), previously known as the American Board of Nursing Specialties (ABNS) Accreditation Council, and is the sole accrediting body of organizations for nursing certification. Accreditation by the council is a peer-review process that grants nursing certification to obtain accreditation through compliance "...with the highest quality standards available in the industry" (ABSNC, 2012, p. 2). Other certifying agencies are connected with specific specialty nursing organizations. In 2008, the ANCC and the ANA designated March 19 as Certified Nurses' Day in honor of the birthday of Margretta Madden Styles, a world-famous expert on nurse credentialing, a long-time dedicated advocate for nursing standards and certification, and a forefront advocate on behalf of advanced practice nursing practice and regulation for more than 20 years (ANCC, 2012a).

HISTORY AND BACKGROUND OF CERTIFICATION IN TRANSCULTURAL NURSING

Dr. Madeleine Leininger originally founded the field of TCN in the mid-1950s. Since that time, Leininger and her followers have contributed more than 400 scientific studies to the field of TCN (Glittenberg, 2004) accumulating a vast, impressive body of knowledge about caring for people from different cultures. The need for TCN certification became evident during the 1970s when nurses were struggling to care for immigrants, refugees, and other groups of people from diverse cultures (McFarland & Leininger, 2002).

The Transcultural Nursing Certification *Committee* (TCNCC) was established in 1987 (Transcultural Nursing Society [TCNS], 2013); it offered its initial examination in 1988 at the TCNS annual conference and meeting in Edmonton, Alberta, Canada (Andrews & Boyle, 2012). The major purpose of certification was the protection of clients of various cultures from "… negligent, offensive, harmful, unethical, nontherapeutic, or inappropriate care practices" (McFarland & Leininger, 2002, p. 544). To prove eligibility, every applicant prepared a portfolio documenting academic and experiential theory, concepts, and research in TCN (Andrews & Boyle, 2012). The certification format consisted of a multiple-choice test followed by an oral examination conducted by the Certification Committee. Thereafter, the certification examination continued to be administered during the annual international TCNS conferences (TCNS, 2013). McFarland and Leininger (2002) reported a total of about 100 certified and recertified transcultural nurses. This number decreased to approximately 85 CTNs worldwide by 2009; based on data from the TCNS website (www.tcns.org, 2013), a more recent count of transcultural nurses includes 22 with basic certification ([CTN-B]; all in the United States except for one in Canada) and 59 who hold advanced certification ([CTN-A]; all in the United States except for one each in Australia, Israel, and Saudi Arabia). Eighty-one transcultural nurses are far too few to answer the need for caring, educating, mentoring, and role modeling in the vast arenas of nursing practice, education, administration, and research.

To update standards and policies of certification and recertification, the Transcultural Nursing Certification *Committee* (TCNCC) was reorganized in 2000 with Dr. Jeanne Hoffer as chair. The format of the examination remained a combination of multiple-choice questions and a verbal examination. In comparison, certification examinations by the ANCC and other nursing specialties were all in multiple-choice formats; some organizations also offered computerized testing.

The TCNS Board of Trustees appointed a Certification Task Force in 2004. The main goals of the Certification Task Force were "…to review current certification practices and make recommendations for future directions in certification" (TCNS, 2013, para 1). The Task Force completed its work in 2006. The TCNS Board of Trustees established its Certification *Commission* [TCNCC] in the same year with Dr. Marilyn McFarland as chair. However, the Commission was not chartered and functioned as a *committee* with the following appointed as sub-committee chairs: Curriculum (Dr. Susan Mattson); evaluation (Dr. Mary Simpson); eligibility and credentialing (Dr. Priscilla Sagar); finance and grants (Dr. Patricia Vint); marketing and public relations (first, Dr. Beth Rose; later, Dr. Hiba Wehbe-Alamah); and recertification evaluation (Maj. Helen Nyback). The Transcultural Nursing Certification Commission held its initial meeting in Detroit,

Michigan on July 8, 2006 (TCNCC, 2007). The TCNCC abolished the oral examination and decided to base the examination solely on multiple-choice questions to establish parity with other certification examinations (Sagar, 2012). Furthermore, the TCNCC decided to use online versus paper-and-pencil testing; the online examination was made available at testing locations nationwide during multiple test periods throughout the year (Andrews & Boyle, 2012; Sagar, 2012).

Between 2007 and 2009, Dr. Mary Simpson, Dr. Priscilla Sagar, Dr. Marilyn McFarland, and Dr. Hiba Wehbe-Alamah developed the *advanced certification* exam based on an outline developed by the Core Curriculum Committee. In 2011, an ad hoc committee composed of Dr. Marty Douglas, Dr. Dula Pacquiao, Dr. Scollan-Koliopolus, and Dr. Arlene Farren developed the *basic certification* examination (personal communication, M. R. McFarland, October 17, 2011). The basic exam was based on the Core Curriculum for Transcultural Nursing and Health Care that had been published in 2010 as a supplement to the *Journal of Transcultural Nursing* (Douglas & Pacquiao, 2010).

Test questions were requested from TCNS scholars and divided into seven domains (Andrews et al., 2011; TCNCC, 2007):

I: Foundations for Transcultural Care
II: Culturally-based Health, Caring, and Healing Practices
III: Assessment of Cultural Information Relevant to Health Care
IV: Culturally-based Nursing Care
V: Evaluation of Care Outcomes
VI: Research
VII: Professionalism

In November 2011, nineteen examinees took the basic certification pilot exam consisting of 139 items (Andrews et al., 2011).

The TCNCC had received full support from a 3-year (2008–2011) project called *Developing Cultural Competencies for Nurses: Evidence-Based Best Practices* (http://www.ojccnh.org/project/index.shtml) funded by a U.S. Department of Health and Human Services, Health Resources and Services Administration (HRSA) grant written and directed by Dr. Margaret Andrews, Director of Nursing, School of Health Professions Studies at the University of Michigan–Flint (UMF). The project was co-directed by Dr. Teresa Cervantez Thompson from Madonna University, Livonia, Michigan, and was subsequently extended for an additional 2-year period (2012–2013). This grant-funded support enabled the TCNCC to hire statisticians to determine the reliability and validity of both basic and advanced certification examinations and the remuneration of committee members for attending TCNCC meetings or national preparatory precertification train-the-trainer workshops.

The University of Michigan–Flint, Madonna University, and the Transcultural Nursing Society, in collaboration with other organizations that share the mission of promoting cultural competency in nursing and health care, offered a series of online and face-to-face educational programs. The purpose of these programs was to utilize transcultural nursing as "…a framework for developing the cognitive, affective, and psychomotor cultural competencies of nursing faculty, practicing nurses, and nursing students" (Andrews et al., 2011, p. 300) "…[to] develop their skills in addressing individuals, groups, and communities that are diverse, with special emphasis on those at risk for health disparities" (Andrews & Thompson, 2008, para 2) and to relate nurses' cultural competencies with the "…reduction or elimination of [these] health disparities across the life span" (para 3). Particular emphasis was given to the *Healthy People 2010* indicators of "… obesity, depression, low-birthweight infants, diabetes mellitus, hypertension, human immune deficiency virus/acquired immunodeficiency syndrome (HIV/AIDS), and cancer" (para 3).

The educational program series used a train-the-trainer approach with faculty that included national transcultural nursing leaders, authors, and experts. More importantly, the project aimed to prepare nurses to become Certified Transcultural Nurses (CTNs). The project also began publication of the peer-reviewed *Online Journal of Cultural Competence in Nursing and Healthcare* (*OJCCNH*) and established a website (http://www.ojccnh .org) that provided free, current, extensive online, print, and audiovisual (AV) resources on cultural competence and health disparities, including full-text articles from the *OJCCNH* in portable document file (pdf) format. Online and face-to-face classes and workshops, print materials, and AV resources provided opportunities for acquiring TCN knowledge, skills, and competencies in all areas of nursing, and thus a foundational preparation for certification.

The first advanced certification *pilot exams* comprised solely of multiple-choice questions were offered in January and February 2009; the second exams were given in June and July 2009. The new eligibility requirements for the *advanced certification* examination went into effect in December 2009 and the *basic certification* examination was piloted in November 2011 (TCNS, 2013). By implementing the basic certification, the TCNCC acknowledged that cultural competence must be practiced by all nurses (Andrews & Boyle, 2012) and that all 3,063,163 registered nurses in the United States (USDHHS, HRSA, 2010) must heed the call for cultural knowledge, skills, and competencies in TCN and apply them at all levels and settings of practice (Sagar, 2012).

RESEARCH ON THE VALUE OF SPECIALTY CERTIFICATION

Specialty nursing certification boards need to promote recognition of certified nurses and encourage minority nurses to obtain certification; noncertified nurses need to overcome barriers and seek certification. Multiple studies have been conducted to explore the value of specialty certification. The American Board of Nursing Specialties (ABNS) Accreditation Council (2006) administered the Value of Certification Survey using the Perceived Value of Certification Tool ([PVCT], Competency and Credentialing Institute, 2006). Containing 18 value statements related to certification, the PVCT was determined to be a reliable tool (ABNS, 2006). Twenty (83%) ABNS member organizations took part in the online survey hosted by Professional Examination Service from March 31 to June 10, 2005. This Value of Certification survey had a total of 94,768 respondents including 8,615 (75%) certified nurses and 2,812 (25%) noncertified nurses (ABNS, 2006). Of the noncertified nurses, 1,608 (14%) were nurse managers. The respondents' educational preparation by degree was as follows: Baccalaureate (43.4%), master's (21.5%), associate (20.4%), diploma in nursing (13.4%), and doctoral (1.3%). Respondents were 91.6% female and 92.1% Caucasian. Seeking certification was voluntary for 72.5% of the nurses (ABNS, 2006).

The ABNS (2006) study found that certified nurses, noncertified nurses, and nurse managers showed high level of agreement on the value of certification. For respondents who have never held certification, the main barriers were the cost of the exams and a lack of institutional rewards and support. Nurses who let their certification lapse cited reasons such as not practicing in the specialty, minimal or no compensation for certification, and lack of recognition. Cited rewards and benefits for obtaining certification were reimbursement of examination costs, being able to display credentials, and compensation for continuing education (ABNS, 2006). Only 18.6% of respondents indicated receiving a salary increase and 21.4% reported not receiving any incentive for certification. Certified and noncertified nurses showed similar rates of job retention and work absences in a 1-year period (ABNS, 2006).

The ABNS (2006) outlined the following implications of this survey: Healthcare organizations need to support nurses to overcome barriers to certification and to offer incentives for certification; specialty nursing certification boards need to promote recognition of certified nurses and encourage minority nurses to obtain certification; and, noncertified nurses need to overcome barriers and seek certification (p. 4). It is imperative that certified nurses serve as role models and collaborate with "...professional nursing organizations, specialty nursing certification boards, and their employers to advocate for meaningful incentives and rewards that foster certification" (ABNS, 2006, p. 4).

Piazza, Donohue, and Dykes (2006) conducted a descriptive comparative study among 457 nurses in a 174-bed acute care hospital in Connecticut to validate the overall value of certification. Of the 265 nurse respondents, 259 met the criteria for inclusion in the study; 103 (39%) had obtained national certification. The Conditions of Work Effectiveness Questionnaire II ([CWEQ], Laschinger, n. d.) was used in the final sample. Piazza et al. (2006) used five out of six of the CWEQ-II subscales: Four empowerment structures and the job activities scale (measures informal power). Comprised mostly of women (n = 252 [97.3%]), the nurses' ages ranged from 23 to 77 years with a mean age of 44.05 years. The respondents worked as staff nurses (72.2%), administrators (12%), and advanced practice nurses (3.5%), with 69% working on the day shift (Piazza et al., 2006). Registered nurses (RNs) in the Connecticut study had a total CWEQ-II score of 21.28 out of 30 which indicated moderate levels of empowerment. Administrator scores showed high levels of empowerment while those of advanced practice registered nurses (APRNs) and staff nurses indicated moderate empowerment. The findings of this study indicated a positive effect on nurses' empowerment levels as a result of nursing specialty certification which may then enhance work effectiveness. As their work effectiveness is enhanced, nurses will become further empowered to care for clients more effectively, including those whose cultures differ from their own (Piazza et al., 2006).

Another study connected nurse specialty certification among baccalaureate-prepared nurses and higher proportions of baccalaureate-prepared nurses on staff with improved patient outcomes (Kendall-Gallagher, Aiken, Sloane, & Cimiotti, 2011). Kendall-Gallagher et al. used secondary data from this nurse survey in conjunction with data from the American Hospital Association (AHA) and de-identified hospital abstracts of 1,283,241 surgical patients from 652 hospitals in California, Florida, New Jersey, and Pennsylvania. An important finding was the correlation of nurse specialty certification among nurses with BSN or higher degrees with decreased surgical mortality (p. 192).

McFarland and Leininger (2002) asserted that transcultural nurses gain "...respect, status, public recognition, and often advancement in their employment" (p. 545) from certification and recertification. Recertification ensures maintenance of transcultural competence by the requisite updating of nursing knowledge and skills (McFarland & Leininger, 2002).

Research studies about *transcultural certification* substantiating the value of certification and contributing to the body of knowledge in the discipline of transcultural nursing are long overdue. Studies are needed to evaluate the motivations nurses may have for seeking basic or advanced certification; factors influencing when initial certification is sought; number of renewals; perceived value of certification; satisfaction of certified nurses; influence of certification on nurse self-confidence; roles that mentoring and role modeling play toward facilitating initial certification and renewals; and certification benefits to nurses such as opportunities for leadership, advancement, recognition, and monetary rewards. There is an especially urgent need for CTN certification research that explores the effects of certification on patient outcomes. Research among certified nurses in general and transcultural nurses in particular could uncover a heretofore hidden and untapped body of knowledge. Questions that might be asked include: *Is there satisfaction in having obtained the CTN? Is there empowerment in having a particular certification? Are there differences in perception among nurses from various specialty certifications?*

There are gaps in the body of knowledge about the cultural competence of nursing faculty, students, and graduates of nursing schools. Mixer (2008) used the CCT to explore teaching of cultural care by nursing faculty. Her research revealed three themes: *Faculty provided generic and professional care to nursing students; faculty did not use an organizing conceptual framework;* and *care is essential for faculty health and wellbeing* (p. 32). Based on these findings, Mixer recommended conducting larger-scale studies to support, substantiate, and build new *caring* nursing knowledge in the area of nursing education using the culture care theory (p. 34). More studies are needed to actually measure cultural competence of faculty, students, and graduates of nursing schools (Kardong-Edgreen & Campinha-Bacote, 2008; Sargent, Sedlak, & Martsolf 2005). There is also a paucity of research about African American, Hispanic, and Native American nurses who elect to stay in their own communities. Many studies used standards based from the perspective of Anglo American participants; those standards may not apply to the more culturally diverse U.S. population.

ELIGIBILITY REQUIREMENTS

Advanced Certification

Eligibility criteria for advanced certification in TCN (CTN-A) include: current active registered nurse (RN) license in a state or territory of the United States or legally recognized equivalent in another country; master's, post-master's, or doctorate in nursing or a related field or legally recognized equivalent in another country; completion of one 3-credit academic course or the equivalent of 42 continuing education contact hours or units in cultural competence; and completion of 2,400 hours of TCN practice as an RN (TCNCC, 2011). The CTN-A certification and each subsequent recertification are valid for a period of 5 years.

Basic Certification

For basic certification in TCN (CTN-B), the eligibility criteria include: current active RN registered nurse (RN) license in a state or territory of the United States or legally recognized equivalent in another country; diploma, associate, or baccalaureate degree in nursing or related field or legally recognized equivalent in another country; completion of one 3-credit academic course or the equivalent of 42 continuing education contact hours or units in cultural competence; and completion of 2,400 hours of TCN practice as an RN (TCNCC, 2007). The CTN-B certification and each subsequent recertification is valid for a period of five years.

The TCNS website contains all information for CTN initial and recertification at the advanced and basic levels (http://www.tcns.org).

ROLES OF CERTIFIED TRANSCULTURAL NURSES IN HEALTH CARE

Certified transcultural nurses are qualified to function at local, national, and global levels (McFarland & Leininger, 2002). The promotion of cultural competence has increasingly become a vital area in accreditation standards for both academia and practice (Sagar, 2012), with the contributions of transcultural nurses to health care also being recognized (Curren, 2006). Since the year 2000 there has been greater acceptance and recognition for the field of TCN; accrediting bodies both in practice and academia have added standards, guidelines, and toolkits focused on cultural diversity and culturally competent care (AACN, 2008; NLN, 2009a, 2009b; TJC, 2010).

According to Leininger (as cited in Kalayjian, Marrone, & Vance, 2010), the professional roles of transcultural nurses include client, student, family, healthcare staff, and community member educators in both formal and informal settings; interdisciplinary consultants and colleagues; expert clinicians; researchers; and entrepreneurs. These roles place the CTN at the core of assessment, planning, implementation, and evaluation of culture-specific generic and professional patient care needs and practices.

Certified Transcultural Nurses in Education

As *nurse educators*, transcultural nurses assess, plan and design, implement, and evaluate curricula to meet the culture-specific generic and professional care needs of individuals, groups, communities, and populations. For example, staff development educators are responsible for all staff education within their healthcare institution or practice setting. There are many advocates for the formal teaching of TCN concepts in nursing curricula; however, there are no standard curricular guidelines or mandates for content integration (Lipson & Desantis, 2007; Mixer, 2008; Ryan, Carlton, & Ali, 2000; Sagar, 2012). Furthermore, there is increased evidence that graduates of nursing programs do not have the academic preparation to care for increasingly diverse populations (Kardong-Edgreen & Campinha-Bacote, 2008).

It is imperative, then, that faculty seek educational and experiential opportunities to prepare for this gargantuan task. The very group (nursing faculty) that needs to assume leadership toward ensuring that the next generation of nurses is prepared to manage clients' culture-specific generic and professional care needs are themselves not prepared in this area (Leininger, 2006). Jeffreys (2006) emphasized the informal and formal education requirements of transcultural nurses to ensure initial and continuing cultural competence. As educators, faculty influence on the recruitment, engagement, and retention of culturally diverse students cannot be overemphasized (McFarland, Mixer, Lewis, & Easley, 2006). It is therefore paramount that nursing faculty seek basic or advanced certification as an avenue toward cultural competence.

Certified Transcultural Nurses in Practice

The majority of practicing RNs are from associate programs and provide direct and indirect patient care in clinical and nonclinical settings (USDHHS, 2010). Most institutions still use client admission assessment tools that have limited questions to assess the complex needs of their culturally diverse clients (Curren, 2006). The areas most commonly addressed in this type of assessment tool are dietary, religious, and communication needs. Although communication assessment includes inquiry into language(s) spoken, many times the tool does not include clarification as to the *preferred* language or *fluency* with reading or writing which are important for receiving patient education. The TJC study (2010) involving Florida hospitals was eye-opening; findings revealed that despite the availability of interpretation and translation services, healthcare professionals still used family members as interpreters.

Transcultural nurses need to not only disseminate certification information but also encourage certification and recertification; they must examine how basic certification could be a stepping stone for further educational and employment opportunities for diploma-, associate-, and baccalaureate-prepared nurses. Some nurses may need more tangible incentives such as salary differentials or reimbursement for exam costs and/or continuing education.

Whether nurse practitioners, clinical specialists, nurse–midwives, or nurse-anesthetists, advanced practice nurses (APNs) are at the forefront of the healthcare delivery system in the United States. Advanced practice CTNs are valuable as providers, consultants, entrepreneurs, advocates, and role models. Truly, APNs are in position to ensure that clients' culture-specific generic and professional care needs are consistently met. Certification and recertification in TCN will promote acquisition and delivery of culturally congruent knowledge, skills, and competencies when providing care for clients from diverse cultures.

Biological variations and their implications regarding drug metabolism; health education; and disparities in the ability to access and receive quality care are concepts that need to be threaded into the educational preparation of APNs. One method of increasing the number of nurses certified in TCN would be for the TCNCC to invite nurses from specialty organizations who are members of the ABNS to apply for basic and advanced CTN certification (Sagar, 2014).

More consultations from TCN experts and certified transcultural nurses are predicted to take place in the future as more and more healthcare institutions, organizations, and practice settings move toward compliance with accreditation guidelines regarding cultural competence. The number of CTN entrepreneurs may also increase as providers of continuing education (CE) programs, consultants, and disseminators of TCN information. All of these elements will contribute to the increased demand for certification by advanced practice nurses.

Certified transcultural nurses knowledgeable in transcultural theory, research, and evidence-based practice are invaluable to enhancing positive staff relationships and promoting improved client outcomes (Andrews & Boyle, 2012; Curren, 2006; Sagar, 2012; TCNS, 2013). Role modeling and mentoring by CTNs promotes excellence in nursing practice and improves patient satisfaction.

Certified Transcultural Nurses in Administration

The value and necessity for role modeling by CTNs as *nurse administrators* cannot be overemphasized. Certified transcultural nurses often work in hospitals and community settings with staff and administrators not prepared in TCN (Curren, 2006). Leininger's Theory of Culture Care Diversity and Universality can be used to assess various employment issues such as discrimination given that minority nurses, especially African Americans, Hispanic Americans, and Native Americans, are underrepresented in the workforce (The Sullivan Commission, 2004). Medicine and other healthcare professions reflect the same lack of diversity (The Sullivan Commission, 2004). Ludwig-Beymer (2013), a long-time advocate of culturally competent organizations, illustrated use of the CCT in assessing and implementing culturally competent nursing initiatives in healthcare organizations. She also stated that the CCT is highly applicable for conducting organizational assessments which are key to the quest for organizational cultural competence.

The individual and organizational journeys toward cultural competence need a supportive climate (Giger, Davidhizar, Purnell, Harden, Phillips, & Strickland, 2007) and mentoring (Purnell, 2007). A supportive climate is one that nurtures the individual or an administrative milieu that encourages and facilitates growth and excellence among nurses. Mentoring from certified transcultural nurses could be a model whereby a new group of nurses could learn the knowledge, skills, and competencies of culturally congruent care. These mentees, with encouragement and support from mentors, could prepare and review for transcultural certification examination. Mentoring could continue after certification; the mentee could also start mentoring other nurses. This approach is similar to the train-the-trainer approach used by the cultural competence grant at the University of Michigan–Flint (Andrews & Thompson, 2008).

Certified Transcultural Nurses in Research

Another vital role of the CTN is as *nurse-researcher*. This role was pioneered by Dr. Madeleine Leininger in the 1960s and has been carried forward by her followers in order to discover culture care diversities and universalities with the use of Theory of Culture Care Diversity and Universality and the ethnonursing research method (Leininger, 2012). In 1960, Leininger was concerned with nursing's heavy borrowing of research methodology from other disciplines. Leininger (2012) developed the ethnonursing method "…to tease out culture care data" (p. xi) and to study the "…vast wealth of untapped cultural knowledge" (p. x) for application to health care.

Leininger (2012) expressed much hope that the application of findings from the culture care theory and related theories would yield many benefits to patient care. Nurses have choices when selecting a theory or model to use as a framework for research; nurses need to see the fit between the theory and/or model and the research being conducted, being mindful of the gaps in knowledge and lack of research among minority and vulnerable populations. Transcultural nurses are at vantage points to lead much needed research; add to the body of knowledge for evidence-based practice (EBP); discover gaps for needed future research; and promote positive outcomes in patient care (Sagar, 2012).

SCENARIOS AND VISIONS

Certification in advanced and basic transcultural nursing needs to be encouraged and rewarded. Rewards could be in the form of financial incentives; prestige and importance such as names listed in an honors column on bulletin boards or newsletter; and leadership opportunities within or outside of the organization. Certification in transcultural nursing "…demonstrates to nurse colleagues, patients, employers, and others the knowledge, experience, and commitment to transcultural nursing" (TCNS, 2013, para 1). McFarland and Leininger (2002) eloquently referred to certification as an imperative global need to ensure culturally congruent, safe, and quality care.

This author's vision of a partnership between a healthcare system, a school of nursing, and the community is exemplified in the fictional scenario described in **Box 20-1**. In the idealized partnership, there is organizational support to assist nurses in overcoming certification barriers, including incentives for certification and recertification. The scenario demonstrates how nurses who are certified can serve as role models, change agents, and advocates for certification in addition to collaborating with institutions and professional nursing organizations to obtain meaningful incentives for seeking and maintaining certification (Sagar, 2014).

Box 20-1 Envisioned collaborative partnership

Sunrise Care (SC) has a 500-bed acute hospital; two skilled nursing homes with 200 beds each; a rehabilitation center offering cardiac, physical, and occupational therapies; and a home care agency. Sunrise Care's chief nursing officer (CNO) is also the vice president. SC prides itself on being a Magnet Hospital, having just received status renewal after its initial Magnet designation 5 1/2 years ago. SC is located in Mount Pleasant, an extremely poor, underserved community along the Hudson River with a very ethnically and culturally diverse population consisting of African Americans, Mexican Americans, and Southeast Asians (Filipinos, Vietnamese, Hmong, Cambodians). The remaining 50% of the Mount Pleasant's population consists of second- and third-generation Italian Americans, Irish Americans, and Polish Americans and their descendants.

Box 20-1 Envisioned collaborative partnership (*continued*)

> One hundred and fifty out of Sunrise Care's 700 registered nurses hold certifications in their specialty areas, including TCN with 13 basic (CTN-B) and 8 advanced (CTN-A) certifications. Other areas of certification are case management, critical care, emergency, oncology, medical-surgical, nursing administration, home health, informatics, nurse executives, and professional development. Sunrise Care's advanced practice nurse practitioners and clinical specialists are certified in gerontology, pain management, perinatalogy, pediatrics, and psychiatric/mental health.
>
> SC has been successful in its goal to encourage initial certification and sustain renewal of certification by offering incentives for its certified nurses. SC pays its nurses a full wage on the day of the examination. Every nurse is eligible to apply for $2,500 per year for airfare, hotel, and food to attend and present at conferences. In addition to receiving a pay differential of $6,000 per year, every certified nurse is listed on the organizational honor roll bulletin boards, newsletter, and intranet throughout all the SC facilities as well as in the SC press releases to outside media. When leadership opportunities arise, eligible CTNs are given hiring priority.
>
> Nurses with baccalaureate degrees or higher are members of Delta Mu, the Sigma Theta Tau International Honor Society for Nursing (STTI) chapter at Sunshine University School of Nursing (SUSN), one of the hospital's community partners; master's- and doctorally-prepared nurses hold dual appointments as faculty at SUSN. SC nurses have partnered with community organizations in Mount Pleasant to jointly sponsor various health promotion events for the public; a weekly farmer's market; a support group for pregnant teenagers; weekly yoga classes at the community center; and a nurse job-shadowing program for elementary school children.

CONCLUSION

It is vitally important that CTNs lead the way toward applying holistic TCN theory and models in whatever educational, clinical practice, or administrative setting of their employment. Moreover, CTNs need to explore the "fit" and congruence of such theories and models to not only their specific settings but also with regard to any current governmental mandates, guidelines, and accrediting body standards (Sagar, 2012). Engaging approximately 3,063,163 registered nurses (USDHHS, 2010) in this call to develop knowledge, skills, and competencies in TCN and applying these across settings to care "…for patients in homes, in communities, and in institutions; teaching and preparing the next generations of nurses; and in leading in academia and organizations" (Sagar, 2012, p. 135) will be a formidable yet an achievable task.

DEDICATION

This chapter is wholeheartedly dedicated to Dr. Madeleine Leininger whose mentorship and support inspired, inspires, and will continue to inspire my work in transcultural nursing.

APPENDIX 20-A: NATIONAL STANDARDS ON CULTURALLY AND LINGUISTICALLY APPROPRIATE SERVICES (CLAS)

The CLAS standards are primarily directed at health care organizations; however, individual providers are also encouraged to use the standards to make their practices more culturally and linguistically accessible. The principles and activities of culturally and linguistically appropriate services should be integrated throughout an organization and undertaken in partnership with the communities being served.

The 14 standards are organized by themes: Culturally Competent Care (Standards 1–3), Language Access Services (Standards 4–7), and Organizational Supports for Cultural Competence (Standards 8–14). Within this framework, there are three types of standards of varying stringency—mandates, guidelines, and recommendations—as follows:

- CLAS **mandates** are current federal requirements for all recipients of federal funds (Standards 4, 5, 6, and 7).
- CLAS **guidelines** are activities recommended by OMH for adoption as mandates by federal, state, and national accrediting agencies (Standards 1, 2, 3, 8, 9, 10, 11, 12, and 13).
- CLAS **recommendations** are suggested by OMH for voluntary adoption by healthcare organizations (Standard 14).

> **Standard 1:** Health care organizations should ensure that patients/consumers receive from all staff members effective, understandable, and respectful care that is provided in a manner compatible with their cultural health beliefs and practices and preferred language.
>
> **Standard 2:** Health care organizations should implement strategies to recruit, retain, and promote at all levels of the organization a diverse staff and leadership that are representative of the demographic characteristics of the service area.
>
> **Standard 3:** Health care organizations should ensure that staff at all levels and across all disciplines receive ongoing education and training in culturally and linguistically appropriate service delivery.
>
> **Standard 4:** Health care organizations must offer and provide language assistance services, including bilingual staff and interpreter services, at no cost to each patient/consumer with limited English proficiency at all points of contact, in a timely manner during all hours of operation.
>
> **Standard 5:** Health care organizations must provide to patients/consumers in their preferred language both verbal offers and written

notices informing them of their right to receive language assistance services.

Standard 6: Health care organizations must assure the competence of language assistance provided to limited-English-proficient patients/consumers by interpreters and bilingual staff. Family and friends should not be used to provide interpretation services (except on request by the patient/consumer).

Standard 7: Health care organizations must make available easily understood patient-related materials and post signage in the languages of the commonly encountered groups and/or groups represented in the service area.

Standard 8: Health care organizations should develop, implement, and promote a written strategic plan that outlines clear goals, policies, operational plans, and management accountability/oversight mechanisms to provide culturally and linguistically appropriate services.

Standard 9: Health care organizations should conduct initial and ongoing organizational self-assessments of CLAS-related activities and are encouraged to integrate cultural and linguistic competence-related measures into their internal audits, performance improvement programs, patient satisfaction assessments, and outcomes-based evaluations.

Standard 10: Health care organizations should ensure that data on the individual patient's/consumer's race, ethnicity, and spoken and written language are collected in health records, integrated into the organization's management information systems, and periodically updated.

Standard 11: Health care organizations should maintain a current demographic, cultural, and epidemiological profile of the community as well as a needs assessment to accurately plan for and implement services that respond to the cultural and linguistic characteristics of the service area.

Standard 12: Health care organizations should develop participatory, collaborative partnerships with communities and utilize a variety of formal and informal mechanisms to facilitate community and patient/consumer involvement in designing and implementing CLAS-related activities.

Standard 13: Health care organizations should ensure that conflict and grievance resolution processes are culturally and linguistically sensitive and capable of identifying, preventing, and resolving cross-cultural conflicts or complaints by patients/consumers.

Standard 14: Health care organizations are encouraged to regularly make available to the public information about their progress and successful innovations in implementing the CLAS standards and to provide public notice in their communities about the availability of this information.

U.S. Department of Health and Human Services, Office of Minority Health. (2000). Culturally and linguistically appropriate services. http://minorityhealth.hhs.gov/templates/browse .aspx?lvl=2&lvlID=15

DISCUSSION QUESTIONS

1. As the staff development educator and the only transcultural nurse with advanced transcultural nursing certification (CTN-A) in a small community hospital, how would you encourage nurses to seek and maintain CTN certification?

2. You are a newly-hired certified transcultural nurse with advanced certification (CTN-A) at a small community hospital that receives federal funding. There are no language access services (LAS) in the hospital. Discuss your priority initiative.

3. You are a certified transcultural nurse with basic certification (CTN-B). You just overheard a staff nurse saying, "It is a waste of time to get certified; it does not make a difference in patient care." How would you reply to this comment?

4. Despite the availability of language access services (LAS), findings from The Joint Commission (2010) indicate that healthcare professionals often use family members as interpreters. As a transcultural nurse with CTN-A (advanced certification) and the only staff development educator in your hospital, discuss how you would prevent this from happening in your practice setting.

5. Analyze the need for research exploring transcultural nursing certification, nurse satisfaction, and improvement in patient outcomes. Why do you think this type of research will add to TCN body of knowledge? Explain.

REFERENCES

Accreditation Board for Specialty Nursing Certification (ABSNC). (2012). Frequently asked questions. Retrieved from http://www.nursingcertification .org/

American Association of Colleges of Nursing (AACN). (1998). *The essentials of baccalaureate education for professional nursing practice.* Washington, DC: Author.

American Association of Colleges of Nursing (AACN). (2008). *Cultural competency in baccalaureate nursing education.* Washington, DC: Author.

American Board of Nursing Specialties (ABNS). (2006). Value of certification survey executive summary. Retrieved from http://www.nursingcertification.org/pdf/executive_summary.pdf

American Nurses' Association (ANA). (1991). *Position statement on cultural diversity in nursing practice.* Kansas City, MO: Author.

American Nurses' Association (ANA). (1995). *Nursing's social policy statement.* Washington, DC: Author.

American Nurses' Association (ANA). (2003). *Nursing's social policy statement* (2nd ed.). Washington, DC: Nurses Books.

American Nurses' Credentialing Center (ANCC). (2009). Nursing excellence: Your journey, our passion. [ANCC overview brochure]. Retrieved from http://www.nursecredentialing.org/FunctionalCategory/AboutANCC/ANCC-Overview-Brochure.pdf

American Nurses' Credentialing Center (ANCC). (2012a). Certified Nurses Day: A day to recognize certified nurses. Retrieved from http://www.certifiednursesday.org/about.htm

American Nurses' Credentialing Center (ANCC). (2012b). Magnet: Program overview. Retrieved from http://www.nursecredentialing.org/Magnet/ProgramOverview

Andrews, M. M., & Boyle, J. S. (2012). Theoretical foundations of transcultural nursing. In M. M. Andrews & J. S. Boyle (Eds.), *Transcultural concepts in nursing care* (6th ed., pp. 3–16). Philadelphia, PA: Wolters Kluwer/Lippincott, William, & Wilkins.

Andrews, M. M., & Thompson, T. C. (2008). Developing cultural competencies for nurses: Evidence-based best practices. Retrieved from http://www.ojccnh.org/project/objectives.shtml

Andrews, M. M., Thompson, T. L., Wehbe-Alamah, H., McFarland, M. R., Hanson, P. A., Hasenau, S. M., ... Vint, P. A. (2011). Developing a culturally competent workforce through collaborative partnerships. *Journal of Transcultural Nursing, 22*(3), 300–306. doi: 10.1177/1043659611404214

Competency and Credentialing Institute. (2006). *Perceived Value of Certification Tool (PVCT).* Denver, CO: Author.

Curren, D. A. (2006). Culture care needs in the clinical setting. In M. M. Leininger & M. R. McFarland (Eds.), *Culture care diversity and universality: A worldwide nursing theory* (2nd ed., pp. 159–180). Sudbury, MA: Jones and Bartlett.

Douglas, M. K., & Pacquiao, D. F. (Eds.). (2010). *Core curriculum for transcultural nursing and health care.* Thousand Oaks, CA: Dual printing as supplement to *Journal of Transcultural Nursing, 21*(1).

Eisemon, N., & Cline, A. (2006). The value of certification [Guest editorial]. *Gastroenterology Nursing, 29*(6), 428–429.

Fights, S. D. (2012). Lippincott's 2012 nursing directory [Supplement], pp. 10–11. Retrieved from http://www.nursingcenter.com/pdf.asp?AID=1287263

Giger, J. N., Davidhizar, R. E., Purnell, L., Harden, J. T., Phillips, J., & Strickland, O. (2007). American Academy of Nursing expert panel report: Developing cultural competence to eliminate health disparities in ethnic minorities and other vulnerable populations. *Journal of Transcultural Nursing, 18*(2), 95–102.

Glittenberg, J. (2004). A transdisciplinary, transcultural model for health care. *Journal of Transcultural Nursing, 15*(1), 6–10.

Institute of Medicine. (2010, October 5). *The future of nursing: Leading change, advancing health.* Washington, DC: National Academies Press.

Jeffreys, M. (2006). *Teaching cultural competence in nursing and health care.* New York, NY: Springer Publishing.

Kalayjian, A., Marrone, S. R., & Vance, C. (2010). Professional roles and attributes of the transcultural nurse. In M. K. Douglas & D. F. Pacquiao (Eds.), *Core curriculum for transcultural nursing and health care.* Thousand Oaks, CA: Dual printing as supplement to *Journal of Transcultural Nursing, 21*(1), 406S–417S.

Kardong-Edgreen, S., & Campinha-Bacote, J. (2008). Cultural competency of graduating US bachelor of science nursing students. *Contemporary Nurse: Advances in Contemporary Transcultural Nursing, Special Issue* (2nd ed., Australia), *28*(1–2), 37–44.

Kelly-Thomas, K. J. (1998). The nature of staff development practice: Theories, skill acquisition, and research. In K. J. Kelly-Thomas, *Clinical and nursing staff development: Current competence, future focus* (2nd ed., pp. 54–72). Philadelphia, PA: Lippincott.

Kendall-Gallagher, D., Aiken, L. H., Sloane, D. M., & Cimiotti, J. P. (2011). Nurse specialty certification, inpatient mortality, and failure to rescue. *Journal of Nursing Scholarship, 43*(2), 188–194.

Laschinger, H. K. (n. d.). *Conditions of Work Effectiveness Questionnaire-II (CWEQ-II).* London, ON, Canada: Arthur Labatt Family School of Nursing, University of Western Ontario.

Leininger, M. M. (2006). Envisioning the future of culture care theory and ethnonursing method. In M. M. Leininger & M. R. McFarland (Eds.), *Culture care diversity and universality: A worldwide nursing theory* (2nd ed., pp. 389–394). Sudbury, MA: Jones and Bartlett.

Leininger, M. M. (2012). Foreword. In P. L Sagar, *Transcultural nursing theory and models: Application in nursing education, practice, and administration* (pp. ix–xiv). New York, NY: Springer.

Lipson, J. G., & Desantis, L. A. (2007). Current approaches to integrating elements of cultural competence in nursing education. *Journal of Transcultural Nursing, 18*(1), 10S–20S.

Ludwig-Beymer, P. (2013). Creating culturally competent organizations. In M. M. Andrews & J. S. Boyle (Eds.), *Transcultural concepts in nursing care* (6th ed., pp. 211–242). Philadelphia, PA: Wolters Kluwer/Lippincott, William, & Wilkins.

McFarland, M. R., & Leininger, M. M. (2002). Transcultural nursing: Curricular concepts, principles, and teaching and learning activities for the 21st century.

In M. M. Leininger & M. R. McFarland (Eds.), *Transcultural nursing: Concepts, theories, research, & practice* (3rd ed., pp. 527–561). New York, NY: McGraw-Hill.

McFarland, M., Mixer, S., Lewis, A. E., & Easley, C. (2006). Use of the culture care theory as a framework for the recruitment, engagement, and retention of culturally diverse nursing students in a traditionally European American baccalaureate nursing program. In M. M. Leininger & M. R. McFarland (Eds.), *Culture care diversity and universality: A worldwide nursing theory* (2nd ed., pp. 239–254). Sudbury, MA: Jones and Bartlett.

Mixer, S. J. (2008). Use of the culture care theory and ethnonursing method to discover how nursing faculty teach culture care. *Contemporary Nurse, 28*(1–2), 23–36.

National League for Nursing (NLN). (2009a). A commitment ot diversity in nursing and nursing education. Retrieved from http://www.nln.org/aboutnln/reflection_dialogue/rfl_dial3.htm

National League for Nursing (NLN). (2009b). Diversity toolkit. Retrieved from http://www.nln.org/aboutnln/reflection_dialogue/rfl_dial3.htm

Piazza, I. M., Donohue, M., & Dykes, P. (2006). Differences in perceptions of empowerment among nationally certified and noncertified nurses. *Journal of Nursing Administration, 36*(5), 277–283.

Purnell, L. D. (2007). Commentary on "Current approaches to integrating elements of cultural competence in nursing education." *Journal of Transcultural Nursing, 18*(1), 25S–27S.

Ryan, M., Carlton, K. H., & Ali, N. (2000). Transcultural nursing concepts and experiences in nursing curricula. *Journal of Transcultural Nursing, 11*(4), 300–307.

Sagar, P. L. (2014). Integrating transcultural concepts in staff development: Preparing for credentialing. In P. L. Sagar (Ed.), *Transcultural nursing education strategies.* New York, NY: Springer.

Sagar, P. L. (2012). *Transcultural nursing theory and models: Application in nursing education, practice and administration.* New York, NY: Springer.

Sargent, S. E., Sedlak, C. A., & Martsolf, D. S. (2005). Cultural competence among nursing students and faculty. *Nurse Education Today, 25*(3), 214–221.

The Joint Commission (TJC). (2010). *Cultural and linguistic care in area hospitals.* Oakbrook Terrace, IL: Author.

The Sullivan Commission. (2004). *Missing persons: Minorities in the health professions: A Report of The Sullivan Commission on diversity in the health care workforce.* Durham, NC: Duke University School of Medicine.

Transcultural Nursing Certification Commission (TCNCC). (2007, March 23–25). *Transcultural nursing certification revision.* [Personal archive of minutes from Transcultural Nursing Certification Committee meeting, Fenton, MI].

Transcultural Nursing Certification Commission (TCNCC). (2011, fall). Transcultural nursing certification revision. [Personal archive of minutes from Transcultural Nursing Certification Committee meeting, Fenton, Michigan].

Transcultural Nursing Society (TCNS). (2013). Transcultural nursing certification. Retrieved from http://www.tcns.org/Certification.html

U.S. Department of Health and Human Services, Health Resources Services Administration (HRSA). (2010). The registered nurse population: Initial findings from the 2008 National Sample Survey of registered nurses. Retrieved from bhpr.hrsa.gov/healthworkforce/rnsurveys/rnsurveyinitial2008.pdf

U.S. Department of Health and Human Services, Office of Minority Health (OMH). (2000). Culturally and linguistically appropriate services. Retrieved from http://minorityhealth.hhs.gov/templates/browse.aspx?lvl=2&lvlID=15

Wolgin, F. (1998). Competence assessment systems and measurement strategies. In K. J. Kelly-Thomas, *Clinical and nursing staff development: Current competence, future focus* (2nd ed., pp. 92–120). Philadelphia, PA: Lippincott.

Index

Note: Page numbers followed by *b*, *f*, or *t* indicate materials in boxes, figures, and tables respectively.

A